Incidental Findings
of the Nervous System

Mehmet Turgut · Fuyou Guo
Ahmet Tuncay Turgut · Sanjay Behari
Editors

Incidental Findings of the Nervous System

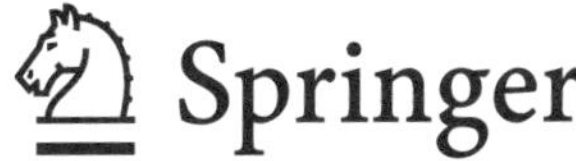

Springer

Editors
Mehmet Turgut
Department of Neurosurgery
Aydın Adnan Menderes University
Faculty of Medicine
Aydın, Turkey

Ahmet Tuncay Turgut
Department of Radiology
Ankara Medipol University
Faculty of Medicine
Çankaya, Ankara, Turkey

Fuyou Guo
Department of Neurosurgery
First Affiliated Hospital of Zhengzhou
Hena, China

Sanjay Behari
Department of Neurosurgery
Sanjay Gandhi
Postgraduate Institute of
Medical Sciences
Lucknow, Uttar Pradesh, India

ISBN 978-3-031-42597-4   ISBN 978-3-031-42595-0   (eBook)
https://doi.org/10.1007/978-3-031-42595-0

This Springer imprint is published by the registered company Springer Nature Switzerland AG
The registered company address is: Gewerbestrasse 11, 6330 Cham, Switzerland

Paper in this product is recyclable.

Introduction

Written and edited by leading international authorities in the field, this book provides an in-depth review of knowledge of the incidental findings of the nervous system, with emphasis on asymptomatic brain and spinal lesions that have the potential to cause illness. It includes very informative chapters, organized into four main groups: firstly, incidental findings of the brain and cranium, including intracranial, intraventricular, and skull base lesions, infarcts, and calcification; secondly, incidental findings of the spine and spinal cord, including spinal cord tumors, syringomyelia, arteriovenous malformations, and craniovertebral junction anomalies; thirdly, incidental findings of the spinal nerves and peripheral nerves, including tumors of the plexi and peripheral nerves; and fourthly, other lesions, including acquired incidental lesions of the brain and spine as well as medicolegal and psychiatric aspects related to these lesions. The uniqueness of this compilation lies in the fact that several abnormalities exist in the nervous system that have the potential to cause life-threatening illness; yet, because they are asymptomatic and incidental, this leads to major management dilemmas related to whether or not to surgically remove the lesion. The proponents of an early surgical management subscribe to the philosophy that getting rid of an entity earlier on when it is asymptomatic leads to an early cure and obviates any risk of it becoming aggressive and incurable later on; those opting for a "wait-and-watch" policy subscribe to the view that no intervention (as well as subjecting the patient to the risk of surgery) is mandated until the lesion becomes symptomatic. This may subject a person to a lifetime of anxiety related to how that lesion is going to evolve, when in all likelihood, the subject may remain asymptomatic throughout his/her life. The psychological aspects of the patient who is extremely disturbed by the presence of this incidental lesion, and who cannot adjust to the reality that the treating doctor actually does not have a well-defined plan for it, are issues that are adequately addressed with clinical illustrations and examples. This comprehensive reference book will be an ideal source for neuroscientists at all levels, from graduate students to researchers in specific disciplines studying this region, including neurosurgeons, neurologists, neuroradiologists, neuropathologists, and psychiatrists, who seek both basic and more advanced information regarding the incidental findings of the nervous system.

Contents

About the Authors

Mehmet Turgut MD, PhD, is Professor of Neurosurgery at Aydın Adnan Menderes University School of Medicine, Aydın, Turkey. He graduated from the Ege University School of Medicine, İzmir, Turkey, and later specialized in neurosurgery in Hacettepe University Hospitals, Ankara, Turkey. In 2004, he received the PhD degree from the Department of Embryology and Histology, Ege University Health Sciences Institute, İzmir, Turkey. His fields of expertise and research interests are broad and include developmental neuroscience, pediatric neurosurgery, infectious diseases of the central nervous system, and peripheral nerve surgery. Dr. Turgut is an editorial board member for 25 international journals, including *European Spine Journal, Surgical Neurology International, Journal of Neurological Surgery Part A: Central European Neurosurgery, Journal of Spine, Journal of Pediatric Neurology, Journal of Brachial Plexus and Peripheral Nerve Injury, Journal of Spine & Neurosurgery, and Journal of Neurosciences in Rural Practice*, and a reviewer for a wide range of international journals and research programs. Dr. Turgut is the lead or co-author of more than 300 papers in peer-reviewed journals and about 78 book chapters, and he is one of the editors in 17 books including *Pituitary Apoplexy; Hydatidosis of the Central Nervous System: Diagnosis and Treatment; Complications of CSF Shunting in Hydrocephalus: Prevention, Identification, and Management; The Chiari Malformations; The Sutures of the Skull: Anatomy, Embryology, Imaging, and Surgery; and Subdural Hematoma: Past to Present to Future Management; Arachnoid Cysts: State-of-the-Art.*

Fuyou Guo MD, is Professor of Neurosurgery at The First Affiliated Hospital of Zhengzhou University, PR China. He graduated from Henan Medical University, Zhengzhou, PR China, and obtained the MD degree from the Department of West China Medical Center of Sichuan University, Chengdu, PR China, in 2005. He underwent post-doctoral research in the University of Michigan, Ann Arbor, USA, in 2008. His fields of expertise and research interests are broad and include cerebrovascular diseases, brain tumor, congenital malformations of the central nervous system, pediatric neurosurgery, and peripheral nerve surgery. Dr. Fuyou is an editorial board member for two international journals including *Glioma* and *Brain & Heart*. He is a reviewer for a wide range of international journals including *Cancer Biology & Medicine, Neurocritical Care, Aging-US, Neurotoxicity Research,* and *Orphanet Journal of Rare Diseases*. Dr. Guo is the lead or co-author of more than 100 papers in peer-reviewed journals, and he is one of the editors in four Chinese books including *Chiari Malformation, Nervous System Tumors, Perioperative Management in Neurosurgery,* and *Precise Operation for Chiari Malformation.*

Ahmet T. Turgut MD, is Professor of Radiology at Ankara Medipol University in Ankara, Turkey. He has nearly 25 years' experience in the field of radiology with key roles in diagnostics, academics, and administration. Dr. Turgut's research interests include diagnostic and interventional oncologic imaging and use of hybrid imaging techniques for the diagnosis and treatment of cancers in particular. He has published more than 100 original papers in peer-reviewed journals and has authored 60 chapters in several textbooks in English including many on neuroradiology. He is editor of three reference books published by Springer. Dr. Turgut has given more than 90 invited lectures at distinguished scientific meetings including *the European Congress of Radiology, International Congress of Radiology and Annual Meetings of the American Institute of Ultrasound in Medicine (AIUM), European Federation of Societies for Ultrasound in Medicine and Biology*

(EFSUMB), Asian Oceanian Society of Radiology, and European Society of Urogenital Radiology (ESUR). He served as the Congress President in ESUR 2013, 20th Annual Meeting of the ESUR held in Istanbul, Turkey. He has been honored as an elected fellow of the ESUR in 2006. He served as executive board member and general secretary of the *Turkish Society of Radiology* from 2011 to 2013. He was given Honorary Membership by the *Iranian Society of Radiology* and *Georgian Association of Radiology*, respectively.

Sanjay Behari MBBS, MS, MCh, DNB, IFAANS, FRCS (Edin), FAMS, is the Director of Sree Chitra Tirunal Institute for Medical Sciences and Technology, Thiruvananthapuram, India, an Institute of National Importance under the Department of Science and Technology, Government of India. He has been a member of the Department of Neurosurgery, Sanjay Gandhi Postgraduate Institute of Medical Sciences (SGPGIMS), Lucknow, for 30 years, as faculty for 28 years, as a professor for 11 years, and as its head for 6 years. He has been an editor of 15 books; has 360 peer-reviewed publications (Google Scholar H index 43, i10 index 163) and 142 chapters in books to his credit; has guided several MCh neurosurgery and neurotology senior residents and PhD and MD students; and has been an examiner for 32 Indian universities and the country examiner for Sudan as well as thesis examiner of South Africa. He has been a "Sugita International Fellow" at the Department of Neurosurgery, Nagoya University School of Medicine, Nagoya, Japan; an International Scholar at the Department of Neurosurgery, Fujita Health University, Aichi, Japan; International Union Against Cancer ICRETT Fellow at the Department of Neurosurgery, University of Erlangen-Nürnberg, Germany; Fellow at the Department of Neurosurgery, Universities of Geneva and Lausanne, Switzerland; Commonwealth Academic Staff Clinical Fellow at the Department of Neurosurgery, Newcastle General Hospital, UK; and Association of Spinal Surgeons of India and Dartmouth Fellow at the Department of Orthopedics, Dartmouth Hitchcock Medical Centre, New Hampshire, USA. His focused area of interest is skull base, spinal, and cerebrovascular surgery. He has been a Visiting Professor to Nagoya and Fukushima University, Japan; Cantonal University, Geneva, Switzerland; Medical University of South Carolina, Charleston, USA; and Hospital Garcia de Orta, Almada, Lisbon, Portugal. He is on the editorial board of 12 journals and is a reviewer for 30 journals. During his 6-year tenure as Chief Editor of *Neurology India*, its Thomson Reuters impact factor reached 2.708, the highest ever in 65 years and among one of the highest among international neurosurgical journals. He has 4 filed patents, has taken several national orations, and has conducted 6 live operative demonstrations and 237 guest presentations. He has won several institutional awards, including being the Best Institutional Researcher and Guide in Best Institutional Research Awards; being a part of a team with IIT Kanpur won the James Dyson National Award for Best Biomedical Invention in India in 2017 and the Best Publication Award at the World Federation of Neurosurgical Societies in 2022. He is also on the governing body and Board of Studies of several national institutes, as well as National Government Health and Medical Education Committees in India.

Part I

Incidental Findings of the Brain and Cranium

Benign Enlargement of the Subarachnoid Spaces and Subdural Collections

Saurav Samantray, Chandrashekhar Deopujari, Sheena Ali, and Foram Gala

1.1 Introduction

Benign extracerebral collections are commonly found in infants, especially with the availability and growing use of various imaging modalities. Most of these collections, presenting as dilated subarachnoid spaces on imaging, are the most common cause of macrocephaly [1–3] in infancy. Though this disorder has been named as benign enlargement of subarachnoid space (BESS) in recent literature, there is great confusion surrounding the nature of this entity demonstrated by the various names used for its description like benign external hydrocephalus (BEH), extraventricular hydrocephalus, benign subdural effusion, benign extracellular fluid collection, extraventricular obstructive hydrocephalus, subdural hygroma, pseudo-hydrocephalus, benign extra-axial collections, subarachnomegaly, and subdural effusions of infancy [4, 5].

S. Samantray
Neurosurgery, NH, SRCC Children's Hospital, Mumbai, India

C. Deopujari (✉)
Neurosurgery, Bombay Hospital
(Institute of Medical Sciences), Mumbai, India

S. Ali
Neurosurgery, B.J. Wadia Children's Hospital, Mumbai, India

F. Gala
Radiology, B.J. Wadia Children's Hospital, Mumbai, India

The variety in nomenclature reflects the differing views on their being considered one entity and difficult neuroimaging differentiation [3]. The anatomical substrate, whether subdural fluid or cerebrospinal fluid (CSF) in the subarachnoid space, has been a subject of disagreement amongst researchers [6, 7]. This review will try to address various issues about BESS viz. clinical manifestation, incidence and progression of macrocephaly, long-term prognosis, need for shunting, association with subdural collections, relation to non-accidental injury(NAI) and finally will discuss whether all cases are truly benign. The terms BESS and BEH will be used interchangeably throughout this review.

1.2 Definition

In 1918, external hydrocephalus was first defined by Dandy as a condition with increased intracranial pressure and dilated subarachnoid spaces in infancy. He had also subclassified hydrocephalus in several ways including division into internal and external hydrocephalus [8, 9].

In current literature, external hydrocephalus is commonly defined as a large or rapidly growing head circumference in infants combined with enlarged subarachnoid spaces and moderate to no ventricular enlargement on neuroimaging [10–12]. Kumar recommended additional criteria of the absence of "clinicoradiological features of

M. Turgut et al. (eds.), *Incidental Findings of the Nervous System*,
https://doi.org/10.1007/978-3-031-42595-0_1

raised intracranial pressure," e.g., ventriculomegaly without periventricular lucency, and nontense fontanels [4].

Macrocephaly, an essential component of BESS, is defined as head circumference more than two standard deviations above the population mean or above the 98th centile [13].

1.3 Epidemiology

A Norwegian retrospective population based study found an incidence of BESS to be 0.4 per 1000 live births [14]. In this study (86.4%) of the patients were male, and mean age at referral was 7.3 months.

A tertiary pediatric neurology center in Pennsylvania, USA, in a review of incidental findings, found that 0.6% of the children had external hydrocephalus [15]. Two thirds of these infants were found to be boys in another study [16]. BEH was associated with prematurity in many studies [10, 17].

Several studies have reported a familial predisposition in BEH [6, 18] with a 40% chance of a family member being macrocephalic while two reports have found this coherence as high as 80–90% [10, 19].

An autosomal dominant mode of transmission for the non-syndromic macrocephaly cases has been assumed by many [20–22], although a multifactorial model of inheritance with a polygenic genetic base was proposed by a 1996 study [23]. This group's findings challenged the assumption of autosomal dominant inheritance for BESS since risk of recurrence appears to be much lower than it should have been if the assumption was true. There are many genetic conditions, on the other side of the spectrum, which are associated with dilatation of subarachnoid spaces like Mucopolysaccharidoses types I, II and III, Achondroplasia, Soto's syndrome, Glutaric aciduria type I [24].

1.4 Etiology

Most cases are without a known cause and hence termed "idiopathic." However, numerous conditions such as prematurity and intraventricular hemorrhage [16, 25, 26], meningitis [25, 27], metabolic disorder [28], steroid therapy [29], chemotherapy [30], neurosurgery [31], and trauma [25, 27] may be responsible for its causation. Many premature infants can have intraventricular hemorrhage and subarachnoid hemorrhage which can go undetected due to lack of symptoms, thereby rendering the idiopathic nature of BESS uncertain in those cases [32, 33].

1.5 Pathophysiology

1.5.1 Physiological Development of the Subarachnoid Spaces

The major seat of cerebrospinal fluid (CSF) production are the four choroid plexuses in the ventricles. After production, the CSF exits into the basal cisterns, entering the subarachnoid space over the surface of the cortex [34]. The secretory epithelium of the choroid plexus is formed by 6 weeks of gestation [35]. There is uncertainty around the time CSF production begins, but circulation is established from the ventricles to the subarachnoid space by 2 months of age [36]. The separation of the arachnoid membrane from the primitive dura mater leads to the formation of the subarachnoid space. This process then spreads from the ventral portion of the mesorhombencephalon to the spinal cord caudally and to the prosencephalon cranially [37]. CSF is absorbed from the subarachnoid space into the cerebral venous system through herniations of the arachnoid membrane into the dural venous sinuses [38, 39]. Microscopic arachnoid villi are first formed by the microtubular invaginations of the subarachnoid space into the lumen of the dural venous sinuses in utero [34]. This embryological step probably correlates with the decrease in size of the arachnoid space after 32 weeks of gestation and demonstrable on fetal magnetic resonance imaging studies [40]. Arachnoid villi can be found in the fetus and newborn, and the granulations develop between 6 and 18 months of age [41, 42].

Infants can have varying functional maturity of the arachnoid villi which can result in absorption not keeping pace with CSF production for a period of time. CSF accumulates as a result, preferentially in the subarachnoid space until skull sutures are unfused. The ventricles remain undilated till the bulk of CSF absorption occurs through the subarachnoid channels that cover the cerebral hemispheres [43]. After 2 years of age, the capacity for CSF absorption exceeds the normal rate of production by two to four times [36]. Further growth of the arachnoid villi and granulations leads to the formation of macroscopic Pacchionian bodies which are visible by 3 years of age [34]. This process of evolution of a CSF absorption system can be variable in its timeline thereby leading to the variability in the size of the subarachnoid spaces in normal children [44] and providing a physiologic basis for benign enlargement of the subarachnoid spaces.

1.5.2 Pathogenesis

There are various theories that have been proposed to explain the pathogenesis of BESS.

1. *Delayed maturation of arachnoid villi*: This is the most common theory which suggests that the defective CSF absorption due to immature arachnoid villi leads to CSF accumulation causing dilatation of the subarachnoid spaces and ventricles [43]. As the brain and skull are compliant, it does not lead to an increase in Intracranial pressure [25]. The maturation of villi around 18 months of age ends the CSF accumulation and consequent subarachnoid space dilatation.

2. *Arachnoid tear*: This leads to a one way valve mechanism causing CSF accumulation [45]. This mechanism generally leads to subdural fluid collection but can also cause localized subarachnoid space dilatation.

3. *Loculation of CSF* causing accumulation in the localized subarachnoid space [46].

4. *Subdural fluid impairing CSF absorption* [47].

5. *Communicating hydrocephalus theory*: Some believe external hydrocephalus is a step towards developing internal hydrocephalus [12]. If immature arachnoid villi are the cause, there may be restoration of CSF absorption around 18 months of age leading to resolution of BEH. However, children whose arachnoid villi are absent/grossly underdeveloped end up needing a shunt [48].

6. *Cranio-encephalic disproportion*: When the skull grows faster than the brain, it leads to transient subarachnoid space enlargement [10, 49].

7. *Dural venous sinus patency and positional plagiocephaly*: Cinalli et al. proposed that decreased patency of the venous sinuses and consequent increased venous outflow resistance contributes to the development of BEH in the first 3 years of life. The same authors found that positional plagiocephaly, found to be associated with BEH, contributed to the decreased patency of the homolateral dural sinus [50].

1.6 Clinical Manifestations

1.6.1 Macrocephaly

Hellbusch found 28 (71.8%) out 39 patients with BESS to have macrocephaly which meant that 28.2% of the cases had a normal head circumference [16]. The usual presentation of BESS is an otherwise normal infant presenting with increasing head circumference typically around 6 months of age which stabilizes around 18 months of age [51–53]. There might be marked frontal bossing as a result of the typical frontal subarachnoid space enlargement [54]. Head circumference measured after this period generally stays above but parallel to the 95th–98th centile [17, 18, 43]. On long-term follow-up, 11–87% of children with BESS end up with macrocephaly [6, 55, 56].

Most studies report no signs and symptoms of increased intracranial pressure (irritability, leth-argy, vomiting, tense and bulging anterior fontanel) though they can be seen occasionally [1, 2, 4]. Rarely studies reported a tense anterior fontanel [18, 57], dilated scalp veins [58], hypotonia [59], ataxia [4], and seizures [6]. However, the sunset sign is not reported in any study [3]. The children generally achieve normal developmental milestones though mild motor delay has been reported attributable to the large head [4, 10].

1.7 Neuroimaging Findings

The classic Neuroimaging picture of BESS is that of enlarged frontal subarachnoid spaces beyond the upper limit with normal to moderately enlarged ventricles [3]. Concurrent findings include wide interhemispheric fissure, enlarged basal cisterns and third ventricle, no flattening of underlying gyri, CSF following gyral pattern and normal sulci posteriorly [4, 60, 61] (Fig. 1.1a, b).

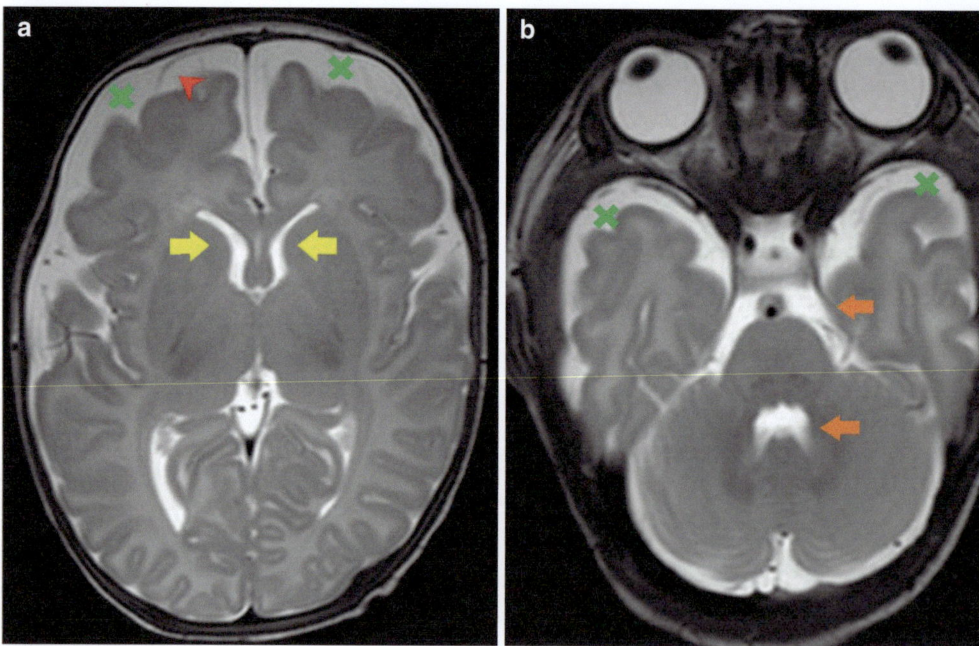

Fig. 1.1 A 1-month-old boy with incidental classical findings of enlarged subarachnoid spaces on axial T2W images. (**a**) The CSF spaces are seen following the gyral contour with no flattening of adjacent gyri. There is an increase in bifrontal subarachnoid spaces (green cross), while the lateral ventricles appear normal (yellow arrow). a distinctive feature of BESS, "cortical vein sign" is noted, comprising of elongated flow voids of bridging veins (red arrow). (**b**) In lower cuts, an enlargement of basal cisterns and fourth ventricle is noted (orange arrow) with conspicuous temporal subarachnoid spaces (green cross)

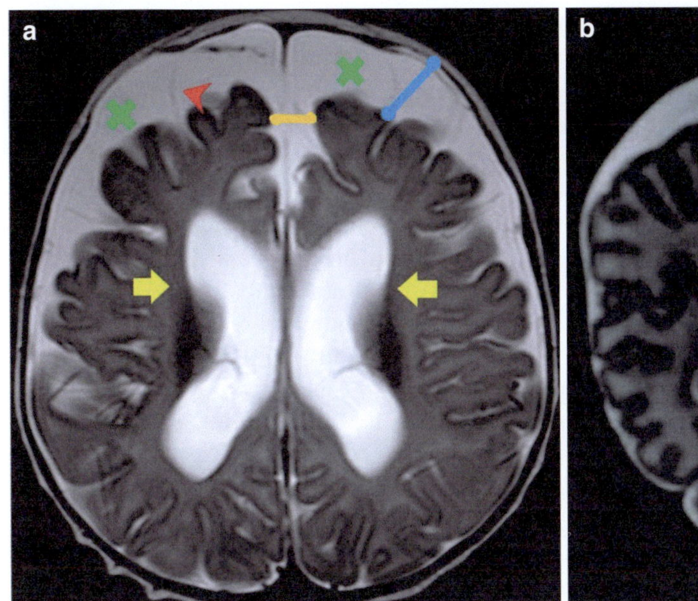
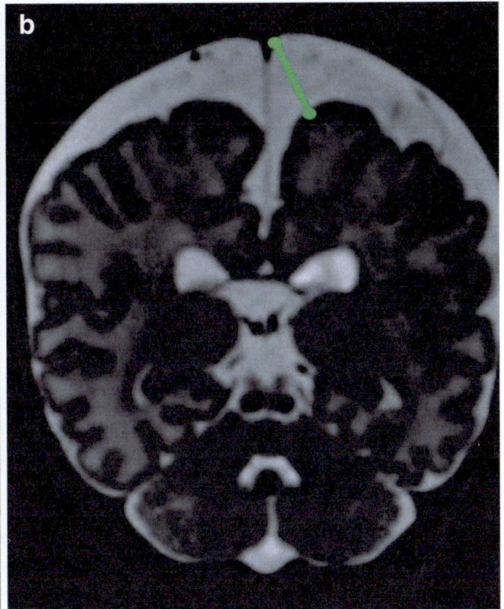

Fig. 1.2 A 5-month-old male with incidental findings of BESS. (**a**) A small variation in imaging showing some prominence of lateral ventricles (yellow arrow) and enlarged subarachnoid spaces in bilateral fronto-temporal regions (green cross), as seen on axial T2W image. The flow voids of bridging cortical veins are prominent, ratifying the "cortical vein sign" (red arrow). there is a classical increase in the interhemispheric distance (yellow line) and cortico cranial width (blue line). (**b**) A coronal T2W view showing an increased sino-cortical width (SCW) (green line)

Some degree of ventricular enlargement is reported in most studies but there are no studies with exact measurements [62, 63]. There is a possible correlation between ventricular size and width of interhemispheric fissure [64]. Maytal et al. [65] found that the sequence of enlargement in BESS was the interhemispheric fissure followed by the frontoparietal convexity subarachnoid space with basal cistern and ventricular enlargement being a late radiological finding (Figs. 1.2a, b and 1.3).

1.7.1 Normal Range [66–69]

The measurements used to quantify BESS are craniocortical width (CCW), interhemispheric fissure width (IFW) and sino-cortical width (SCW). Sinocortical width is defined as the distance from the lateral wall of the superior sagittal sinus to the cerebral cortex (Fig. 1.2a, b). There is no consensus on the cut-off values for any radiological measurement [5, 70]. The range of upper limits for the CCW is 4–10 mm (infants <1 year of age) and

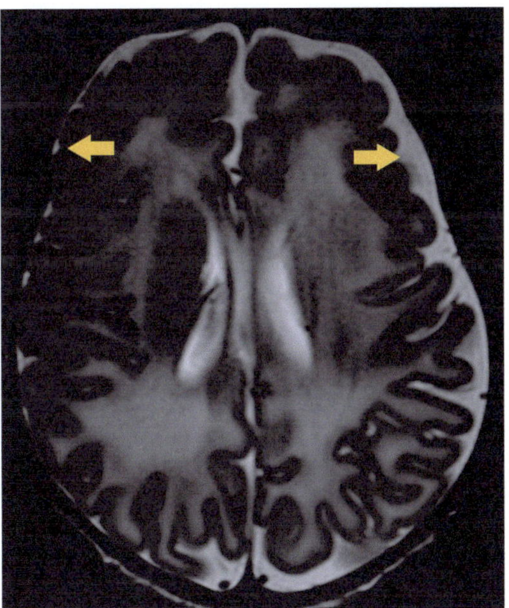

Fig. 1.3 Another child with small variation in imaging with T2W axial view showing BESS presenting as an unilateral asymmetrical enlargement of the left subarachnoid space (left frontotemporo parietal) compared to the right side (orange arrows)

3.3–5 mm (neonates). Upper limit ranges for IHW and SCW are 6–8.5 mm and 2–10 mm respectively. Tucker et al. suggested a grading system for BESS based on the depth of subarachnoid space as Grade 0 (<5 mm), Grade 1 (5–9 mm), Grade 2 (5–9 mm) and found association of incidental subdural collections with higher grades [71].

1.7.2 Imaging Modalities

1. Cranial ultrasound (US)—Often the first procedure as it is easy to perform on an open fontanel. However limited posterior fossa visualization makes it difficult to rule out important causes of obstructive hydrocephalus in a macrocephalic child [72].
2. Computerized tomography (CT)—Good visualization of neuroanatomy but risk of ionizing radiation leading to 0.07% increased lifetime risk of cancer mortality per scan [73, 74].
3. Magnetic resonance imaging (MRI): Maximizes visualization and minimizes risk of radiation. Imaging modality of choice.
4. CSF flow studies: Either by injection of an isotope or a contrast medium intrathecally. Studies have reported slow to no flow especially over cerebral convexities [18, 75].

1.7.3 Long-Term Neuroimaging Outcomes

Most studies show that the frontal subarachnoid space enlargement disappears within 2–3 years of age [4, 55]. Longest follow-up study of 19 years by Muenchberger showed that all patients eventually had a normal MRI [63].

1.8 Differential Diagnosis

There are some conditions that have to be differentiated from BESS on clinical and radiological grounds.

1. Cerebral atrophy: It does not present with increasing head circumference in contrast to BESS. Radiologically, the presence of global widening of cerebral sulci points towards atrophy as BESS typically presents with enlargement of frontal subarachnoid spaces and interhemispheric fissure [76] (Fig. 1.4a, b).
2. Subdural fluid collections: These can be differentiated from BESS by the "cortical vein sign" on MRI or US [77, 78]. A positive sign suggests that the fluid collection is caused by an enlarged subarachnoid space and not a subdural collection which would compress the subarachnoid space and the veins traversing it. On intrathecal injection of dye, the immediate influx of a contrast medium from CSF into a fluid collection suggests external hydrocephalus, whereas no influx indicates a subdural effusion [79]. Ment et al. observed that the enlargement of the basal cisterns often were seen in external hydrocephalus but not in subdural hygromas [54].
3. Convexity and Galassi I arachnoid cyst: These can sometimes masquerade as a loculated extra-axial collection like BESS or subdural effusion as it follows CSF on all sequences [80] (Fig. 1.5). This may be more widespread over convexity in rare instances of ruptured arachnoid cyst [81].

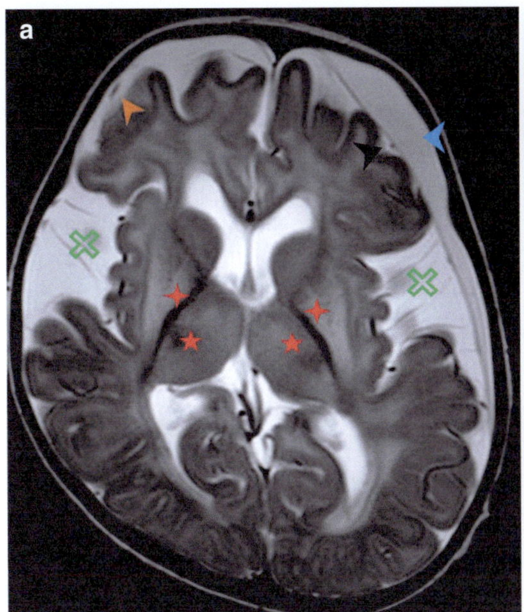 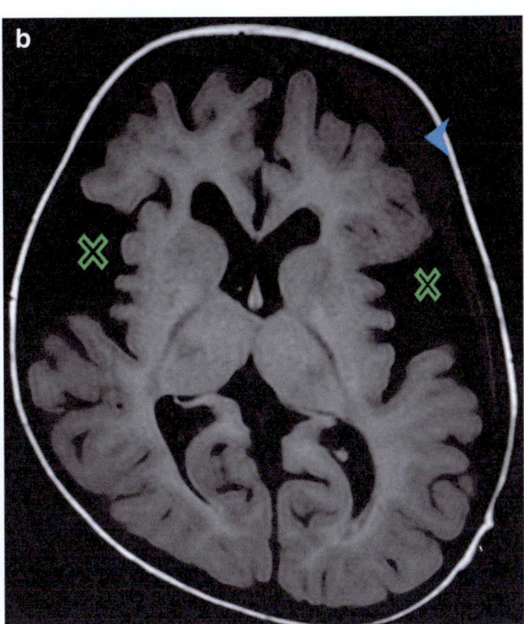

Fig. 1.4 Eight-month-old child with global developmental delay and macrocephaly. Bilateral incomplete opercularization of slyvian fissures and prominent CSF spaces in bitemporal regions, with a left subdural collection due to volume loss and signal changes in bilateral basal ganglia and thalami consistent with glutaric aciduria type 1 noted on T2W axial (**a**) and T1W axial imaging (**b**). (**a**) Cerebral atrophy with resultant temporal subarachnoid space enlargement with widening of Sylvian fissures (green cross) along with bilateral symmetrical hyperdensities in Globus Pallidus (red cross) and subthalamic nucleus (red star). There is the presence of a left subdural collection (blue arrow) showing displacement and compression of the traversing cortical veins (black arrowhead), in stark contrast to the right widened temporal and Sylvian subarachnoid spaces with prominent cortical vein flow voids (orange arrowhead). (**b**) A T1W axial image showing a thin left subdural collection due to volume loss (blue arrow) and enlargement of temporal subarachnoid spaces with widening of Sylvian fissures

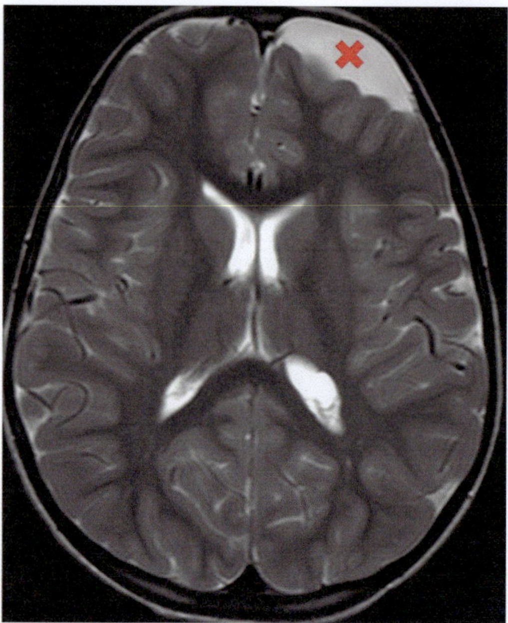

Fig. 1.5 A 3-year-old male showing a left frontal convexity arachnoid cyst on T2W axial image, which can mimic a localized subarachnoid space enlargement following the CSF spaces (red arrow)

1.9 Natural History

A developmental delay is commonly seen at some stage in infancy. Short-term outcomes have been reported by studies which generally found transient developmental delay, primarily gross motor delay and to a lesser extent delay in language development which decreased and corrected by 1–4 years [4, 58, 82]. A study by Muenchberger et al. [63] followed 15 children with BESS, nine of them had detailed neuropsychological assessment up to school with a mean final follow-up of 19 years. Though the final neurological assessment was normal and neuropsychological assessment found normal intellectual ability, several patients showed reduced performance on two tests associated with attention, and two patients with speech delay at 2 years of age performed at below-average levels in most psychological tests at long-term follow-up. Specific learning problems in reading and mathematics or a diagnosis of a psychiatric disease were found in 10 out of 15 patients and eight children had to repeat grades or go to special classes.

In another study, Laubscher et al. [58] did a long-term follow-up on 22 megalencephalic children with "dilated pericerebral subarachnoid spaces." Twelve of them were developmentally delayed). Eleven of these 12 children who had reached school age at the time that the study ended had a normal school outcome. When compared with 22 children without BESS, looking at psychomotor development and school outcome, there was no significant difference between the two groups.

1.10 Treatment

There is no Class I evidence in literature comparing treatment (medical/surgical) versus no treatment, i.e., observation. As BESS is a condition which is by definition benign, it implicitly means that it does not require any treatment and resolves with time. Therefore, observation is the only form of treatment that is required for most cases. The reported modes of treatment, when required, are surgical and medical and the indications, though varied, are generally signs and symptoms of raised intracranial pressure like bulging fontanel, irritability, vomiting accompanied by a growing head circumference. The various forms of surgical treatment reported are direct shunting or burr hole drainage/prolonged external drainage followed by shunting if necessary.

Robertson and Gomez treated two out of six patients with shunts (one lumboperitoneal and one ventriculoperitoneal) because of excessive head growth, ventricular dilatation, and other signs of increased intracranial pressure [12]. One of them was followed for 7 years and developed normally. Ten out of the 14 patients reported by Tsubokawa et al. had macrocephaly and bulging fontanels [83]. All ten underwent surgery with temporary shunt insertion. At 4–6 months after surgery, neuroimaging normalization was seen, although the ventricle enlargement seemed to retract slower. Seven of the ten children operated had a developmental quotient (DQ) of more than 100 at follow-up, indicating normal development, while two of the four non-operated patients had a DQ of less than 39.

Temporary (48 h) bilateral burr hole drainage of the frontal subarachnoid spaces in a 6-month-old girl with external hydrocephalus and developmental delay was reported by Eidlitz-Markus et al. [84]. The head circumference and psychomotor development normalized within a few months and was sustained till the last follow-up at 2 years of age. However, only modest reduction in the size of the CSF spaces was noted. Similarly, Stroobandt et al. [85] suggested treatment with external drainage of pericerebral collections for a week followed by a shunt if the effusion did not resolve.

1.11 Benign Dilatation of Subdural Spaces

Benign enlargement of subdural spaces (BESDS) has been described by many authors using various terminologies like benign subdural effusion [86], benign subdural collection [47], subdural hygroma [87], etc. This entity has been used without clear differentiation to describe clinico-radiological features identical to BESS in many reviews thus adding to the confusion regarding its existence as a separate entity [47, 86].

Many of these studies were done primarily using CT and clinical findings with or without subdural taps to diagnose subdural collections. However, with the advances in imaging, the radiological differentiation between BESS and BESDS is more distinct. There are certain differentiating radiological criteria favoring BESS over BESDS which include (1) bi-hemispheric extracerebral fluid collections: anterior > posterior, (2) widening of the anterior interhemispheric fissure, (3) enlarged subarachnoid spaces, (4) no evidence of cortical atrophy, (5) enlarged or prominent basal cisterns, (6) mild to moderate ventriculomegaly without periventricular lucency, and (7) absence of restriction of blood flow in the cortex adjacent to fluid collection on diffusion-weighted MRI (DW MRI) [87].

There are various factors contributing to its causation like non-accidental injury (NAI), minor/major traumatic injury, meningitis, encephalitis, tumor, following a VP shunt, and without any specific cause (idiopathic) [88].

Interestingly, many studies have reported that BESS can be complicated by subdural hemorrhage (SDH) either spontaneously or following accidental injury [89–92]. The proposed theory is the stretching of bridging veins in the dilated subarachnoid space [92]. There is a mathematical model of the cranial vault suggested by Papasian and Frim [89] which explains the relationship between bridging vein stretching and width of the extra-axial spaces thereby supporting the above theory. The scenario of BESS predisposing to SDH also needs to be very clearly differentiated from SDH secondary to NAI due to obvious medicolegal implications. Clinically, infants with NAI have a very morbid neurological course and risks of mortality whereas those with SDH in pre-existing BESS have a benign course [92–95]. Radiologically, absence of associated intraparenchymal contusions and presence of features of BESS help differentiating from NAI. Caution should therefore be exercised while dealing with an infant with SDH in a scenario of BESS and presumptive diagnosis of NAI should be avoided when other evidence of NAI like long bone fractures, retinal hemorrhages, etc., are absent.

In their study of 20 patients with subdural effusions following minor head injury, Kumar et al. [87] reported that 55% had macrocephaly, 25% had tense AF, 83% presented with seizures, 30% with overt neurological findings like papilloedema, cranial nerve palsies, etc., and 70% with subtle neurological findings with irritability being the most common symptom. The infants with subtle features could mimic the features of BESS.

The various treatment options are observation, subdural needle aspirations, burr hole evacuation, subduro-peritoneal shunt (unilateral/bilateral), and craniotomy for drainage and excision of neo-membranes [87]. It has been suggested that collections with thickness less than 7 mm on CT scan may have a better chance of resolving spontaneously, and hence non-operative approach may be sufficient [96]. Needle aspirations and burr hole drainage may need multiple procedures and are prone to infection. Subduroperitoneal shunts have a very high reported success rate in eliminating subdural collections between 80%

and 100% [97–99]. Unilateral shunt is usually effective in controlling bilateral collections and an unvalved shunt is used in most reports [98, 100, 101]. Subdural shunts, though, have a reported obstruction rate of up to 14% and an infection rate of 5% [98, 99, 102]. Craniotomy is needed only in complex cases.

1.12 Is Benign Enlargement of Subarachnoid Spaces Really Benign?

The usual assumption about BESS is that of an infant presenting with macrocephaly and typical neuroimaging features who has some developmental delay transiently but finally catches up with its peers. This self-limiting nature of the disorder leads to it being perceived as "benign." Many studies reporting a long-term normal outcome are based on clinical and neurological assessments.

However, studies using standardized neuropsychological tests have reported deficits in children with BEH on long-term follow-up. Alvarez et al. using the Denver Developmental Screening Test in 36 children found 14 children with delayed gross motor development, five with delayed language development, and one with global developmental delay at last follow-up at 30 months of age [10]. The same test used by Alper et al. revealed two out of 13 children with fine motor delay. The Peabody picture-vocabulary test used by the same authors showed expressive language delay in two out of seven children older than 2.5 years [6].

Zahl et al., in a retrospective population based study, reported that children and adolescents who were diagnosed with BEH during infancy generally do well. However, for some patients, there appear to be various developmental, social, and cognitive problems, and they seem to struggle more in school than their healthy peers [103]. In addition, various problems like mental retardation [58], epilepsy [104], social behavioral problems [103], autism spectrum disorders [105], and learning disabilities [58, 63] have been reported to be associated in children diagnosed with BEH on long-term follow-up.

In the light of the above evidence, it might be worth questioning the "benign" nature of this condition. However, this does not change the fact that probably most children presenting with this condition will show near resolution of imaging findings and halted progression of macrocephaly without any treatment and will achieve normal development in gross scores of assessment when done by neurologists and neurosurgeons. A more precise and specific outcome assessment by developmental pediatricians and neuropsychologists will be paramount to help establish subtle deficits and the actual impact of this disorder on the quality of life. The impact of timely intervention on long-term outcome is a subject which needs to be analyzed critically with prospective long-term studies. Prophylactic intervention in selected patients in this presumed self-limiting condition will also be a topic of interest and curiosity for future research.

1.13 Conclusion

Benign Enlargement of Subarachnoid spaces and Subdural collections are the most common forms of extracerebral collections found in infancy. Literature is abound with a variety of nomenclature describing these entities. Most cases of BESS present with typical neuroimaging findings and macrocephaly which is expected to settle down within the second year of life. The natural history of BESS favours grossly normal development though long term follow up and detailed neuropsychological tests have unveiled subtle or specific problems in various studies. Most cases do not require any treatment except few which may present with signs of raised intracranial pressure (ICP) warranting some form of surgical intervention. Subdural collections need to be differentiated from BESS. It is also essential to define the etiology of subdural collections as NAI is a significant cause and has profound medical and legal implications. Like BESS, subdural collections also warrant treatment when they present with raised ICP symptoms though many will be asymptomatic.

References

1. Haws ME, Linscott L, Thomas C, Orscheln E, Radhakrishnan R, Kline-Fath B. A retrospective analysis of the utility of head computed tomography and/or magnetic resonance imaging in the management of benign macrocrania. J Pediatr. 2017;182:283–289.e1 [cited 2022 Feb 22]. Available from: https://linkinghub.elsevier.com/retrieve/pii/S0022347616312628.

2. Kuruvilla L. Benign enlargement of subarachnoid spaces in infancy. J Pediatr Neurosci. 2014;9(2):129 [cited 2022 Feb 22]. Available from: http://www.pediatricneurosciences.com/text.asp?2014/9/2/129/139309.

3. Zahl SM, Egge A, Helseth E, Wester K. Benign external hydrocephalus: a review, with emphasis on management. Neurosurg Rev. 2011;34(4):417–32 [cited 2022 Feb 22]. Available from: http://link.springer.com/10.1007/s10143-011-0327-4.

4. Kumar R. External hydrocephalus in small children. Childs Nerv Syst. 2006;22(10):1237–41 [cited 2022 Feb 22]. Available from: http://link.springer.com/10.1007/s00381-006-0047-1.

5. Marino MA, Morabito R, Vinci S, Germanò A, Briguglio M, Alafaci C, et al. Benign external hydrocephalus in infants: a single centre experience and literature review. Neuroradiol J. 2014;27(2):245–50 [cited 2022 Feb 22]. Available from: http://journals.sagepub.com/doi/10.15274/NRJ-2014-10020.

6. Alper G, Ekinci G, Yilmaz Y, Ankan Ç, Telyar G, Erzen C. Magnetic resonance imaging characteristics of benign macrocephaly in children. J Child Neurol. 1999;14(10):678–82 [cited 2022 Feb 22]. Available from: http://journals.sagepub.com/doi/10.1177/088307389901401010.

7. Bodensteiner JB. Benign macrocephaly: a common cause of big heads in the first year. J Child Neurol. 2000;15(9):630–1 [cited 2022 Feb 22]. Available from: http://journals.sagepub.com/doi/10.1177/088307380001500913.

8. Dandy WE. An experimental, clinical and pathological study: part 1—experimental studies. Am J Dis Child. 1914;VIII(6):406 [cited 2022 Feb 22]. Available from: http://archpedi.jamanetwork.com/article.aspx?doi=10.1001/archpedi.1914.02180010416002.

9. Dandy WE. Extirpation of the choroid plexus of the lateral ventricles in communicating hydrocephalus. Ann Surg. 1918;68(6):569–79 [cited 2022 Feb 22]. Available from: http://journals.lww.com/00000658-191812000-00001.

10. Alvarez LA, Maytal J, Shinnar S. Idiopathic external hydrocephalus: natural history and relationship to benign familial macrocephaly. Pediatrics. 1986;77(6):901–7.

11. Pettit RE. Macrocephaly with head growth parallel to normal growth pattern: neurological, developmental, and computerized tomography findings in full-term infants. Arch Neurol. 1980;37(8):518 [cited 2022 Feb 22]. Available from: http://archneur.jamanetwork.com/article.aspx?doi=10.1001/archneur.1980.00500570066011.

12. Robertson WC. External hydrocephalus: early finding in congenital communicating hydrocephalus. Arch Neurol. 1978;35(8):541 [cited 2022 Feb 22]. Available from: http://archneur.jamanetwork.com/article.aspx?doi=10.1001/archneur.1978.00500320061014.

13. DiLiberti JH. Inherited macrocephaly-hamartoma syndromes. Am J Med Genet. 1998;79(4):284–90 [cited 2022 Feb 23]. Available from: https://onlinelibrary.wiley.com/doi/10.1002/(SICI)1096-8628(19981002)79:4<284::AID-AJMG10>3.0.CO;2-N.

14. Wiig US, Zahl SM, Egge A, Helseth E, Wester K. Epidemiology of benign external hydrocephalus in Norway—a population-based study. Pediatr Neurol. 2017;73:36–41 [cited 2022 Feb 23]. Available from: https://linkinghub.elsevier.com/retrieve/pii/S088789941730070X.

15. Asch AJ, Myers GJ. Benign familial macrocephaly: report of a family and review of the literature. Pediatrics. 1976;57(4):535–9.

16. Hellbusch LC. Benign extracerebral fluid collections in infancy: clinical presentation and long-term follow-up. J Neurosurg Pediatr. 2007;107(2):119–25 [cited 2022 Feb 23]. Available from: http://thejns.org/doi/abs/10.3171/PED-07/08/119.

17. Al-Saedi SA, Lemke RP, Debooy VD, Casiro O. Subarachnoid fluid collections: a cause of macrocrania in preterm infants. J Pediatr. 1996;128(2):234–6 [cited 2022 Feb 24]. Available from: https://linkinghub.elsevier.com/retrieve/pii/S0022347696703967.

18. Andersson H, Elfverson J, Svendsen P. External hydrocephalus in infants. Pediatr Neurosurg. 1984;11(6):398–402 [cited 2022 Feb 23]. Available from: https://www.karger.com/Article/FullText/120203.

19. Segal-Kuperschmit D, Cozacov C, Luder A. [Idiopathic external hydrocephalus]. Harefuah. 1995;128(3):150–2, 199.

20. Nogueira GJ, Zaglul HF. Hypodense extracerebral images on computed tomography in children: external hydrocephalus: a misnomer? Childs Nerv Syst. 1991;7(6):336–41 [cited 2022 Feb 24]. Available from: http://link.springer.com/10.1007/BF00304833.

21. Palencia Luaces R, Aldana Gómez J, Tresierra Unzaga F. [Idiopathic external hydrocephaly and familial macrocephaly in infancy]. An Esp Pediatr. 1992;36(3):186–8.

22. Wilms G, Vanderschueren G, Demaerel PH, Smet MH, Van Calenbergh F, Plets C, et al. CT and MR in infants with pericerebral collections and macrocephaly: benign enlargement of the subarachnoid spaces versus subdural collections. AJNR Am J Neuroradiol. 1993;14(4):855–60.

23. Arbour L, Watters GV, Hall JG, Fraser FC. Multifactorial inheritance of non-syndromic macrocephaly. Clin Genet. 2008;50(2):57–62 [cited 2022 Feb 24]. Available from: https://onlinelibrary.wiley.com/doi/10.1111/j.1399-0004.1996.tb02349.x.

24. Paciorkowski AR, Greenstein RM. When is enlargement of the subarachnoid spaces not benign? A genetic perspective. Pediatr Neurol. 2007;37(1):1–7 [cited 2022 Feb 24]. Available from: https://linkinghub.elsevier.com/retrieve/pii/S0887899407001518.

25. Kendall B, Holland I. Benign communicating hydrocephalus in children. Neuroradiology. 1981;21(2):93–6 [cited 2022 Feb 23]. Available from: http://link.springer.com/10.1007/BF00342987.

26. Lorber J, Bhat US. Posthaemorrhagic hydrocephalus: diagnosis, differential diagnosis, treatment, and long-term results. Arch Dis Child. 1974;49(10):751–62 [cited 2022 Feb 23]. Available from: https://adc.bmj.com/lookup/doi/10.1136/adc.49.10.751.

27. Rekate HL, Blitz AM. Hydrocephalus in children. In: Handbook of clinical neurology. Elsevier; 2016 [cited 2022 Feb 23]. p. 1261–73. Available from: https://linkinghub.elsevier.com/retrieve/pii/B9780444534866000648.

28. Bhasker B, Raghupathy P, Nair TM, Ahmed SR, deSilva V, Bhuyan BC, et al. External hydrocephalus in primary hypomagnesaemia: a new finding. Arch Dis Child. 1999;81:505–50.

29. Gordon N. Apparent cerebral atrophy in patients on treatment with steroids. Dev Med Child Neurol. 2008;22(4):502–6 [cited 2022 Feb 23]. Available from: https://onlinelibrary.wiley.com/doi/10.1111/j.1469-8749.1980.tb04355.x.

30. Enzmann DR, Lane B. Enlargement of subarachnoid spaces and lateral ventricles in pediatric patients undergoing chemotherapy. J Pediatr. 1978;92(4):535–9 [cited 2022 Feb 23]. Available from: https://linkinghub.elsevier.com/retrieve/pii/S0022347678802832.

31. Hoppe-Hirsch E, Rose CS, Renier D, Hirsch J-F. Pericerebral collections after shunting. Childs Nerv Syst. 1987;3(2):97–102 [cited 2022 Feb 23]. Available from: http://link.springer.com/10.1007/BF00271133.

32. Burstein J, Papile L, Burstein R. Intraventricular hemorrhage and hydrocephalus in premature newborns: a prospective study with CT. Am J Roentgenol. 1979;132(4):631–5 [cited 2022 Feb 23]. Available from: http://www.ajronline.org/doi/10.2214/ajr.132.4.631.

33. Govaert P, Oostra A, Matthys D, Vanhaesebrouck P, Leroy J. How idiopathic is idiopathic external hydrocephalus? Dev Med Child Neurol. 1991;33(3):274–6 [cited 2022 Feb 23]. Available from: https://onlinelibrary.wiley.com/doi/10.1111/j.1469-8749.1991.tb05121.x.

34. Davson H, Segal M. Introduction. In: Davson H, Segal MB, editors. Physiology of the CSF and blood-brain barriers. 1st ed. Boca Raton, FL: CRC Press; 1996. p. 3–7.

35. Volpe J. Neural tube formation and prosencephalic development. In: Volpe JJ, editor. Neurology of the newborn. 4th ed. Philadelphia: W.B. Saunders Co.; 2001. p. 3–44.

36. Sarnat H. Neuroembryology, genetic programming, and malformations of the nervous system. In: Menkes JH, Sarnat HB, Maria BL, editors. Child neurology. 7th ed. Philadelphia: Lippincott Williams & Wilkins; 2006. p. 330–47.

37. Girard NJ, Raybaud CA. Ventriculomegaly and pericerebral CSF collection in the fetus: early stage of benign external hydrocephalus? Childs Nerv Syst. 2001;17(4–5):239–45 [cited 2022 Feb 24]. Available from: http://link.springer.com/10.1007/PL00013727.

38. Greitz D. Radiological assessment of hydrocephalus: new theories and implications for therapy. Neurosurg Rev. 2004;27(3):145–165 [cited 2022 Feb 24]. Available from: http://link.springer.com/10.1007/s10143-004-0326-9.

39. Han CY, Backous DD. Basic principles of cerebrospinal fluid metabolism and intracranial pressure homeostasis. Otolaryngol Clin North Am. 2005;38(4):569–76 [cited 2022 Feb 24]. Available from: https://linkinghub.elsevier.com/retrieve/pii/S003066650500006X.

40. Watanabe Y, Abe S, Takagi K, Yamamoto T, Kato T. Evolution of subarachnoid space in normal fetuses using magnetic resonance imaging. Prenat Diagn. 2005;25(13):1217–22 [cited 2022 Feb 24]. Available from: https://onlinelibrary.wiley.com/doi/10.1002/pd.1315.

41. Fishman R. Anatomical aspects of the cerebrospinal fluid. In: Fishman RA, editor. Cerebrospinal fluid in diseases of the nervous system. Philadelphia: W.B. Saunders Co; 1980. p. 6–18.

42. Upton ML, Weller RO. The morphology of cerebrospinal fluid drainage pathways in human arachnoid granulations. J Neurosurg. 1985;63(6):867–75 [cited 2022 Feb 24]. Available from: https://thejns.org/view/journals/j-neurosurg/63/6/article-p867.xml.

43. Barlow CF. CSF dynamics in hydrocephalus—with special attention to external hydrocephalus. Brain Dev. 1984;6(2):119–27 [cited 2022 Feb 24]. Available from: https://linkinghub.elsevier.com/retrieve/pii/S0387760484800601.

44. Kleinman PK, Zito JL, Davidson RI, Raptopoulos V. The subarachnoid spaces in children: normal variations in size. Radiology. 1983;147(2):455–7 [cited 2022 Feb 24]. Available from: http://pubs.rsna.org/doi/10.1148/radiology.147.2.6601281.

45. Dandy WE. Treatment of an unusual subdural hydroma (external hydrocephalus). Arch Surg. 1946;52(4):421 [cited 2022 Feb 24]. Available from: http://archsurg.jamanetwork.com/article.aspx?doi=10.1001/archsurg.1946.01230050428003.

46. Snyder R, Snyder RD. Benign "subdural" collections. J Pediatr. 1979;95:499–500.

47. Robertson WC, Chun RWM, Orrison WW, Sackett JF. Benign subdural collections of infancy. J Pediatr. 1979;94(3):382–5 [cited 2022 Feb 24]. Available from: https://linkinghub.elsevier.com/retrieve/pii/S0022347679805752.

48. Gomez D, DiBenedetto A, Pavese A, Firpo A, Hershan D, Potts D. Development of arachnoid villi and granulations in man. Acta Anat Basel. 1982;111:247–58.

49. Girard N, Gire C, Sigaudy S, Porcu G, d'Ercole C, Figarella-Branger D, et al. MR imaging of acquired fetal brain disorders. Childs Nerv Syst. 2003;19(7–8):490–500 [cited 2022 Feb 24]. Available from: http://link.springer.com/10.1007/s00381-003-0761-x.

50. Cinalli G, di Martino G, Russo C, Mazio F, Nastro A, Mirone G, et al. Dural venous sinus anatomy in children with external hydrocephalus: analysis of a series of 97 patients. Childs Nerv Syst. 2021;37(10):3021–32 [cited 2022 Mar 7]. Available from: https://link.springer.com/10.1007/s00381-021-05322-5.

51. Carolan PL, McLaurin RL, Towbin RB, Towbin JA, Egelhoff JC. Benign extra-axial collections of infancy. Pediatr Neurosurg. 1985;12(3):140–4 [cited 2022 Feb 24]. Available from: https://www.karger.com/Article/FullText/120236.

52. Khosroshahi N, Nikkhah A. Benign enlargement of subarachnoid space in infancy: "a review with emphasis on diagnostic work-up". Iran J Child Neurol. 2018;12(4):7–15.

53. Pascual-Castroviejo I, Pascual-Pascual SI, Velázquez-Fragua R. [A study and follow-up of ten cases of benign enlargement of the subarachnoid spaces]. Rev Neurol. 2004;39(8):701–6.

54. Ment LR, Duncan CC, Geehr R. Benign enlargement of the subarachnoid spaces in the infant. J Neurosurg. 1981;54(4):504–8 [cited 2022 Feb 24]. Available from: https://thejns.org/view/journals/j-neurosurg/54/4/article-p504.xml.

55. Castro-Gago M, Pérez-Gómez C, Novo-Rodríguez MI, Blanco-Barca O, Alonso-Martin A, Eirís-Puñal J. [Benign idiopathic external hydrocephalus (benign subdural collection) in 39 children: its natural history and relation to familial macrocephaly]. Rev Neurol. 2005;40(9):513–7.

56. Gherpelli JLD, Scaramuzzi V, Manreza MLG, Diament AJ. Follow-up study of macrocephalic children with enlargement of the subarachnoid space. Arq Neuropsiquiatr. 1992;50(2):156–62 [cited 2022 Feb 24]. Available from: http://www.scielo.br/scielo.php?script=sci_arttext&pid=S0004-282X1992000200004&lng=en&tlng=en.

57. Gooskens RH, Willemse J, Faber J, Verdonck AF. Macrocephalies—a differentiated approach. Neuropediatrics. 1989;20(3):164–9 [cited 2022 Feb 24]. Available from: http://www.thieme-connect.de/DOI/DOI?10.1055/s-2008-1071284.

58. Laubscher B, Deonna T, Uske A, van Melle G. Primitive megalencephaly in children: natural history, medium term prognosis with special reference to external hydrocephalus. Eur J Pediatr. 1990;149(7):502–7 [cited 2022 Feb 24]. Available from: http://link.springer.com/10.1007/BF01959405.

59. Azais M, Echenne B. [Idiopathic pericerebral swelling (external hydrocephalus) of infants]. Ann Pediatr (Paris). 1992;39(9):550–8.

60. El-Feky M, Di Muzio B. Benign enlargement of the subarachnoid space in infancy. In: Radiopaedia.org. 2011 [cited 2022 Mar 6]. Available from: http://radiopaedia.org/articles/13118.

61. Kapila A, Trice J, Spies WG, Siegel BA, Gado MH. Enlarged cerebrospinal fluid spaces in infants with subdural hematomas. Radiology. 1982;142(3):669–72 [cited 2022 Feb 24]. Available from: http://pubs.rsna.org/doi/10.1148/radiology.142.3.6977789.

62. Medina LS, Frawley K, Zurakowski D, Buttros D, DeGrauw AJ, Crone KR. Children with macrocrania: clinical and imaging predictors of disorders requiring surgery. AJNR Am J Neuroradiol. 2001;22(3):564–70.

63. Muenchberger H, Assaad N, Joy P, Brunsdon R, Shores EA. Idiopathic macrocephaly in the infant: long-term neurological and neuropsychological outcome. Childs Nerv Syst. 2006;22(10):1242–8 [cited 2022 Feb 24]. Available from: http://link.springer.com/10.1007/s00381-006-0080-0.

64. Prassopoulos P, Cavouras D, Golfinopoulos S, Nezi M. The size of the intra- and extraventricular cerebrospinal fluid compartments in children with idiopathic benign widening of the frontal subarachnoid space. Neuroradiology. 1995;37(5):418–21 [cited 2022 Feb 24]. Available from: http://link.springer.com/10.1007/BF00588027.

65. Maytal J, Alvarez L, Elkin C, Shinnar S. External hydrocephalus: radiologic spectrum and differentiation from cerebral atrophy. Am J Roentgenol. 1987;148(6):1223–30[cited 2022 Feb 24]. Available from: http://www.ajronline.org/doi/10.2214/ajr.148.6.1223.

66. Fessell DP, Frankel DA, Wolfson WP. Sonography of extraaxial fluid in neurologically normal infants with head circumference greater than or equal to the 95th percentile for age. J Ultrasound Med. 2000;19(7):443–7 [cited 2022 Feb 24]. Available from: http://doi.wiley.com/10.7863/jum.2000.19.7.443.

67. Frankel DA, Fessell DP, Wolfson WP. High resolution sonographic determination of the normal dimensions of the intracranial extraaxial compartment in the newborn infant. J Ultrasound Med. 1998;17(7):411–5 [cited 2022 Feb 24]. Available from: http://doi.wiley.com/10.7863/jum.1998.17.7.411.

68. Fukuyama Y, Miyao M, Ishizu T, Maruyama H. Developmental changes in normal cranial measurements by computed tomography. Dev Med Child Neurol. 2008;21(4):425–32 [cited 2022 Feb 24]. Available from: https://onlinelibrary.wiley.com/doi/10.1111/j.1469-8749.1979.tb01645.x.

69. Libicher M, Tröger J. US measurement of the subarachnoid space in infants: normal values. Radiology. 1992;184(3):749–51 [cited 2022 Feb 24]. Available from: http://pubs.rsna.org/doi/10.1148/radiology.184.3.1509061.

70. Yew AY, Maher CO, Muraszko KM, Garton HJL. Long-term health status in benign external hydrocephalus. Pediatr Neurosurg. 2011;47(1):1–6 [cited 2022 Mar 6]. Available from: https://www.karger.com/Article/FullText/322357.

71. Tucker J, Choudhary AK, Piatt J. Macrocephaly in infancy: benign enlargement of the subarachnoid spaces and subdural collections. J Neurosurg Pediatr. 2016;18(1):16–20 [cited 2022 Feb 27]. Available from: https://thejns.org/view/journals/j-neurosurg-pediatr/18/1/article-p16.xml.

72. Enríquez G, Correa F, Lucaya J, Piqueras J, Aso C, Ortega A. Potential pitfalls in cranial sonography. Pediatr Radiol. 2003;33(2):110–7 [cited 2022 Feb 24]. Available from: http://link.springer.com/10.1007/s00247-002-0836-y.

73. Brenner DJ, Elliston CD, Hall EJ, Berdon WE. Estimated risks of radiation-induced fatal cancer from pediatric CT. Am J Roentgenol. 2001;176(2):289–96 [cited 2022 Feb 24]. Available from: http://www.ajronline.org/doi/10.2214/ajr.176.2.1760289.

74. Martin DR, Semelka RC. Health effects of ionising radiation from diagnostic CT. Lancet. 2006;367(9524):1712–4 [cited 2022 Feb 24]. Available from: https://linkinghub.elsevier.com/retrieve/pii/S0140673606687485.

75. Briner S, Bodensteiner J. Benign subdural collections of infancy. Pediatrics. 1981;67(6):802–4 [cited 2022 Feb 24]. Available from: https://publications.aap.org/pediatrics/article/67/6/802/39072/Benign-Subdural-Collections-of-Infancy.

76. Lorber J, Priestley BL. Children with large heads: à practical approach to diagnosis in 557 children, with special reference to 109 children with megalencephaly. Dev Med Child Neurol. 2008;23(5):494–504 [cited 2022 Feb 27]. Available from: https://onlinelibrary.wiley.com/doi/10.1111/j.1469-8749.1981.tb02023.x.

77. Kuzma BB, Goodman JM. Differentiating external hydrocephalus from chronic subdural hematoma. Surg Neurol. 1998;50(1):86–8.

78. Chen CY, Chou TY, Zimmerman RA, Lee CC, Chen FH, Faro SH. Pericerebral fluid collection: differentiation of enlarged subarachnoid spaces from subdural collections with color Doppler US. Radiology. 1996;201(2):389–92 [cited 2022 Feb 27]. Available from: http://pubs.rsna.org/doi/10.1148/radiology.201.2.8888229.

79. Pietil TA, Palleske H, Distelmaier PM. Subdural effusions: determination of contrast medium influx from CSF to the fluid accumulation by computed tomography as an aid to the indications for management. Acta Neurochir (Wien). 1992;118(3–4):103–7 [cited 2022 Feb 27]. Available from: http://link.springer.com/10.1007/BF01401294.

80. Botz B, Weerakkody Y. Subdural hygroma. In: Radiopaedia.org. 2012 [cited 2022 Mar 3]. Available from: http://radiopaedia.org/articles/18609.

81. Donaldson JW, Edwards-Brown M, Luerssen TG. Arachnoid cyst rupture with concurrent subdural hygroma. Pediatr Neurosurg. 2000;32(3):137–9 [cited 2022 Mar 8]. Available from: https://www.karger.com/Article/FullText/28918.

82. Nickel RE, Galtenstein JS. Developmental prognosis for infants with benign enlargement of the subarachnoid spaces. Dev Med Child Neurol. 2008;29(2):181–6 [cited 2022 Mar 1]. Available from: https://onlinelibrary.wiley.com/doi/10.1111/j.1469-8749.1987.tb02133.x.

83. Tsubokawa T, Nakamura S, Satoh K. Effect of temporary subdural-peritoneal shunt on subdural effusion with subarachnoid effusion. Pediatr Neurosurg. 1984;11(1):47–59 [cited 2022 Mar 2]. Available from: https://www.karger.com/Article/FullText/120159.

84. Eidlitz-Markus T, Shuper A, Constantini S. Short-term subarachnoid space drainage: a potential treatment for extraventricular hydrocephalus. Childs Nerv Syst. 2003;19(5–6):367–70 [cited 2022 Mar 2]. Available from: http://link.springer.com/10.1007/s00381-003-0751-z.

85. Stroobandt G, Evrard P, Thauvoy C, Laterre C. [Subdural or sub-arachnoid pericerebral effusions in the infant with subdural or subarachnoid localisation (author's transl)]. Neurochirurgie. 1981;27(1):49–57.

86. Mori K, Handa H, Itoh M, Okuno T. Benign subdural effusion in infants. J Comput Assist Tomogr. 1980;4(4):466–71 [cited 2022 Mar 3]. Available from: http://journals.lww.com/00004728-198008000-00009.

87. Kumar R, Singhal N, Mahapatra AK. Traumatic subdural effusions in children following minor head injury. Childs Nerv Syst. 2008;24(12):1391–6 [cited 2022 Mar 3]. Available from: http://link.springer.com/10.1007/s00381-008-0645-1.

88. Tolias C, Sgouros S, Walsh AR, Hockley AD. Outcome of surgical treatment for subdural fluid collections in infants. Pediatr Neurosurg. 2000;33(4):194–7 [cited 2022 Mar 3]. Available from: https://www.karger.com/Article/FullText/55952.

89. Papasian NC, Frim DM. A theoretical model of benign external hydrocephalus that predicts a predisposition towards extra-axial hemorrhage after minor head trauma. Pediatr Neurosurg. 2000;33(4):188–93 [cited 2022 Mar 6]. Available from: https://www.karger.com/Article/FullText/55951.

90. Pittman T. Significance of a subdural hematoma in a child with external hydrocephalus. Pediatr Neurosurg. 2003;39(2):57–9 [cited 2022 Mar 6].

Available from: https://www.karger.com/Article/FullText/71315.

91. Ravid S, Maytal J. External hydrocephalus: a probable cause for subdural hematoma in infancy. Pediatr Neurol. 2003;28(2):139–41 [cited 2022 Mar 6]. Available from: https://linkinghub.elsevier.com/retrieve/pii/S0887899402005003.

92. McNeely PD, Atkinson JD, Saigal G, O'Gorman AM, Farmer J-P. Subdural hematomas in infants with benign enlargement of the subarachnoid spaces are not pathognomonic for child abuse. AJNR Am J Neuroradiol. 2006;27(8):1725–8.

93. Hoskote A, Richards P, Anslow P, McShane T. Subdural haematoma and non-accidental head injury in children. Childs Nerv Syst. 2002;18(6–7):311–7.

94. Duhaime AC, Alario AJ, Lewander WJ, Schut L, Sutton LN, Seidl TS, et al. Head injury in very young children: mechanisms, injury types, and ophthalmologic findings in 100 hospitalized patients younger than 2 years of age. Pediatrics. 1992;90(2 Pt 1):179–85.

95. Jayawant S, Rawlinson A, Gibbon F, Price J, Schulte J, Sharples P, et al. Subdural haemorrhages in infants: population based study. BMJ. 1998;317(7172):1558–61.

96. Rothenberger A, Brandl H. Subdural effusions in children under two years—clinical and computer-tomographical data. Neuropediatrics. 1980;11(02):139–50 [cited 2022 Mar 3]. Available from: http://www.thieme-connect.de/DOI/DOI?10.1055/s-2008-1071384.

97. Morota N, Sakamoto K, Kobayashi N, Kitazawa K, Kobayashi S. Infantile subdural fluid collection: diagnosis and postoperative course. Childs Nerv Syst. 1995;11(8):459–66 [cited 2022 Mar 3]. Available from: http://link.springer.com/10.1007/BF00334966.

98. Litofsky NS, Raffel C, McComb JG. Management of symptomatic chronic extra-axial fluid collections in pediatric patients. Neurosurgery. 1992;31(3):445–50 [cited 2022 Mar 3]. Available from: https://academic.oup.com/neurosurgery/article/31/3/445/2752096.

99. Vinchon M, Noulé N, Soto-Ares G, Dhellemmes P. Subduroperitoneal drainage for subdural hematomas in infants: results in 244 cases. J Neurosurg. 2001;95(2):249–55 [cited 2022 Mar 3]. Available from: https://thejns.org/view/journals/j-neurosurg/95/2/article-p249.xml.

100. Aoki N, Masuzawa H. Bilateral chronic subdural hematomas without communication between the hematoma cavities: treatment with unilateral subdural-peritoneal shunt. Neurosurgery. 1988;22(5):911–3.

101. Aoki N, Mizutani H, Masuzawa H. Unilateral subdural-peritoneal shunting for bilateral chronic subdural hematomas in infancy. Report of three cases. J Neurosurg. 1985;63(1):134–7.

102. Mircevski M, Boyadziev I, Ruskov P, Mircevska D, Davkov S. Surgical treatment of acute subdural hygroma in children. Childs Nerv Syst. 1986;2(6):314–6 [cited 2022 Mar 3]. Available from: http://link.springer.com/10.1007/BF00271946.

103. Zahl SM, Egge A, Helseth E, Skarbø A-B, Wester K. Quality of life and physician-reported developmental, cognitive, and social problems in children with benign external hydrocephalus—long-term follow-up. Childs Nerv Syst. 2019;35(2):245–50 [cited 2022 Mar 6]. Available from: http://link.springer.com/10.1007/s00381-018-4016-2.

104. Syvertsen M, Nakken KO, Edland A, Hansen G, Hellum MK, Koht J. Prevalence and etiology of epilepsy in a Norwegian county—a population based study. Epilepsia. 2015;56(5):699–706 [cited 2022 Mar 6]. Available from: https://onlinelibrary.wiley.com/doi/10.1111/epi.12972.

105. Surén P, Bakken IJ, Aase H, Chin R, Gunnes N, Lie KK, et al. Autism spectrum disorder, ADHD, epilepsy, and cerebral palsy in Norwegian children. Pediatrics. 2012;130(1):e152–8 [cited 2022 Mar 6]. Available from: https://publications.aap.org/pediatrics/article/130/1/e152/29870/Autism-Spectrum-Disorder-ADHD-Epilepsy-and.

Incidental Intracranial Calcifications

Bal Krishna Ojha (ID), Chhitij Srivastava (ID), and Anit Parihar

2.1 Introduction

Intracranial calcifications are calcifications within the brain parenchyma or its vasculature. They are common radiographic finding and their etiology varies from benign physiological processes to multiple pathological processes. Brain calcifications have been reported in up to 72% in autopsy cases but their clinical prevalence ranges from 1% in young individuals to up to 20% in elderly [1]. Due to its high sensitivity in the visualization of bone tissue and calcifications, computed tomography (CT) scan has replaced the use of conventional radiography and CT scan is even considered superior to magnetic resonance imaging (MRI) in detection and characterization of intracranial calcifications [2].

Physiological intracranial calcifications can develop in pineal gland, habenula, choroid plexus, basal ganglia, and dura matter. Pathological intracranial calcifications can be grouped under congenital (genetic/developmental) disorders, infections (congenital and acquired), vascular disorders, neoplastic disorders, metabolic/endocrine disorders, inflammatory disorders, and posttreatment/posttraumatic/ some neurotoxicity disorders [3, 4].

2.2 Physiologic Intracranial Calcifications

Physiologic intracranial calcifications are usually age related incidental findings on non-contrast CT (NCCT) scan and usually found in following locations.

2.2.1 Pineal Calcifications

Before the age of 50 years, the pineal gland is most common site of physiological calcification (71.6%) and most of the time, these are less than 1 cm and described as course and compact [5]. Pineal calcifications if more than 1 cm in size and if they are numerous should be further investigated with assessment of pineal gland volume as well as clinical and biochemical investigations [6–8] (Fig. 2.1).

2.2.2 Choroid Plexus Calcification

Choroid plexus calcification has been reported as most common site of physiological calcification after 50 years of age [5]. They are most com-

B. K. Ojha (✉) · C. Srivastava
Department of Neurosurgery, King George's Medical University, Lucknow, Uttar Pradesh, India

A. Parihar
Department of Radiodiagnosis, King George's Medical University, Lucknow, Uttar Pradesh, India

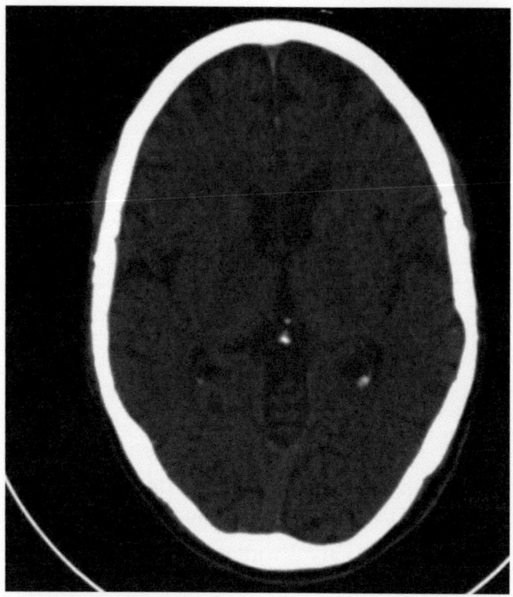

Fig. 2.1 Pineal gland calcification

monly found in ventricular atria where higher concentration of choroid plexus is found (choroidal glomus) and usually described as punctuate [4]. If they are found in atypical locations such as body of lateral ventricles, roof of third ventricle or interventricular foramen or fourth ventricle, may need further evaluation for any underlying pathology [7] (Fig. 2.2).

2.2.3 Habenula Calcification

Habenula calcification has been reported to be found in 10–15% of adults. They are usually curvilinear and found few millimeters anterior to pineal body [7, 8]. Association of schizophrenia and learning disorders and habenular calcification has been reported in literature [9, 10].

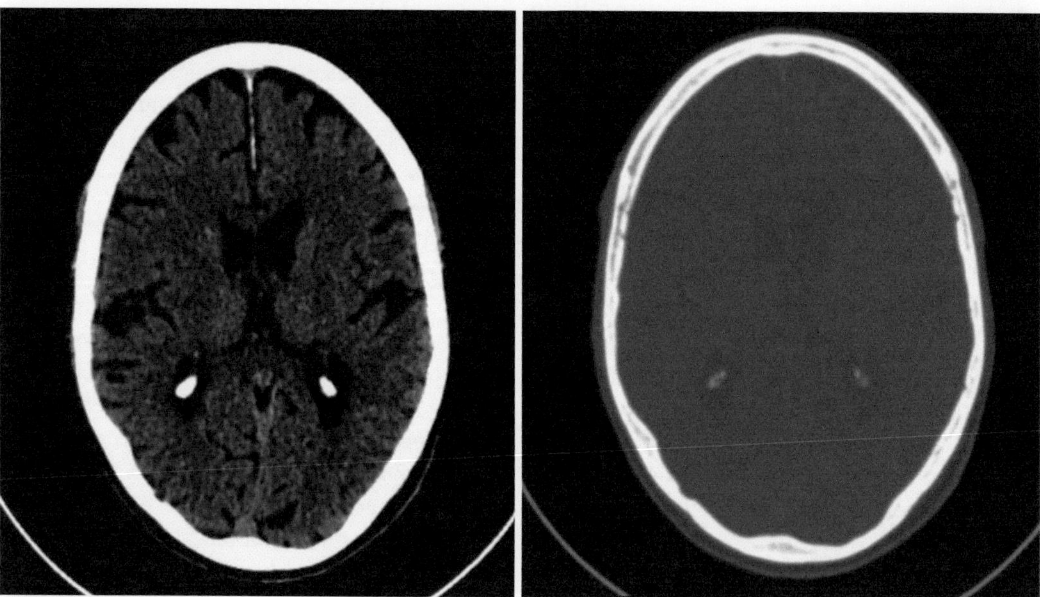

Fig. 2.2 Choroid plexus calcifications

2.2.4 Dura Matter Calcifications

Dura matter calcifications are most commonly seen in tentorium cerebelli (laminar pattern) and falx cerebri (dense flat plates in the midline) and they occur with frequency ranging from 2% to 20% [10, 11]. As with other physiological intracranial calcifications, their frequency increases with advancing agem but if they are observed in young population, sebaceous nevus syndrome should be ruled out [4] (Fig. 2.3).

2.2.5 Basal Ganglia Calcifications

Basal ganglia calcifications have been reported in 0.3–1.5% individuals and have been reported to be found more commonly in female [8]. Majority of these calcifications are found in globus pallidus and if they appear in patients younger than 30 years of age, a metabolic pathology should be ruled out [5].They are found in a fine dotted or thick symmetrical and conglomerate pattern [4] (Fig. 2.4).

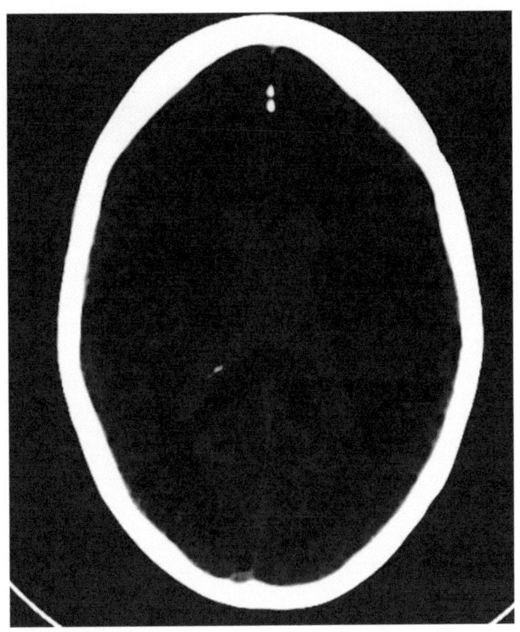

Fig. 2.3 Dural (falx) calcifications

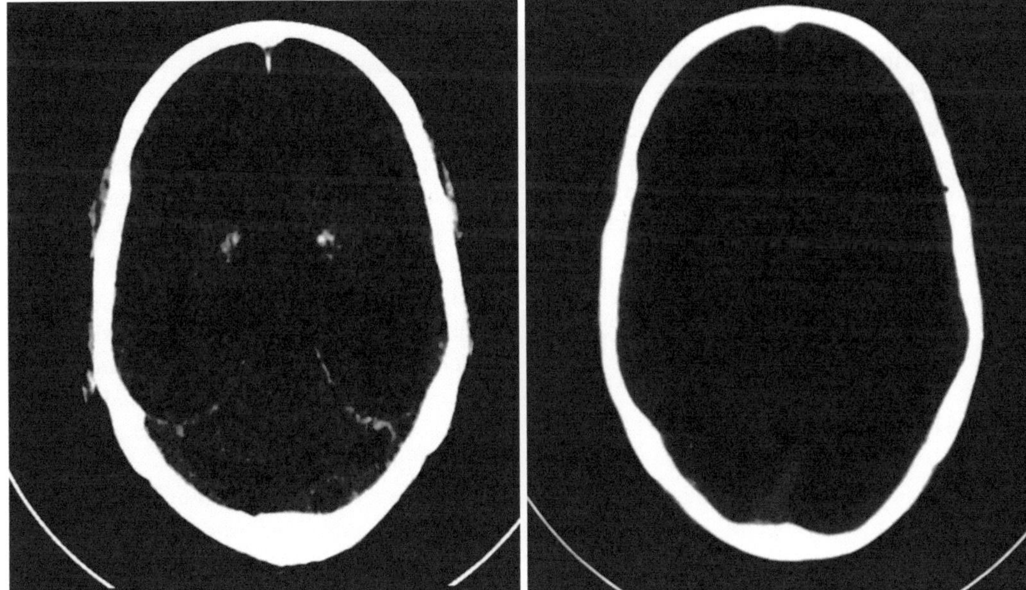

Fig. 2.4 Bilateral basal ganglia calcifications

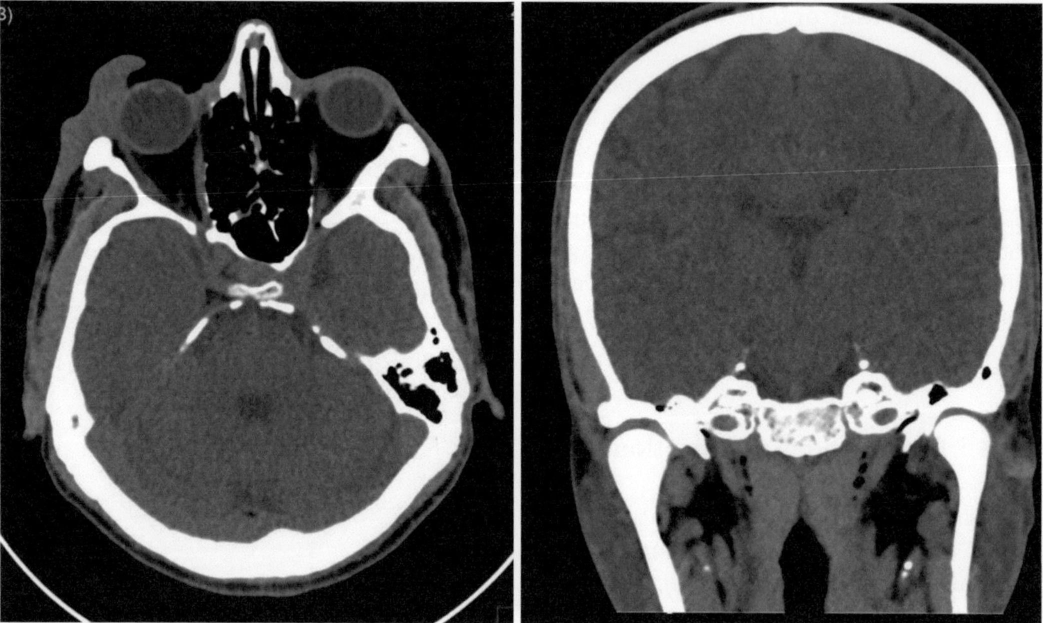

Fig. 2.5 Posterior clinoid calcifications

2.2.6 Petroclenoid Ligament and Sagittal Sinus Calcification

Petroclenoid ligament and sagittal sinus can develop calcification in a laminar or discreetly nodular pattern with advancing age [4] (Fig. 2.5).

2.3 Pathological Intracranial Calcifications

2.3.1 Congenital/Genetic or Development Disorders

2.3.1.1 Sturge-Weber Syndrome

Sturge-Weber syndrome also known encephalotrigeminal angiomatosis is a neurocutaneous syndrome with a prevalence of 1 in 50,000 live births, characterized by port wine stain on face, ipsilateral leptomeningeal vascular malformations and congenital glaucoma, presenting with seizures, visual field defects, hemiparesis, and mental retardation [4, 12–14]. These patients can develop cortical calcifications with a linear pattern in a double or curvilinear contour predominating in convolutions of parietal and occipital lobes (tram track appearance) [8] (Fig. 2.6).

2.3.1.2 Tuberous Sclerosis

Tuberous sclerosis also known as Bourneville's disease is an autosomal dominant neurocutaneous disorder with prevalence of 1 in 6000–12,000 live births [15]. Hamartomas may be found in brain, kidney, eyes, skin, and other organs. Most common intracranial findings are cortical tubers, sub ependymal nodules, giant cell astrocytomas, and abnormalities of the white matter. Most common clinical presentation is with clinical triad of Vogt: mental retardation, epilepsy and subcutaneous adenoma [16]. Sub ependymal nodules show calcification in up to 54–88% of individuals and they are most commonly found in atrium and along the caudothalamic groove, less commonly cortical tubers may also show calcifications [3, 4] (Fig. 2.7).

2.3.1.3 Neurofibromatosis Type 1

Neurofibromatosis type 1 also known as von Recklinghausen disease is an autosomal dominant disorder with incidence of 1 per 2000 live

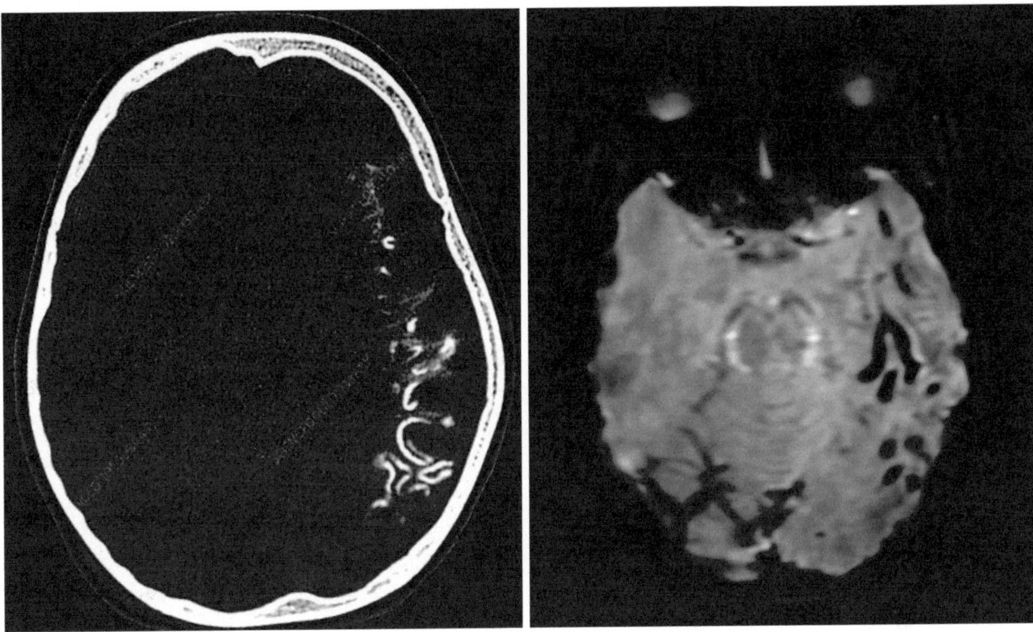

Fig. 2.6 Tram track calcifications—Sturge-Weber syndrome

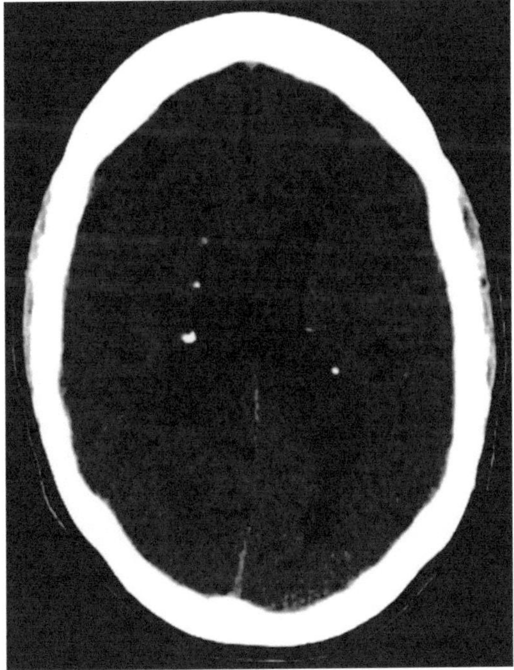

Fig. 2.7 Subependymal calcified tubers in tuberous sclerosis

births [4]. Tumors associated with neurofibromatosis type 1 (NF1) include peripheral nerve sheet tumors, leukemia, pheochromocytoma, gastrointestinal stromal tumors, and intracranial lesions. The intracranial lesions are gliomas, dysplasias, and hamartomas that affect the global palidus [17, 18]. Calcifications may be seen in choroid plexus of lateral ventricles and sometimes nodular calcifications of the cerebellum. Tumor-related calcifications may also be present [7].

2.3.1.4 Cockayne Syndrome

Cockayne syndrome is an autosomal recessive disorder characterized by cachectic dwarfism, wrinkled skin, loss of subcutaneous fat, beaked nose stooped pasture with some patients exhibiting severe photosensitivity [3]. This disorder is often associated with brain calcifications which are characterized by their subcortical location, in basal ganglia (rock or spot calcification) and dentate nuclei (thick pattern) [11, 19, 20].

2.3.1.5 Intracranial Lipomas

Intracranial lipomas are benign congenital malformations located in the midline. Occasionally a peripheral curvilinear or focal calcification may be seen [21].

2.3.1.6 Krabbe Disease

Krabbe disease is an autosomal recessive disorder characterized by early clinical symptoms before 4 months of age. Symptoms include irritability, hypersensitivity to stimulation, startle response, spasticity, poor feeding, unexplained recurrent high fever, and microcephaly [22]. Brain calcifications are noted at the level of the internal capsule and corona radiata in areas of abnormal white matter and globoid cells accumulation [23].

2.3.1.7 Aicardi-Goutières Syndrome

Aicardi-Goutières syndrome is an autosomal recessive disorder that presents either during neonatal or infantile period. The neonatal form presents as fever, seizures, hepatosplenomegaly, thrombocytopenia, and anemia with or without microcephaly. However, the infantile form presents as irritability, fever, loss of skills, and acquired microcephaly. Brain calcification associated with Aicardi-Goutières syndrome has been described as symmetrical, spot-like calcification at the level of the basal ganglia and deep white matter of both frontal and parietal lobes. Other sites have been implicated as well and include the dentate, cerebellar cortex, brainstem, and deep and superficial cerebral cortex [23].

2.3.1.8 Fahr Disease

Fahr disease is a rare neurodegenerative condition with more than 35 different names used in publications including bilateral striopallidodentate calcification and idiopathic basal ganglia calcification. Indeed, Fahr disease exhibits a wide range of clinical presentations ranging from asymptomatic to severe movement and neuropsychological disorders [23, 24]. Intracranial calcifications in Fahr disease usually involve the grey matter structures and to less extent the white matter. They are typically described as symmetrical, involving the caudate, putamen, globus pallidus, thalamus, deep cortex, and dentate [23] (Fig. 2.8).

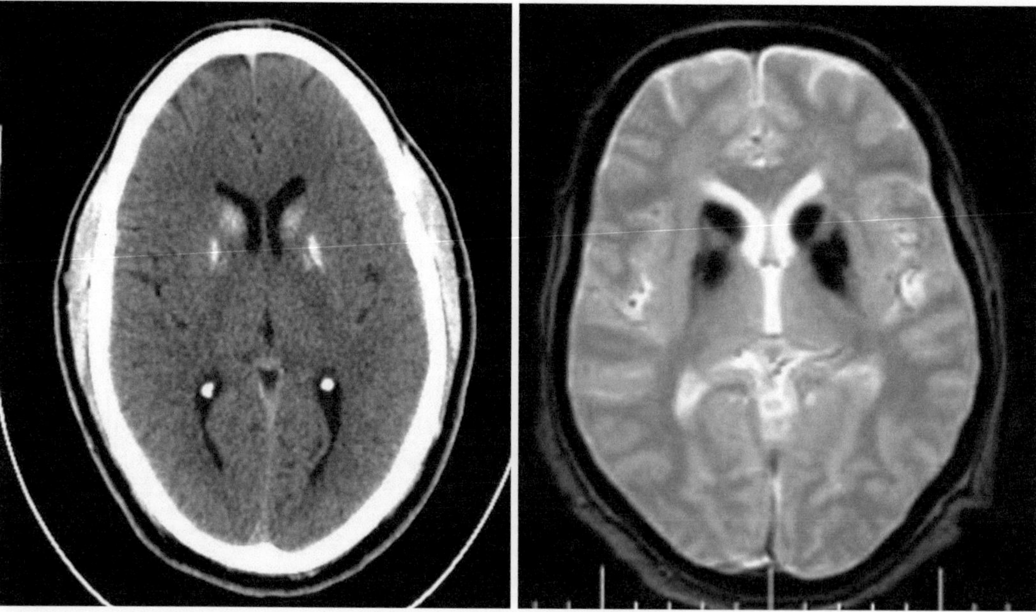

Fig. 2.8 Bilateral basal ganglia calcifications—Fahr disease

2.3.2   Congenital Infections

Congenital infections like toxoplasmosis, rubella, cytomegalovirus, herpes simplex (TORCH) infections, congenital Zika infection, and congenital HIV encephalitis can be associated with intracranial calcifications.

2.3.2.1 Congenital Toxoplasmosis

Congenital toxoplasmosis (transplacental spread) has incidence of 0.1–0.6%. It is generally associated with hydrocephalus and intracranial calcifications. Calcifications may be found in periventricular area and cortex where they are nodular in shape and they may also be found in thalamus and basal ganglia where they are curvilinear in shape [7, 8, 25]. Size of calcifications correlates with time of infection. It is also reported that calcifications related to toxoplasmosis tend to decrease or may even resolve after treatment [2, 26] (Fig. 2.9).

2.3.2.2 Congenital Rubella Infection

Congenital rubella infection (transplacental spread) has become rare and less prevalent since

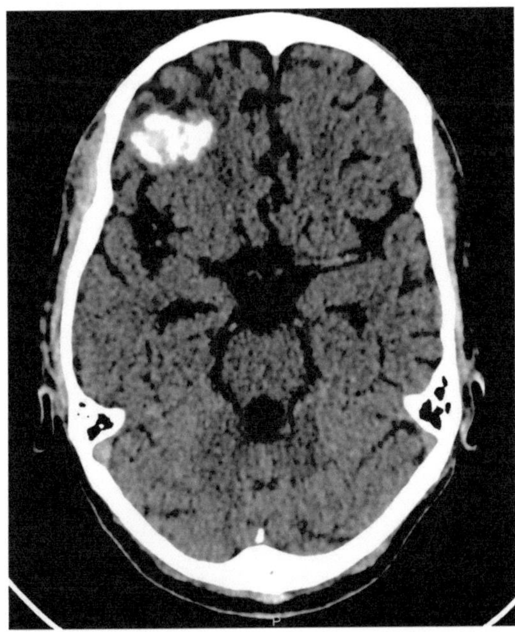

Fig. 2.9 Known case of HIV positive—toxoplasmosis (chronic)

the availability of rubella vaccine. It is associated with meningitis, ventriculitis, ventriculomegaly, encephalitis, seizures, cataract, hearing loss, cardiac defects, and intracranial calcifications [25]. Calcifications may be found in periventricular white matter basal ganglia and brain stem [8, 25].

2.3.2.3 Congenital Cytomegalo Virus

Congenital cytomegalo virus (transplacental spread) infection is the most common among the torch infections with prevalence of 0.6–0.7% [25]. It is usually associated with choreoretinitis, microcephaly, hydrocephalus, periventricular pseudo cysts, malformations of cortical development, development delay, mental retardation, and intracranial calcifications [8]. Calcifications are seen in periventricular region and brain parenchyma where they are thick and chunky in appearance and also in basal ganglia where they are faint and punctate [25].

2.3.2.4 Congenital or Neonatal Harpese

Congenital or neonatal harpes (intrapartum spread during birth from cutaneous lesions in the mother, rarely transplacental) is the second most common TORCH infection after cytomegalo virus infection with a prevalence of 1 in 5000 live births [25]. It is associated with extensive neuronal destruction, multicystic encephalmalacia, and scattered calcifications in thalamic, periventricular as well as in the convolutions [8].

2.3.2.5 Congenital Zika Infection

Congenital Zika infection (trans placental spread) leads to destruction of developing brain microcephaly and craniofacial disproportion. Calcifications are most commonly found in between the cortex and subcortical white matter. They may be thick and sometimes coarse [27, 28].

2.3.2.6 Congenital HIV Infection

Congenital human immunodeficiency virus (HIV) infection (most commonly trans placental or intrapartum spread) along with other manifestations of central nervous system invasion of HIV like microcephaly, ventriculomegaly, and cerebral atrophy, there can be symmetrical calcification in basal ganglia and subcortical white matter [25] (Fig. 2.9).

2.3.3 Acquired Infections

Viral encephalitis (herpes, HIV, etc.), neurocysticercosis, hydatid cyst of brain, neurotuberculosis, and opportunistic fungal infections of brain may be associated with intracranial calcification.

2.3.3.1 Viral Encephalitis (Herpes, HIV, etc.)

Encephalmalacia following viral encephalitis may lead to residual calcifications [4].

2.3.3.2 Neurocysticercosis and Hydatid Cyst of the Brain

Upon death, the larvae of the neurocystecercus are seen as an eccentric calcified nodule within a peripherally calcified cyst (Fig. 2.10). Similarly when hydatid cyst of the brain dies, the dead parasite is observed as single septate or multiloculated calcification [4, 7, 8].

2.3.3.3 Neurotuberculosis

Neurotuberculosis can take various forms including intra cranial tuberculoma. Tuberculomas may calcify in the center producing pathogonomic "target sign" or "sign of white" with a surrounding ring enhancement [7] (Fig. 2.11).

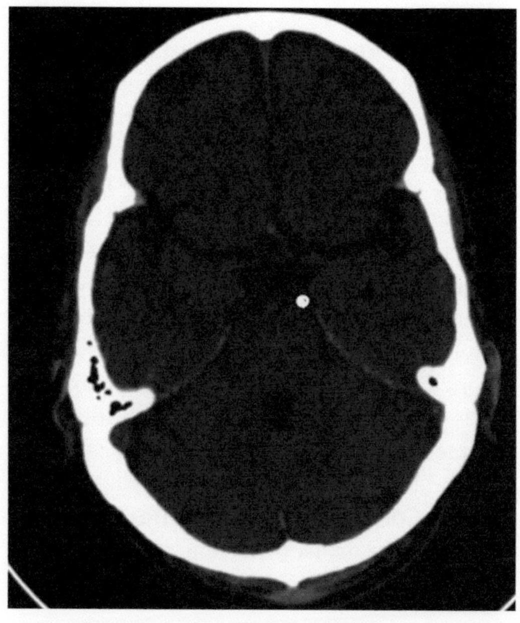

Fig. 2.11 Calcified granuloma (tuberculoma) in a known case of tuberculosis brain

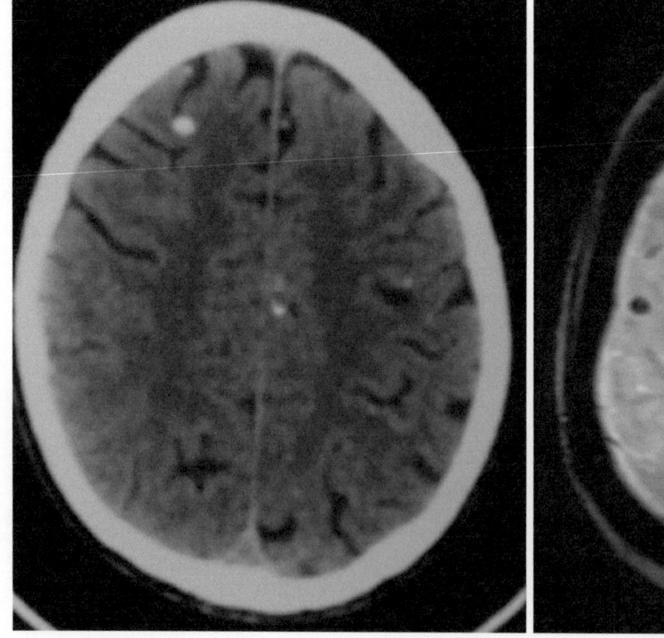

Fig. 2.10 Calcified NCC

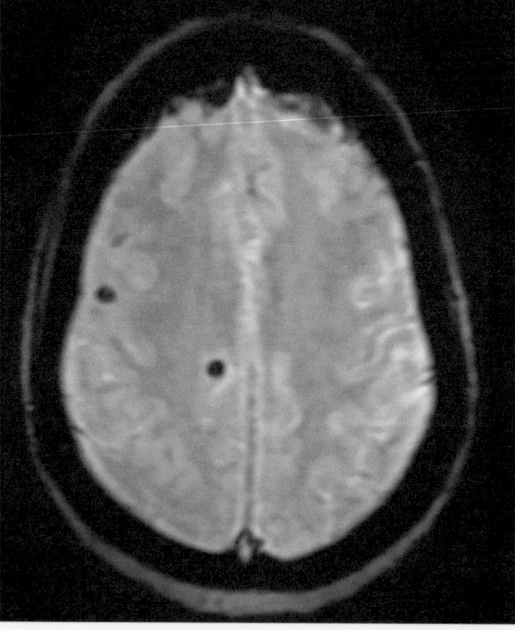

2.3.3.4 Opportunistic Fungal Infections

Opportunistic fungal infections primary affect patients with advanced HIV or other immuno deficiency disorder. Rarely punctuate calcifications in the brain parenchyma and leptomeninges may be seen. Leptomeningeal calcifications may represent sequlae of epidural empyema and chronic subdural hematoma [7, 29].

2.3.4 Vascular Calcification

Vascular causes of intracranial calcification include calcification in atherosclerotic walls of intracranial arteries, cavernous angiomas, arteriovenous malformations, dural arteriovenous (AV) fistulas, and aneurysms.

2.3.4.1 Calcification in Atherosclerotic Walls of Intracranial Arteries

These are seen more frequently found in internal carotid (60%), vertebral (20%), middle cerebral (5%), and basilar arteries (5%). The incidence of these calcifications increases with age and peaks in individuals older than 65 [5, 19] (Fig. 2.12).

2.3.4.2 Calcifications in Cavernous Angioma

These are seen in up to 33% of cases [7]. They look like scattered dots or stippled in the vessel wall or adjacent parenchyma ("corn popcorn" appearance). They are more commonly found in the lesions which have not yet bled [17] (Fig. 2.13).

2.3.4.3 Calcifications in Arteriovenous Malformations

Two types of calcifications may be seen in arteriovenous malformations. Primary serpentine distribution calcification may be seen in up to 30% cases along the tortuous veins or the nidus. Secondary dystrophic calcification may be seen away from the malformation due to hypoxic injury [20].

2.3.4.4 Calcifications in AV Fistulas

A non-specific pattern of bilateral symmetrical subcortical calcifications similar to Fahr disease may be seen. But, unlike the Fahr disease, calcifications are not seen in other areas [7].

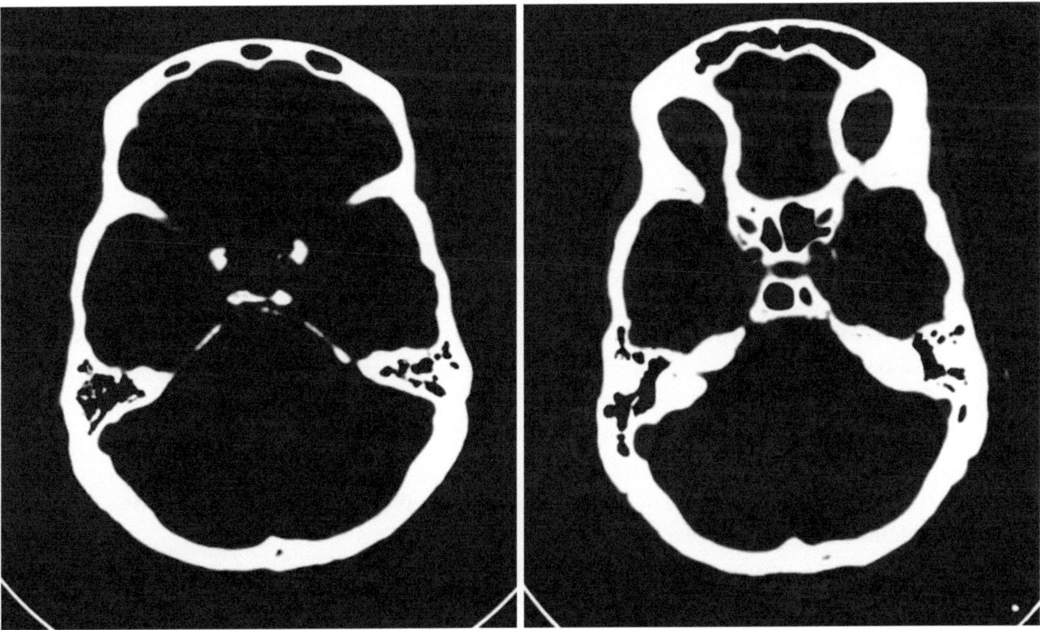

Fig. 2.12 Vascular calcifications

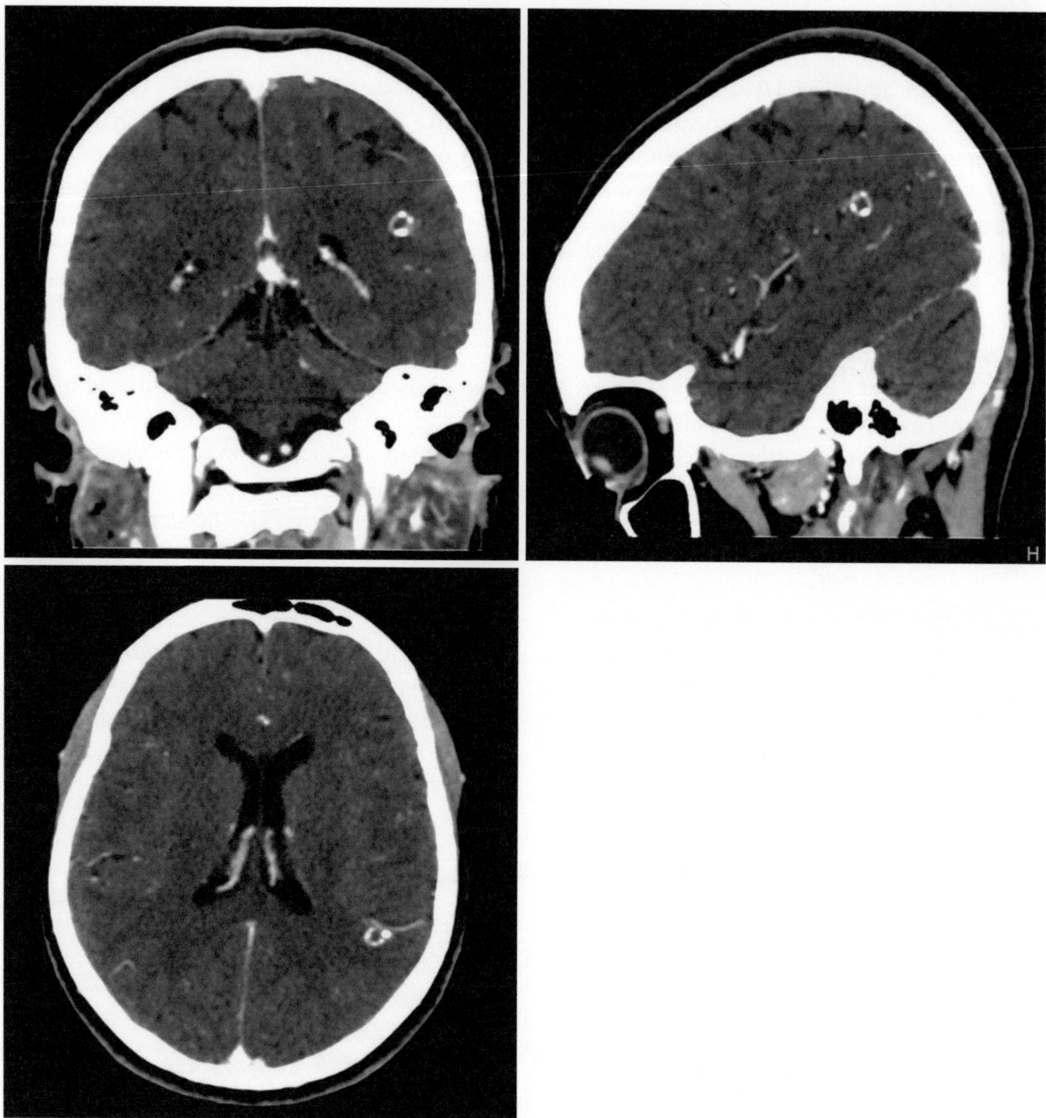

Fig. 2.13 Cavernoma with calcifications

2.3.4.5 Calcifications in Brain Aneurysms

Aneurysms may develop mural calcifications when partially or completely thrombosed. Sometimes non-thrombosed aneurysms especially the fusiform variety may show development of calcification in the wall [20, 30]. Dissecting aneurysms, especially in pediatric population, may also develop calcific plaque.

Mineralization of lanticulostriate arteries on CT scan has been reported among children with basal ganglia ischemic strokes [31, 32].

2.3.5 Neoplastic Calcifications

Many of the intracranial neoplasm can show calcification which is of no pathological signifi-

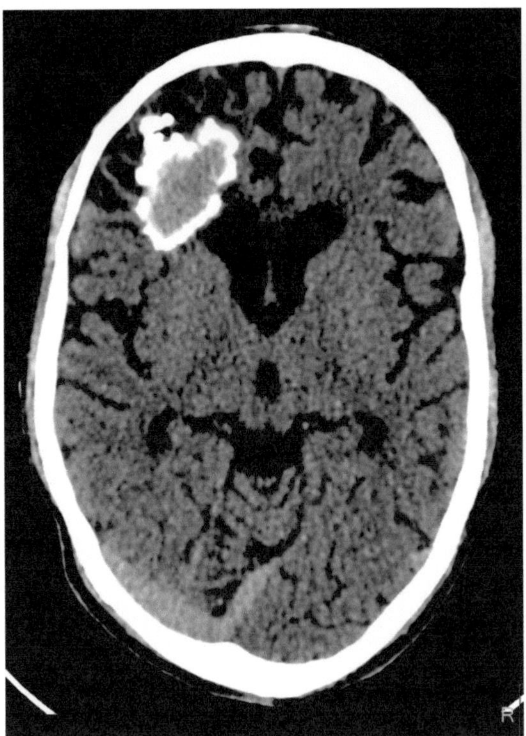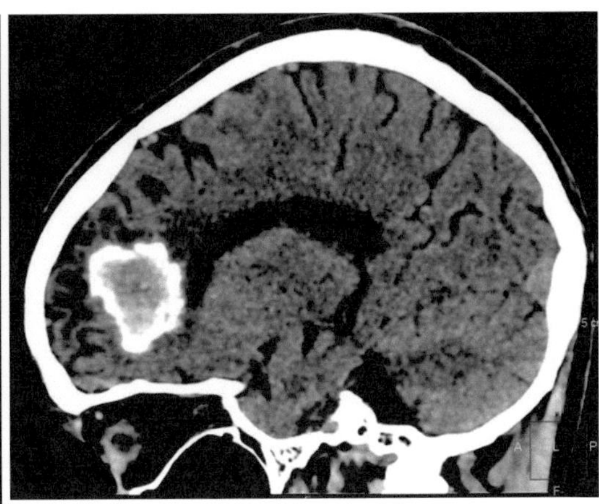

Fig. 2.14 Oligodendrioglioma

cance, but along with consideration of age of the patient and location of the tumor, it helps in narrowing diagnostic possibilities.

2.3.5.1 Intraxial Tumors

Intraxial tumors such as astrocytomas, oligodendrogliomas, gangliogliomas, medulloblastoma, and metastatic lesions may show calcifications. These are associated with hemorrhage by combination of neovascularization, arteriovenous shunts, and rapid tumor growth leading to necrosis and disruption of intracellular calcium regulation, which ultimately leads to calcium deposition.

2.3.5.1.1 Astrocytomas

Calcification may be seen in up to 20% of astrocytomas (up to 25% in pilocytic variety, up to 40% in xanthoastrocytoma, and up to 70% in subependymal giant cell astrocytoma) [7, 25].

2.3.5.1.2 Oligodendrogliomas

Oligodendrogliomas may show calcification in 40% of pediatric patients and up to 90% in adults. These calcifications may be described as central, microcalcifications, or lumpy calcifications [7, 25] (Fig. 2.14).

2.3.5.1.3 Gangliogliomas

Gangliogliomas may show mural calcification in up to 41% patients [7, 25].

2.3.5.1.4 Medulloblastomas

Medulloblastomas may show scattered dots of calcification or clumped calcification in up to 30% of cases [25, 30].

2.3.5.1.5 Metastatic Lesions

Metastatic lesions to brain especially from lung, breast, osteogenic sarcoma, and mucinous adenocarcinoma may show calcifications. Calcifications

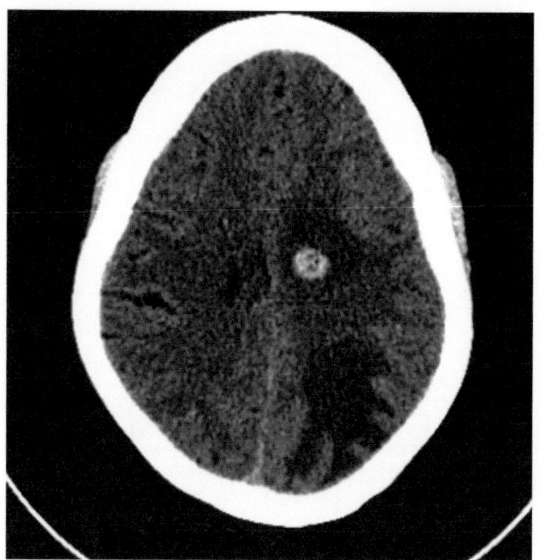

Fig. 2.15 Known case of carcinoma breast—brain metastasis with calcifications

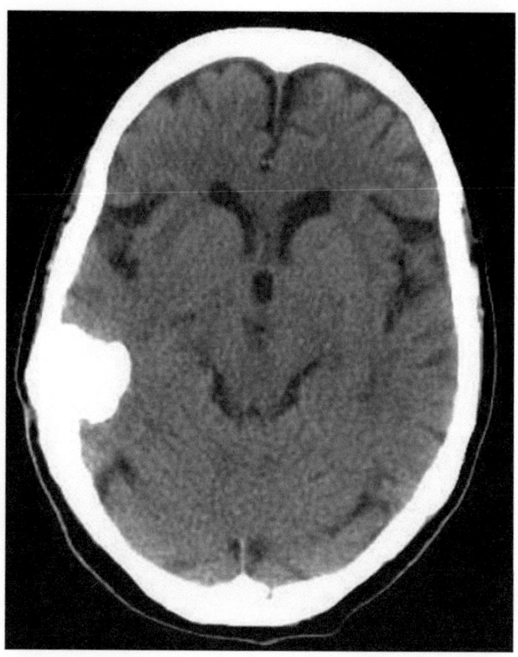

Fig. 2.16 Calcified meningioma

may also develop secondary to radiation and chemotherapy [7, 33] (Fig. 2.15).

2.3.5.2 Extra Axial Tumors

Extra axial tumors like meningiomas, craniopharyngiomas, pineal tumors, germ cell tumors, and lipomas commonly show calcifications. Schwannomas, pituitary adenomas, dermoids, and epidermoids rarely calcify.

2.3.5.2.1 Meningiomas

Meningiomas may show calcification in 20–69% cases and display a variety of patterns including sunburst, sand like, rim, and globular calcifications [7, 25] (Fig. 2.16).

2.3.5.2.2 Craniopharyngiomas

Craniopharyngiomas may show calcification in up to 93% in the pediatric population and are less likely to calcify in adults [7, 25]. Calcification may range from thin and circumferential to amorphous and lobulated in appearance [25].

2.3.5.2.3 Pineal Tumors

Pineal tumors may exhibit calcification in up to 50% of cases. They exhibit two types of calcification, it may occur in a peripheral fashion leading to so called exploded pattern of calcification which is supposed to be arising from the pineal gland itself and other is centrally located calcification which are produced by the pineal tumor [7, 25].

2.3.5.2.4 Germ Cell Tumors

Germ cell tumors of pineal region especially teratoma may also show calcifications [7, 25].

2.3.5.2.5 Schwannomas, Pituitary Adenomas, Dermoids, and Epidermoids

Schwannomas, pituitary adenomas, dermoids and epidermoids may also show occasional calcifications [3].

2.3.5.3 Intraventricular Tumors

Intraventricular tumors like ependymomas, choroid plexus tumors, central neurocytoma, and intraventricular meningiomas may also show calcification.

2.3.5.3.1 Intraventricular Ependymomas

Intraventricular ependymomas may show calcifications in up to 50% cases and they appear in form of dots or mass/rock like [34].

2.3.5.3.2 Choroid Plexus Papilomas and Carcinomas

Choroid plexus papilomas and carcinomas may show calcification in up to 25% of cases and they appear in form of dots [34].

2.3.5.3.3 Central Neurocytoma

Central neurocytoma show calcification in up to 50% of cases that take form of dots to large masses of calcification [34].

2.3.5.3.4 Intraventricular Meningiomas

Intraventricular meningiomas may show calcification in up to 50% of cases which may display of variety of patterns including sand like, sunburst, rim, or globular calcifications all over the tumor [8].

2.3.6 Metabolic Endocrine Disorders

Metabolic endocrine disorders like hypoparathyroidism, hyperparathyroidism, and hypothyroidism may lead to brain calcifications. In these disorders calcifications develop in bilateral basal ganglia. They may also occur in the dentate nucleus, corona radiata, subcortical white matter, and thalamus [25].

2.3.7 Inflammatory Disorders

Inflammatory disorders like systemic lupus erythematosus and cerebral sarcoidosis may be associated with intracranial calcifications.

2.3.7.1 Systemic Lupus Erythematosus

In systemic lupus erythematosus (SLE), calcifications are found to be symmetrical and bilateral, involving cerebellum followed by centrum semiovale, globus pallidus, putamen, head of caudate, and thalamus. In this disease, intracranial calcifications may be found as isolated finding or along with brain atrophy or cerebral infarcts [35].

2.3.7.2 Cerebral Sarcoidosis

In cerebral sarcoidosis calcifications have been found to be present in suprasellar location, hypothalamus and cerebellum [36, 37].

2.3.8 Posttreatment or Posttrauma Calcifications

Rarely acquired calcifications may develop in scarring produced after surgical treatment or after radiotherapy or posttrauma [4] (Fig. 2.17).

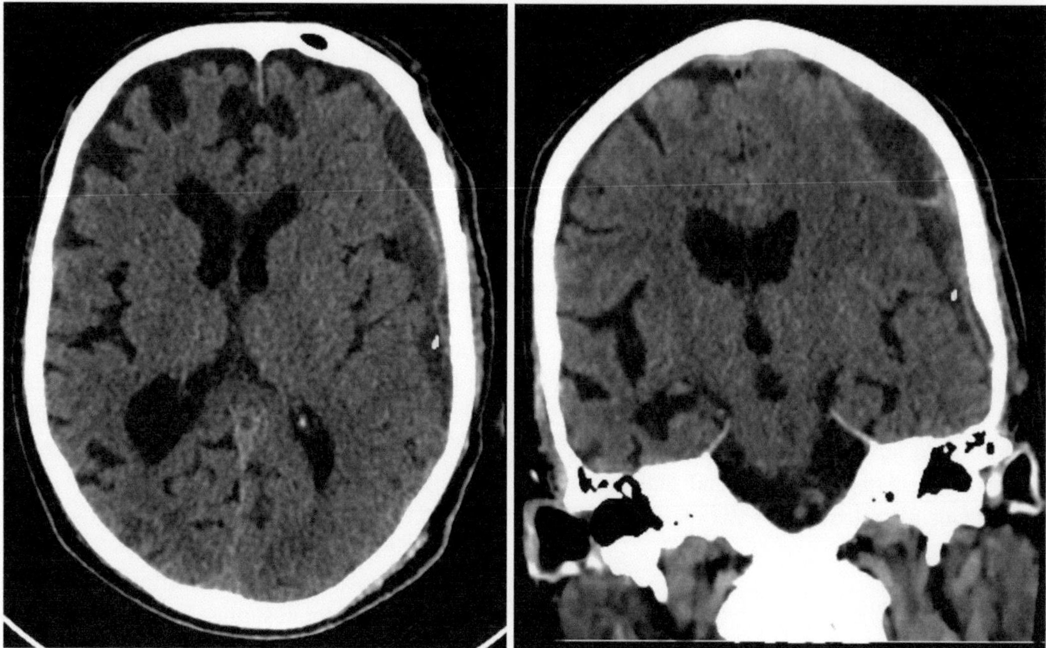

Fig. 2.17 Chronic subdural hematoma with specks of calcification

2.3.9 Neurotoxicity

Chronic lead exposures may lead to calcifications in subcortical area, basal ganglia, vermis, cerebellum, hippocampus, deep white matter, and cerebral cortex [38].

2.4 Conclusion

Intracranial calcifications are common findings in NCCT scan of the head and they may be found in both pediatric and adult populations. They present with a wide spectrum of presentations and may be physiological or pathological. Their location, pattern, morphology along with the available clinical information are essential clues to approach proper diagnosis.

References

1. Deng H, Zheng W, Jankovic J. Genetics and molecular biology of brain calcification. Ageing Res Rev. 2015;22:20–38.
2. Celzo FG. Brain stones revisited—between a rock and a hard place. Insights Imaging. 2013;4:625–35.
3. Saade C, Najem E, Asmar K, Salman R, El Achkar B, Naffaa L. Intracranial calcifications on CT: an updated review. J Radiol Case Rep. 2019;13(8):1–18. https://doi.org/10.3941/jrcr.v13i8.3633.
4. Taborda KNN, Wilches C, Manrique A. A diagnostic algorithm for patients with intracranial calcifications. Rev Colomb Radiol. 2017;28:4732–9.
5. Yalcin A, Ceylan M, Bayraktutan OF, Sonkaya AR, Yuce I. Age and gender related prevalence of intracranial calcifications in CT imaging; data from 12,000 healthy subjects. J Chem Neuroanat. 2016;78:20–4.
6. Deepak S, Jayakumar B, Shanavas. Extensive intracranial calcifications. J Assoc Physicians India. 2005;53:948.

7. Grech R, Grech S, Mizzi A. Intracranial calcifications: a pictorial review. Neuroradiol J. 2012;25(4):427–51.
8. Kiroglu Y, Çalli C, Karabulut N, Öncel Ç. Intracranial calcifications on CT. Diagn Interv Radiol. 2010;16(4):263.
9. Kunz D, Schmitz S, Mahlberg R, Mohr A, Stöter C, Wolf K, et al. A new concept for melatonin deficit: on pineal calcification and melatonin excretion. Neuropsychopharmacology. 1999;21(6):765–72.
10. Whitehead MT, Oh C, Raju A, Choudhri AF. Physiologic pineal region, choroid plexus, and dural calcifications in the first decade of life. Am J Neuroradiol. 2015;36(3):575–80.
11. Kendall B, Cavanagh N. Intracranial calcification in paediatric computed tomography. Neuroradiology. 1986;28(4):324–30.
12. Agrawal PJ, et al. Spectrum of CT and MR findings in Sturge-Weber syndrome: a case report. Med J Dr. D.Y. Patil Univ. 2014;7(4):497–501.
13. Bose SC. A case report of Sturge Weber syndrome. Univ J Med Med Spec. 2018;4(2). ISSN: 2455-2852.
14. Pilli VK, Behen ME, Hu J, Xuan Y, Janisse J, Chugani HT, Juhász C. Clinical and metabolic correlates of cerebral calcifications in Sturge-Weber syndrome. Dev Med Child Neurol. 2017;59(9):952–8.
15. Baron Y, Barkovich AJ. MR imaging of tuberous sclerosis in neonates and young infants. AJNR Am J Neuroradiol. 1999;20:907–16.
16. Umeoka S, Koyama T, Miki Y. Pictorial review of tuberous sclerosis in various organs. Radiographics. 2008;28(7):e32.
17. Arts WF, Van Dongen KJ. Intracranial calcified deposits in neurofibromatosis. J Neurol Neurosurg Psychiatry. 1986;49:1317–20.
18. Fortman BF, et al. Neurofibromatosis type 1: a diagnostic mimicker at CT 1. Radiographics. 2001;21(3):601–12.
19. Chen XY, Lam WW, Ng HK, Fan YH, Wong KS. The frequency and determinants of calcification in intracranial arteries in Chinese patients who underwent computed tomography examinations. Cerebrovasc Dis. 2006;21(1–2):91–7.
20. Gezercan Y, Acik V, Çavuş G, Ökten AI, Bilgin E, Millet H, Olmaz B. Six different extremely calcified lesions of the brain: brain stones. Springerplus. 2016;5(1):1941.
21. Yilmaz N, Unal O, Kiymaz N, Yilmaz C, Etlik O. Intracranial lipomas — a clinical study. Clin Neurol Neurosurg. 2006;108:363–8.
22. Elitt CM, Volpe JJ. Degenerative disorders of the newborn. In: Volpe's neurology of the newborn. Elsevier; 2018. p. 823–58. ISBN: 9780323531764.
23. Livingston JH, Stivaros S, Warren D, Crow YJ. Intracranial calcification in childhood: a review of aetiologies and recognizable phenotypes. Dev Med Child Neurol. 2014;56(7):612–26.
24. Savino E, Soavi C, Capatti E, Borrelli M, Vigna GB, Passaro A, Zuliani G. Bilateral strio-pallido-dentate calcinosis (Fahr's disease): report of seven cases and revision of literature. BMC Neurol. 2016;16(1):165.
25. Dinizio AM, Vincent JK, Nickerson JP. Intracranial calcifications in the pediatric age group: an imaging review. J Pediatr Neuroradiol. 2015;4(3):49–59. ISSN: 1309-6680.
26. Patel DV, Holfels EM, Vogel NP, Boyer KM, Mets MB, Swisher CN, Roizen NJ, Stein LK, Stein MA, Hopkins J, Withers SE. Resolution of intracranial calcifications in infants with treated congenital toxoplasmosis. Radiology. 1996;199(2):433–40.
27. Aragao MD, van der Linden V, Brainer-Lima AM, Coeli RR, Rocha MA, da Silva PS, de Carvalho MD, van der Linden A, de Holanda AC, Valenca MM. Clinical features and neuroimaging (CT and MRI) findings in presumed Zika virus related congenital infection and microcephaly: retrospective case series study. BMJ. 2016;353:i1901.
28. Cavalheiro S, López A, Serra S, Da Cunha A, Devanir M, Costa S, et al. Microcephaly and Zika virus: neonatal neuroradiological aspects. Childs Nerv Syst. 2016;32:2–5.
29. Offiah CE, Naseer A. Spectrum of imaging appearances of intracranial cryptococcal infection in HIV/AIDS patients in the anti-retroviral therapy era. Clin Radiol. 2016;71(1):9–17.
30. Makariou E, Patsalides AD. Intracranial calcifications. Appl Radiol. 2009;38(11):48. ISSN: 0160-9963.
31. Lingappa L, Varma RD, Siddaiahgari S, Konanki R. Mineralizing angiopathy with infantile basal ganglia stroke after minor trauma. Dev Med Child Neurol. 2014;56(1):78–84.
32. Gowda VK, Manjeri V, Srinivasan VM, Sajjan SV, Benakappa A. Mineralizing angiopathy with basal ganglia stroke after minor trauma: case series including two familial cases. J Pediatr Neurosci. 2018;13(4):448.
33. Concha T, Moriones AB, Trueba HV. Calcificaciones intracraneales en el TC de urgencias: Manual para el residente: Objetivo docente; 2012. p. 1–19.
34. Crawford SC, Boyer RS, Harnsberger HR, Pollei SR, Smoker WR, Osborn AG. Disorders of histogenesis: the neurocutaneous syndromes. Semin Ultrasound CT MR. 1988;9(3):247–67.
35. Raymond AA, Zariah AA, Samad SA, Chin CN, Kong NC. Brain calcification in patients with cerebral lupus. Lupus. 1996;5(2):123–8.
36. Herring AB, Urich H. Sarcoidosis of the central nervous system. J Neurol Sci. 1969;9(3):405–22.
37. Lawrence WP, El Gammal T, Pool WH, Apter L. Radiological manifestations of neurosarcoidosis: report of three cases and review of literature. Clin Radiol. 1974;25(3):343–8.
38. Reyes PF, Gonzalez CF, Zalewska MK, Besarab A. Intracranial calcification in adults with chronic lead exposure. Am J Roentgenol. 1986;146(2):26770.

Intracranial Arachnoid Cysts

3

Mehmet Turgut, Kaan Özalpay, and Walter A. Hall

3.1 Introduction

In a study conducted for intracranial arachnoid cysts (ACs), which are generally detected incidentally, the prevalence was found to be 1.4% when magnetic resonance imaging (MRI) scans were examined retrospectively [1]. ACs, which are more common in men, are primarily located in the anterior cranial fossa, middle cranial fossa, and posterior to the cerebellum. They usually do not cause any symptoms, even with large cysts. Surgical treatment has been shown to be beneficial in those ACs with symptoms due to the mass effect that they cause [2].

3.2 Etiology

Let's consider a question that doesn't have a definite answer, what causes ACs [3]? In general, the most accepted developmental theory is that the arachnoid, which is congenital, forms a cyst by trapping the cerebrospinal fluid (CSF) internally due to the misfolding of the arachnoid. Not all ACs seem to follow this theory. They may also be associated with structural changes in the brain parenchyma, such as agenesis, heterotopies, and neural tube closure defects. ACs usually arise within and expand the margins of the CSF cisterns which have abundant arachnoid (i.e. Sylvian fissures, suprasellar, quadrigeminal, cerebellopontine angle and posterior infratentorial midline cisterns) [4].

3.3 Clinical Findings

Incidences of symptomatic and asymptomatic cysts are variable and they depend largely on the population for which it was determined. The location of the AC is highly variable and there is a marked predominance of lesions that are commonly present in the middle cranial and posterior spaces to the cerebellum, called "retrocerebellar." Furthermore, there are fewer cysts over the cerebral convexity and in the suprasellar region [4]. The lowest frequency of the AC is reported in cerebellopontine angle, supracerebellar cistern,

M. Turgut (✉)
Department of Neurosurgery, Aydın Adnan Menderes University Faculty of Medicine, Efeler, Aydın, Turkey

Department of Histology and Embryology, Aydın Adnan Menderes University Health Sciences Institute, Efeler, Aydın, Turkey

K. Özalpay
Department of Neurosurgery, Aydın Adnan Menderes University Faculty of Medicine, Efeler, Aydın, Turkey

W. A. Hall
Department of Neurosurgery, SUNY Upstate University Hospital, Syracuse, NY, USA
e-mail: Hallw@upstate.edu

quadrigeminal cistern, intraventricular region, and near the brain stem.

The location of the ACs is associated with both their symptoms and the required treatment. While the small ACs in the middle fossa do not usually cause symptoms, the larger ones may show various symptoms from headache to epileptic seizures. It should not be ignored that what we consider an AC may also represent a different structure such as a dermoid cyst, abscess, epidermoid cyst, and cystic neurocysticercosis.

Of course, you should not think that the treatment of the disease where the pathology is so controversial will be undisputed. There is almost a consensus on one treatment issue. In asymptomatic ACs, radiographic follow-up is the best way to manage that AC. For those cysts that cause symptoms, there are some surgical options. Open fenestration with ventriculoperitoneal shunt placement, microsurgical open fenestration, endoscopic fenestration, endoscopic third ventriculostomy, and cystoperitoneal shunting are the surgical procedures used for treatment. While some studies have suggested that endoscopic fenestration results in more complications [5], other studies have reported more complications after open craniotomy. The average success rate of endoscopic fenestration has been documented as 78% [6].

In one study, while endoscopic fenestration provided the best results in midline ACs, it may be necessary to add a cystoperitoneal shunt to the surgical options for infratentorial ACs with hydrocephalus. In addition, when fenestrating the cyst, it was observed that it was necessary to open a minimum of 10–15 mm of the wall of the cyst in order to prevent it from closing again; otherwise, it will appear that the cyst re-formed [7]. As can be seen, the treatment chosen will vary depending on the localization of the AC. This consequence makes us ask an important question, where are arachnoid cysts located?

3.3.1 Middle Cranial Fossa

About 50–65% of ACs are found in the middle cranial fossa or Sylvian cistern, as unilateral or bilateral space-occupying lesion. According to the Galassi classification, they are classified as three types [8]:

Type I is the mildest form. The temporal end is compressed posteriorly and there is no displacement of the ventricles or midline structures (Fig. 3.1). Out of 31 patients, three had mild intracranial pressure elevation, three had epileptic seizures, and one had unilateral optic nerve atrophy.

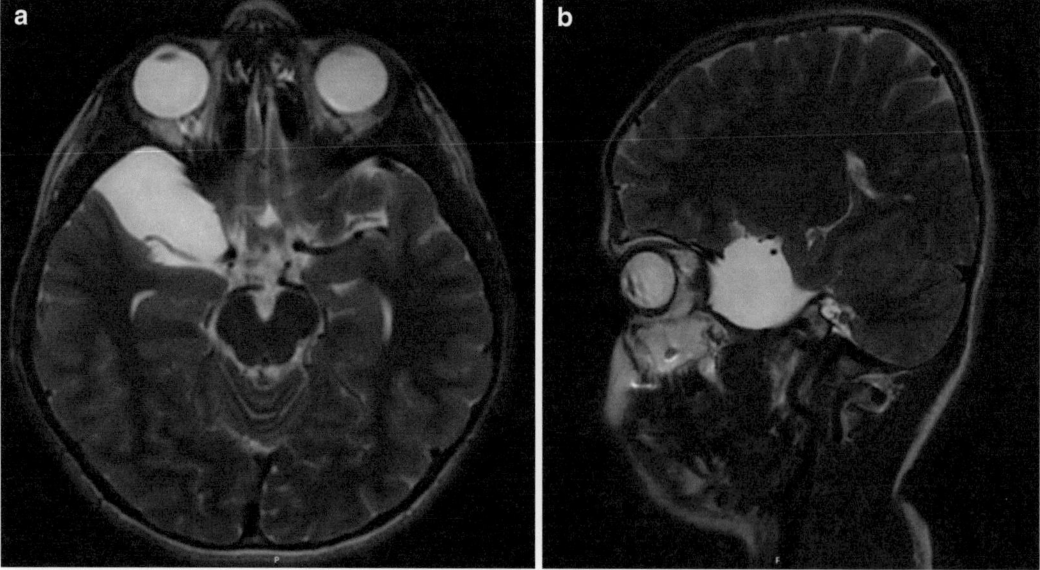

Fig. 3.1 Brain magnetic resonance imaging (MRI) T2-weighted axial (**a**) and sagittal (**b**) sequences demonstrating Galassi Type-I right anterior temporal fossa arachnoid cysts (AC)

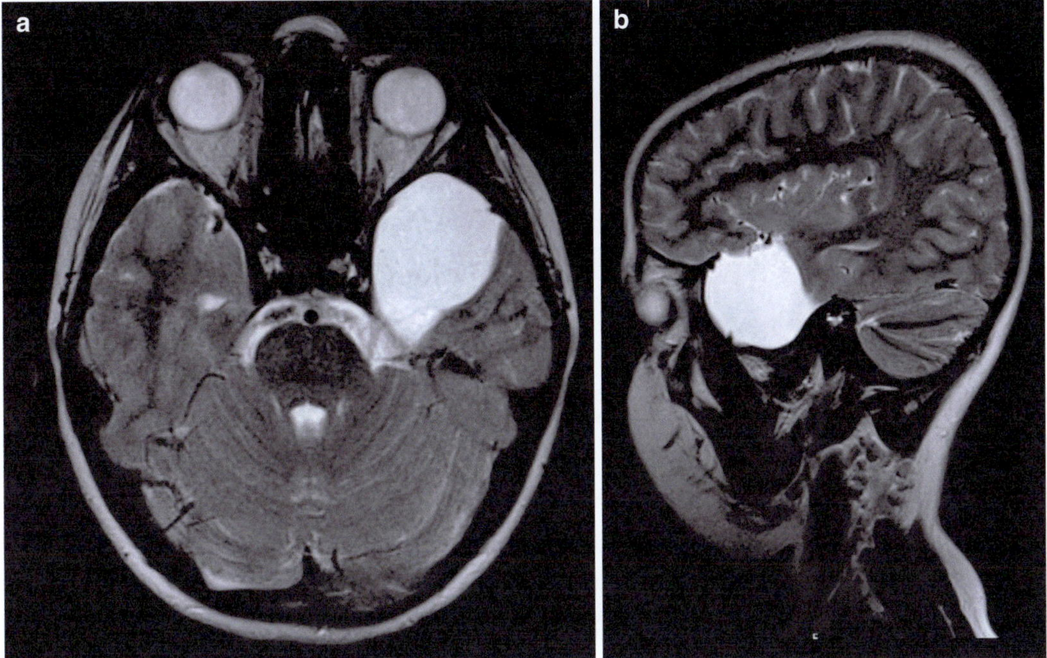

Fig. 3.2 Brain MRI T2-weighted axial (**a**) and sagittal (**b**) sequences showing left temporal AC, Galassi Type-II

Type II, the lesion is medium-sized, occupies the anterior and middle part of the temporal fossa; thus the volume of the temporal lobe is clearly reduced (Fig. 3.2). Although not severe, mass effect is present in half of the patients. Out of 14 cases, increased intracranial pressure was present in eight patients, epileptic seizures in five patients, mental retardation in two patients, and two had the acute onset of ictal symptoms.

Type III is the most severe form. The cyst is very large and oval or round. It covers almost the entire temporal fossa and protrudes into large areas of the cerebral hemispheres. The temporal lobe is severely atrophic. The ventricles and midline are deviated to the opposite side. Along with these findings, cranial deformities and angiographic pathologies are present. Out of 11 patients who were found to have Type III, symptoms of increased intracranial pressure were found in six patients, epileptic seizures in two patients, and optic atrophy in one patient.

It is controversial to fenestrate the medial wall of this type of arachnoid cyst at surgery because there is the Sylvian fissure adjacent to the wall containing important arterial structures. Because the arachnoid cyst wall is usually thick with collagen, it should be opened using sharp-tipped instruments. Here, fenestration is sometimes inadequate, particularly when performed endoscopically. There are also publications recommending microsurgery in this region [9]. However despite all these approaches and the result of a meta-analysis, endoscopic fenestration is the recommended first treatment option for the arachnoid cyst seen in this region. If positive results are not obtained, then other options should be considered [10].

3.3.2 Quadrigeminal

Quadrigeminal (also known as superior *cistern* or *cistern* of the great cerebral vein) ACs are rare and constitute approximately 5–10% of all intracranial arachnoid cysts [11]. These cysts are more likely to cause hydrocephalus than other cysts [12]. Quadrigeminal ACs are classified as follows:

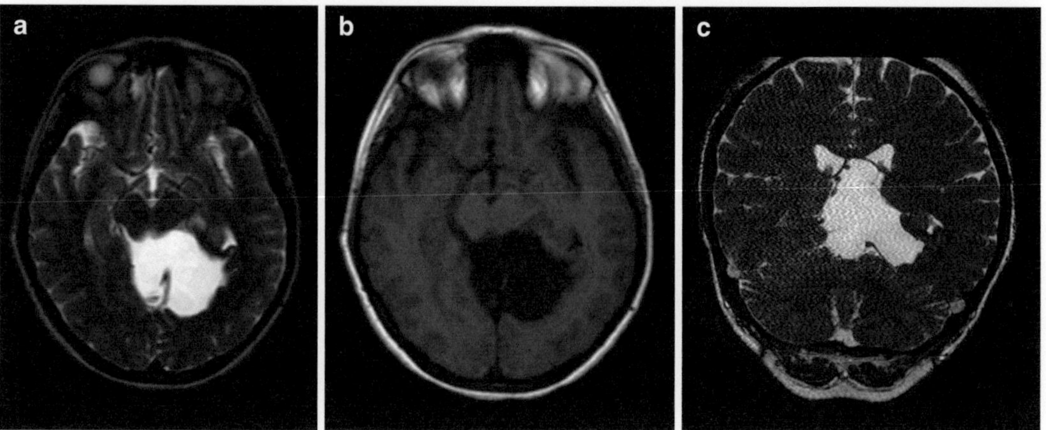

Fig. 3.3 Brain MRI T2-weighted axial (**a**) and coronal (**c**) as well as T1-weighted axial (**b**) sequences showing left quadrigeminal AC type I with extensions of supratentorial and infratentorial compartments

Quadrigeminal AC type I with extensions of supratentorial and infratentorial compartments (Fig. 3.3).

Quadrigeminal AC type II with infratentorial extension (supracerebellar or supra-retrocerebellar).

Quadrigeminal AC type III with lateral extension toward the temporal lobe.

As symptomatic quadrigeminal ACs are usually associated with hydrocephalus because they compress or distort the Aqueduct of Sylvius at an early stage [5]. Clinically, symptoms are headaches, vomiting, lethargy, papilledema, macrocrania, impairment of upward gaze and other ocular disorders, and hemifacial spasm [13].

Quadrigeminal ACs, unlike other cysts due to their location, are usually symptomatic and require some form of surgical intervention. We believe that the type of surgery to be performed is endoscopic. Fenestration of quadrigeminal AC by various surgical techniques sch as cystocisternostomy or cystoventriculostomy plus third ventriculostomy is indicated for these patients. If expertise or clinical acumen precludes such a procedure, craniotomy and fenestration or cystoperitoneal shunting is preferable [14]. It is not recommended to place only a ventriculoperitoneal shunt as it does not solve the cause of the problem completely. It has been observed that 80% of them are successfully treated independently without using a shunt [11, 15].

3.3.3 Suprasellar

Suprasellar ACs usually compress the third ventricle and may progress with hydrocephalus as a result (Fig. 3.4). This cyst is usually treated with an approach called a ventriculo-cystocysternomy. Open surgery for cysts in this location is generally not preferred because the morbidity is more than 70%. With the endoscopic method, the apical membrane is initially torn, performed at the level of the foramen Monroe, and a basilar fenestration is created. Opening these cysts into both the ventricles and the basal cisterns is of great importance in order to prevent cyst recurrence [16, 17].

3.3.4 Interhemispheric

Interhemispheric ACs occur in two locations, midline and parasagittal [18] (Fig. 3.5). They are rare congenital abnormalities and only a few cases have been reported. Out of the 696 ACs discovered incidentally in adults, only four were

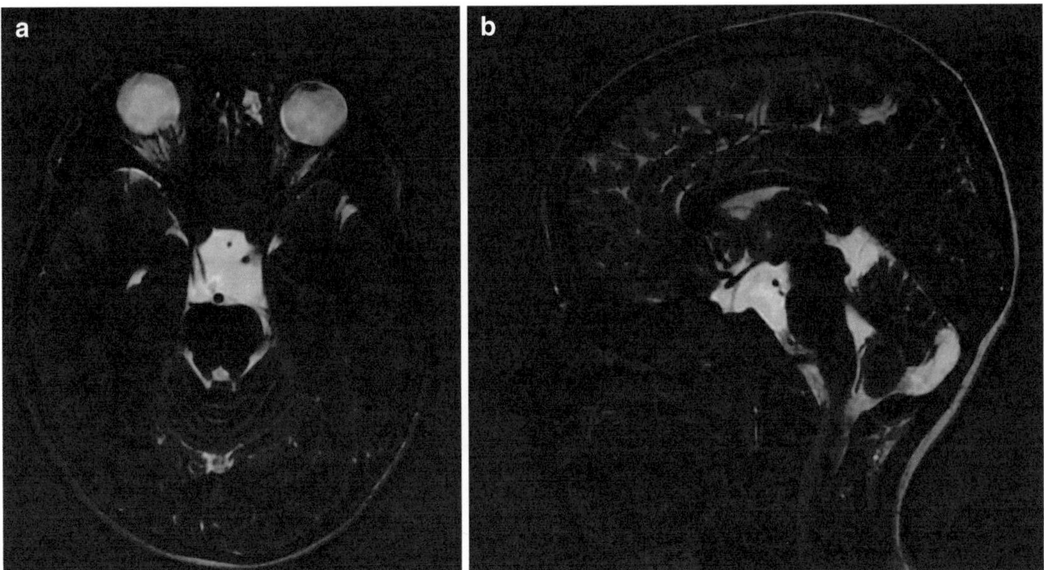

Fig. 3.4 Brain MRI T2-weighted axial (**a**) and sagittal (**b**) sequences showing suprasellar AC

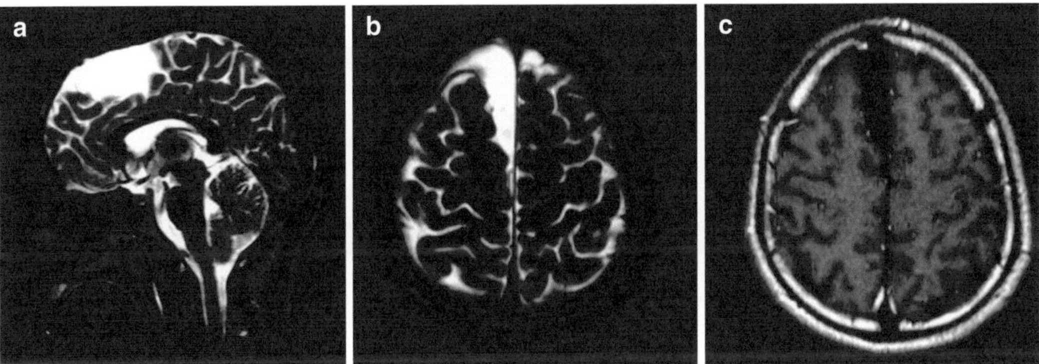

Fig. 3.5 Brain MRI T2-weighted sagittal (**a**) and axial (**b**) sequences as well as T1-weighted axial (**c**) sequences showing interhemispheric AC of a patient with recurrent headache

located in the interhemispheric fissure. They are usually diagnosed in children with other midline neurodevelopmental disorders. Macrocrania, headache, seizures, and psychomotor retardation are the most common symptom presentations [19].

In addition, good clinical or radiological results were reported in 89% of patients with interhemispheric ACs who underwent craniotomy and cyst excision, and in 75% of patients who underwent endoscopic fenestration. As we

have described in the previous pages, endoscopic fenestration was successful in other types, while microsurgery was more successful in interhemispheric ACs [20].

3.3.5 Convexity

Convexity locations are the third most common type of AC [2, 4, 5] (Fig. 3.6). One of the most common presenting symptoms seen in the frontal

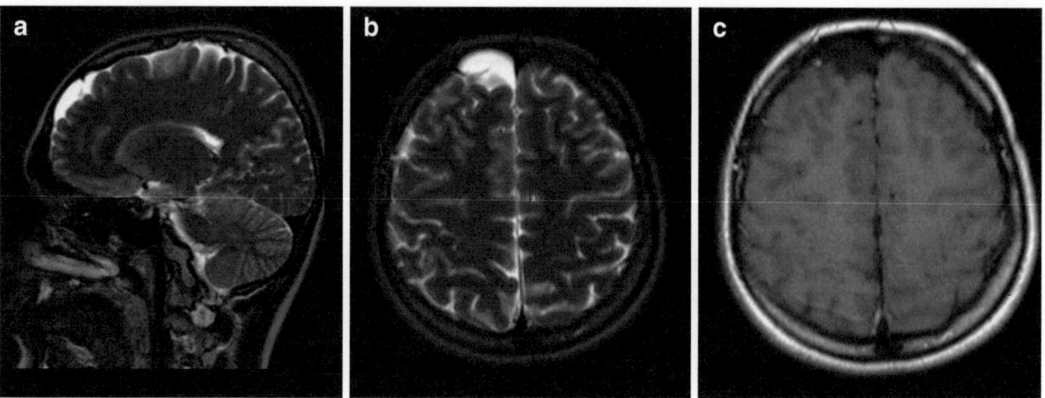

Fig. 3.6 Brain MRI T2-weighted sagittal (**a**) and axial (**b**) as well as T1-weighted axial (**c**) sequences showing right frontal convexity AC

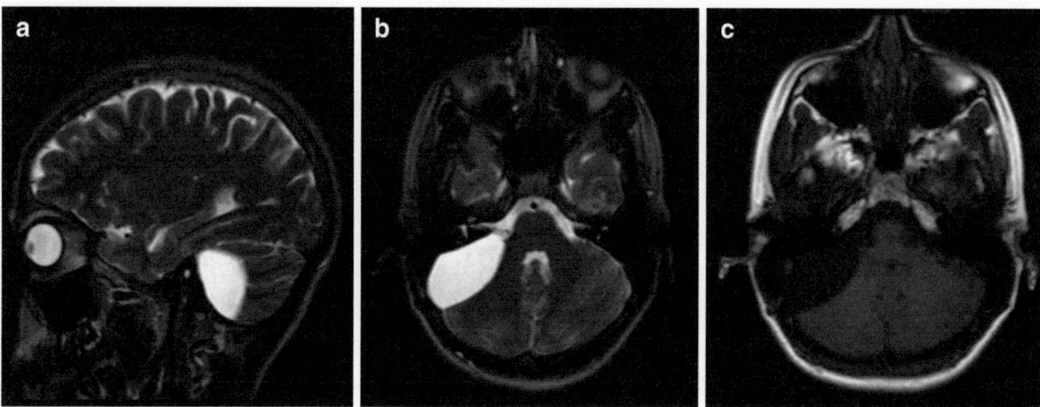

Fig. 3.7 Brain MRI T2-weighted sagittal (**a**) and axial (**b**) as well as T1-weighted axial (**c**) sequences showing right cerebellopontine angle AC

location is depression, which we may find difficult to associate with discomfort [21]. Although the symptoms are generally headache and seizures, there may be pain localized to the AC region, which can be seen in these patients and defined as a nummular headache. It is possible to explain that the cause of this headache was meningeal irritation [22].

3.3.6 Cerebellopontine Angle

The incidence of ACs detected in the cerebellopontine angle out of all arachnoid cysts is 7% (Fig. 3.7). As with other ACs, in this type, apart from headache and other general symptoms (intracranial hypertension, etc.), symptoms related to the involvement of some cranial nerves (CNs) can also be seen. Trigeminal neuralgia (Vth CN), diplopia (VIth CN), hemifacial spasm (VIIth CN), hearing loss, dizziness, and tinnitus (VIIIth CN) are some of these symptoms. In symptomatic patients, endoscopic or microscopic fenestration of the cyst wall, cyst excision, or cysto-peritoneal shunt operations are surgical options [23].

3.3.7 Retrocerebellar

Retrocerebellar ACs are the second most common type comprising 33% of all ACs [1]. They are usually asymptomatic (Fig. 3.8). Headache, dizziness, and gait disturbance can be seen as

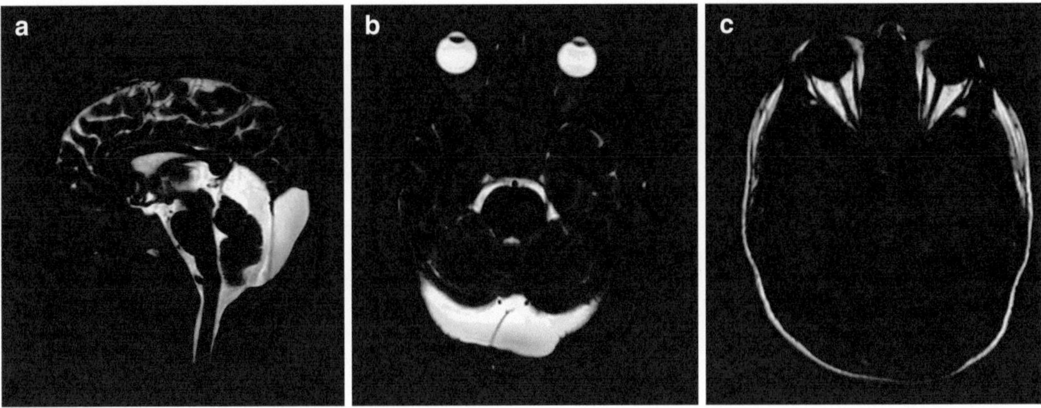

Fig. 3.8 Brain MRI T2-weighted sagittal (**a**) and axial (**b**) as well as T1-weighted axial (**c**) sequences showing bilateral retrocerebellar AC

symptoms with retrocerebellar ACs. It should be kept in mind that hydrocephalus can also be seen in these patients. In symptomatic patients, surgery should be considered in select cases. Cyst-peritoneal shunt placement or endoscopic fenestration is primarily recommended for treatment of cases with retrocerebellar ACs [24].

3.4 Conclusion

ACs are usually asymptomatic and detected incidentally, but surgical treatment options should be considered in symptomatic patients. These surgical treatment options for ACs include microsurgery, endoscopic cyst fenestration, endoscopic third ventriculostomy, and shunt placement. The endoscopic approach is particularly useful for those ACs located in the suprasellar, quadrigeminal, and middle cranial fossa locations. In addition, a third ventriculostomy can be performed if necessary in order to provide better fluid circulation. However, the result obtained with microsurgery is more adequate and microsurgery should be used in cases with interhemispheric ACs, as the first surgical choice.

References

1. Al-Holou WN, Terman S, Kilburg C, Garton HJ, Muraszko KM, Maher CO. Prevalence and natural history of arachnoid cysts in adults. J Neurosurg. 2013;118(2):222–31.
2. Hayes MJ, TerMaath SC, Crook TR, Killeffer JA. A review on the effectiveness of surgical intervention for symptomatic intracranial arachnoid cysts in adults. World Neurosurg. 2019;123:e259–72.
3. García-Conde M, Martín-Viota L. Quistes aracnoideos: embriología y anatomía patológica [Arachnoid cysts: embryology and pathology]. Neurocirugia (Astur). 2015;26(3):137–42. Spanish.
4. White ML, Das JM. Arachnoid cysts [updated 2022 Mar 7]. In: StatPearls. Treasure Island, FL: StatPearls Publishing; 2022. Available from: https://www.ncbi.nlm.nih.gov/books/NBK563272/.
5. Mustansir F, Bashir S, Darbar A. Management of arachnoid cysts: a comprehensive review. Cureus. 2018;10(4):e2458.
6. Lee YH, Kwon YS, Yang KH. Multiloculated hydrocephalus: open craniotomy or endoscopy? J Korean Neurosurg Soc. 2017;60:301–5.
7. Ahn JY, Chio JU, Yoon SH, Chung SS, Lee KC. Treatment and outcome of intracranial arachnoid cysts. J Korean Neurosurg Soc. 1994;23:194–203.
8. Galassi E, Tognetti F, Gaist G, Fagioli L, Frank F, Frank G. CT scan and metrizamide CT cisternography in arachnoid cysts of the middle cranial fossa: classification and pathophysiological aspects. Surg Neurol. 1982;17(5):363–9.

9. Cinalli G, Cappabianca P, de Falco R, Spennato P, Cianciulli E, Cavallo LM, Esposito F, Ruggiero C, Maggi G, de Divitiis E. Current state and future development of intracranial neuroendoscopic surgery. Expert Rev Med Devices. 2005;2(3):351–73.
10. Chen Y, Fang HJ, Li ZF, et al. Treatment of middle cranial fossa arachnoid cysts: a systematic review and meta-analysis. World Neurosurg. 2016;92:480–90.
11. El-Ghandour NM. Endoscopic treatment of quadrigeminal arachnoid cysts in children. J Neurosurg Pediatr. 2013;12(5):521–8.
12. Salem-Memou S, Boukhrissi N. Quadrigeminal cistern arachnoid cyst causing hydrocephalus. Pan Afr Med J. 2020;35:27.
13. Takaki Y, Tsutsumi S, Teramoto S, Nonaka S, Okura H, Suzuki T, Ishii H. Quadrigeminal cistern arachnoid cyst as a probable cause of hemifacial spasm. Radiol Case Rep. 2021;16(6):1300–4.
14. Garg K, Tandon V, Sharma S, Suri A, Chandra PS, Kumar R, Mahapatra AK, Sharma BS. Quadrigeminal cistern arachnoid cyst: a series of 18 patients and a review of literature. Br J Neurosurg. 2015;29(1):70–6.
15. Cinalli G, Spennato P, Columbano L, Ruggiero C, Aliberti F, Trischitta V, Buonocore MC, Cianciulli E. Neuroendoscopic treatment of arachnoid cysts of the quadrigeminal cistern: a series of 14 cases. J Neurosurg Pediatr. 2010;6(5):489–97.
16. Wang JC, Heier L, Souweidane MM. Advances in the endoscopic management of suprasellar arachnoid cysts in children. J Neurosurg. 2004;100:418–26.
17. Gui SB, Wang XS, Zong XY, Zhang YZ, Li CZ. Suprasellar cysts: clinical presentation, surgical indications, and optimal surgical treatment. BMC Neurol. 2011;11:52.
18. Mori K. Giant interhemispheric cysts associated with agenesis of the corpus callosum. J Neurosurg. 1992;76:224–30.
19. Albakr A, Sader N, Lama S, Sutherland GR. Interhemispheric arachnoid cyst. Surg Neurol Int. 2021;12:125.
20. Gangemi M, Seneca V, Colella G, Cioffi V, Imperato A, Maiuri F. Endoscopy versus microsurgical cyst excision and shunting for treating intracranial arachnoid cysts. J Neurosurg Pediatr. 2011;8:158–64.
21. Hayes MJ, et al. A review on the effectiveness of surgical intervention for symptomatic intracranial arachnoid cysts in adults. World Neurosurg. 2019;123:e259–72.
22. Guillem A, Barriga FJ, Giménez-Roldán S. Nummular headache associated to arachnoid cysts. J Headache Pain. 2009;10:215–7.
23. Cincu R, Agrawal A, Eiras J. Intracranial arachnoid cysts: current concepts and treatment alternatives. Clin Neurol Neurosurg. 2007;109(10):837–43.
24. Srinivasan U, Lawrence R. Posterior fossa arachnoid cysts in adults: surgical strategy: case series. Asian J Neurosurg. 2015;10(01):47.

Choroid Plexus Cyst

Kanwaljeet Garg, Deepak Agrawal, and Ajay Garg

4.1 Introduction

Neuroepithelial cysts are rare benign lesions of the brain and they can be intraventricular or intraparenchymal [1, 2]. Choroid plexus cysts (CPC) are one of the commonest intraventricular neuroepithelial cysts [3]. CPCs are a relatively common incidental finding seen on magnetic resonance imaging (MRI) done for some unrelated indication. Before the era of MRI, they were detected on postmortem examination and were reported to be present in up to 50% of autopsy specimens [4]. The prevalence of CPC has been reported to vary between 0.6% and 2.35% in the literature [5, 6]. The commonest location of CPC is the glomus of the lateral ventricles, though they can occur in any part of the lateral ventricles [3]. CPCs contain cerebrospinal fluid (CSF) with a slightly higher protein concentration.

4.2 Age Group

CPCs are more common in children than in adults [7]. It has been reported that CPCs can be found in upto 34% of fetuses or neonates [3].

K. Garg · D. Agrawal (✉)
Department of Neurosurgery, All India Institute of Medical Sciences, New Delhi, India

A. Garg
Department of Neuroradiology, All India Institute of Medical Sciences, New Delhi, India

CPCs can also be found in older age groups. The pathogenesis of CPCs in these two groups is different.

4.3 Size and Location of Choroid Plexus Cysts

CPCs are usually located on the trigonal area of the lateral ventricles [4, 8, 9]. CPCs located in the anterior part of the lateral ventricle are very rare [10]. They are usually small, less than 1 cm in size [8]. CPCs have been reported to be bilateral in two thirds of the cases [9].

4.4 Radiological Appearance (Figs. 4.1, 4.2 and 4.3)

CPC are not as common on MRI as on postmortem examination as the standard MRI techniques cannot detect all the intracranial cysts [11–13]. Due to their content, which is CSF, it is difficult to identify CPC on the computed tomography (CT) and standard T1 sequences. Protein content of the cyst may be slightly high, as seen in some of the surgically excised cysts but the content is not so high for them to be seen on CT or T1 sequences [2, 12]. CPCs can be visualized on T2 weighted MRI sequence. However, the wall of the cyst may not be seen on T2WI. FLAIR images may better delineate the cyst by suppressing the signal of

M. Turgut et al. (eds.), *Incidental Findings of the Nervous System*,
https://doi.org/10.1007/978-3-031-42595-0_4

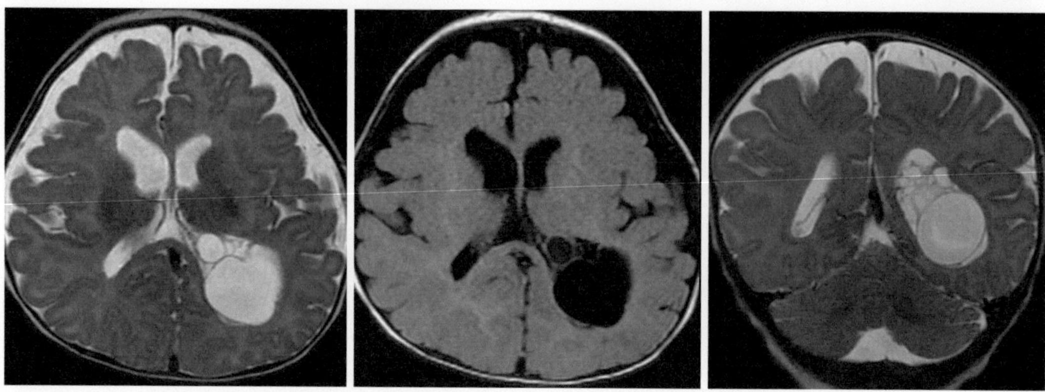

Fig. 4.1 T2WI (axial), T1WI (axial), and T2WI (coronal) magnetic resonance imaging (MRI) sequences showing choroid plexus cyst (CPC) in the left lateral ventricle

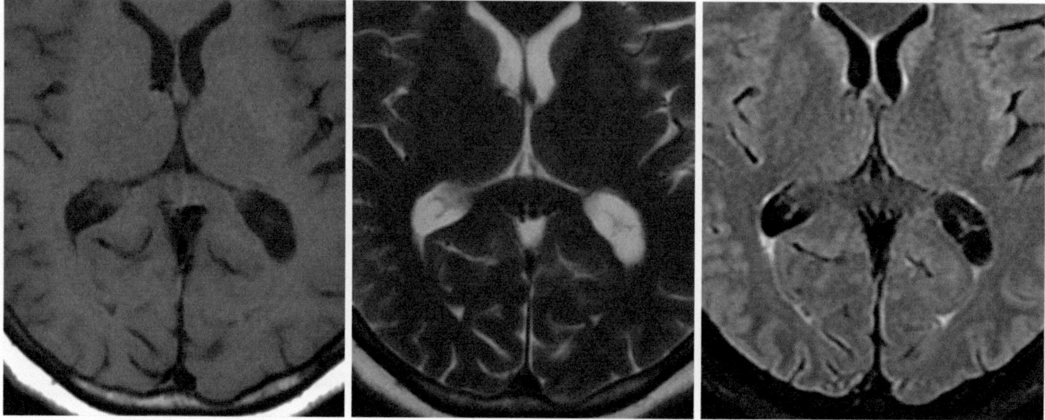

Fig. 4.2 T1WI, T2WI, and FLAIR MRI sequences showing CPC in the left lateral ventricle

CSF. FLAIR sequence may differentiate the signal of a cyst containing proteinaceous material from that of one containing only CSF. However, the size of a CPC may appear smaller due to the prominence of choroid plexus on FLAIR sequence [3].

The wall of a CPC is also very thin and closely opposed to the ependymal lining of the ventricles [2, 14]. Hence, it is difficult to appreciate it on CT. Cyst wall may be seen occasionally on T1WI and T2WI. Postcontrast MRI images show a well demarcated cyst wall or outer cyst margin [15].

Diffusion weighted imaging may reveal the CPCs as high signal intensity areas due to the restricted motion of the water molecules in the cyst as a result of the slightly high proteinaceous content [9]. It corresponds to cysts lined by connective tissue and containing mucinous material.

Kinoshita et al. confirmed these findings on MRI pathological correlation on an autopsy [8]. Due to contrast offered, diffusion weighted MRI can identify small cysts [11, 12].

Cakir et al. reviewed the MRI of around 1000 patients who had undergone MRI at their center [3]. They identified 90 high signal intensity lesions suggestive of CPC in the atria of the lateral ventricles on DTI images. The standard MRI sequences could identify only 18 of these 90 CPCs as the cysts had the same signal intensity as that of CSF. Most of these cysts had signal intensity more than that of CSF on fast FLAIR sequences. The size of the majority of the cysts (80%) varied from 0.5 cm to 1 cm. Nine of these 90 cysts caused focal ventricular expansion.

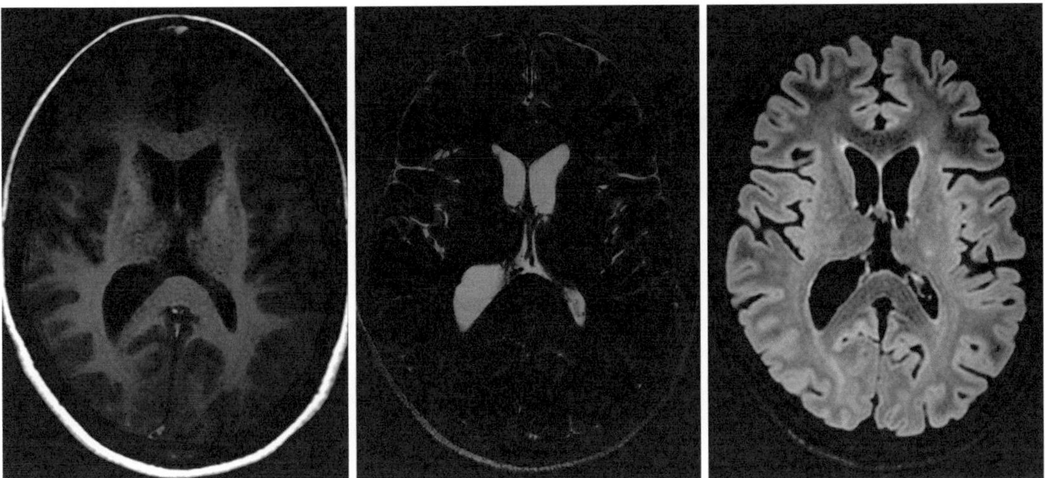

Fig. 4.3 T1WI, T2WI, and FLAIR MRI sequences showing CPC in the right lateral ventricle

4.5 Radiological Differential Diagnosis

A close radiological differential of CPC is choroid plexus xanthogranuloma [9]. They are usually bilateral and symmetrical. They may represent degenerating cystic glomera [3]. These two pathologies may appear identical on MRI but the latter has peripheral calcium deposits on pathological examination [16]. Moreover, there may be high signal intensity in choroid plexus xanthogranuloma on T1 WI due to the presence of fat [17]. Other differential diagnoses of CPC include the other neuroepithelial cysts like colloid cysts, epithelial cysts, intraventricular arachnoid cysts, and choroidal epithelial cysts [3]. It may be difficult to differentiate between an ependymal and intraventricular arachnoid cyst on MRI. The wall of ependymal cyst is closely attached to the ventricular lining, appears to be thinner, and is less consistently seen on T1-weighted images.

4.6 Pathogenesis of Choroid Plexus Cysts

The common origin of all neuroepithelial cysts is the primitive neuroepithelium that lines the neural tube [18]. The pathogenesis of CPC may involve altered histogenesis of the choroid plexus resulting in formation of fluid filled folds in the stroma. They most commonly contain CSF [12].

The most commonly accepted theory suggests that a small cyst is formed by a folding of the neuroepithelium into the choroid's matrix and of the stroma into the ventricle [9]. This results in the formation of choroidal villi, which are finger-like projections, and the neck of the latter may get pinched off to separate it from the ventricle [9]. The accumulation of secretions from the secretory activity of these epithelial cells in the congenitally formed cyst and the fluid activity transported from the exterior will produce a clear CSF-like substance [9]. Hyaline degeneration of the connective tissue stroma, deposition of calcium salts and pigment, vacuolation of the epithelial lining, and formation of small cysts in the body of the choroid plexus can even be found in early childhood [4]. Choroid plexus can undergo physiological regression with advancing age [10]. The common pathogenesis of CPCs seen in elderly patients is the degeneration of the choroid plexus [4].

4.7 Histological Findings of Choroid Plexus Cysts

Histologically, they are lined by a layer of compressed epithelium or connective tissue [8]. The outer fibrous membrane is lined by an inner cuboidal choroid plexus epithelium [19]. Connective tissue lined cysts can result from regressive changes in the choroid plexus. These cysts are age related and all filled with mucin secreted by the connective tissue lining. CPC and other cysts which are radiological differentials can be differentiated using the immunohistochemistry markers as these cysts will show immunoreactivity of the structures from which they are derived. Choroid plexus epithelium can be identified using its positivity for transthyretin while the ependyma will get stained with glial fibrillary acidic protein. Colloid cyst expresses epithelial markers like mucin. Staining with these markers lend support to the origin of these neuroepithelial cysts [20, 21].

4.8 Natural History of Choroid Plexus Cysts

Most of the CPCs remain stable over time. Occasionally, CPCs can grow in size and cause obstructive hydrocephalus [22]. Rarely, CPCs may disappear completely [23]. Spontaneous hemorrhage in a CPC has also been reported [24]. Binning et al. reported asymptomatic enlargement of bilateral CPCs following cerebral hypotension secondary to ventriculoperitoneal shunt [25]. However, the patient remained asymptomatic.

4.9 Choroid Plexus Cysts in Fetus

CPC can also be commonly seen on antenatal ultrasonography (USG) in the second trimester [26]. The reported incidence of CPC in second trimester USG is around 1% of fetuses who undergo a routine screening USG [27, 28]. Usually, they are transient and most of them regress by 26 postmenstrual weeks. The CPCs which do not regress during pregnancy can even regress shortly after birth [26, 28].

They can be associated with fetal aneuploidy, particularly trisomy 18, and hence CPC seen on antenatal imaging studies can be significant and require further work up [5, 28]. An isolated CPC in the absence of other fetal anomalies and low risk biochemical screening for aneuploidy does not require any specific intervention [27, 28]. Maher et al. reported that most of the CPCs seen on antenatal examination regress [26]. However, a rare cyst may persist and even enlarge requiring surgical intervention [26, 29].

4.10 Symptoms

The CPCs are usually asymptomatic, and an incidental finding seen on MRI done for some unrelated reason [9]. Rare cases of symptomatic CPC requiring surgical intervention have been reported in literature [10, 15, 30–33]. Usually, the symptomatic cysts are larger than 1 cm and can lead to episodic blockage of normal CSF circulation.

4.11 Which Choroid Plexus Cysts Require Follow-Up

CPCs larger than 1 cm or those in areas other than the trigone of the lateral ventricle should be carefully followed. These cysts have a tendency to result in raised intracranial pressure due to blockage of the normal CSF flow because of their large size or proximity to foramen of Monro. CPC located in the trigone are unlikely to cause symptoms unless large. However, CPC located in the anterior and middle part of the lateral ventricle can be symptomatic even when small.

References

1. Sherman JL, Camponovo E, Citrin CM. MR imaging of CSF-like choroidal fissure and parenchymal cysts of the brain. AJNR Am J Neuroradiol. 1990;11:939–45.
2. Czervionke LF, Daniels DL, Meyer GA, Pojunas KW, Williams AL, Haughton VM. Neuroepithelial cysts of the lateral ventricles: MR appearance. AJNR Am J Neuroradiol. 1987;8:609–13.
3. Cakir B, Karakas HM, Unlu E, Tuncbilek N. Asymptomatic choroid plexus cysts in the lateral ventricles: an incidental finding on diffusion-weighted MRI. Neuroradiology. 2002;44:830–3.
4. Baker GS, Gottlieb CM. Cyst of the choroid plexus of the lateral ventricle causing disabling headache and unconsciousness: report of case. Proc Staff Meet Mayo Clin. 1956;31:95–7.
5. Geary M, Patel S, Lamont R. Isolated choroid plexus cysts and association with fetal aneuploidy in an unselected population. Ultrasound Obstet Gynecol. 1997;10:171–3.
6. Reinsch RC. Choroid plexus cysts—association with trisomy: prospective review of 16,059 patients. Am J Obstet Gynecol. 1997;176:1381–3.
7. Kennedy KA, Carey JC. Choroid plexus cysts: significance and current management practices. Semin Ultrasound CT MR. 1993;14:23–30.
8. Kinoshita T, Moritani T, Hiwatashi A, Numaguchi Y, Wang HZ, Westesson P-LA, et al. Clinically silent choroid plexus cyst: evaluation by diffusion-weighted MRI. Neuroradiology. 2005;47:251–5.
9. Maekawa T, Hori M, Murata K, Feiweier T, Andica C, Fukunaga I, et al. Choroid plexus cysts analyzed using diffusion-weighted imaging with short diffusion-time. Magn Reson Imaging. 2019;57:323–7.
10. Parízek J, Jakubec J, Hobza V, Nemecková J, Cernoch Z, Sercl M, et al. Choroid plexus cyst of the left lateral ventricle with intermittent blockage of the foramen of Monro, and initial invagination into the III ventricle in a child. Childs Nerv Syst. 1998;14:700–8.
11. Duda V, Juhnke I. [Persistent cysts of the choroid plexus as sonographic indications of a genetic defect]. Z Geburtshilfe Perinatol. 1990;194:236–9.
12. Odake G, Tenjin H, Murakami N. Cyst of the choroid plexus in the lateral ventricle: case report and review of the literature. Neurosurgery. 1990;27:470–6.
13. Riebel T, Nasir R, Weber K. Choroid plexus cysts: a normal finding on ultrasound. Pediatr Radiol. 1992;22:410–2.
14. Kjos BO, Brant-Zawadzki M, Kucharczyk W, Kelly WM, Norman D, Newton TH. Cystic intracranial lesions: magnetic resonance imaging. Radiology. 1985;155:363–9.
15. Numaguchi Y, Foster RW, Gum GK. Large asymptomatic noncolloid neuroepithelial cysts in the lateral ventricle: CT and MR features. Neuroradiology. 1989;31:98–101.
16. Hinshaw DB, Fahmy JL, Peckham N, Thompson JR, Hasso AN, Holshouser B, et al. The bright choroid plexus on MR: CT and pathologic correlation. AJNR Am J Neuroradiol. 1988;9:483–6.
17. Pear BL. Xanthogranuloma of the choroid plexus. AJR Am J Roentgenol. 1984;143:401–2.
18. Shuangshoti S, Roberts MP, Netsky MG. Neuroepithelial (colloid) cysts: pathogenesis and relation to choroid plexus and ependyma. Arch Pathol. 1965;80:214–24.
19. Hanbali F, Fuller GN, Leeds NE, Sawaya R. Choroid plexus cyst and chordoid glioma. Report of two cases. Neurosurg Focus. 2001;10:E5.
20. Coca S, Martínez A, Vaquero J, Moreno M, Martos JA, Rodríguez J, et al. Immunohistochemical study of intracranial cysts. Histol Histopathol. 1993;8:651–4.
21. Lach B, Scheithauer BW, Gregor A, Wick MR. Colloid cyst of the third ventricle. A comparative immunohistochemical study of neuraxis cysts and choroid plexus epithelium. J Neurosurg. 1993;78:101–11.
22. Radaideh MM, Leeds NE, Kumar AJ, Bruner JM, Sawaya R. Unusual small choroid plexus cyst obstructing the foramen of monroe: case report. AJNR Am J Neuroradiol. 2002;23:841–3.
23. Heilman CB, Zerris VA. Transient choroid plexus cysts and benign asymmetrical ventricles: a case suggesting a possible link: case report. Neurosurgery. 2003;52:213–5. discussion 215
24. Baka JJ, Sanders WP. MRI of hemorrhagic choroid plexus cyst. Neuroradiology. 1993;35:428–30.
25. Binning MJ, Couldwell WT. Choroid plexus cyst development and growth following ventricular shunting. J Clin Neurosci. 2008;15:79–81.
26. Maher CO, Piatt JH, Section on Neurologic Surgery, American Academy of Pediatrics. Incidental findings on brain and spine imaging in children. Pediatrics. 2015;135:e1084–96.
27. Shah N. Prenatal diagnosis of choroid plexus cyst: what next? J Obstet Gynaecol India. 2018;68:366–8.
28. Society for Maternal-Fetal Medicine (SMFM), Yeaton-Massey A, Monteagudo A. Intracranial cysts. Am J Obstet Gynecol. 2020;223:B42–6.
29. Becker S, Niemann G, Schöning M, Wallwiener D, Mielke G. Clinically significant persistence and enlargement of an antenatally diagnosed isolated choroid plexus cyst. Ultrasound Obstet Gynecol. 2002;20:620–2.
30. Nahed BV, Darbar A, Doiron R, Saad A, Robson CD, Smith ER. Acute hydrocephalus secondary to obstruction of the foramen of monro and cerebral aqueduct caused by a choroid plexus cyst in the lateral ventricle. Case report. J Neurosurg 2007 [cited 2022 Jun 5];107. Available from: https://pubmed.ncbi.nlm.nih.gov/17918533/.
31. Jeon JH, Lee SW, Ko JK, Choi BG, Cha SH, Song GS, et al. Neuroendoscopic removal of large choroid plexus cyst: a case report. J Korean Med Sci. 2005;20:335–9.
32. Tamai S, Hayashi Y, Sasagawa Y, Oishi M, Nakada M. A case of a mobile choroid plexus cyst presenting with different types of obstructive hydrocephalus. Surg Neurol Int. 2018;9:47.
33. Azab WA, Mijalcic RM, Aboalhasan AA, Khan TA, Abdelnabi EA. Endoscopic management of a choroid plexus cyst of the third ventricle: case report and documentation of dynamic behavior. Childs Nerv Syst. 2015;31:815–9.

Choroidal Fissure Cyst

5

Meng Wang and Fuyou Guo

5.1 Introduction

Choroidal fissure cyst (CFC) is a rare embryological entity at the level of the choroidal fissure (Fig. 5.1) [1]. With the improvement and availability of radiological imaging, an increasing number of incidental asymptomatic CFCs are being diagnosed. Computed tomography (CT) and magnetic resonance imaging (MRI) are used to differentiate between the CFC and other differential diagnoses of cysts located at the choroidal fissures including cystic neoplasm, dermoid/epidermoid cysts, and enlargement of the choroidal fissure due to focal temporal lobe atrophy [2].

Patients with CFCs are usually asymptomatic or show symptoms that do not correlate with anatomical location. Very few patients can present with seizure and headache, but the cysts do not reflect the location of the epileptogenic focus [3, 4]. These patients could be managed successfully with antiepileptic therapy and did not require an operation [5]. Surgical intervention is indicated only in accompanying life-threatening conditions such as massive hemorrhage [6]. Regular follow-up is recommended since small proportion cysts can grow gradually over time [7].

M. Wang (✉) · F. Guo
Department of Neurosurgery, The First Affiliated
Hospital of Zhengzhou University,
Zhengzhou, Henan Province, China

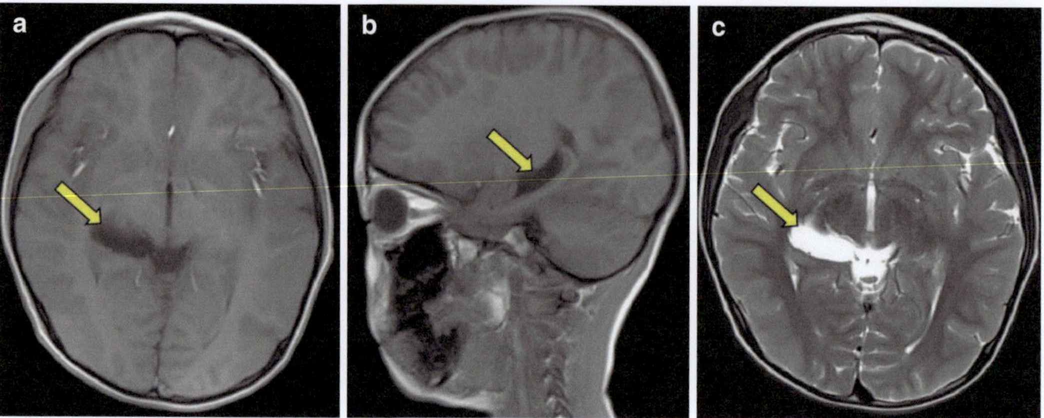

Fig. 5.1 Right choroidal fissure cyst (CFC) in a 6-year-old boy (yellow arrows). Axial T1 (**a**), sagittal T1 (**b**), and axial T2 magnetic resonance imaging (MRI) (**c**)

5.2 Embryology and Anatomy

The primitive brain consists of a lateral ventricle during the earliest stage of embryonic development. At the eighth week of pregnancy, the vascular pia meningeal lapses into the medial side of the cerebral hemisphere, leading to the formation of choroid cleft. Choroid fissure extends the posterior system of the original ventricle by the interventricular foramen [8]. Mesodermal tissue, mainly comprised of vascular structures, migrates into the newly formed ventricular cavity through the choroidal fissure to become the tela choroidea which will then mature and become more vascularized in order to form the choroid plexus.

The choroidal fissure is the fissure between the tenia fornicis and tenia choroidea, and is located between the fornix and the thalamus in the medial part of the lateral ventricle. It is divided into three parts: (a) a corpus portion located in the corpus of the lateral ventricle between the corpus of the fornix and the thalamus, (b) an atrial part situated in the atrium of the lateral ventricle between the crus of the fornix and the pulvinar, and (c) a temporal part located in the temporal horn between the fimbriae of the fornix and the posterior part of the internal capsule [8]. The tela choroidea arises from the teniae, invaginates through the choroidal fissure, and passes into the temporal horn, where it gives rise to the choroid plexus [9].

5.3 Imaging Characteristics and Differential Diagnosis

The clinical presentation and preoperative neuroimaging evaluation are essential factors that enhance our ability to determine the best therapeutic plan for each case. When a cystic lesion at the level of the choroidal fissure is observed on imaging, the main objective is the differentiation between benign cysts and lesions with an operation indication (cystic neoplasm or infectious cysts) [8]. Cystic lesions at the level of the choroidal fissure can be divided into three groups according to their intensities on MRI: low intensity pattern suggesting presence of cerebrospinal fluid (CSF); intermediate intensity pattern suggesting presence of protein; and high intensity pattern suggesting presence of colloid cyst or hemorrhage [10]. CSF-containing cysts can be differentiated from other cystic lesions through the above-mentioned method. Other significant characteristics of CSF-containing cysts include absence of contrast enhancement, lack of surrounding edema, undetectable wall, or associated soft tissue mass [10]. The position of the choroid plexus relative to the cyst can be used to identify CFCs and temporal intraventricular cysts. Intraventricular cysts will displace the choroid plexus medially, whereas choroidal fissure cysts will displace the choroid plexus laterally (Fig. 5.2) [11].

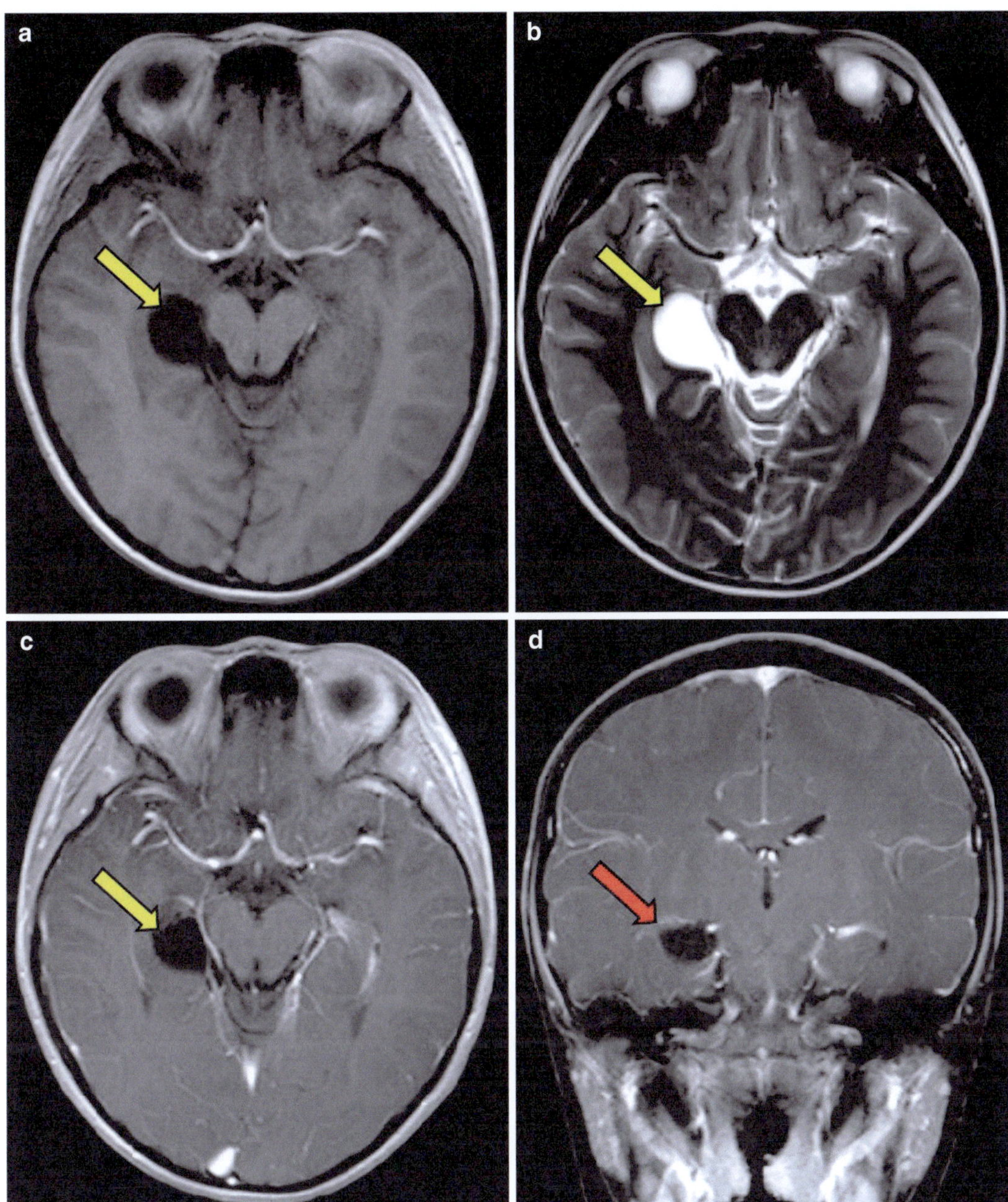

Fig. 5.2 Right CFC in an 11-year-old girl (yellow arrows). Axial T1 (**a**), T2 (**b**), enhanced T1-weighted (**c**), and coronal enhanced T1-weighted MRI (**d**). Coronal enhanced T1-weighted MRI showing the cyst medial to the right choroid plexus (red arrow) excluding an intraventricular cyst

5.4 Histology and Pathology

Although histology and pathology of CFCs have never been described previously, many reports are available describing arachnoid cysts at other locations. The wall of an arachnoid cyst consists of meningothelial cells lining a fibrous connective tissue membrane. The expression of epithelial membrane antigen is positive, but acidic protein and S-100 are negative [12].

The pathogenetic mechanism intracranial arachnoid cysts is still unclear. Several theories about the pathogenesis of primary arachnoid cysts have been reported. Starkman et al. hypothesized that arachnoid cysts were caused by aberrant splitting and duplication in the arachnoid membrane [13]. Rengachary et al. found that splitting of the arachnoid membrane at the margin of the cyst, which indicated that the structural of the arachnoid cyst wall, is different from the normal arachnoid membrane [14]. Other pathogenetic mechanisms have been hypothesized as for intraventricular arachnoidal cysts. Yeates et al. suggested that intraventricular arachnoidal cyst may originate from the arachnoid tissue in the choroid plexus and bulged into the lateral ventricle [15]. Nakase et al. stated that intraventricular cysts may arise from the arachnoid layer when it invaginates via the choroidal fissure [11]. Hence, CFCs may be a special type of arachnoidal cysts, which did not migrate into the temporal horn.

5.5 Therapeutic Principles and Preoperative Evaluation

Just as mentioned above, patients with CFCs are usually asymptomatic and do not require surgical treatment. There are limited reports about CFC being treated via surgery. Tubbs et al. reported a case series of symptomatic enlargement of CFCs that were surgically treated [16]. Based on the authors' experience, surgical fenestration of such cysts has good long-term results. Hamit et al. reported a case of growing and hemorrhagic CFC which was treated surgically, and considered that operation was indicated only in accompanying life-threatening conditions [6].

Sporadically, CFCs may be found in patients with complex partial epileptic seizures [3]. Arroyo et al. described a series of nine patients with seizure and CFC, and found that there was usually no relationship between the seizure focus and the cyst [4]. Sherman et al. reported five patients with seizures, and confirmed that the cysts were probably unrelated to the seizures since there were no focal electroencephalographic signs or physical manifestations of the seizure disorders that corresponded to the cysts [2]. Based on the above research findings, we can get the conclusion that the preferred treatment for patients with seizure is conservative treatment instead of operation.

5.6 Surgical Therapy for Choroidal Fissure Cysts

There are limited reports in previous literatures of CFCs being treated surgically on account of the cysts are usually small and asymptomatic. The main purpose of surgery is to establish communication between the cyst and the subarachnoid space [17]. Tubbs et al. demonstrated that CFCs could be effectively treated with fenestration through a retrospective analysis of four patients with symptomatic enlargement of CFCs that were surgically treated [16]. Because small proportion choroidal fissure cysts can grow gradually over time, regular follow-up with neuroimaging is recommended.

5.7 Conclusion

CFCs are related to this fissure and are often found incidentally on imaging. The differential diagnoses of CFCs include neuroepithelial cysts, cystic neoplasm, dermoid cysts, parasitic cysts, and temporal intraventricular cysts. CFCs are often incidental findings and frequently asymptomatic. Surgical treatment is unnecessary for asymptomatic patients, and should be carefully assessed for symptomatic cases because the cysts are generally considered not responsible for the symptoms. Regular follow-up is recommended since small proportion cysts can grow gradually over time.

References

1. Al-Saadi T. The dilemma of choroidal fissure cyst and seizure. J Epilepsy Res. 2020;10:1–2.
2. Sherman JL, Camponovo E, Citrin CM. MR imaging of CSF-like choroidal fissure and parenchymal cysts of the brain. AJR Am J Roentgenol. 1990;155:1069–75.
3. Morioka T, Nishio S, Suzuki S, Fukui M, Nishiyama T. Choroidal fissure cyst in the temporal horn associated with complex partial seizure. Clin Neurol Neurosurg. 1994;96:164–7.
4. Arroyo S, Santamaria J. What is the relationship between arachnoid cysts and seizure foci? Epilepsia. 1997;38:1098–102.
5. Achour A, Mnari W, Miladi A, Hmida B, Maatouk M, Golli M, Zrig A. Temporal choroidal fissure cyst: a rare cause of temporal lobe epilepsy. Pan Afr Med J. 2020;36:120.
6. Karatas A, Gelal F, Gurkan G, Feran H. Growing hemorrhagic choroidal fissure cyst. J Korean Neurosurg Soc. 2016;59:168–71.
7. Altafulla JJ, Suh S, Bordes S, Prickett J, Iwanaga J, Loukas M, Dumont AS, Tubbs RS. Choroidal fissure and choroidal fissure cysts: a comprehensive review. Anat Cell Biol. 2020;30:121–5.
8. de Jong L, Thewissen L, van Loon J, Van Calenbergh F. Choroidal fissure cerebrospinal fluid-containing cysts: case series, anatomical consideration, and review of the literature. World Neurosurg. 2011;75:704–8.
9. Wen HT, Rhoton AL Jr, De Oliveira E. Transchoroid approach to the third ventricle: an anatomic study of the choroidal fissure and its clinical application. Neurosurgery. 1998;42:1205–19.
10. Kjos BO, Brant-Zawadzki M, Kucharczyk W, Kelly WM, Norman D, Newton TH. Cystic intracranial lesions: magnetic resonance imaging. Radiology. 1985;155:363–9.
11. Park SW, Yoon SH, Cho KH, Shin YS. A large arachnoid cyst of the lateral ventricle extending from the supracerebellar cistern—case report. Surg Neurol. 2006;65:611–4.
12. Boockvar JA, Shafa RBA, Forman MS, O'Rourke DM. Symptomatic lateral ventricular ependymal cysts: criteria for distinguishing these rare cysts from other symptomatic cysts of the ventricles: case report. Neurosurgery. 2000;46:1229–33.
13. Nakano H, Ogashiwa M. Complete remission of narcolepsy after surgical treatment of an arachnoid cyst in the cerebellopontine angle. J Neurol Neurosurg Psychiatry. 1995;58:264.
14. Rengachary SS, Watanabe I. Ultrastructure and pathogenesis of intracranial arachnoid cysts. J Neuropathol Exp Neurol. 1981;40:61–83.
15. Yeates A, Enzmann D. An intraventricular arachnoid cyst. J Comput Assist Tomogr. 1979;3:697–700.
16. Tubbs RS, Muhleman M, McClugage SG, Loukas M, Miller JH, Chern JJ, Rozzelle CJ, Oakes WJ, Cohen-Gadol AA. Progressive symptomatic increase in the size of choroidal fissure cysts. J Neurosurg Pediatr. 2012;10:306–9.
17. Eymann R, Kiefer M. Relevance and therapy of intracranial arachnoidal cysts. Radiologe. 2018;58:135–41.

Dermoid and Epidermoid Cyst

6

Fuyou Guo

6.1 Introduction

Intracranial dermoid cyst (DC) is benign tumor with an average prevalence between 0.4% and 0.6% of all intracranial tumors [1]. Unlike their slightly more common epidermoid counterparts, DC tend to occur in the midline. The most common locations for intracranial DC are the posterior fossa cisterns (Fig. 6.1); occasionally DC can also be found in cisterns surrounding the suprasellar region or in the fourth ventricle [2]. In addition, this lesion is solitarily described by rupture based on previous literature; rupture of intracranial DC is a rare event and can lead to a variety of clinical presentations [3–6].

Intracranial epidermoid cyst (EC), also known as pearoma and cholesteatoma, is rare benign congenital lesion and account for approximately 0.2–1.8% of all intracranial brain tumors [7]. Unlike DC, intracranial EC is located off-midline and the incidence rate of intracranial EC is also more common than that of DC. They frequently occur at the cerebellopontine angles (CPAs) and parasellar regions, insinuating between brain structure [8]. Occasionally intracranial EC involved in the brainstem was reported as extremely rare case in previous literatures [9, 10]. Intracranial EC, as an uncommon benign lesion with slow growth, the clinical manifestations are often occult and atypical. With the widespread usage of magnetic resonance imaging (MRI) examination, many asymptomatic DC/EC are being discovered incidentally. Although many authors advocate conservative management for small or asymptomatic cysts, surgical resection is recommended in selected patients with obvious symptoms.

F. Guo (✉)
Department of Neurosurgery, First Affiliated Hospital
of Zhengzhou University,
Zhengzhou, Henan Province, China

International Joint Laboratory of Nervous System
Malformations, First Affiliated Hospital of
Zhengzhou University,
Zhengzhou, Henan Province, China

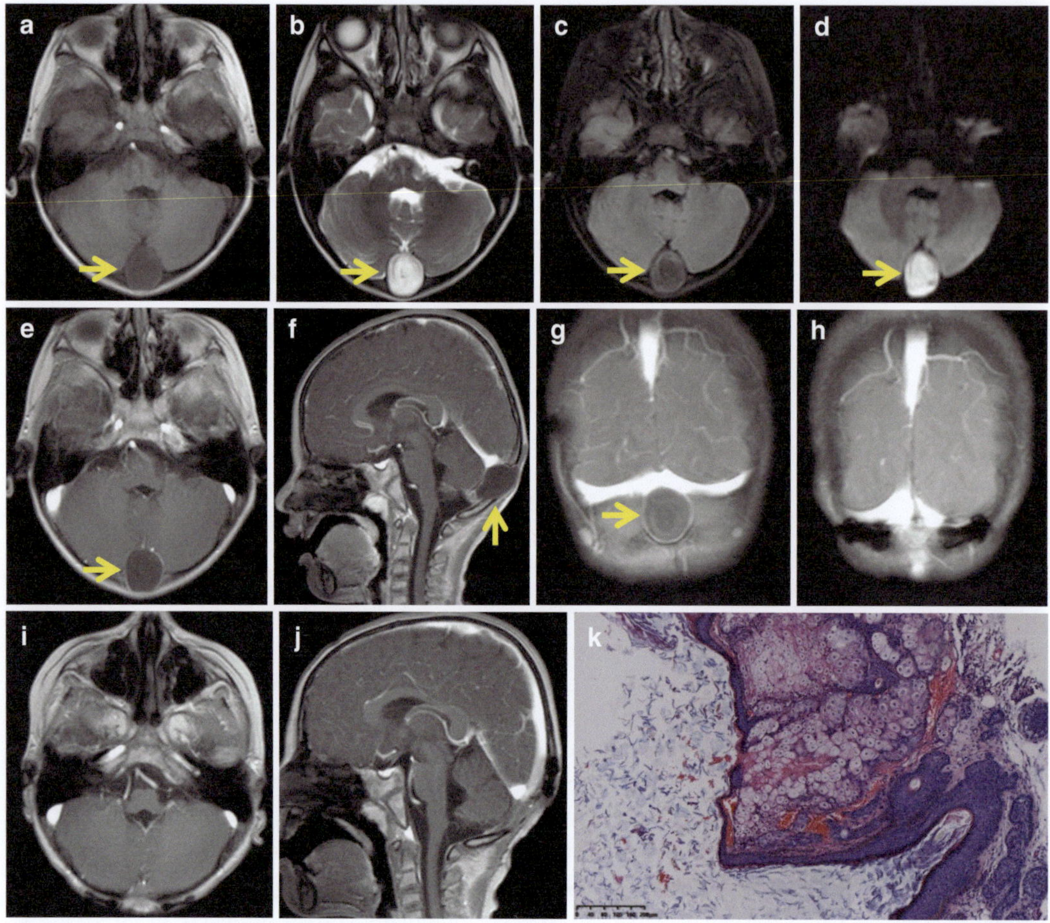

Fig. 6.1 A three-year-old child was admitted with slow-growing lump in occipital for 3 years. Axial T1-weighted image showing a hyperintense oval lesion (**a**) and inhomogeneous hyperintensity on T2-weighted image (**b**). Fluid attenuated inversion recovery (FLAIR) sequence showing slightly hyperintense (**c**), diffusion-weighted magnetic resonance imaging (MRI) revealing strong restricted diffusion of the lesion (**d**). The capsule of lesion exhibiting moderate enhancement on axial, sagittal, and coronal MRI with gadolinium (**e–g**), Yellow arrow indicating lesion. The lesion was totally removed at 6 month follow-up on enhanced coronal, axial and sagittal MRI (**h–j**). H-E staining showing dermal appendage with sebaceous and sweat glands (**k**, ×10)

6.2 Clinical Features

Intracranial DC are rare congenital lesions of the brain that account for less than 1% of all intracranial tumors. The distributions of intracranial DC are predominantly involved in the midline location; they have been reported in the vermis and the fourth ventricle, or suprasellar cistern and occasionally in the subfrontal areas. The common initial symptoms present as headache, epilepsy, nausea, vomiting, and so on. However, there are some DC that, depending on the location, can cause a variety of symptoms [11]. Other factors such as lesion size, growth rate, with or without rupture also contribute to the onset of symptoms. Based on the report of Kahilogullari et al. [12], patients with cyst rupture can be asymptomatic or otherwise present

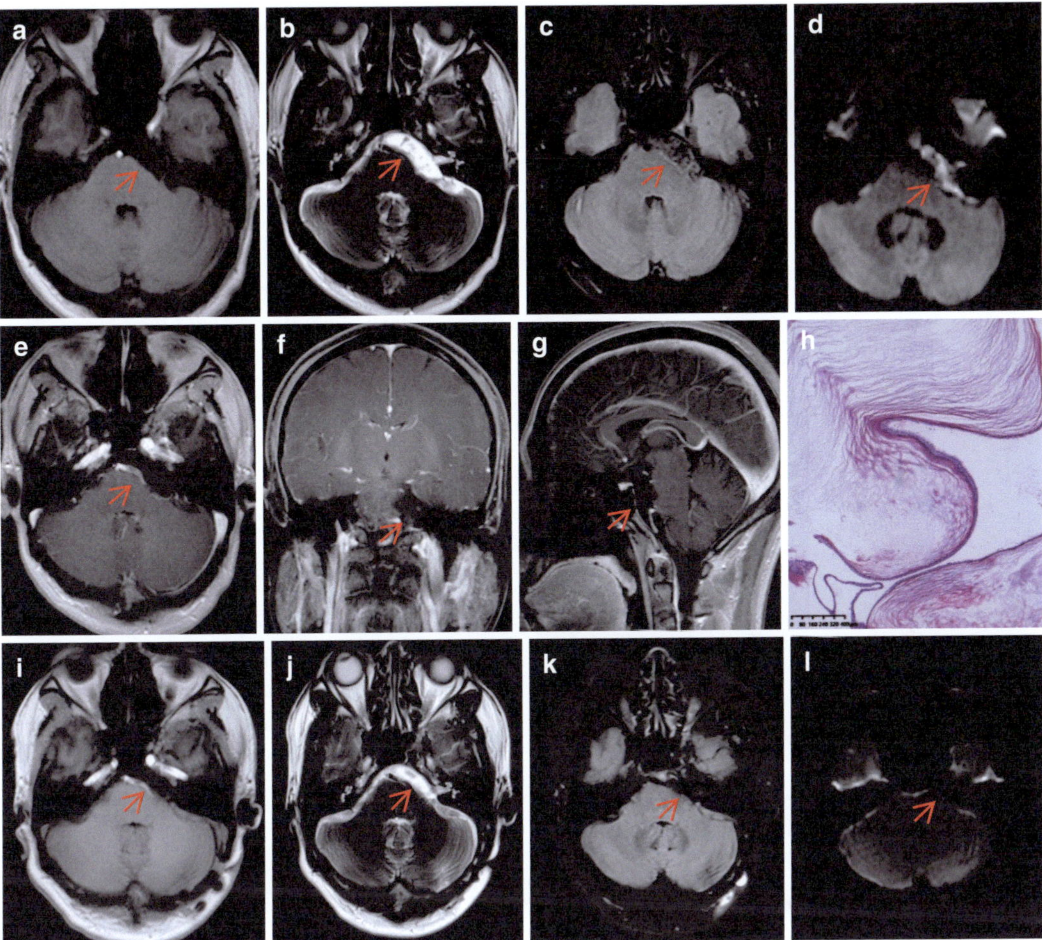

Fig. 6.2 One male patient aged 38 was admitted with intermittent trigeminal neurolgia for 15 days. The lesion appeared hyperintense on axial T1 and mixed signal on T2 MRI respectively in the left cerebellopontine angle (CPA) (**a, b**), FLAIR showing hyperintense signal and remarkable restriction on DWI (**c, d**), no enhancement was observed in axial, coronal, and sagittal contrast MRI (**e–g**), photomicrographs showing squamous epithelium and stratified keratin debris (**h**: H-E ×4). Postoperative MRI revealed that no residual tumor was found in axial T1 and T2-weighted MRI (**i, j**), FLAIR showing no signal and restriction on DWI respectively (**k, l**)

with various clinical symptoms as headache, seizure, aseptic meningitis, hydrocephalus, vasospasm, neuropsychiatric symptoms, cerebral ischemia, signs of cavernous sinus involvement, and olfactory delusion. Consequently, DC are usually identified due to complications such as meningitis, obstructive hydrocephalus, local mass effects, or increased intracranial pressure. The most common complication after the rupture of the cyst was aseptic meningitis. In addition, the rupture of the cyst may result in long-term spillage of lipid droplets, which may pose a potential embolic risk.

The most common intradural locations of EC are CPA (60%) (Figs. 6.2, 6.3, 6.7, and 6.8), fourth ventricle (5–18%), parasellar area, and middle cranial fossa (15%) (Fig. 6.4); less frequently, they are located within ventricles and brain parenchyma [13]. Intracranial EC is a congenital lesion with a slow, long clinical course

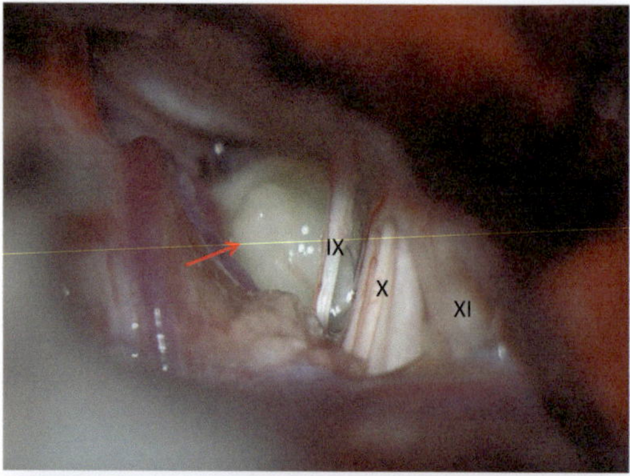

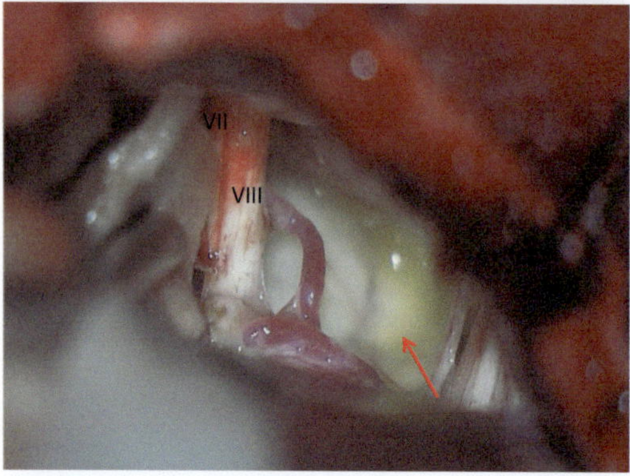

Fig. 6.3 Operative view under the operative microscope: red arrow indicating EC located in CPA and surrounding cranial nerve. Figure 6.2 and this figure was the same patient

and an average age at diagnosis around 30–40 years. There are several dramatical clinical characteristics of ECs as follows: (1) The most common intracranial location is CPA, followed by the fourth ventricle and sellar and/or parasellar region. (2) This lesion is occasionally observed in frontal lobe, parietal lobe, occipital lobe skull plate barrier, even extremely in brainstem. (3) Intradiploic epidermoid cyst is involved in local mass of skull and could lead to penetrating destruction of the bone or present as a small lump under the scalp (Fig. 6.5). (4) Due to its slow growth, half of the patients with EC are found by physical examination accidentally. However, some patients are defined by EC rupture (Fig. 6.6). (5) The clinical symptoms of the patients vary with the compression of the surrounding tissue by the tumor size. Patients with CPA ECs presented predominantly with trigeminal neuralgia (35%) and hearing loss (29%), while patients with fourth ventricle ECs have features of raised intracranial pressure and gait ataxia (69.2% respectively) [14]. The key points of differential diagnosis between EC and DC are obtained in Table 6.1.

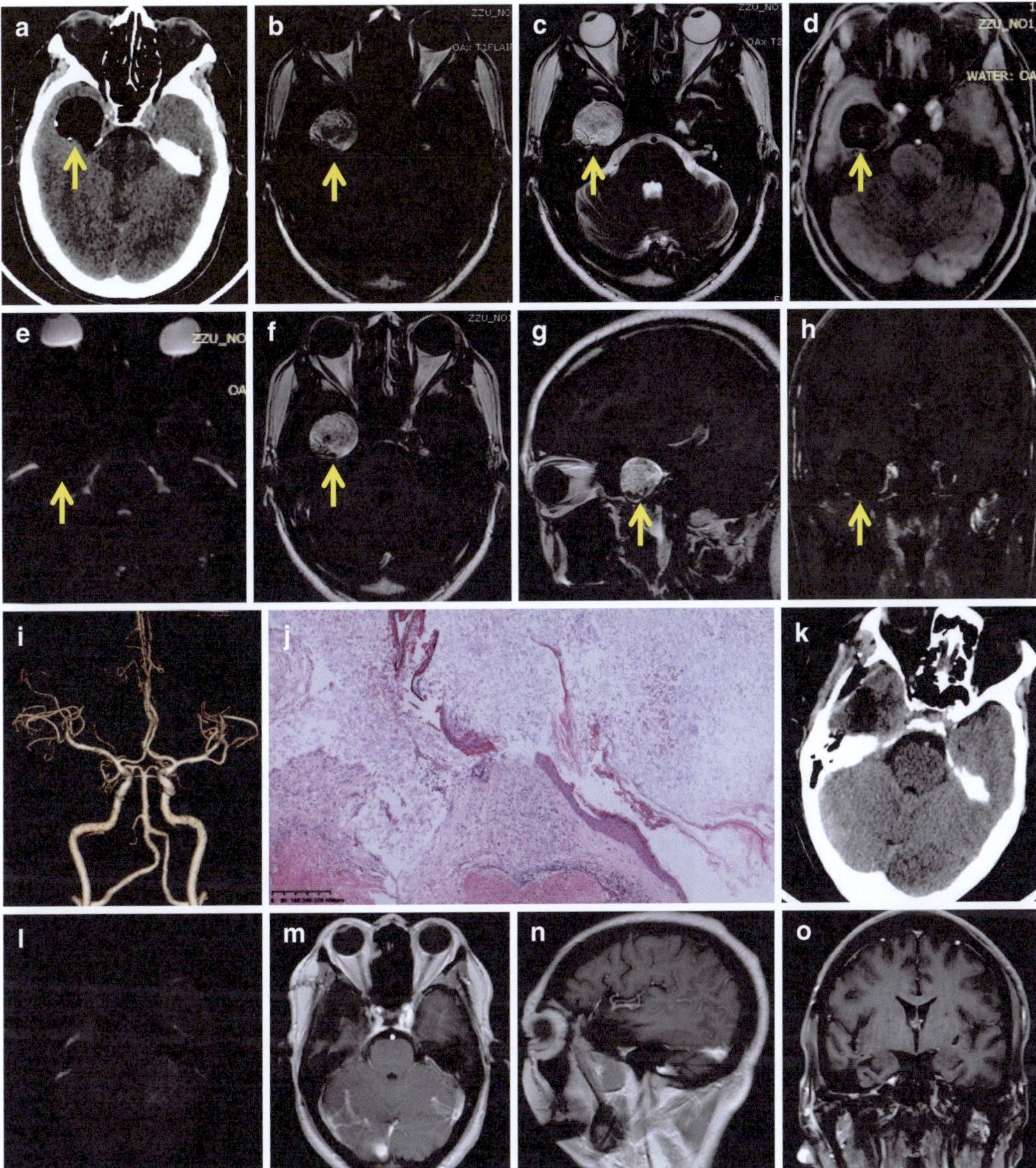

Fig. 6.4 A 43-year-old male presented with headache for 1 month. CT showed a fat density lesion at the base of the middle cranial fossa with well-defined margin and multiple high-density spots around it (**a**). MRI showed mixed hyperintense signal on T1WI and T2WI (**b**, **c**), and hypointense signal on lipid pressure imaging (**d**). DWI showed high signal intensity with mild diffusion limitation (**e**). Contrast-enhanced MRI showed no significant enhancement (**f–h**), yellow arrow indicating lesion. The preoperative CTA showing no aneurysm (**i**), photomicrographs of tissue samples obtained for pathological examination revealing fresh and old hemorrhage, as well as cholesterol crystals within granulation (**j**: H-E ×4), postoperative CT demonstrated that the epidermoid cyst was removed totally (**k**). No recurrent tumor occurred on DWI and enhanced MRI 3 years after operation (**l–o**)

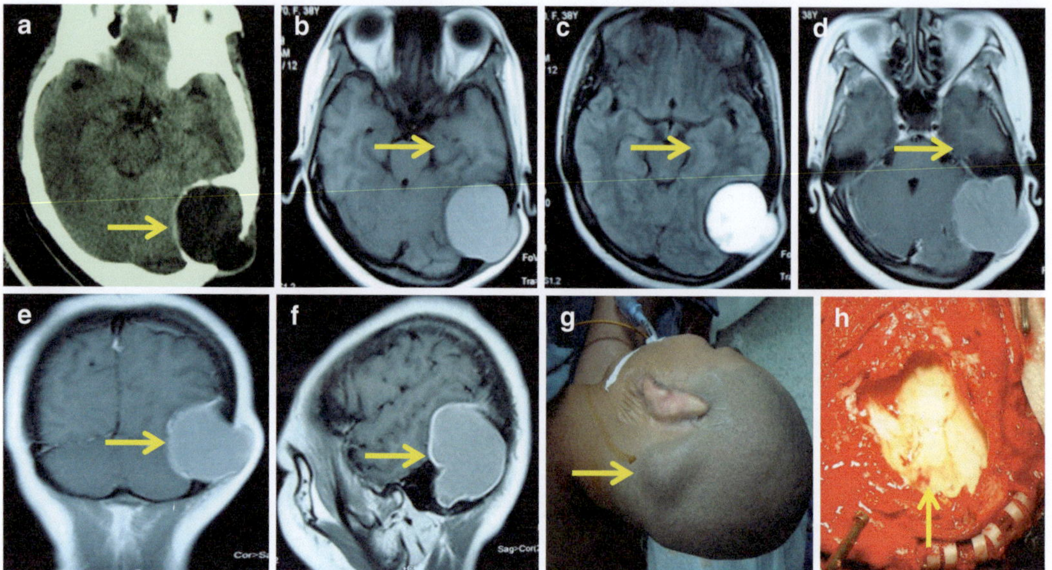

Fig. 6.5 Intradiploic epidermoid cysts involved in the left temporal skull. Computed tomography (CT) demonstrating a hypodense mass and penetrating skull in the left temporal-occipital lobe (**a**). MRI showed a well-circumscribed mass with brain compression (**b–f**). There was an obvious lump at the left temporal-occipital scalp (**g**). Operative view demonstrated a firm extra-axial mass with pearly white tumor wrapped in capsule and bone erosion (**h**)

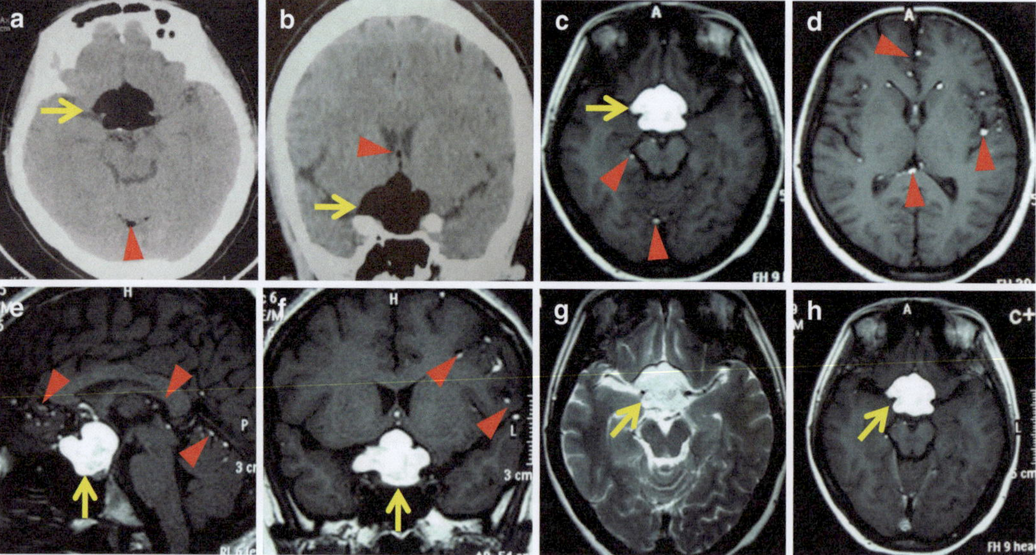

Fig. 6.6 A 33-year-old female patient was admitted with headache and decreased vision for 3 days. Axial and coronal CT demonstrating a hypodense mass in sellar region and ruptured droplets (**a**, **b**). On MRI, there was an hyperintense signal on T1WI with multiple hyper-intense fat droplets in the supresellar area, pineal region, and left frontal lobe (**b–f**). Axial MRI showing hyperintense signal on T2WI (**g**). Contrast-enhanced MRI showed no obvious enhancement of the lesion (**h–j**), yellow arrow showing lesion, red triangle indicating droplet. After surgery 1 month, the tumor was completely removed on follow-up MRI examination (**k–m**), and photomicrograph of tumor displaying a kelrin-containing tumor with squamous epithelium lining (**n**, **o**: H-E ×10)

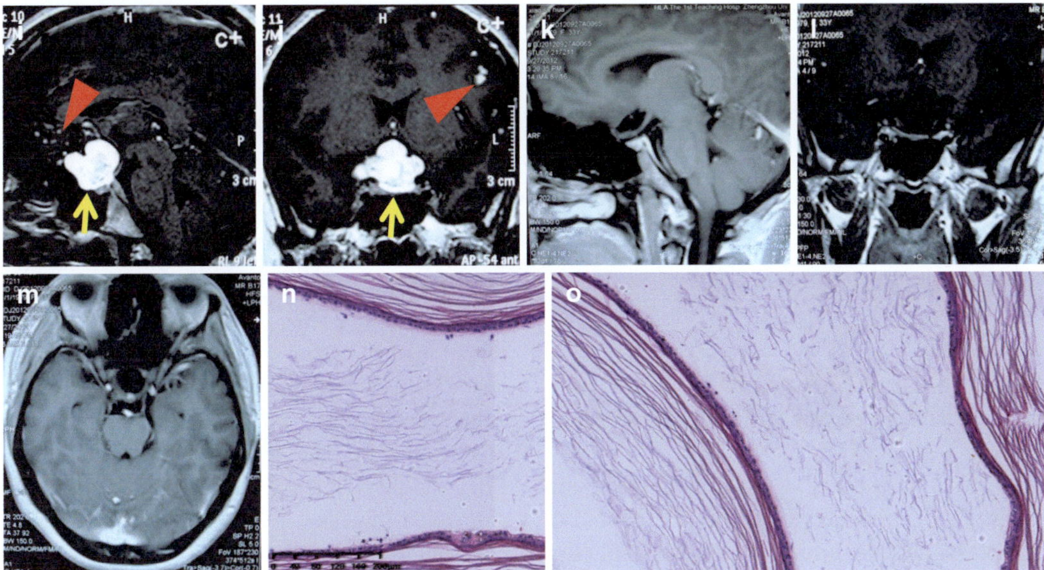

Fig. 6.6 (continued)

Table 6.1 Differential diagnosis between intracranial epidermoid and dermoid cyst

Differential points	Epidermoid cyst (EC)	Dermoid cyst (DC)
Incidence [17]	0.2–1.8% of all primary intracranial tumors, 4–9 times more than dermoid cysts	0.2–0.7% of all primary intracranial tumors
Age [10]	30–40 years	At an earlier age of development (predominance to children)
Male/female	Males are more commonly affected	Slightly higher predominance in female
Distributions	Off midline in location Cerebellopontine angle cistern (40–50%) Followed by the fourth ventricle (17%) Sellar and/or parasellar region (10–15%)	Frequently midline in location Children lesion prone to posterior fossa adult locations were sellar, parasellar, frontonasal regions
Combined malformation	Uncommon	50% of patients with congenital abnormality such as dermoid sinus
CT features	Hypodense on CT	Hypodense on CT, with some hyperdense areas of calcium deposit
MRI features [18]	Hypointense on T1-weighted Hyperintense on T2-weighted FLAIR with hyperintense restriction on DWI	T1-hyperintense regions and heterogeneous on T2 due to the presence of fat and show facilitated diffusion
Cyst capsule	Squamous epithelium solely	Squamous epithelium and dermal appendages
Cyst content	Desquamated anucleate squamae and cholesterol	Hair follicles, sebaceous glands, and apocrine glands
Rupture	Considerable rare due to thick layer of stratified squamous epithelium, epidermoid cyst rupture is less than dermoid cyst	Incidence of 0.18%, rupture is generally spontaneous, occasionally due to head trauma or surgery
Concurrent meningitis	Aseptic meningitis	Recurrent bacterial meningitis

(continued)

Table 6.1 (continued)

Differential points	Epidermoid cyst (EC)	Dermoid cyst (DC)
Hemorrhage	Occasionally occur	Considerably rare
Malignant transformation	Occasionally occur	Extremely uncommon
Pathological distinction	Absence of skin appendages in the cyst wall	Presence of skin appendages in the cyst wall

DWI diffusion-weighted imaging, *FLAIR* fluid-attenuated inversion recovery, *CT* computed tomography, *MRI* magnetic resonance imaging

6.3 Patient Selection and Preoperative Evaluation

Prior to any successful treatment, the initial diagnosis of intracranial DC and EC should be suspected and confirmed promptly. The clinical presentation and neuroimaging evaluation are essential factors that enhance our ability to determine the best therapeutic plan for individual case. DC usually occur clinically at a younger age than EC; moreover, the incidence of DC rupture is more frequently than EC. If intradural dermoids rupture, their contents may spill into the ventricular or subarachnoid space and cause chemical meningitis even death, which is a very serious complication usually requiring emergency treatment. Intracranial DC and EC should be clinically differentiated from arachnoid cysts, teratomas, lipomas, gliomas, and cystic craniopharyngiomas.

CT and MRI play an important role in the diagnosis of intracranial DC and EC. On CT scans, intracranial DC show a round low-density non-enhancing image with well-defined boundary and no edema around it. The cyst wall shows a high-density calcification. Intracranial DC exhibits increased signal intensity on T1-weighted sequences. The appearance of DC on T2-weighted sequences is highly variable and ranges from decreased signal to heterogeneously increased signal, which is attributed to the presence of fluid and fat components as well as intraluminal hair follicles or sweat glands. The cyst on DWI is hyperintense. Meanwhile, the cyst is not usually enhanced, but the capsule may be enhanced after contrast administration [15, 16]. CT scans of intracranial EC show a homogeneous hypodense lesion with irregular borders and without contrast enhancement but indistinguishable from an arachnoid cyst. The striking features of EC on MRI shows isointense to CSF; however, fluid-attenuated inversion recovery (FLAIR) MRI or echo-planar diffusion-weighted imaging (DWI) is superior to conventional MRI in detecting EC. There are often a heterogeneous signal higher than CSF. DWI sequence is still a very valuable diagnostic and differential method, because of the high viscosity of the capsule contents and the limited diffusion of water molecules, the EC is obviously high signal [17]. Edema, tissue infiltration, rapid growth, and new contrast-enhanced imaging may indicate the presence of cyst rupture or malignancy [18]. In addition, the intensity of mixed signal on preoperative T1WI in patients with intracranial epidermoid cyst may be associated with a higher risk of postoperative delayed hemorrhage [19].

The choice of management for intracranial DC or EC should be treated for individually. A small, asymptomatic DC or EC may not necessitate immediate excision as it can be stable for years, especially for those lesions are identified by accidently or physical examination. On the other hand, the presence of intracranial DC grow over time and can further lead to meningitis or develop into an brain abscess; complete surgical excision without disruption of the cyst wall by an experienced surgeon is advocated before the development of such complications. Surgical treatment is also recommended if there are remarkably cranial compression and hydrocephalus duet to cysts growing gradually.

6.4 Surgical Principles

Surgical resection is the first choice of treatment for DC. Aspiration or biopsies of DC have the potential to cause infection, further leading to osteomyelitis, meningitis, or cerebral abscess. Complete resection is sought in cases where the lesion is easy to access and there is no adherence to vital structures. It is not recommended in cases where the capsule is attached to neurovascular or vital structures such as the brain stem, because of its association with higher morbidity. Raghunath et al. [20] described that posterior fossa DC associated with congenital anomalies which was treated surgically in 15 patients. Seven patients had a dermal sinus and tract in the suboccipital region (47%), eight cases was concurrent with hydrocephalus (53%). Satisfactory outcome was achieved only dermal sinus tract was also excised to prevent infection and recurrence. If the hydrocephalus don't dissolve after cyst resection, ventriculoperitoneal shunt or endoscopic third ventriculostomy should be further performed.

DC are more adherent to arachnoid compared with EC, which makes the tumor capsule is strongly adherent to surrounding neurovascular structures, subtotal resection should be considered for patients safety. In addition, the patient's cosmetic concerns must be taken into account when discussing treatment options. Four criteria should be fulfilled when considering an ideal surgical approach to midline nasofrontal DC: (1) provide adequate access to a midline cyst; (2) allow a possible corridor to the skull base; (3) provide excellent window for reconstruction when needed; (4) result in a cosmetically satisfactory scar [21]; the principles of nasofrontal DC are suitable for intracranial DC in selected patients.

Ideal treatment of choice for EC is removal of cystic components with complete resection of capsule as to avoid recurrence. However, total resection can be more challenging sometimes as the capsule can be densely adherent to eloquent areas. Based on previous literatures, there are still no consensus regarding to optimal surgery for intracranial EC. Yaşargil et al. [22] favored aggressively total excision of cyst lesions to avoid recurrence. However, some authors favored the relatively less radical attitude for total resection so as to preserving nerve function [23]. In our opinion, the risks and benefits of operating surrounding key vascular structures must be carefully balanced before operation; total removal is often obtained under neuromonitoring in selected cases with meticulous dissection for capsule from arachnoid layers. In addition, endoscopic assistance may help to remove maximally tumors in otherwise inaccessible areas in view of adequate exposure and vascularized tissue [24, 25] (Figs. 6.7 and 6.8).

The majority of DC/EC are located in the subarachnoid space. Enlargement of the subarachnoid space because of the presence of tumor inside it creates large highways through which remove the tumor possible. The key surgical technique is to keep subarachnoid intact, no matter what DC or EC, spilling of cyst contents is carefully avoided during the operation; the surgical field is irrigated by excessive normal saline with dexamethasone so as to reducing aseptic meningitis once operation completion. Dura is closed in a watertight way and the suture line reinforced with fibrin glue or a tissue dural patch.

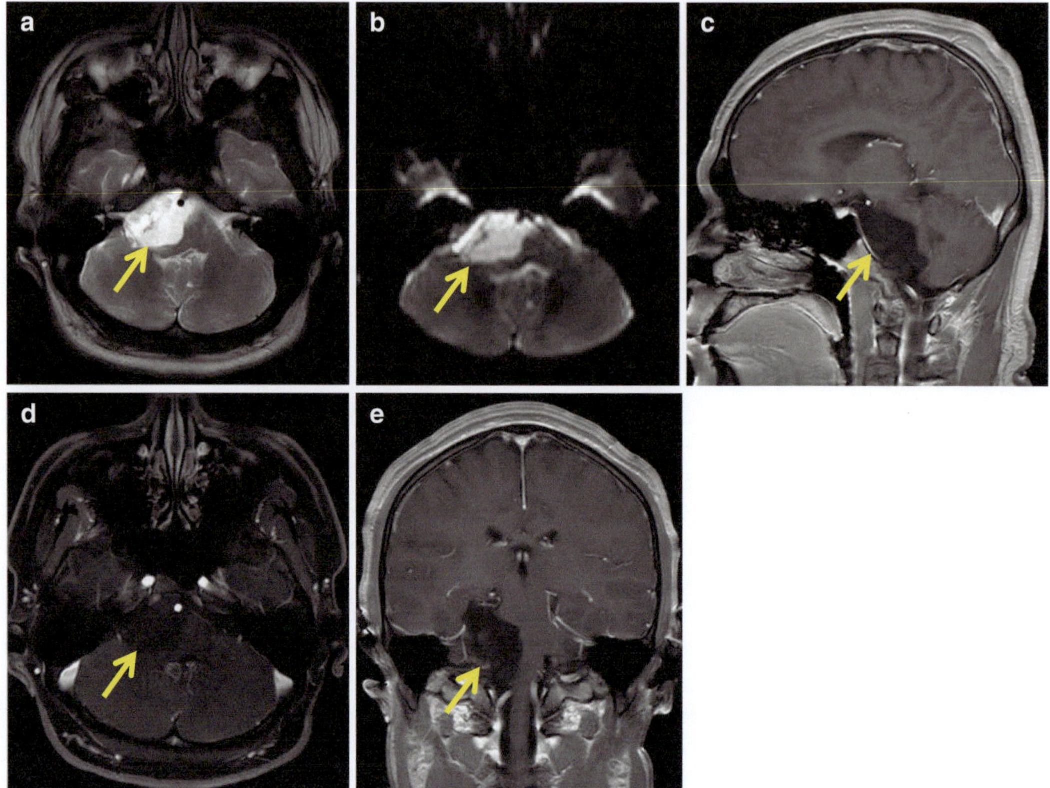

Fig. 6.7 Huge epidermoid cysts (EC) involved in right CPA, preoperative axial MRI showing hyperintense signal on T2WI (**a**), DWI showed high signal intensity with diffusion limitation (**b**). Contrast-enhanced MRI showed no significant enhancement (**c–e**), yellow arrow indicating lesion

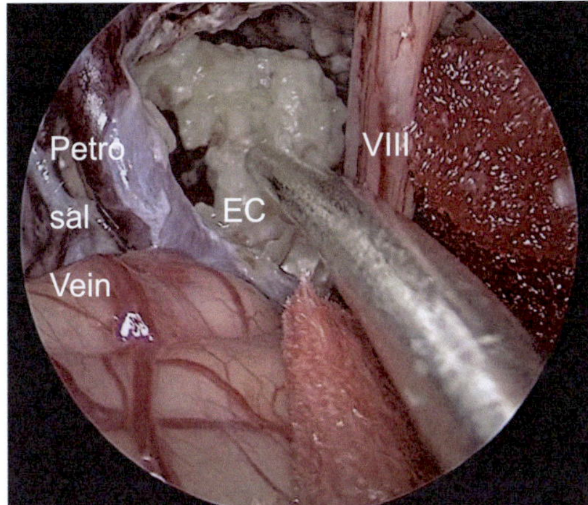

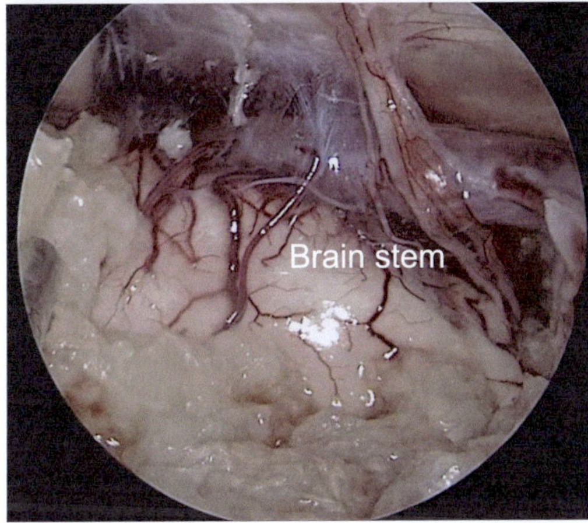

Fig. 6.8 Operative view under the endoscopic assistance: indicating EC surrounding petrosal vein and VIII cranial nerve as well as brain stem

6.5 Surgical Therapy for DC

Surgical therapy for DC is indicated if the patient demonstrates as follows: (1) Obvious neurological deficits caused by brain compression or skull erosion due to the DC growing in size of the lesion; (2) DC concurrent with dermal sinus and tract results in potential risk of intracranial infection and abscess formation even if lesion is small; (3) Increased intracranial pressure of acute hydrocephalus which results from CSF obstruction owing to DC or DC rupture; (4) Highly susception of malignant transformation of DC.

Although DC with histologically benign, in term of its tendency for growth and possible complications especially in pediatric patient, early

surgical intervention for DC is recommended. The earlier signs and symptoms of DC are identified; the better is the patient's surgical outcome. Surgical timing is adopted as early as possible, even emergency operation is performed if patients develop acute hydrocephalus. Early correct diagnosis and timely management result in better outcome in majority of DC. Additionally, surgical therapy may not be essential in all patients with ruptured intracranial DC. In a few selected patients who do not manifest increased intracranial pressure and show no change in the size of the lesion on sequential radiologic follow-up, conservative management may be advocated, especially when the ruptured intracranial dermoid is involved in deeply eloquent areas and with wide dissemination of contents [26].

Gross-total resection whenever possible remains the mainstay of treatment for DC. Rapid neurosurgical intervention is indicated to curb neurological deficit or treat systemic complications and prevent the development of severe intracranial infections. The radical surgical treatment is a complete resection of the dermal sinus and related tissues besides DC, incomplete resection can be complicated by recurrent infections. Maaloul et al. [27] described a 2-year-old girl was hospitalized for meningitis whose diagnosis was established as DC associated with dermal sinus; the excellent outcome was obtained in this patient after radical excision of both the occipital cyst and the dermal sinus as well as systemic antibiotic therapy. However, subtotal removal should be considered if the capsule of DC is adherent to the vital structure.

DCs are usually found at the midline of posterior fossa; they occur even less frequently in supratentorial location. Supratentorial DC was occasionally described as an exquisitely rare entity in previous literatures [28–30]. No matter what its location in infratentorial or supratentorial area, satisfactory outcomes are achieved after meticulously surgical treatment for DC. It should be highlighted that special care is taken to prevent spreading of content inside the ventricle during operation; the capsule is dissected sharply after removal of the cystic content; moreover, subtotal resection was recommended if the DC is located in close adhesion to the brainstem, hypothalamus, or vital vessels.

6.6 Surgical Therapy for EC

Surgical strategy for EC is indicated when patient presents neurological deficit due to mass effect. Choosing the optimal approach will mainly depend on the location, the size of the lesion, and the surgeon's preference and experience. The most common location of infratentorial EC is CPA, followed by fourth ventricle. Consequently, suboccipital retrosigmoid approach is most suitable to remove as much tumor and capsule for EC located in CPA, and midline subocciptal craniotomy is the best approach for EC in fourth ventricle. However, if patients with giant EC occasionally have supratentorial extension and is involving the middle fossa, the modified Kawase approach or combined approach (subtemporal and retromastoid) is used to achieve a wide exposure.

Total removal should be the standard goal when operating on posterior fossa ECs [14]. The epithelial capsule has to be peeled from the structures to prevent recurrence, as this is the live portion of the tumor. However, the surgeon must be cognizant of the tumor capsule's adherence to vital neural and vascular structures, and the severe neurological deficits following surgery must be taken into account. In addition, the tumor contents should not be allowed to spill into the subarachnoid space as they are intensely irritant and can cause aseptic meningitis. The surgical field should be slowly irrigated to ensure the removal of any remnants and to avoid dispersing remnants to other areas of the brain.

Intraoperative usage of multiple modality also contributes to excellent outcomes. Aboud et al. [31] reported one series of giant EC which surgery performed under intraoperative neurophysiological monitoring including somatosensory evoked potentials and brainstem auditory evoked responses and accurate neuronavigation; total removal of the capsule of giant epidermoid tumors was achieved in 73% of patients with de novo tumors; moreover, obvious function improvement and low morbidity/mortality as well as lower recurrence were observed in this series of patients.

Supratentorial EC is predominantly located in medial base of middle crania fossa. Thirty-one patients with cavernous sinus EC were surgically treated in previous literature, excellent results including symptoms remained stable or improved in 90.3% of patients, which was related with the proper surgical approach including extradural, intradural, and combined approach for best exposure. In addition, aggressive attitude toward total tumor capsule resection was up for 51.6% of the all patients [32]; similar conception regarding surgical therapy was adopted for intracranial EC [22].

Supratentorial EC, infrequently be found in the interhemispheric and Sylvian fissure, besides parasellar area. Das et al. [33] reported 22 consecutive patients with interhemispheric EC were treated surgically. The extent of excision was total in 17 (77.3%), near total in three (13.6%), and subtotal in two (9%) patients. No tumor recurrence was found after mean follow-up of 32 months. Following surgical techniques play an important role in excellent outcomes: The bridging veins protection by utilizing a more horizontal rather than a vertical trajectory of surgery may be a good maneuver to avoid the veins damage. Surgical excision of tumor capsule should be meticulous and conservation so as to avoid anterior cerebral artery or its branches injury. Prevention of ventricles opening due to extreme thinning of the corpus callosum dissection also exerts positive role in good results.

6.7 Surgical Therapy for Rupture of DC/EC

DCs rupture more frequently than EC. The most common signs of rupture are headaches (31.8%), seizures (29.5%), transient hemiparesis (15.9%), chemical meningitis (6.9%), psychosyndrome (4.5)%, visual disturbance (4.5%), and death (2.3%) [34]. If intradural dermoids rupture, their contents may spill into the ventricular or subarachnoid space and cause chemical meningitis, which is a very serious complication usually requiring surgical treatment.

Ramdasi et al. [35] reported one unusual DC situated in the interdural Meckel's cavity which ruptured into five intracranial spaces including interdural, extradural (foramen ovale), subdural, subarachnoid, and intraventricular spaces. This patient underwent right retrosigmoid craniectomy with total excision of the lesion under neurophysiological monitoring. Steroids was administrated subsequently for 21 days and then slowly tapered. This patient recovered from all her symptoms, at 1 year follow-up she was symptom-free with no neurodeficits. In addition, hydrocephalus and ventriculitis was caused from scattered fat droplets from ruptured DC; good outcome was obtained after early surgery, thorough ventricular wash with ringer lactate, postoperative extraventricular drain and steroid cover to manage ruptured cyst and chemical meningitis [36].

Shashidhar et al. [37] described that ruptured intracranial DC presented dominantly with either headache or seizures in a series of nine cases. Ruptured DC demonstrated with a various of clinical features; decision for mode of management has to be decided based on case-by-case basis. Treatment of patients varied from medical management in four cases to cerebrospinal fluid diversion in two cases and surgery resection for the lesion in three cases. Surgery is frequently contemplated in cases of ruptured DC, it requires fully decompression of the lesion with extensive irrigation of the surrounding subarachnoid space during the surgery to wash out the debris and reduce the incidence of postoperative fat dissemination and aseptic meningitis; however, medical management is a reasonable option in patients with eloquent lesions which pose high risk of morbidity by surgery.

Rarely, an EC rupture may leak keratin into the surrounding cisterns and cause aseptic or chemical meningitis. Trikamji et al. [38] described one adult case of recurrent chemical meningitis secondary to a ruptured EC in the sella. Meningitis secondary to meningeal irritation from the keratin can also contribute to the development of hydrocephalus [39].

It is emphasized that sudden onset of neurological symptoms should be considered due to rare rupture of DC/EC. While close observation with serial imaging is a reasonable management option with high surgical risk in deep and eloquent area in selected patients, surgery is usually the mainstay in majority of ruptured DC/EC. Timely detection, early surgical intervention, and steroids usage as well as watchful follow-ups can lead to full recovery from devastating complication caused by DC/EC rupture.

6.8 Minimally Invasive Techniques

In order to reduce some surgical complications such as vital neurovascular injury, postoperative deficits, and diminished cyst recurrence, minimally invasive techniques including endoscopic assistance, intraoperative neurophysiological monitoring, intra-operative MRI guidance, and awake craniotomy are recommended to use in DC/EC surgery. Furthermore, those techniques improve visualization and total resection of the cystic lesion.

Vaz-Guimaraes et al. [40] favored that endoscopic assistance was helpful for maximally cyst remove. In 21 patients who underwent endoscopic assisted endonasal surgery for EC and DC resection, total resection (total removal of cyst contents and capsule) was achieved in eight patients (38.1%), near-total resection (total removal of cyst contents, incomplete removal of cyst capsule) in nine patients (42.9%), and subtotal resection (incomplete removal of cyst contents and capsule) in four patients (19%). The noticeable advantages of endoscopic assistance could provide a more direct surgical corridor with less manipulation of neurovascular structures compared with open transcranial approaches; moreover, endoscope could supply better illumination which easily visualize the blind spots, remnant tumor lobules, and a better understanding of the nature and degree of tumor capsule-blood vessel adherence.

Intraoperative neurophysiological monitoring (IONM) is an essential tool for avoid vital structures injury. Monitoring including somatosensory evoked potentials and brainstem auditory evoked responses. IONM-aided resection of intracranial DC/EC is necessary when lesion is giant or located in eloquent area such as brain stem. Satisfactory outcomes were achieved under the guidance of IONM in previous literatures [31, 41].

Recently, Kondo et al. [42] reported three patients with EC were treated by surgery under the guidance of intra-operative magnetic resonance imaging (iMRI). No complications were observed in those patients, and all symptoms were resolved within 3 months. In this study, the images obtained through iMRI were clear representations of remnant tumors, and iMRI proved to be a useful and safe tool for total EC resection.

Other technique such as awake craniotomy also contributes to complete resection of the capsule and avoid postoperative neurologic deficits. de Macêdo Filho et al. [43] reported one 45-year-old patient presented with a generalized seizure episode due to intraparenchymal EC close to Broca area. The author performed a left frontal awake craniotomy under local anesthesia so as to map both languages, using the motor task and a test for language monitoring. Although the lesion showed peripheral coarse calcifications involved in Broca area, gross total resection was achieved and no neurologic deficits were found in this patient.

6.9 Postoperative Complications

The most common complication after surgery for DC is hydrocephalus. Another relatively common complication is aseptic meningitis, which caused by rupture of multiple cysts or inadequate intraoperative protection of the contents of the cysts into the subarachnoid space and the ventricular system. The risk of recurrence and malignant transformation is considerably low in dermoid cysts. Radiotherapy or radiosurgery were seldom recommended for cranial dermoid cysts, probably due to the non-neoplastic characteristic of the lesions.

Aseptic meningitis such as headache and fever is the leading postoperative complication following surgery for EC but could be cured by steroid administration. Postoperative delayed hemorrhage is the most disastrous complication after operation. The potential mechanism of delayed hemorrhage is the erosion and destruction of the blood vessels in the capsule by inflammation. Another uncommon complication is transformation into squamous-cell carcinoma following EC resection. When patient present with symptoms including rapid progression of clinical symptoms, edema around the cyst, and enhancement of imaging, it should keep in mind that rare malignant transformation from benign cyst, the mechanism of malignancy may be the recurrent inflammatory stimulation of the residual tumor. Moreover, repeated cystic rupture may be another explanation for the malignant transformation of ECs. Consequently, close follow-up should be performed for those who did not achieve gross total resection of benign intracranial ECs [44].

6.10 Conclusion

Intracranial DC are congenital, benign, slow-growing lesions that arise in the midline and are usually associated with the sinus tract. However, the incidence of intracranial EC is more 4–9 time than that of DC; the predominant location is involved in the posterior fossa usually arise in the lateral subarachnoid cisterns. Majority of intracranial DC are located in posterior fossa cisterns. Although histopathological confirmation remains the gold standard in diagnosing DC/EC, imaging modalities especially MRI may be useful in excluding other differential diagnoses. The histopathological features of DC are anomalies comprising of hair follicles, sweat glands, sebaceous glands, and lined by stratified squamous epithelium; EC presents as a pearly lesion of the squamous keratinized epithelium and capsule containing cell debris, keratin, and cholesterol. Conservative treatment is selected in asymptomatic lesions that have been incidentally diagnosticated for intracranial DC/EC. However, surgical resection is the first choice of treatment for DC/

EC. The primary goal of surgical treatment for DC is a complete resection of the dermal sinus and cyst related tissues; incomplete resection can be complicated by recurrent infections. Ideal treatment of choice for EC is removal of cystic components with complete resection of capsule as to avoid recurrence. Unfortunately, total resection can be more challenging sometimes as the capsule can be densely adherent to eloquent areas such as neurovascular structures. It should be highlighted that neurological deficits usually occur when a neurosurgeon pursues of complete resection of capsule. Minimally invasive techniques including endoscopic assistance, intraoperative neurophysiological monitoring, intra-operative magnetic resonance imaging guidance, and awake craniotomy were recommended to use in DC/EC surgery.

References

1. Tolebeyan AS, Kuruvilla DE. Headache in ruptured intracranial dermoid cysts. Curr Pain Headache Rep. 2020;24(7):31.
2. Fanous AA, Gupta P, Li V. Analysis of the growth pattern of a dermoid cyst. J Neurosurg Pediatr. 2014;14(6):621–5.
3. Skovrlj B, Mascitelli JR, Steinberger JM, Weiss N. Progressive visual loss following rupture of an intracranial dermoid cyst. J Clin Neurosci. 2014;21(1):159–61.
4. Thakker C, Milinis K, Sahu A, Gunawardana B. Ruptured intracranial dermoid cyst causing headache and meningism. BMJ Case Rep. 2016; https://doi.org/10.1136/bcr-2015-213527.
5. Ak R, Doğanay F, Doğan M. Rare cause of seizures: ruptured intracranial dermoid cyst. Clin Exp Emerg Med. 2019;6(1):89–90.
6. Jin H, Guo ZN, Luo Y, Zhao R, Sun MS, Yang Y. Intracranial dermoid cyst rupture-related brain ischemia: case report and hemodynamic study. Medicine (Baltimore). 2017;96(4):e5631.
7. Khan AB, Goethe EA, Hadley CC, Rouah E, North R, Srinivasan VM, Gallagher KK, Fuentes A, Vaz-Guimaraes F. Infundibular epidermoid cyst: case report and systematic review. World Neurosurg. 2019;130:110–4.
8. Jain N, Tadghare J, Patel A. Epidermoid cyst of the cerebellopontine angle presenting with contralateral trigeminal neuralgia: extremely rare case and review of literature. World Neurosurg. 2019;122:220–3.
9. Singh SK, Jain K, Jain VK. Intrinsic epidermoid of the brain stem: case report and review of the literature. Childs Nerv Syst. 2018;34(8):1589–92.
10. Patibandla MR, Yerramneni VK, Mudumba VS, Manisha N, Addagada GC. Brainstem epidermoid cyst: an update. Asian J Neurosurg. 2016;11(3):194–200.
11. Ochoa A, Saenz A, Argañaraz R, Mantese B. Ruptured dermoid cyst in the Meckel's cave presenting with trigeminal neuralgia in a pediatric patient: a case report. Childs Nerv Syst. 2020;36(12):3141–6.
12. Kahilogullari G, Yakar F, Bayatli E, Erden E, Meco C, Unlu A. Endoscopic removal of a suprasellar dermoid cyst in a pediatric patient: a case report and review of the literature. Childs Nerv Syst. 2018;34(8):1583–7.
13. Mangraviti A, Mazzucchi E, Izzo A, et al. Surgical management of intracranial giant epidermoid cysts in adult: a case-based update. Asian J Neurosurg. 2018;13(4):1288–91.
14. Gopalakrishnan CV, Ansari KA, Nair S, Menon G. Long term outcome in surgically treated posterior fossa epidermoids. Clin Neurol Neurosurg. 2014;117:93–9.
15. Kato N, Radke J, Vajkoczy P, Schneider UC. [Intrasylvian dermoid cysts of the pediatric patient: a case report and review]. No Shinkei Geka. 2014;42(10):925–9.
16. Muçaj S, Ugurel MS, Dedushi K, Ramadani N, Jerliu N. Role of MRI in diagnosis of ruptured intracranial dermoid cyst. Acta Inform Med. 2017;25(2):141–4.
17. Manzo G, De Gennaro A, Cozzolino A, Martinelli E, Manto A. DWI findings in a iatrogenic lumbar epidermoid cyst. A case report. Neuroradiol J. 2013;26(4):469–75.
18. Roh TH, Park YS, Park YG, Kim SH, Chang JH. Intracranial squamous cell carcinoma arising in a cerebellopontine angle epidermoid cyst: a case report and literature review. Medicine (Baltimore). 2017;96(51):e9423.
19. Deng X, Li J, Ke D, Liu L, Ma J, Cheng J, Hui X. Mixed signal intensity on preoperative T1 MRI might be associated with delayed postoperative hemorrhage in patients with intracranial epidermoid cyst. World Neurosurg. 2020;133:e218–24.
20. Raghunath A, Indira Devi B, Bhat DI, Somanna S. Dermoid cysts of the posterior fossa—morbid associations of a benign lesion. Br J Neurosurg. 2013;27(6):765–71.
21. El-Fattah AM, Naguib A, El-Sisi H, Kamal E, Tawfik A. Midline nasofrontal dermoids in children: a review of 29 cases managed at Mansoura University hospitals. Int J Pediatr Otorhinolaryngol. 2016;83:88–92.
22. Yaşargil MG, Abernathey CD, Sarioglu AC. Microneurosurgical treatment of intracranial dermoid and epidermoid tumors. Neurosurgery. 1989;24(4):561–7.
23. Czernicki T, Kunert P, Nowak A, Wojciechowski J, Marchel A. Epidermoid cysts of the cerebellopontine angle: clinical features and treatment outcomes. Neurol Neurochir Pol. 2016;50(2):75–82.
24. Tuchman A, Platt A, Winer J, Pham M, Giannotta S, Zada G. Endoscopic-assisted resection of intracranial epidermoid tumors. World Neurosurg. 2014;82(3–4):450–4.

25. Singh I, Rohilla S, Kumar P, Krishana G. Combined microsurgical and endoscopic technique for removal of extensive intracranial epidermoids. Surg Neurol Int. 2018;9:36.
26. Singla N, Kapoor A. Ruptured intracranial dermoid: is surgery indispensible: 11-year follow-up of a rare entity. World Neurosurg. 2016;88:693.e23–4.
27. Maaloul I, Hsairi M, Fourati H, Chabchoub I, Kamoun T, Mnif Z, Hachicha M. Occipital dermoid cyst associated with dermal sinus complicated with meningitis: a case report. Arch Pediatr. 2016;23(2):197–200.
28. Schneider UC, Koch A, Stenzel W, Thomale UW. Intracranial, supratentorial dermoid cysts in paediatric patients-two cases and a review of the literature. Childs Nerv Syst. 2012;28(2):185–90.
29. Garces J, Mathkour M, Beard B, Sulaiman OA, Ware ML. Insular and Sylvian fissure dermoid cyst with giant cell reactivity: case report and review of literature. World Neurosurg. 2016;93(491):e1–5.
30. Obled L, Peciu-Florianu I, Perbet R, Vannod-Michel Q, Reyns N. Rare case of giant supratentorial dermoid cyst. World Neurosurg. 2020;135:72–5.
31. Aboud E, Abolfotoh M, Pravdenkova S, Gokoglu A, Gokden M, Al-Mefty O. Giant intracranial epidermoids: is total removal feasible? J Neurosurg. 2015;122(4):743–56.
32. Zhou F, Yang Z, Zhu W, Chen L, Song J, Quan K, Li S, Li P, Pan Z, Liu P, Mao Y. Epidermoid cysts of the cavernous sinus: clinical features, surgical outcomes, and literature review. J Neurosurg. 2018;129(4):973–83.
33. Das KK, Honna RM, Attri G, Khatri D, Gosal JS, Dixit P, Singh S, Verma PK, Maurya VP, Bhaisora KS, Sardhara J, Mehrotra A, Srivastava AK, Jaiswal AK, Behari S. A single-center surgical experience of interhemispheric epidermoids and proposal of a new radiological classification. World Neurosurg. 2020;141:e606–14.
34. Youmans JR, Winn HR, editors. Youmans & Winn neurological surgery. 7th ed. Elsevier; 2017.
35. Ramdasi R, Thorve S, Karnavat C. Explosion of dermoid cyst into five intracranial spaces—a rare event. Br J Neurosurg. 2020;34(6):667–8.
36. Bishnoi I, Bishnoi S, Gahlawat N, Bhardwaj L, Duggal G, Singal G, Singh P. Management of a rare case of intraventricular ruptured dermoid cyst and chemical meningitis. Br J Neurosurg. 2023;37:630–3. https://doi.org/10.1080/02688697.2018.1530728.
37. Shashidhar A, Sadashiva N, Prabhuraj AR, Narasingha Rao K, Tiwari S, Saini J, Shukla D, Devi BI. Ruptured intracranial dermoid cysts: a retrospective institutional review. J Clin Neurosci. 2019;67:172–7.
38. Trikamji B, Morrow M. Recurrent chemical meningitis due to parasellar epidermoid cyst. Cureus. 2018;10(10):e3496.
39. Fernández-de Thomas RJ, Vicenty-Padilla JC, Sánchez-Jiménez JG, Labat EJ, Carballo-Cuello CM, De Jesús O, Vigo-Prieto JA. Obstructive hydrocephalus and chemical meningitis secondary to a ruptured spinal epidermoid cyst. World Neurosurg. 2019;132:173–6.
40. Vaz-Guimaraes F, Koutourousiou M, de Almeida JR, Tyler-Kabara EC, Fernandez-Miranda JC, Wang EW, Snyderman CH, Gardner PA. Endoscopic endonasal surgery for epidermoid and dermoid cysts: a 10-year experience. J Neurosurg. 2018;1:1–11. https://doi.org/10.3171/2017.7.JNS162783.
41. Cohen AR, Stone SSD. Endoscope-assisted microsurgical resection of intrinsic brainstem epidermoid: technical note and review of the literature. J Neurosurg Pediatr. 2020;26(6):654–60.
42. Kondo A, Akiyama O, Aoki S, Arai H. Application of intra-operative magnetic resonance imaging for intracranial epidermoid cysts. Br J Neurosurg. 2023;37:507–11.
43. de Macêdo Filho LJM, Aguiar GCM, Pessoa FC, Diógenes GS, Borges FS, Joaquim AF, de Albuquerque LAF. Intraparenchymal epidermoid cyst close to Broca area-awake craniotomy and gross total resection. World Neurosurg. 2020;141:367–72.
44. Zuo P, Sun T, Wang Y, Geng Y, Zhang P, Wu Z, Zhang J, Zhang L. Primary squamous cell carcinomas arising in intracranial epidermoid cysts: a series of nine cases and systematic review. Front Oncol. 2021;11:750899. https://doi.org/10.3389/fonc.2021.750899.

Prakash Nair, Sanjay Honavalli Murali,
Gowtham Matham, Darshan Hirisave Ravi,
and Easwer Harihara Venkat

7.1 Introduction

Tumors detected incidentally on imaging without any clinical symptoms, signs, or suspicion are called incidentalomas. The ever increasing availability and performance of central nervous system (CNS) imaging has led to the overwhelming number of incidentally detected lesions within the brain [1–4]. These lesions present an unexpected dilemma to both the patient and the surgeon. Both the patient and the surgeon are faced with the "what if" regarding the risk of future complications when managed conservatively. While aphorisms like "If it ain't broken, don't fix it" have often guided surgical management of these tumors, a better understanding of the natural history of these diseases has resulted in certain guidelines on individualized management of these incidentalomas.

The easy availability and access to diagnostic imaging facilities has resulted in a greater number of incidentalomas. The total number of magnetic resonance imaging (MRI) scans doubled in Norway from 2002 to 2008 [5]. The incidence of vestibular schwannomas (VSs) increased nearly six fold in Denmark over a 30 year period up to 2008. The average size at diagnosis dropped from 3 to 1 cm [6].

In the population based Rotterdam scan study of 5800 participants, 9.5%, i.e., 549 participants with incidental findings on brain MRIs were followed over a period of 9 years. Most common incidental findings were meningiomas (2.5%) and cerebral aneurysms (2.3%). One hundred forty-four of the 188 (3.2%) patients referred to medical specialists were managed conservatively. The study concluded that MRIs picked up just over 3% incidental findings of enough significance for referral and further work up, most of which are amenable for conservative management [7].

The current evidence regarding the management of incidentalomas makes this topic very relevant in the era of ever increasing diagnostic imaging modalities.

7.2 Vestibular Schwannoma

Acoustic schwannomas were detected at a frequency of 0.02–1.6% [8–10]. VS commonly presents with hearing loss, tinnitus, ataxia, and occasionally facial palsy or trigeminal neuralgia. Larger VS may present with cerebellar signs, long tract signs, or features of hydrocephalus. An incidental VS is diagnosed in an otherwise

P. Nair (✉) · S. H. Murali · G. Matham
D. H. Ravi · E. H. Venkat
Department of Neurosurgery, Sree Chitra Tirunal
Institute for Medical Science and Technology,
Trivandrum, Kerala, India

asymptomatic patients who undergo radiological imaging for an unrelated clinical indication not related to VS.

The incidence of VSs in autopsy studies is around 1% [11]. From an MRI database 46,414 patients, Lin et al. calculated that the estimated VS prevalence was around 0.02% from an MRI database of patients [9]. Even though the number appears small, it provides a significant proportion of VS patients in daily practice. Average tumor size at the time of diagnosis was 13.8 mm (Fig. 7.1).

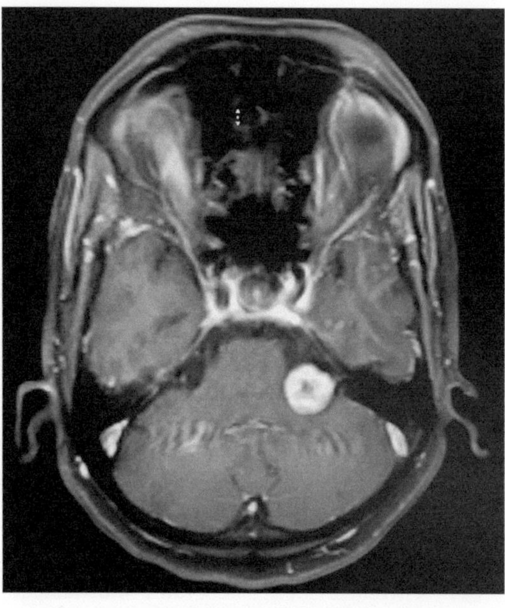

Fig. 7.1 This 49-year-old female patient underwent magnetic resonance imaging (MRI) for evaluation of a transient ischemic episode from which she recovered without any neurological deficits. Clinical examination was unremarkable. MRI (axial gadolinium enhanced T1W image) showing a left cerebellopontine angle vestibular schwannoma (VS) extending into the interval auditory meatus with increased perioptic cerebrospinal fluid (CSF) intensity and optic nerve sheath thickening with an empty sella. There was no associated ventriculomegaly. She was placed on imaging follow-up. Eight months later, she developed visual blurring. Examination revealed bilateral papilledema and 6/36 vision in the left eye. Lumbar puncture revealed high opening CSF pressure (220 mm of water) and was diagnosed with increased intracranial hypertension. Patient underwent a thecoperitoneal shunt and the VS was kept on imaging follow-up

7.2.1 Growth Patterns and Natural History

Incidental VS pose a challenge to the physician where unified management protocols are sparse. For patients who are on conservative management, this poses a certain amount of psychological burden. Efforts have been made to understand the rate of growth of these incidental VS and to see whether the growth pattern and behavior of incidental tumors differs from symptomatic VS.

Hoa et al. reviewed literature on incidental VS from English literature and concluded that around 2/3 of incidental VS did not progress over an observation period of 5 years; however, VS that were larger than 1.5–2 cm in their largest dimension at diagnosis had a greater probability to grow [12, 13].

Meta-analysis conducted by Nikolopoulos et al. showed that rate of tumor growth varies significantly among patients who are managed conservatively. Also the number of tumors demonstrating growth varied from 6% to 73%, with the rate of individual tumor growth varying significantly as well, from 0.3 to 4.8 mm/year, while the mean growth rate varied between 1 and 2 mm/year for all tumors [13]. This study also observed that cystic tumors had a higher growth rate (approximately 3.7 mm/year) when compared to solid counterparts, but the tumors showing continuous growth constituted only 15–25% of the tumors.

There is poor consensus regarding hearing loss in natural course of disease. In VS hearing disturbances happens because of ischemia of the inner ear or protein shedding from the tumor [14]. Another study by Carlson et al. which exclusively studied incidental VS growth pattern showed that there is no significant difference in their pattern of growth from the routine symptomatic VS [10]. Stangerup et al. also demonstrated that while nearly 50% patients with incidental VS maintained hearing over a period of 5 years, initial hearing loss at diagnosis, predicted a greater chance of progressive hearing loss [15] (Fig. 7.2).

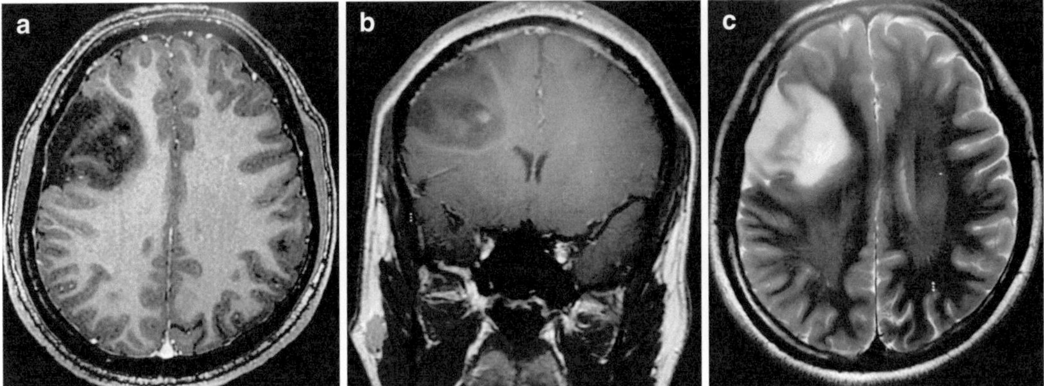

Fig. 7.2 This 28-year-old gentlemen got into a physical altercation in an inebriated state at a local pub. He sustained blows to the head following which he had two episodes of vomiting. (**a**) Computed tomography (CT) scan of the head was taken in the emergency room to rule out a head injury. The scan revealed a hypo density in the right frontal lobe. (**b**, **c**) MRI with diffusion, perfusion, and spectroscopy studies was performed which revealed a low grade glioma in the right frontal lobe. Patient was offered surgery but opted for conservative management with serial imaging. He is asymptomatic 2 years after the initial imaging

7.2.2 Management

The natural history of these incidentally found lesions must be weighed against the potential morbidity associated with intervention. There are three treatment options available-conservative management, stereotactic radiosurgery, and surgical decompression.

Conservative management (wait and watch) while following the tumor with serial imaging studies in asymptomatic patients is based on the observation that a large percentage of tumors do not progress. In contrast, surgery or radiotherapy can result in significant complications and is best avoided unless the patient is symptomatic while being followed up.

An initial MRI done after 6 months and yearly thereafter should be adequate to assess the growth pattern of the tumor [16]. Patients who have slow tumor growth rates may be kept on imaging follow-up with MRI repeated every year. A growth rate of >2 mm/year is a strong predictor of failed conservative management and these patients must be offered surgical resection of the tumor [12]. Apart from radiological progression, clinically it is also important to see for development of symptoms and also obtain audiometry studies to identify deterioration of hearing.

7.2.2.1 Tumors with Progression

Tumors that progress while on yearly imaging follow-up (>2 mm/year) should be offered intervention. While microsurgical resection and stereotactic radiosurgery have both been used for managing smaller VS, the scope of this chapter does not extend to discussing the indication of these modalities.

Patients without serviceable hearing and a VS that is increasing in size, may undergo either retrosigmoid or translabyrinthine approach for microsurgical resection. On the other hand, tumors with serviceable hearing can be approached through the retrosigmoid corridor in an attempt to preserve hearing. For small tumors (≤1.5 cm) located laterally in the internal auditory canal, a middle fossa approach may be used.

Patient's with a selected group of indications may be considered for conservative wait and watch approach; this includes patient age (>60 years), poor health or significant medical risks for surgery, small tumor size (less than 2 cm), and Koos Grade 1 or 2 tumours, with minimal or no incapacitating symptoms [17] (Figs. 7.3 and 7.4).

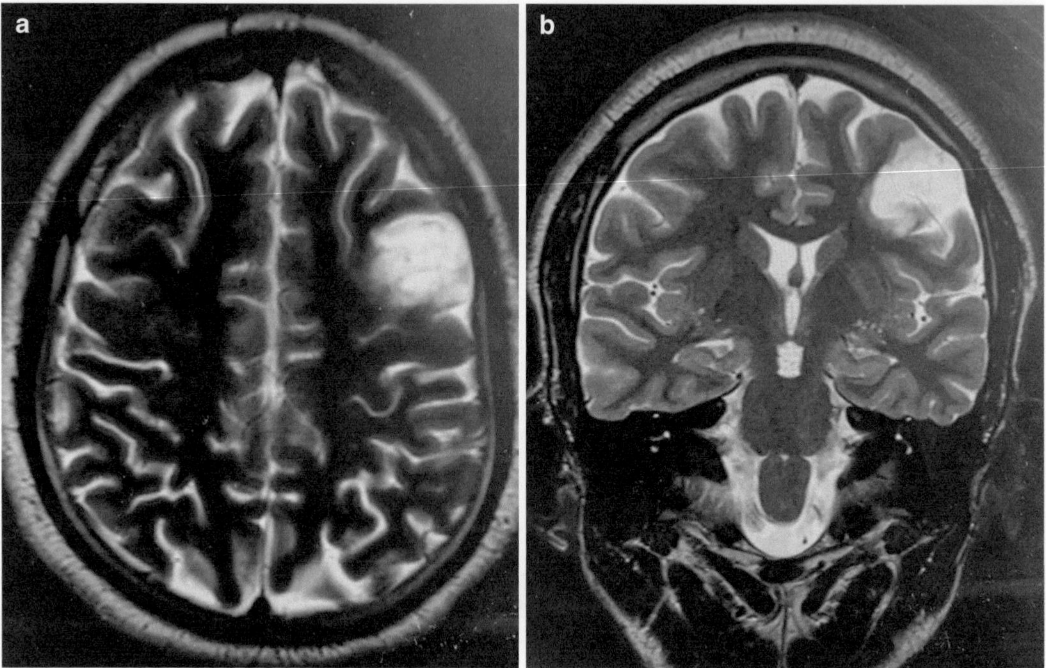

Fig. 7.3 This 32-year-old male patient working at the hospital was recruited as a control for an imaging study by a radiology resident for his post-doctoral dissertation. He was completely asymptomatic. (**a**) MRI revealed a left frontal cortical lesion with a typical soap bubble appearance which is characteristic of a dysplastic neuroepithelial tumor. (**b**) He was managed conservatively in view of absence of symptoms. He is on follow-up and doing well 2 years after the initial imaging

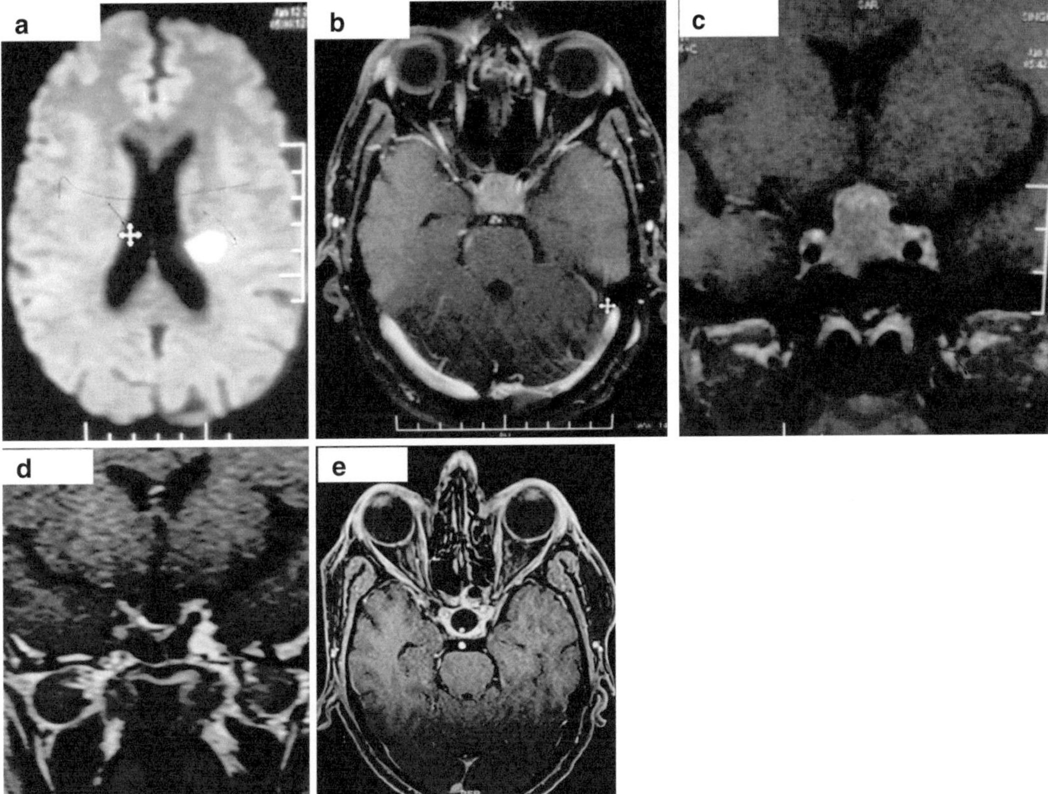

Fig. 7.4 This 57-year-old male patient presented with complaints of sudden onset right hemiparesis and was evaluated in the emergency for stroke. On (**a**) diffusion weighted imaging (DWI) MRI, he was diagnosed to have had an acute ischemic stroke in the left capsuloganglionic region. He was also found to have an (**b**, **c**) incidentally detected sellar mass with "snow-man" shaped suprasellar extension, and chiasmal compression. The sella was found to be enlarged and the lesion was brightly enhancing on contrast; the imaging was suggestive of a pituitary ade-noma. He was initiated on anti-platelet medications in view of cerebrovascular accident. Patient did not have any visual complaints However, 3 months later, he was found to have evolving bitemporal hemianopia and was offered surgery. He underwent transnasal transsphenoidal endo-scopic resection of the tumor. Patient was discharged on the fourth postoperative day with improvement in visual complaints. Post-operative MRI (**d**, **e**) shows complete exclsion of the pituitary adenoma

7.3 Low Grade Gliomas

The natural history of incidentally detected low grade gliomas (iLGG) is poorly understood. iLGG are commonly detected following imaging for unrelated complaints, trauma, or research. The incidence of iLGG has been shown to range from 0.025% to 0.3% in population-based imaging studies and they comprise of 3–5% of all LGG [18–21].

LGGs tend to progress, and they may undergo transformation to a higher grade and grow rapidly in the future. Studies have described a median growth rate of 3.5 mm/year and tend to become symptomatic at a median interval of 2 years from radiological discovery [18, 22]. A large number of recent studies have demonstrated that maximal safe resection improves the overall survival in patients with symptomatic glioma.

Hence, while surgery is indicated in symptomatic low grade gliomas (sLGG), incidentally detected low grade gliomas present a significant dilemma on whether surgery is indicated or not (Figs. 7.5 and 7.6).

7.3.1 Epidemiology

Early literature on LGG favors the principle of "primum non nocere"—first, do no harm, and suggests that patients may not lose much by waiting and a >2 mm/year growth on MRI is reasonable justification for surgery [18, 23]. This treatment paradigm has been called into questions following the observation that iLGG's have similar growth rates to sLGG, have similar median Ki67 proliferative, and there were no differences in the molecular profile (IDH1/2 or 1p/19q) and O6-methylguanine-DNA-

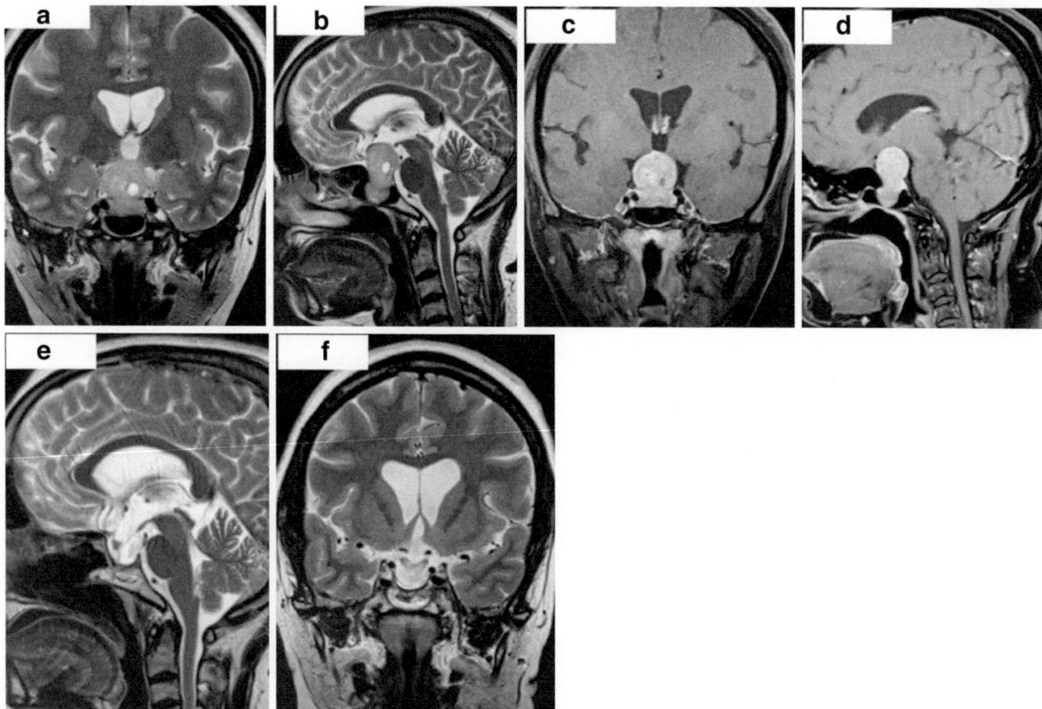

Fig. 7.5 This 47-year-old female patient presented with history of low back ache. Patient underwent imaging of the spine with a screening MRI of the brain. The screening MRI brain (**a–d**) revealed a pituitary adenoma with suprasellar extension and compression of the chiasm. Perimetry revealed bitemporal hemianopia. She had not been symptomatic for the same. In view of an existing visual deficit, she was advised surgical resection of the pituitary adenoma. Patient underwent trans-nasal endoscopic surgery and was discharged on the third postoperative day after an uneventful surgery. Post-operative MRI (**e, f**) shows complete excision of the pituitary adenoma

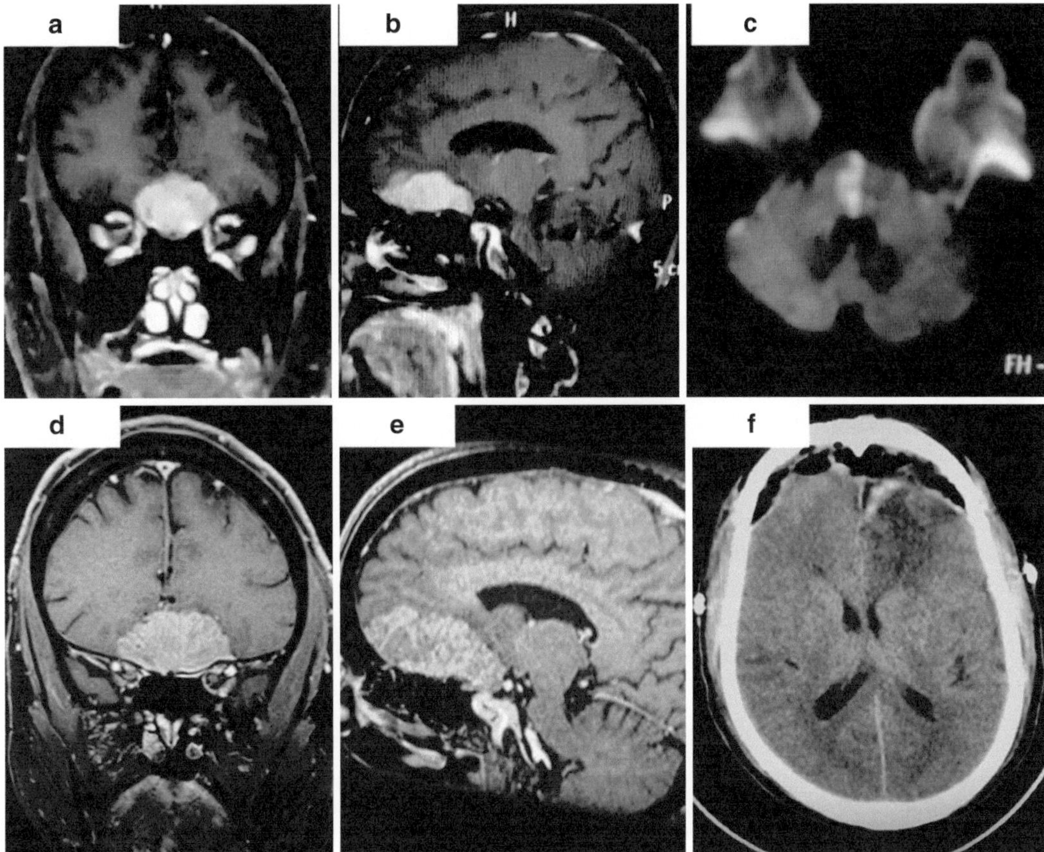

Fig. 7.6 A 69-year-old gentleman with history of hypertension and diabetes presented with sudden onset left hemiparesis. Stroke protocol imaging revealed a vertebrobasilar stroke with right pontine infarct. MRI also showed an incidental anterior skull base meningioma, which was kept on imaging follow-up. Patient recovered from the stroke and was on imaging follow-up with occasional history of headache. MRI at the end of the second year revealed a progressive increase in the size of the lesion. Patient was offered surgery for the same but opted for conservative management in view of his age, paucity of symptoms, and risks associated with surgery. Patient however returned 3 months later with history of seizures. He underwent bifrontal craniotomy and Simpson's grade 2 resection of the meningioma. (**a**, **b**) Coronal and sagittal T1W images showing the meningioma at initial diagnosis. (**c**) Axial DWI showing diffusion restriction in the right side of the brainstem (**d**, **e**) Coronal and sagittal show the increase in the size of the lesion 2 years later. (**f**) Shows an axial contrast CT which shows complete excision of the lesion

methyltransferase promoter methylation between iLGG and sLGG [23, 24].

The extent of neuropsychological dysfunction may not be adequately qualified in iLGG; Cochereau et al. showed that nearly 60% of the iLGG patients in their study had cognitive dysfunction like changes in executive function, memory disturbances, or impaired attention. Pallud et al. suggest a median interval of 48 months between imaging diagnosis and onset of symptoms in iLGG. The median duration for malignant transformation was 5.7 years following imaging diagnosis [18, 25].

Endothelial micro proliferation in the middle of the tumor was found in 27% of the cases during histopathological examination which is a harbinger of malignant transformation justifying further early surgical excision [26].

7.3.2 Management Options

The literature suggests that early identification of LGG is associated with improved outcomes as it is easier to operate on a smaller lesion [24, 27–29]. iLGG detected may have longer overall survival following diagnosis compared to those diagnosed with clinical symptoms, probably due to smaller tumor volume and less midline shift at diagnosis [18]. Outcomes measured in terms of survival was better for incidentally detected LGG than symptomatic LGG [18, 22, 30]. Duffau et al. [23] in their series of 11 incidentally detected LGG were able to perform gross total resection in 33% cases and a supramarginal resection (corresponding to fluid-attenuated inversion recovery hyperintensity) in 27% cases owing to smaller size of tumor, even in eloquent regions.

Potts et al. [22] in their study noted that LGGs diagnosed incidentally had a lower tumor volume (20.2 vs 53.9 cm^3 for symptomatic LGGs) and were less often found in eloquent areas. They also found that iLGGs have a higher rate of gross total resection (GTR) and had overall better score on Kaplan Meier analysis. In eloquent cortex supramaximal resection was possible in many cases with techniques of awake craniotomy and electrocorticography (ECOG) monitoring. An optimal resection based on functional boundaries, based on direct stimulation, i.e., functional mapping was possible and had better morbidity profiles than image guided resections [27]. The estimated 5- and 10-years progression-free survival of the iLGG and sLGG groups were 90.91% and 51.65%, and 36.38% and 5.47%, respectively [24].

Thus, in view of recent literature, iLGG probably represent an earlier phase in the natural history of LGGs. Early surgery achieves a greater percentage of GTR, and improves overall survival. Surgical resection for this cohort should be performed in centers with clinical expertise in managing LGG. Surgical adjuncts like functional mapping, awake craniotomy, and ECOG increase the extent of GTR and reduce the rates of permanent neurological deficits (Figs. 7.7 and 7.8).

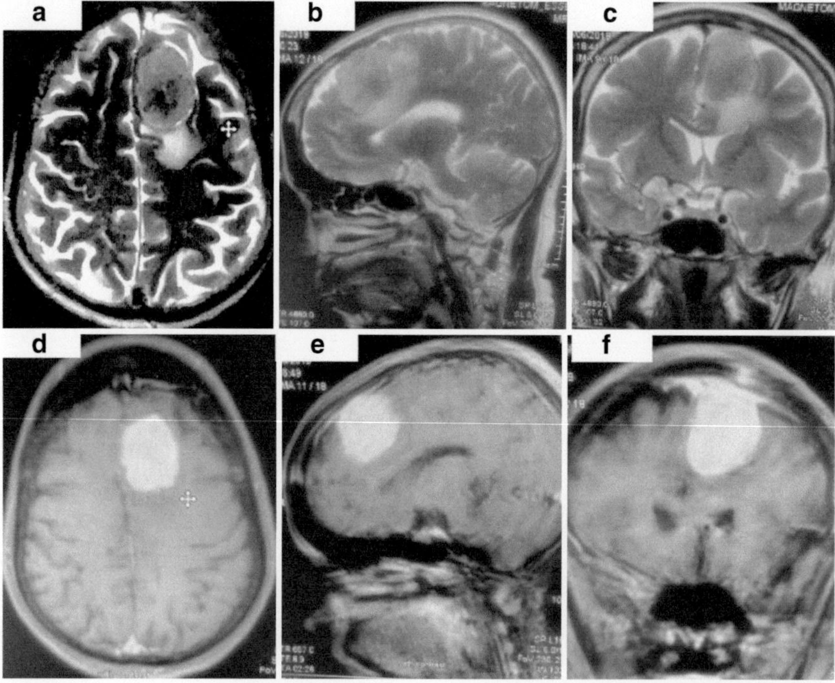

Fig. 7.7 This 60-year-old female patient came with history of fall from a two-wheel motor vehicle with brief history of loss of consciousness. Patient regained consciousness within 5 min, she was taken to an emergency room where CT head was performed to rule out a head injury. Imaging revealed an incidental left frontal high convexity meningioma. Further imaging was performed to a certain the diagnosis. On MRI, (a–f), an extra axial dural based contrast enhancing meningioma was seen, there was perilesional edema in the adjacent brain parenchyma. In view of perilesional edema and mild mass effect, patient was offered surgery which proceeded uneventfully. Patient was discharged on the third postoperative day and remains on follow-up

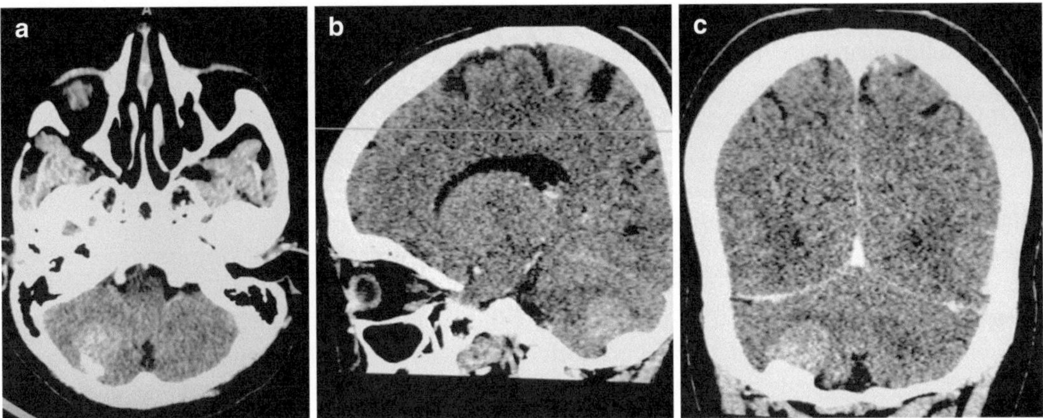

Fig. 7.8 This 32-year-old female patient presented with a history of left hemicranial headache which was intermittent, mild in intensity without any history of vomiting in association with the headache. CT imaging (**a–c**) showed a hyper dense dura-based lesion with hyperostosis of the underlying bone, suggestive of a right cerebellar convex-ity meningioma to which the patient's symptoms did not correlate. The patient was managed conservatively with follow-up imaging. Patient is currently on follow-up for the past 10 years with no new complaints. Headaches are no longer present

7.4 Pituitary Incidentalomas

The Endocrine Society defines pituitary incidentalomas as those tumors of the pituitary gland which are discovered incidentally when imaging is performed in order to evaluate symptoms which are not related to a sellar lesion. The average incidence frequency in combined autopsy data was around 10.6% [31]. Microincidentalomas are seen in around 10–38% in MRI in adults who were evaluated with imaging for varied reasons [32].

7.4.1 Evaluation

7.4.1.1 Hormonal

All patients with a pituitary incidentaloma need to undergo hormonal evaluation. This is of paramount importance in incidentalomas to diagnose either existing hormonal disturbance or to diagnose any hormonal disturbance which can arise during follow-up. Incidence of hormone hyposecretion and hypersecretion both are documented. Assessment of prolactin, growth hormone (GH), and adrenocorticotropic hormone should be done in evaluation of hypersecretion.

Diluted prolactin levels in patients of large macroincidentalomas is in order to counteract the Hook effect which may result in spuriously low values [33]. Subclinical hypercortisolism has been regularly reported in studies with incidentalomas and hence a thorough clinical evaluation and further hormonal evaluation should be done for the possibility of Cushing's disease.

Hypopituitarism has been documented quite extensively in these patients. Gonadotropin deficiency was seen in up to 30% of patients whereas thyroid axis deficiency in about 28% patients. Cortisol axis was affected in up to 18% of these patients whereas GH axis in about 8% [34–36].

The initial hormonal assessment therefore includes screening of thyroid stimulating hormone, luteinizing hormone, follicle stimulating hormone, and morning cortisol levels. Initial evaluation of GH may also be performed.

7.4.1.2 Imaging

MRI has replaced CT as the choice of investigation for evaluation of patients with sellar incidentalomas. It has been recommended that all patients should undergo an MRI even if the incidentaloma is diagnosed in CT. This allows better delineation of the extent and also description of the nature of the lesion [33].

The MRI appearance may vary. A simple cyst with no solid enhancing component, the cyst can have a uniform signal as cerebrospinal fluid (CSF) or T1 hyperintensity in MRI denoting protein content.

Solid lesion: These are mostly indicative of a pituitary lesion, i.e., pituitary adenoma, but differentiating these from other lesions is quite essential. The pseudolesions can be nodular or glandular hyperplasia, fibrous tissue, cell clumping, or even artifacts related to imaging techniques. This is especially true for lesions less than 5 mm in size.

Pituitary protocols routinely use thin slices and smaller field of vision. Imaging noise seen in these techniques can cause apparent glandular heterogeneity [37]. Volume artifacts are particularly notorious due to the presence of adjacent cavernous sinus and carotid arteries.

7.4.1.3 Visual Field

It is recommended also that for all patients with sellar incidentalomas, especially those abutting the chiasm, evaluation should include an objective visual assessment at diagnosis and follow-up as well.

7.4.2 Management

In patients who have visual field defects on evaluation, surgical decompression is recommended. Patients with biochemical features of hormonal hyper secretion also need active management. Prolactin secreting tumors are treated with dopaminergic agonists. Patients with Cushing's disease, acromegaly, or thyrotropinoma will need surgical resection. Conservative treatment is recommended in cases with no visual field defects or features of hormone hyper secretion [33].

7.4.2.1 Cystic Incidental Lesions

Pure cystic lesions with no solid component or mixed intensity are almost always seen to be Rathke's cleft cyst. These lesions seldom grow and hence regular imaging can be avoided unless patient is symptomatic either visually or endocrinologically. Surgery can be offered to symptomatic patients or those with changes in visual fields.

7.4.2.2 Microincidentalomas

Regular hormonal testing is not required in the follow-up period if there is no change in the clinical history or MRI findings. In case of an micro incidentaloma MRI scan after 1 year of the initial scan has been recommended and then every 1–2 years for next 3 years. This frequency can be further reduced [33]. A baseline visual field testing may be done at initial diagnosis and further repeated only if the lesion grows sufficiently to encroach the optic apparatus. Patients with lesions less than 5 mm are highly unlikely to hemorrhage [38].

7.4.2.3 Macroincidentaloma

Macroincidentalomas often present a dilemma on the decision to operate or not, especially due to the risk of hemorrhage in these patients. Imaging has been recommended be done 6 months after initial diagnosis and yearly thereafter [33]. Periodic assessment of visual fields is needed in asymptomatic patients or when a patient complaints of visual symptoms. Hypopituitarism is more common with macroincidentalomas. It has been suggested that this can be either due to stalk compression or increased intrasellar pressure both of which are reversible. Hence hormonal evaluation is recommended in these patients, initially 6 months after initial presentation and yearly thereafter.

In cases where the patient becomes symptomatic with development of new visual field defects, repeat imaging is needed; if this demonstrates increase in size of the tumor or areas of hemorrhage, surgery should be advised. Asymptomatic increase in tumor size during imaging follow-up necessitates closer follow-up (Figs. 7.9 and 7.10).

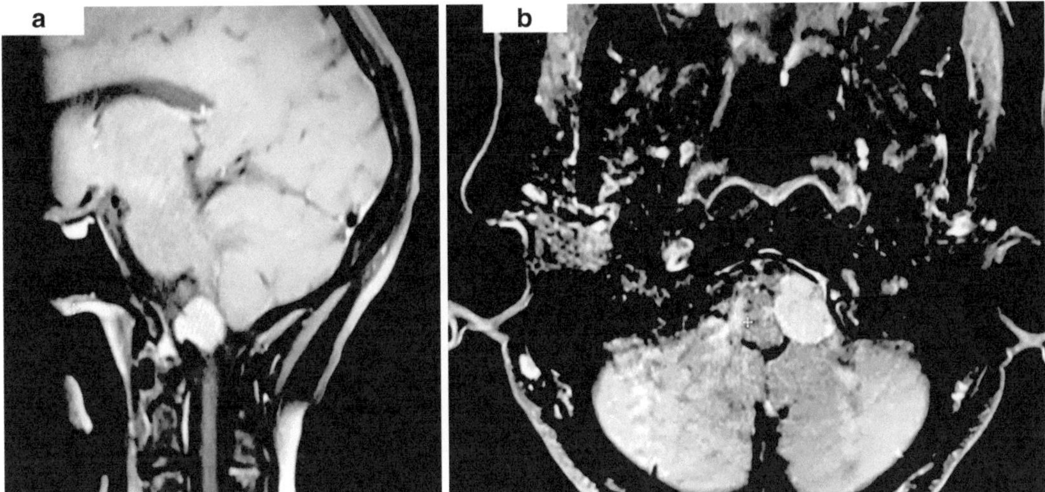

Fig. 7.9 This 49-year-old female patient presented with complaints of low back ache and underwent a screening MRI of the whole spine as part of work up for low back ache. MRI (**a**, **b**) showed a dura-based contrast enhancing tumor near the foramen magnum which was suggestive of a foramen magnum meningioma. The finding was incidental and she was asymptomatic for this tumour. Conservative management for the foramen magnum meningioma was pursued in view of the risks associated with surgery and lack of symptoms. Patient has been on follow-up for 6 years and continues to be asymptomatic

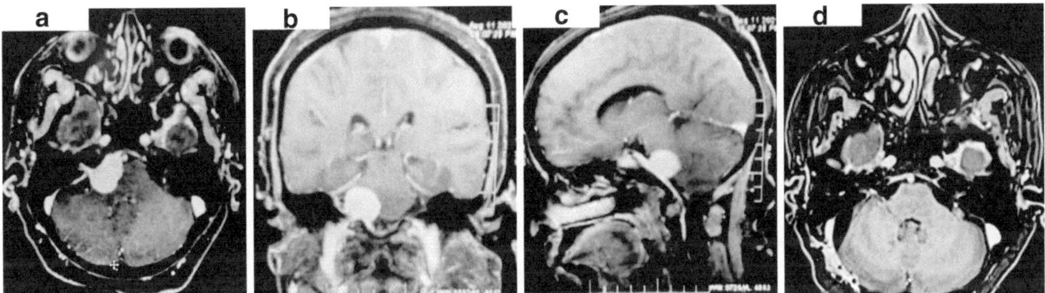

Fig. 7.10 This 55-year-old female patient was diagnosed with multinodular goiter 5 years back for which she underwent a total thyroidectomy. Histopathological examination was suggestive of a papillary carcinoma thyroid. As part of work up CT scan of neck was done which revealed a petroclival meningioma. Follow-up MRI (**a–c**) imaging showed a dura-based lesion involving the anterior part of the petrous bone and the clivus with intense contrast enhancement, which was suggestive of a petroclival meningioma. The patient was initially advised imaging follow-up but the meningioma showed an increase in size over time. In view of a progressively enlarging tumor, she was counselled for surgical resection. Tumor resection was performed by a retrosigmoid approach and Simpson's grade 2 excision was achieved. Histopathological examination revealed fibrous meningioma WHO grade 1 (MIB labelling index 6–8%). Postoperative course was uneventful and patient was discharged on the third postoperative day. The post-operative MRI (**d**) showed complete excision of the meningioma. She is on regular follow-up

7.5 Meningiomas

7.5.1 Epidemiology

Meningiomas are benign tumors of the central nervous system that originate from arachnoid caps cells of the meninges [39]. While meningiomas are benign tumors, and can often remain asymptomatic during a person's life, they do end to progress gradually. They are the second most common primary brain tumor and have been graded into three grade, grade I (begin), grade II (atypical), and grade III (malignant or anaplastic) [40].

Incidentally detected meningiomas are diagnosed on imaging studies performed for unrelated symptoms. Staneczek et al. reported an annual incidence of meningiomas of 1.85 per 100,000 population, with 50% of the meningiomas discovered during autopsy [41].

The Rotterdam study [7] found incidentally detected meningiomas to be 2.5% of the 5800 participants screened for incidental lesions (Fig. 7.11).

7.5.2 Natural History of Progression

Nakamura et al. [42] analyzed the growth pattern of incidentally detected meningiomas via volumetric analysis of CT and MRI in 41 patients. They found the mean growth rate to be 0.796 cm^3/year (0.03–2.62 range), i.e., a 14.6% volume increase per year on average.

The growth pattern of meningiomas also depends on the histology. Benign lesions may be static, grow linearly or exponentially, whereas atypical meningiomas grow exponentially [43, 44]. Pial parasitation features visualized on MRI like broken continuity CSF cleft with ambigu-

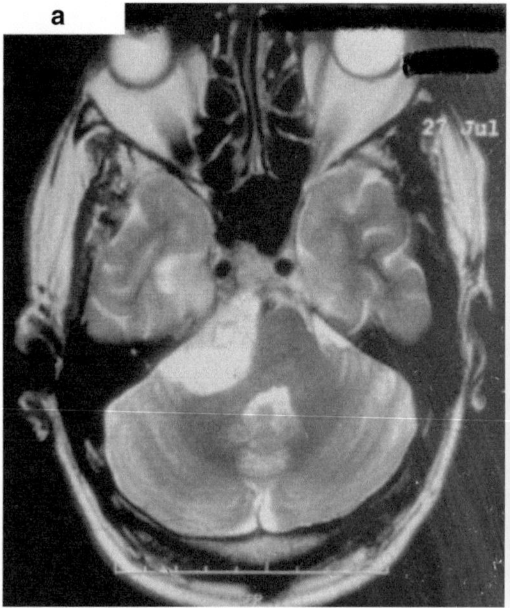
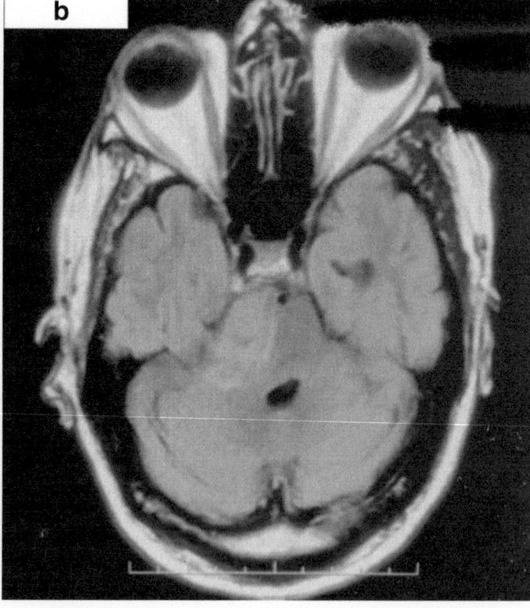
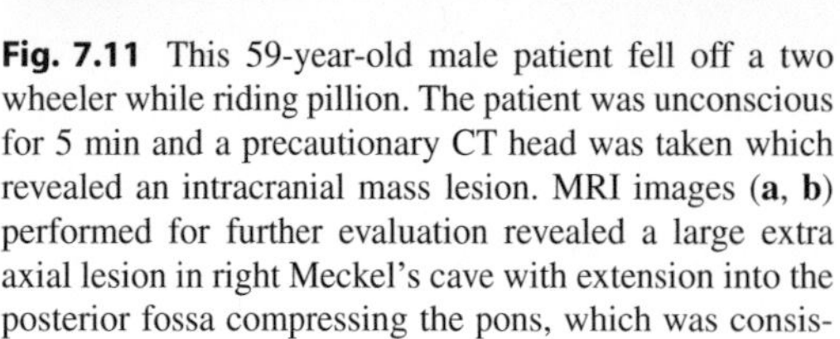

Fig. 7.11 This 59-year-old male patient fell off a two wheeler while riding pillion. The patient was unconscious for 5 min and a precautionary CT head was taken which revealed an intracranial mass lesion. MRI images (**a**, **b**) performed for further evaluation revealed a large extra axial lesion in right Meckel's cave with extension into the posterior fossa compressing the pons, which was consistent with a trigeminal SV. Patient had no history of facial numbness or pain. Considering the size of the lesion and brainstem compression, he was advised surgery. The histopathology was suggestive of a schwannoma. Postoperatively patient had transient numbness over the face and no other deficits

ous brain tumor margins, significant peritumoral edema, and irregular tumor shape may indicate a tendency for rapid growth [44]. Yano et al. [45] reported that 16.4% cases of asymptomatic incidental meningiomas became symptomatic over a mean period of 3.9 years of follow-up. Niiro et al. reported similar rates of 12.5% patients becoming symptomatic after a mean period of 3.2 years [46]. There is a positive correlation between size and symptoms and in general symptomatic meningiomas tend to be larger [47]. The location of the meningioma may also determine the duration in which patients may become symptomatic. For example lesions in the cavernous sinus or CP angle may become symptomatic at much smaller sizes than convexity meningiomas.

Meningiomas may follow the Gompertzian growth model and their growth rate varies over time, possibly being exponential in the early phase and eventually plateau after a certain tumor mass is attained [42–44]. Nevertheless, larger tumors need to be monitored carefully because risk associated with further growth is high. Age is another important factor to predict the growth pattern. Age induced endocrine changes may result a decrease in meningioma growth in patients above 60 years [42].

Assessment of diametric increase may be misleading. Skull base lesions are deceitful in their static diameter on imaging as their irregular shape may result in growth not within the measurement axis [42]. Computer aided volumetric assessment might therefore be a better tool to assess the growth of tumors in interval scans [7].

7.5.3 Radiological Features of Progression

Radiologically T2 hyper-intensity predicts a softer tumor with possibly lesser tumor cell cohesion and hence, higher growth rate. T2 hypo, T1 hyper tumors being more fibrous are slower growing [42]. Similarly, calcification may indicate a slower tumor growth rate [44–46, 48, 49]. Location was not a significant factor influencing the growth rate of meningiomas [45].

7.5.4 Management

In consideration of approach to an incidentally detected intracranial meningioma, it would be prudent to follow up the lesion with serial imaging to assess its rate of growth, unless mass effect or herniation is impending.

Follow-up MRI with and without contrast should first be obtained 3 months after diagnosis, then 9 months after diagnosis, and then every year after diagnosis.

Most incidentally detected meningiomas can be managed with serial MRI follow-up due to their indolent nature. However surgical excision is indicated if the size increase is >1 cm^3/year [45] or if patient is symptomatic with significant mass effect on surrounding neurovascular structures. Location is another important factor in determining need for surgery. Young patients with easily accessible asymptomatic meningiomas to be considered for surgery, especially if the meningioma shows progression on radiological imaging. Skull base meningiomas, on the other hand, have a higher risk of morbidity following surgery, and can be followed up for longer periods with imaging in asymptomatic individuals [50, 51]. Mass effect due to brain invasion and edema is another indication for surgery as this also indicates the possibly of a high grade meningioma [50].

Lastly, meningiomas that become symptomatic, are large at presentation, or irregularly shaped need to be surgically excised.

Age is an important indicator to consider the need for surgery as perioperative morbidity steeply rises with age >70 from 3.5% to 20% [45, 47].

7.5.5 Surgery

Goals of surgery include maximal safe excision and obtaining tissue for pathological diagnosis. In some asymptomatic lesions, surgery can be offered to prevent possible tumor growth that would make further surgery more complicated, i.e., near the sinus/eloquent areas.

Residual tumor attached to sensitive structures can be left during surgery and later treated with radiosurgery.

7.5.5.1 Radiation Therapy
Gamma Knife radiosurgery can be used safely in lesions less than 3 cm in diameter or lesions in locations that are difficult to access surgically. In regard to asymptomatic meningiomas, radiosurgery can be advocated when patients have lesions that are at an increased risk for growth, are located in anatomic locations with high surgical morbidity, have co-morbidities that elevate risk for surgery, or are older than 65 years old.

7.5.6 Conclusion

Incidental meningiomas in asymptomatic patients may be advised an initial follow-up imaging in 3 months with an MRI brain with gadolinium to assess for rapid growth. If initial follow-up imaging is stable, then the intervals for surveillance imaging can be increased to 6 months and then yearly afterward. Surgical resection for meningioma is usually considered for patients who have tumor growth of greater than 1 cm³/year or patients who have a symptomatic meningioma.

7.6 Trigeminal Schwannomas

Trigeminal SVs are more common in middle aged females. While vestibular SVs make up >80% of the intracranial schwannomas, trigeminal SVs are the second most common intracranial SV but still are far less common in comparison (0.8–8%) [52]. This corresponds to 0.07–0.36% of all intracranial tumors [53].

7.6.1 Imaging

CT imaging: they appear iso to hyper dense with intense contrast enhancement, in a majority of patients (33–50%) it causes remodelling of the petrous bone [54, 55]. Erosion of the petrous apex is highly suggestive of a trigeminal SV [53, 56]. On MRI they appear well circumscribed heterogenously enhancing mass lesions which are isointense on T1W and hyper intense on T2W [55, 57–59]. They are located in the region of the fifth cranial nerve, with a non-invasive, encapsulated benign growth pattern. Hemorrhage and cystic changes are common [55, 60].

7.6.2 Management Strategy

Asymptomatic trigeminal SVs are rare; however, their incidence is increasing with the wide-spread availability and use of MRI [61, 62]. These lesions tend to grow more rapidly than sporadic vestibular SVs but less rapidly than vestibular SVs in neurofibromatosis type 2 (NF2). Asymptomatic trigeminal SV may be followed up with yearly imaging. Asymptomatic trigeminal SVs can be followed up with imaging but once symptomatic need to be surgically resected.

7.7 Subependymal Giant Cell Astrocytomas (SEGA)

Subependymal giant cell astrocytomas (SEGAs) are intraventricular seen almost exclusively in tuberous sclerosis (TS). They are typically located near the region of foramen of Monro [63]. They are usually asymptomatic and detected incidentally when a patient is imaged for some other presentation of TS. When they do become symptomatic, it is may be the result of obstruction of the foramen of Monro resulting in hydrocephalus.

SEGAs display a slow expansive growth pattern with little risk of malignant transformation [63]. Complete loss of the tuberin-hamartin complex due to mutation in the TSC gene results in dysregulation of downstream mTOR pathway [64, 65]. A differential diagnosis for a SEGA is the subependymal nodule (SEN) which is a hamartomatous lesion also seen in tuberous sclerosis. While SEGA are in proximity to the foramen of Monro, SEN can be located anywhere in the walls of the ventricle [66]. SEGA tend to increase in size over a period of time, SEN are usually static lesions. SEGA tend to be bigger than 5–12 mm, with incomplete calcification and contrast enhancement when compared to SENs [67–69].

7.7.1 Imaging

CT shows iso to hyper dense lesion with variable degree of contrast enhancement. Areas of cystic degeneration and calcifications may be seen.

MRI: SEGA lesions are well circumscribed non-encapsulated lesions, iso intense on T1W images and hyperintense on T2W images with homogenous contrast enhancement located in the medial wall of lateral ventricle near the foramen of Monro. Calcifications appear as hypointensity on T2W and SWI sequences. There is no transventricular extension. Magnetic resonance spectroscopy (MRS) shows increased choline and reduced N-acetylaspartate and creatine [70].

7.7.2 Management

Incidentally detected asymptomatic SEGA is managed conservatively. Tumors that show an increase in size of on serial imaging may need surgical intervention. Ribaupierre et al. recommended that SEGA larger than 5 mm, located near the foramen of Monro that show an increase in size and incomplete calcification should undergo surgical resection. Surgery is also indicated if there is obstruction to the foramen of Monro resulting in obstructive hydrocephalus [63, 66]. The patients with features suggestive of SEGA on imaging need further work up for other features of tuberous sclerosis [63]. When gross total resection is not possible, subtotal resection is acceptable as they are slow growing

tumors. If surgery is not possible, ventriculo-peritoneal shunting for obstructive hydrocephalus should relieve symptoms. Everolimus is a mTOR pathway inhibitor has found usage in medical management of SEGA's where surgery is not a possibility by causing tumor shrinkage [71, 72].

References

1. Zaazoue MA, Manley PE, Kapur K, Ullrich NJ, Silvera VM, Goumnerova LC. Natural history and management of incidentally discovered focal brain lesions indeterminate for tumor in children. Neurosurgery. 2020;86:357–65.
2. Graf WD, Kayyali HR, Alexander JJ, Simon SD, Morriss MC. Neuroimaging-use trends in non-acute pediatric headache before and after clinical practice parameters. Pediatrics. 2008;122:e1001–5.
3. Perret C, Boltshauser E, Scheer I, Kellenberger CJ, Grotzer MA. Incidental findings of mass lesions on neuroimages in children. Neurosurg Focus. 2011;31:E20.
4. Roth J, Soleman J, Paraskevopoulos D, Keating RF, Constantini S. Incidental brain tumors in children: an international neurosurgical, oncological survey. Childs Nerv Syst. 2018;34:325–1333.
5. Norwegian Radiation Protection Authority. Radiological investigations in Norway as of 2008 (in Norwegian). Available at: http://www.nrpa.no/dav/dc3ba89a7a.pdf. Accessed 19 Sept 2012.
6. Stangerup SE, Caye-Thomasen P. Epidemiology and natural history of vestibular schwannomas. Otolaryngol Clin N Am. 2012;45:257–68.
7. Bos D, Poels M, Adams H, Akoudad S, Cremers L, Zonneveld H, Hoogendam Y, Verhaaren B, Verlinden V, Verbruggen J, Peymani A, Hofman A, Krestin G, Vincent A, Feelders R, Koudstaal P, van der Lugt A, Ikram M, Vernooij M. Prevalence, clinical management, and natural course of incidental findings on brain MR images: the population-based Rotterdam scan study. Radiology. 2016;281(2):507–15.
8. Anderson TD, Loevner LA, Bigelow DC, Mirza N. Prevalence of unsuspected acoustic neuroma found by magnetic resonance imaging. Otolaryngol Head Neck Surg. 2000;122:643–6.
9. Lin D, Hegarty JL, Fischbein NJ, Jackler RK. The prevalence of "incidental" acoustic neuroma. Arch Otolaryngol Head Neck Surg. 2005;131:241–4.
10. Carlson ML, Lees KA, Patel NS, et al. The clinical behavior of asymptomatic incidental vestibular schwannomas is similar to that of symptomatic tumors. Otol Neurotol. 2016;37:1435–41.
11. Selesnick SH, Jackler RK, Pitts LW. The changing clinical presentation of acoustic tumors in the MRI era. Laryngoscope. 1993;103:431–6.

12. Hoa M, Drazin D, Hanna G, Schwartz MS, Lekovic GP. The approach to the patient with incidentally diagnosed vestibular schwannoma. Neurosurgical Focus. 2012;33(3):E2.

13. Nikolopoulos TP, Fortnum H, O'Donoghue G, Baguley D. Acoustic neuroma growth: a systematic review of the evidence. Otol Neurotol. 2010;31:478–85.

14. Hajioff D, Raut VV, Walsh RM, Bath AP, Bance ML, Guha A, et al. Conservative management of vestibular schwannomas: third review of a 10-year prospective study. Clin Otolaryngol. 2008;33:255–9.

15. Stangerup SE, Cayé-Thomasen P, Tos M, Thomsen J. Change in hearing during 'wait and scan' management of patients with vestibular schwannoma. J Laryngol Otol. 2008;122:673–81.

16. Smouha EE, Yoo M, Mohr K, Davis RP. Conservative management of acoustic neuroma: a meta-analysis and proposed treatment algorithm. Laryngoscope. 2005;115:450–4.

17. Bakkouri WE, Kania RE, Guichard JP, Lot G, Herman P, Huy PT. Conservative management of 386 cases of unilateral vestibular schwannoma: tumor growth and consequences for treatment. Clinical article. J Neurosurg. 2009;110:662–9.

18. Pallud J, Fontaine D, Duffau H, Mandonnet E, Sanai N, Taillandier L, Peruzzi P, Guillevin R, Bauchet L, Bernier V, Baron MH, Guyotat J, Capelle L. Natural history of incidental World Health Organization grade II gliomas. Ann Neurol. 2010;68:727–33.

19. Bauchet L, Rigau V, Mathieu-Daude H, Figarella-Branger D, Hugues D, Palusseau L, Bauchet F, Fabbro M, Campello C, Capelle L, Durand A, Trétarre B, Frappaz D, Henin D, Menei P, Honnorat J, Segnarbieux F. French brain tumor data bank: methodology and first results on 10,000 cases. J Neuro-Oncol. 2007;84:189–99.

20. Kamiguchi H, Shiobara R, Toya S. Accidentally detected brain tumors: clinical analysis of a series of 110 patients. Clin Neurol Neurosurg. 1996;98:171–5.

21. Olson JD, Riedel E, DeAngelis LM. Long-term outcome of low-grade oligodendroglioma and mixed glioma. Neurology. 2000;54:1442–8.

22. Potts MB, Smith JS, Molinaro AM, Berger MS. Natural history and surgical management of incidentally discovered low-grade gliomas. J Neurosurg. 2012;116:326–72.

23. Duffau H, Pallud J, Mandonnet E. Evidence for the genesis of WHO grade II glioma in an asymptomatic young adult using repeated MRIs. Acta Neurochir. 2011;153(473–477):9.

24. Ius T, Ng S, et al. The benefit of early surgery on overall survival in incidental low-grade glioma patients: a multicenter study. Neuro-Oncology. 2022;24:624.

25. Katzman GL, Dagher AP, Patronas NJ. Incidental findings on brain magnetic resonance imaging from 1000 asymptomatic volunteers. JAMA. 1999;282:36–9.

26. Catherine Ling MD, et al. Endothelial cell hypertrophy and microvascular proliferation in meningiomas are correlated with higher histological grade and shorter progression-free survival. J Neuropathol Exp Neurol. 2016;75(12):1160–70.

27. Duffau H. Awake surgery for incidental WHO grade II gliomas involving eloquent areas. Acta Neurochir. 2012;154:757–584.

28. Sanai N, Chang S, Berger MS. Low grade gliomas in adults. J Neurosurg. 2011;115(5):948–65.

29. Aghi MK, Nahed BV, Sloan AE, Ryken TC, Kalkanis SN, Olson JJ. The role of surgery in the management of patients with diffuse low grade glioma: a systematic review and evidence-based clinical practice guideline. J Neuro-Oncol. 2015;125(3):503–30.

30. Floeth FW, Sabel M, Stoffels G, Pauleit D, Hamacher K, Steiger HJ, Langen KJ. Prognostic value of 18F-fluroethyl-L-tyrosine PET and MRI in small non-specific incidental brain lesions. J Nucl Med. 2008;49:730–7.

31. Molitch ME. Nonfunctioning pituitary tumors and pituitary incidentalomas. Endocrinol Metab Clin N Am. 2008;37(1):151–71. https://doi.org/10.1016/j.ecl.2007.10.011.

32. Hall WA, Luciano MG, Doppman JL, Patronas NJ, Oldfield EH. Pituitary magnetic resonance imaging in normal human volunteers: occult adenomas in the general population. Ann Intern Med. 1994;120(10):817–20. https://doi.org/10.7326/0003-4819-120-10-199405150-00001.

33. Freda PU, Beckers AM, Katznelson L, Molitch ME, Montori VM, Post KD, Vance ML. Pituitary incidentaloma: an endocrine society clinical practice guideline. J Clin Endocrinol Metabol. 2011;96(4):894–904. https://doi.org/10.1210/jc.2010-1048.

34. Day PF, Guitelman M, Artese R, Fiszledjer L, Chervin A, Vitale NM, Stalldecker G, De Miguel V, Cornaló D, Alfieri A, Susana M, Gil M. Retrospective multicentric study of pituitary incidentalomas. Pituitary. 2004;7(3):145–8. https://doi.org/10.1007/s11102-005-1757-1.

35. Feldkamp J, Santen R, Harms E, Aulich A, Mödder U, Scherbaum WA. Incidentally discovered pituitary lesions: high frequency of macroadenomas and hormone-secreting adenomas—results of a prospective study: incidental pituitary lesions. Clin Endocrinol. 1999;51(1):109–13. https://doi.org/10.1046/j.1365-2265.1999.00748.x.

36. Reincke M, Allolio B, Saeger W, Menzel J, Winkelmann W. The "incidentaloma" of the pituitary gland. Is neurosurgery required? JAMA. 1990;263(20):2772–6.

37. Hoang JK, Hoffman AR, González RG, Wintermark M, Glenn BJ, Pandharipande PV, Berland LL, Seidenwurm DJ. Management of incidental pituitary findings on CT, MRI, and 18F-fluorodeoxyglucose PET: a white paper of the ACR incidental findings committee. J Am Coll Radiol. 2018;15(7):966–72. https://doi.org/10.1016/j.jacr.2018.03.037.

38. Buurman H, Saeger W. Subclinical adenomas in postmortem pituitaries: classification and correlations to clinical data. Exp Clin Endocrinol Diabetes. 2006;114(S1) https://doi.org/10.1055/s-2006-932930.

39. Huntoon K, et al. Meningioma—a review of clinic pathologic and molecular aspects. Front Oncol. 2020;10:579599.

40. Louis DN, et al. The 2021 WHO classification of tumors of the central nervous system: a summary. Neuro-Oncology. 2021;23:1231.

41. Staneczek W, Jänisch W. Epidemiologic data on meningiomas in East Germany 1961-1986: incidence, localization, age and sex distribution. Clin Neuropathol. 1992;11:135–41.

42. Nakamura M, Roser F, Michel J, Jacobs C, Samii M. The natural history of incidental meningiomas. Neurosurgery. 2003;53(1):62–70, discussion 70–1.

43. Braunstein JB, Vick NA. Meningiomas: the decision not to operate. Neurology. 1997;48(5):1459–62.

44. Hashiba T, Hashimoto N, Maruno M, et al. Scoring radiologic characteristics to predict proliferative potential in meningiomas. Brain Tumor Pathol. 2006;23(1):49–54.

45. Yano S, Kuratsu J-I, Kumamoto Brain Tumor Research Group. Indications for surgery in patients with asymptomatic meningiomas based on an extensive experience. J Neurosurg. 2006;105(4):538–43.

46. Niiro M, Yatsushiro K, Nakamura K, Kawahara Y, Kuratsu J. Natural history of elderly patients with asymptomatic meningiomas. J Neurol Neurosurg Psychiatry. 2000;68(1):25–8.

47. Kuratsu J, Kochi M, Ushio Y. Incidence and clinical features of asymptomatic meningiomas. J Neurosurg. 2000;92(5):766–70.

48. Go RS, Taylor BV, Kimmel DW. The natural history of asymptomatic meningiomas in Olmsted County, Minnesota. Neurology. 1998;51(6):1718–20.

49. Nakasu S, Fukami T, Nakajima M, Watanabe K, Ichikawa M, Matsuda M. Growth pattern changes of meningiomas: long-term analysis. Neurosurgery. 2005;56(5):946–55, discussion 946–55.

50. Herscovici Z, Rappaport Z, Sulkes J, Danaila L, Rubin G. Natural history of conservatively treated meningiomas. Neurology. 2004;63(6):1133–4.

51. Bindal R, Goodman JM, Kawasaki A, Purvin V, Kuzma B. The natural history of untreated skull base meningiomas. Surg Neurol. 2003;59(2):87–92.

52. Ostrom QT, et al. CBTRUS statistical report: primary brain and central nervous system tumors diagnosed in the United States in 2007-2011. Neuro-Oncology. 2014;16(Suppl 4):iv1–iv63.

53. Lesoin F, et al. Neurinomas of the trigeminal nerve. Acta Neurochir. 1986;82(3–4):118–22.

54. Al-Mefty O, et al. Trigeminal schwannomas: removal of dumbbell-shaped tumors through the expanded Meckel cave and outcomes of cranial nerve function. J Neurosurg. 2002;96(3):453–63.

55. Pamir MN, et al. Surgical treatment of trigeminal schwannomas. Neurosurg Rev. 2007;30(4):329–37.

56. Palacios E, MacGee EE. The radiographic diagnosis of trigeminal neurinomas. J Neurosurg. 1972;36(2):153–6.

57. Rigamonti D, et al. Magnetic resonance imaging and trigeminal schwannoma. Surg Neurol. 1987;28(1):67–70.

58. VandeVyver V, et al. MRI findings of the normal and diseased trigeminal nerve ganglion and branches: a pictorial review. JBR-BTR. 2007;90(4):272–7.

59. Majoie CB, et al. Primary nerve-sheath tumours of the trigeminal nerve: clinical and MRI findings. Neuroradiology. 1999;41(2):100–8.

60. Asari S, et al. CT and MRI of haemorrhage into intracranial neuromas. Neuroradiology. 1993;35(4):247–50.

61. Yoshida K, Kawase T. Trigeminal neurinomas extending into multiple fossae: surgical methods and review of the literature. J Neurosurg. 1999;91(2):202–11.

62. McCormick PC, et al. Trigeminal schwannoma. Surgical series of 14 cases with review of the literature. J Neurosurg. 1988;69(6):850–60.

63. Louis DN, Ohgaki H, Wiestler OD, et al. The 2007 WHO classification of tumours of the central nervous system. Acta Neuropathol. 2007;114:97–109.

64. Lam C, Bouffet E, Tabori U, et al. Rapamycin (sirolimus) in tuberous sclerosis associated pediatric central nervous system tumors. Pediatr Blood Cancer. 2010;54:476–9.

65. Chan JA, Zhang H, Roberts PS, et al. Pathogenesis of tuberous sclerosis subependymal giant cell astrocytomas: biallelic inactivation of TSC1 or TSC2 leads to mTOR activation. J Neuropathol Exp Neurol. 2004;63:1236–42.

66. Arca G, Pacheco E, Alfonso I, et al. Characteristic brain magnetic resonance imaging (MRI) findings in neonates with tuberous sclerosis complex. J Child Neurol. 2006;21:280–5.

67. de Ribaupierre S, Dorfmuller G, Bulteau C, et al. Subependymal giant-cell astrocytomas in pediatric tuberous sclerosis disease: when should we operate? Neurosurgery. 2007;60:83–9, discussion 89–90.

68. Adamsbaum C, Merzoug V, Kalifa G. Imaging of CNS manifestations of tuberous sclerosis in children [in French]. J Neuroradiol. 2005;32:204–9.

69. Goh S, Butler W, Thiele EA. Subependymal giant cell tumors in tuberous sclerosis complex. Neurology. 2004;63:1457–61.

70. Nabbout R, Santos M, Rolland Y, Delalande O, Dulac O, Chiron C. Early diagnosis of subependymal giant cell astrocytoma in children with tuberous sclerosis. J Neurol Neurosurg Psychiatry. 1999;66:370–5.

71. Franz DN, Belousova E, Sparagana S, et al. Efficacy and safety of everolimus for subependymal giant cell astrocytomas associated with tuberous sclerosis complex (EXIST-1): a multicentre, randomised, placebo-controlled phase 3 trial. Lancet. 2013;381:125–32.

72. Krueger DA, Care MM, Holland K, et al. Everolimus for subependymal giant-cell astrocytomas in tuberous sclerosis. N Engl J Med. 2010;363:1801–11.

Unruptured Incidental Intracranial Aneurysms

8

Qichang Fu and Fuyou Guo

8.1 Introduction

Saccular intracranial aneurysms (IAs) are berry-like vascular malformations that often occur in intracranial arteries [1]. Their formation, growth, and eventual rupture may be related to hemodynamic abnormalities, wall degeneration, etc. [1] About 85% IAs are in the anterior circulation, and 15% are in the posterior circulation [2]. IAs occur in 3–5% of adults regardless of race or location [3]. The occurrence of IAs has a familial aggregation phenomenon. Individuals with two or more relatives suffering from IAs or subarachnoid hemorrhages (SAHs) have an incidence of IAs of about 8–9% [4]. The incidence of IAs is higher in women than in men [2].

Unruptured intracranial saccular aneurysms (UIAs) are IAs without bleeding or pathologically confirmed aneurysm wall rupture. Most UIAs have no specific symptoms, and a few with

symptoms such as headache and ptosis, so asymptomatic UIAs are challenging to find [5]. However, with the advancement of imaging, non-invasive detection techniques such as MRA and CTA have gradually become popular in clinical practice [6]. More and more UIAs have been discovered incidentally [7].

Ruptured saccular intracranial aneurysms (RIAs) cause 80–85% of SAH and account for up to 5–10% of strokes; SAH has a 30-day mortality rate of 30–45%; 50% surviving hemorrhagic patients will be left disabled [8, 9].

8.2 Patient Selection and Preoperative Evaluation

Imaging technology is the cornerstone of the diagnosis and treatment of IAs. Digital Subtraction Angiography is still the "gold standard" for diagnosing IAs. Still, with the advancement of imaging technology, the sensitivity and specificity of magnetic resonanace angiography (MRA) and computed tomography angiography (CTA) for diagnosing IAs have approached digital subtraction angiography (DSA) [6, 10]. CTA scans are fast and therefore have advantages in diagnosing hemorrhagic IAs [10, 11]. MRA is non-invasive and non-radiative, so it has advantages in the follow-up of UIAs [12] (Fig. 8.1). Whether UIAs or RIAs diagnosis and treatment, it is necessary to evaluate the imaging technology

Q. Fu
Department of Magnetic Resonance, The First Affiliated Hospital of Zhengzhou University, Zhengzhou, Henan Province, China

International Joint Laboratory of Nervous System Malformation, Zhengzhou, Henan Province, China

F. Guo (✉)
Department of Neurosurgery, The First Affiliated Hospital of Zhengzhou University, Zhengzhou, Henan Province, China

International Joint Laboratory of Nervous System Malformation, Zhengzhou, Henan Province, China

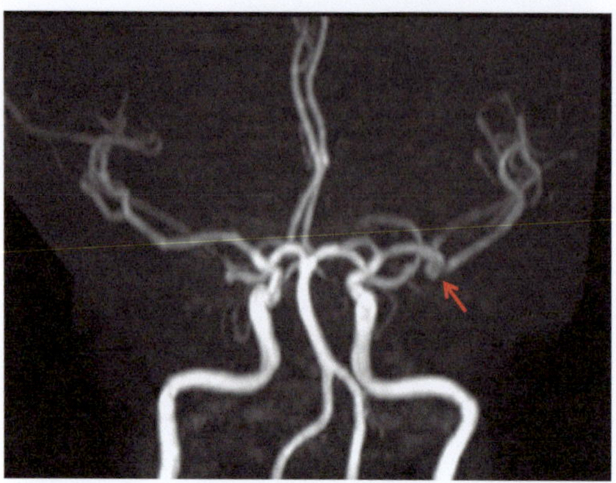

Fig. 8.1 Magnetic resonance angiography demonstrates an aneurysm of the left middle cerebral artery

comprehensively and formulate an individualized diagnosis and treatment plan [3, 9, 13, 14].

8.2.1 Selection and Preoperative Evaluation of Patients with Unruptured UIAs

The risk of spontaneous rupture of UIAs is no more than 1% per year [6]. Risks exist with either surgical or endovascular treatment, with cumulative morbidity and cumulative mortality ranging from 3% to 10%, depending on the technique used [15]. Therefore, a comprehensive assessment of the rupture risk of UIAs is required, and select patients with a higher rupture risk for treatment [16]. The risk factors for rupture of UIAs include two aspects, patient-related risk factors and aneurysm-related risk factors [17, 18].

Patient-related risk factors include geographic location, family history, age, gender, hypertension, smoking, and alcoholism [18, 19]. The risk of aneurysm rupture varies among patients in different regions, and the risk of rupture in Japanese is higher than that of Europeans and Americans [3]. Patients with a family history of IAs had a higher risk of rupture than those without a family history [3, 4]. There are conflicting reports on the role of age in aneurysm risk factors. The ISUIA study concluded that age >59 years was associated with an increased risk of aneurysm rupture [20]. Studies have also shown that the risk of aneurysm rupture decreases with increasing age.

The SUAVe study concluded that age <50 was associated with an increased risk of aneurysm rupture [21]. Women have a higher risk of rupture than men due to differences in estrogen levels [3, 22]. High blood pressure, smoking, and alcohol use may increase the risk of aneurysm rupture [3, 19]. In addition, we should also consider mental factors such as anxiety and depression caused by UIAs in diagnosing and treating UIAs [2, 23–25].

Aneurysm-related risk factors mainly include the structural characteristics, number, symptoms, or previous history of SAH of the aneurysm. The structural features of UIAs include aneurysm size, aneurysm morphology, and aneurysm location [1, 18]. Most current studies suggest that the larger the diameter of the aneurysm, the higher the risk of rupture. The ISUIA-2 study defined the rupture risk of aneurysms at 7 mm, with UIAs smaller than 7 mm in diameter having a lower risk of rupture and aneurysms larger than 7 mm in diameter having a significantly higher risk of rupture [20]. Aneurysms with irregular shapes or accuses had a significantly increased risk of rupture, 1.63 times that of aneurysms with regular shapes [26]. The ISUIA and UCAS studies have found that aneurysms located in the posterior circulation and anterior communicating vessels have a higher risk of rupture than other locations [20, 26]. Studies such as ISUIA and SUAVe suggest that multiple UIAs have a higher risk of rupture than single aneurysms [20, 21]. UIAs with symptoms such as sentinel headache or aneurysm-related oculomotor nerve palsy are at higher risk of rupture [5, 27]. UIAs with a prior history of SAH are at higher risk of rupture [20, 26]. Recent studies suggest that functional features such as aneurysm wall enhancement on vessel wall imaging may also increase rupture risk [28, 29] (Fig. 8.2).

As mentioned above, the rupture risk of UIAs is related to various factors, and it isn't easy to accurately evaluate in routine diagnosis and treatment practice. Some scholars have proposed a scoring system to predict the risk of aneurysm rupture. The PHASES scoring system integrates population, hypertension, age, size of the aneurysm, earlier SAH, and site of the aneurysm for an individualized assessment of the 5-year rupture risk of aneurysms [18]. The ELPSS scoring system combines the history of earlier SAH, location of the aneurysm, age,

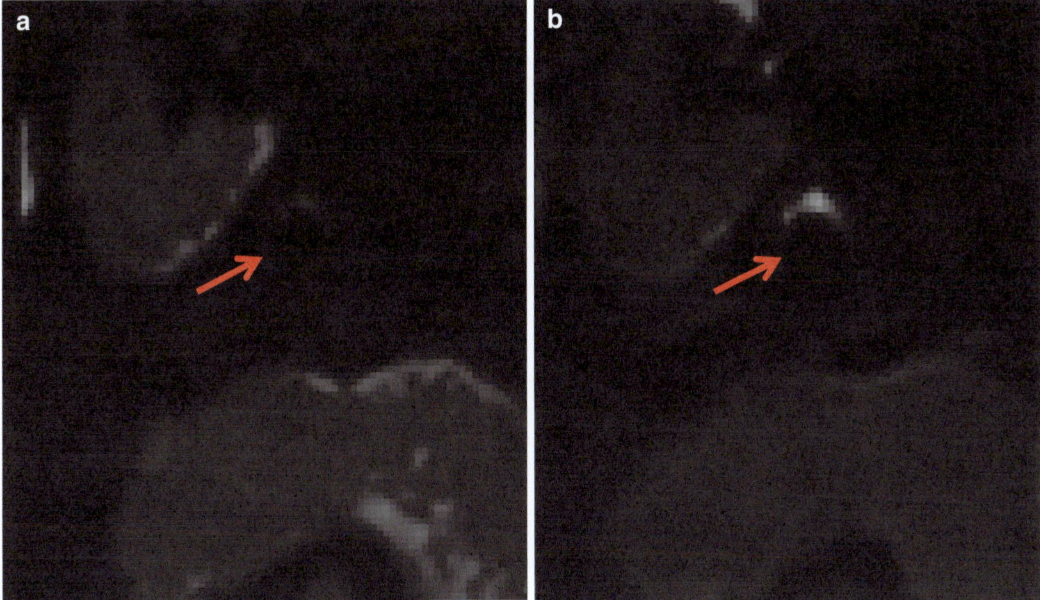

Fig. 8.2 Vessel wall imaging suggested local enhancement of aneurysm wall in different layers (red arrow indicating) (**a**, **b**) of left middle cerebral artery

population, size of the aneurysm, and shape of the aneurysm to calculate the risk of aneurysm growth at 3 and 5 years [30]. However, applying the above scoring systems in clinical practice is still limited due to the complexity of aneurysm rupture risk [31–33]. Therefore, treatment decisions for UIAs need to strike a balance between treatment risk and rupture risk [2, 34].

8.2.2 Selection and Preoperative Evaluation of Patients with Ruptured IAs

Ruptured saccular intracranial aneurysms (RIAs) cause 80–85% of aSAH [9, 13]. RIAs mainly include SAH and IAs [35]. Patients with aSAH have typical "thunderclap-like" headaches, projectile vomiting, and neck stiffness [9, 13, 14, 16]. A few patients have atypical symptoms, which can easily lead to misdiagnosis [13, 14]. Therefore, the high-density shadow in the subarachnoid space detected by head CT is still the cornerstone of diagnosing aSAH. Within 12 h after the onset of SAH, the sensitivity of CT was as high as 98–100%, decreased to 57–85%

Table 8.1 Hunt-Hess grades

1	Asymptomatic, or mild headache, mild neck stiffness
2	Moderate to severe headache, neck stiffness, or cranial nerve paralysis
3	Drowsiness or confusion, mild focal neurological impairment
4	Coma, moderate to severe hemiplegia
5	Deep coma, tonic, near-death state

Note: For severe systemic diseases (such as hypertensive nephropathy, diabetes, severe arteriosclerosis, chronic obstructive pulmonary disease) or severe vasospasm found on angiography, add 1 point to the score

within 6 days [36]. After 10 days of bleeding or when the amount of bleeding is small, CT examination may be negative. Patients with negative CT must clarify SAH through lumbar puncture further. In addition, FLAIR, DWI, SWI, and other magnetic resonance sequences can also help identify suspicious SAH with negative CT [9, 13, 37]. Several versions of the clinical grading scale for SAH patients include the Hunt-Hess grades (Table 8.1) [38], the modified Fisher scale (which mainly assesses the risk of vasospasm) (Table 8.2) [39], etc. Although the choice of the scale is still controversial, it is still recom-

Table 8.2 Modified Fisher scale

Fraction	CT appearance	Vasospasm risk (%)
0	No bleeding or only intraventricular or intraparenchymal hemorrhage	3
1	Only basal cistern hemorrhage	14
2	Peripheral cistern or Sylvian cistern hemorrhage only	38
3	Extensive subarachnoid hemorrhage with parenchymal hemorrhage	57
4	The basal cistern, peripheral cistern, and lateral fissure cistern are thick with hematocele	57

mended for emergency use. Patients are assessed on at least one of the above scales.

DSA remains the "gold standard" for diagnosing IAs. For SAH patients with no aneurysm found on CTA, further DSA is necessary [16, 40]. For SAH patients with no aneurysm found in the first DSA examination, it is essential to consider benign peripheral hemorrhage or vasospasm [13, 40–42]. Benign perimesencephalic hemorrhage is a particular type of spontaneous SAH, and the bleeding is mainly in the midbrain, anterior pons, or quadrigeminal cistern [43]. Vasospasm after SAH may lead to the lack of visualization of distal IAs. Therefore, such patients must re-examine the presence of IAs after remission of vasospasm [44].

The 30-day mortality of SAH due to rupture of IAs is 30–45%, and 50% of surviving bleeding patients will be with a disability [13, 14]. The emergency diagnosis and management of aSAH patients are closely related to the prognosis of the patients [13]. Therefore, once the aneurysm ruptures, emergency treatment is required.

8.3 Principles of Surgery

The primary purpose of the treatment of intracranial aneurysm is to prevent its rupture and hemorrhage [16]. Clipping has been used for decades to treat aneurysms, including ruptured or unruptured brain aneurysms [2]. With the development of technology, the interventional treatment of intracranial aneurysms has gradually become the preferred treatment method for intracranial aneurysms from a candidate means of clipping [20, 23].

The ISAT study is an international, multicenter, prospective, randomized, controlled clinical study funded by the UK Medical Research Council to compare the efficacy of surgical clipping and interventional embolization techniques in patients with ruptured aneurysms [23]. This study lasted from 1994 to 2002, including 2143 patients, and finally found that the interventional embolization group was significantly better than the surgical clipping group. The ISAT study changed the treatment strategy for intracranial aneurysms, making endovascular technology the mainstay of treatment for UIAs.

The 2012 American Stroke Association guidelines for diagnosing and treating aneurysmal subarachnoid hemorrhage indicated that surgical clipping or interventional treatment of the aneurysm for patients with ruptured intracranial aneurysms should be performed as soon as possible. Interventional therapy should be the first choice for patients suitable for clipping or interventional embolization [44].

Interventional treatment of intracranial aneurysms has been widely recognized, but the treatment of intracranial aneurysms still requires individualized evaluation. For patients with intracranial hematoma with significant mass effect, craniotomy to remove the hematoma and aneurysm clipping is still the preferred treatment. Clipping may still be the first choice for middle cerebral artery aneurysms that are refractory to interventional therapy [44].

In addition, interventional therapy needs to choose drugs in the perioperative period to reduce complications, including anticoagulation therapy, antiplatelet therapy, prevention and treatment of vasospasm, management of perioperative blood pressure, and prevention and control aSAH-related epilepsy [45–53].

8.4 Surgical Treatment of Patients with IAs

The exquisite craniotomy technique is one of the key links to the success of aneurysm clipping. Intracranial aneurysm clipping mainly includes seven surgical approaches. Firstly, the classic pterional approach [54]. On the basis of the traditional frontotemporal craniotomy, Yasargil et al. created a pterional approach, which provided a better solution for clipping the anterior segment of the basilar artery and the upper part of the basilar artery and its branches in the circle of Willis [55]. Its branch aneurysm clipping procedure provided good exposure. At present, this surgical approach has been widely used to clip Willis anterior circulation aneurysms, such as proximal internal carotid artery aneurysm (Figs. 8.3, 8.4, 8.5, 8.6, and 8.7), anterior cerebral artery aneurysm, middle cerebral artery aneurysm, basilar artery apical aneurysm, posterior cerebral artery aneurysm, and proximal superior cerebellar artery aneurysm. The pterional approach requires the resection of the lateral bone of the sphenoid ridge. The treatment of the parasellar aneurysm also requires the resection or grinding of the anterior clinoid process, so that the brain tissue is slightly pulled to immediately expose the bottom of the anterior and middle cranial fossa. Second, the mini pterional approach improves the pterional approach [54]. Third, the orbitozygomatic approach, which is an extension of the pterional approach, involves a frontotemporal craniotomy with an additional orbitotomy or zygomaticotomy [56]. The orbitozygomatic approach can increase the exposure angle of anterior and posterior circulation aneurysms, and is more suitable for clipping basilar artery apical aneurysms, especially when the basilar artery bifurcation is high. Instruments and aneurysm clips can only be performed from the bottom up, and the space obtained by removing the zygomatic bone and relaxing the temporalis muscle facilitates visualization of surrounding structures. Surgical instruments and aneurysm clips can only be performed from the bottom up, and the space obtained by removing the zygomatic bone and relaxing the temporalis muscle facilitates visualization of surrounding structures. This approach enables clipping of anterior communicating artery aneurysms. Fourth, the cavernous sinus approach is an exposure method of incising the tentorium edge behind the cavernous sinus and extending downward [57–59]. This approach increases the exposure of the clivus to the inferior tentorial rim. Fifth, the transpetrosal approach, that is, entering

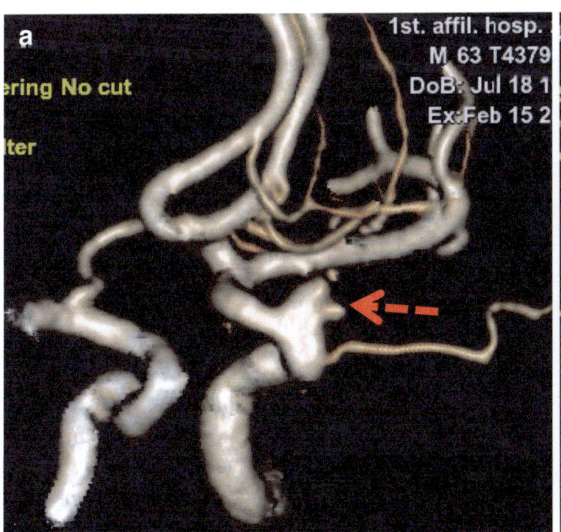

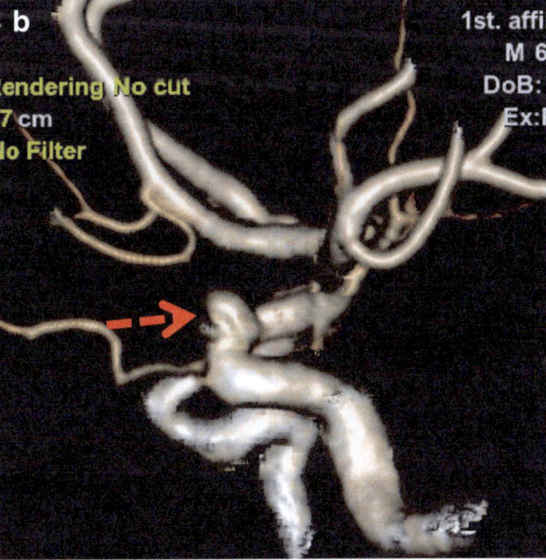

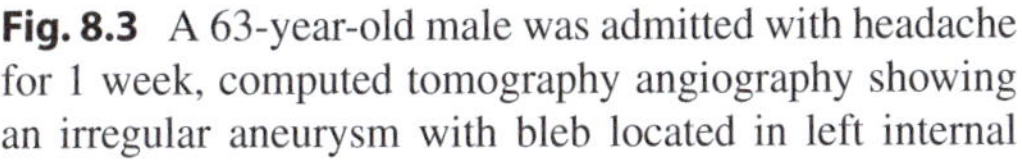

Fig. 8.3 A 63-year-old male was admitted with headache for 1 week, computed tomography angiography showing an irregular aneurysm with bleb located in left internal carotid artery distal to the ophthalmic artery. Broken red arrow indicating aneurysm (**a**, **b**)

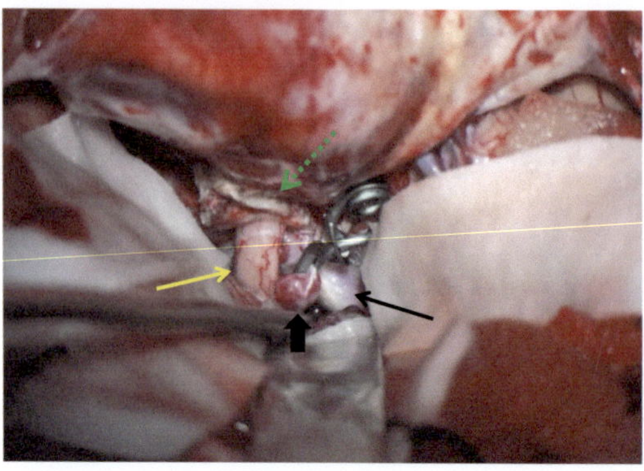

Fig. 8.4 Broken green arrow indicating intradural cli-noidectomy, yellow arrow showing left optic nerve, blue arrow showing the left internal carotid artery, black arrowhead demonstrating aneurysm clipping

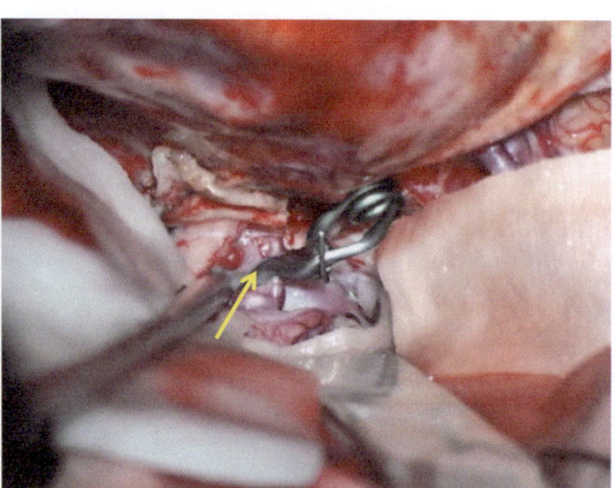

Fig. 8.5 There is a bleb under the left optic nerve, yellow arrow showing aneurysm bleb

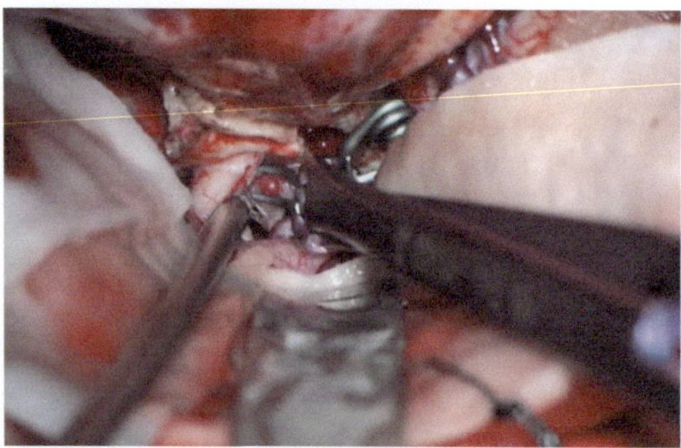

Fig. 8.6 Aneurysm bleb was further obliterated by mini-clip

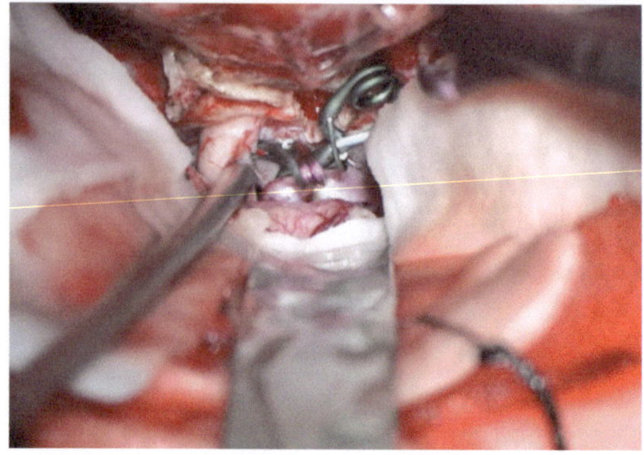

Fig. 8.7 The aneurysm including bleb was totally clipped by two clamps

the posterior cranial fossa from the side of the skull, is a combined approach of the middle and posterior cranial fossa with the petrous bone as the center [60–63]. This method is suitable for clipping aneurysms at the top of the basilar artery. Sixth, the far-lateral suboccipital approach is from the posterolateral aspect of the posterior cranial fossa, and the bone at the foramen magnum is excised into the posteromedial aspect of the occipital condyle, and the pons and basilar artery are exposed between the lateral auditory nerve and the hypoglossal nerve [64–68]. This approach facilitates the clipping of aneurysms close to the midline. Seventh, the interhemispheric approach is beneficial for treating anterior communicating artery aneurysms and aneurysms distal to the anterior cerebral artery [69–73].

Surgical methods for intracranial aneurysms include carotid artery staged ligation, aneurysm clipping, aneurysm isolation, and aneurysm wrapping [74–80]. Before microsurgery and endovascular embolization are used to treat aneurysms, internal carotid artery ligation is one of the important methods for treating giant aneurysms in the cavernous sinus clinoid segments of the internal carotid artery [74]. This surgical method has a high mortality and disability rate, and it has been gradually marginalized in the modern treatment of intracranial aneurysms. Aneurysm clipping removes the threat of aneurysm rebleeding by clipping the neck of the aneurysm, preventing blood from entering the aneurysm sac [75–77]. Aneurysm isolation is the simultaneous occlusion of the proximal and distal ends of the aneurysm parent artery to block blood from entering the aneurysm sac, thereby preventing aneurysm hemorrhage. Simple aneurysm isolation leads to the distal blood supply area of the parent artery to the brain. Complications such as infarction are high, so it is necessary to perform vascular reconstruction surgery such as vascular bypass during the operation [78, 81]. Aneurysm wrapping is a surgical method for surgical treatment such as aneurysm clipping that cannot be performed [79, 80]. Due to the limitation of the anatomical location of the aneurysm, it is difficult for most aneurysms that cannot be clipped to expose the entire aneurysm fully. The range of aneurysms that can be encapsulated is limited and rarely achieves the intended purpose of strengthening the aneurysm wall and preventing bleeding. Therefore, this surgical method has gradually been marginalized in the modern treatment of intracranial aneurysms.

8.5 Interventional Treatment of IAs

In the interventional treatment of intracranial aneurysms (Figs. 8.8, 8.9, and 8.10), an excellent surgical approach is a key to the operation's success. The selection of a reasonable arterial approach is also an important factor for the success or failure of endovascular interventional treatment of aneurysms. The development of existing catheter sheaths and guide catheters has enabled most of the intracranial aneurysms to be completed through the femoral artery approach [82]. In some patients with extreme tortuosity or torsion of the abdominal and descending aorta, a long sheath can be used to improve the support of the delivery system [83, 84]. The radial approach is helpful in the treatment of posterior circulation aneurysms in some patients with aortic arch torsion [85, 86]. Guiding catheters play the role of

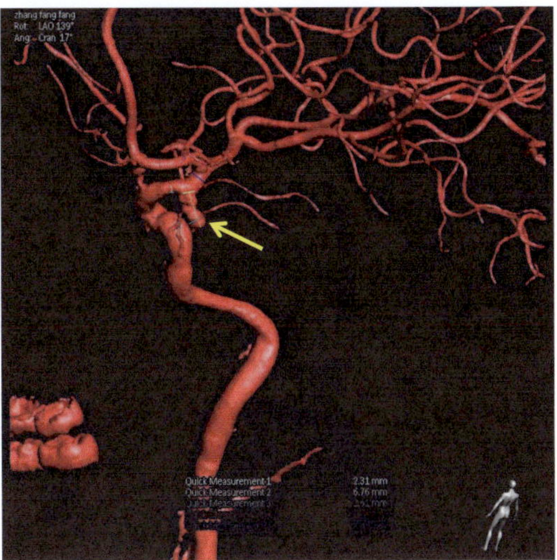

Fig. 8.8 The right posterior communicating aneurysm was defined incidentally by three dimension digital subtraction angiography, the neck of aneurysm was 2.31 mm, the height of aneurysm is 6.76 mm, yellow arrow showing aneurysm

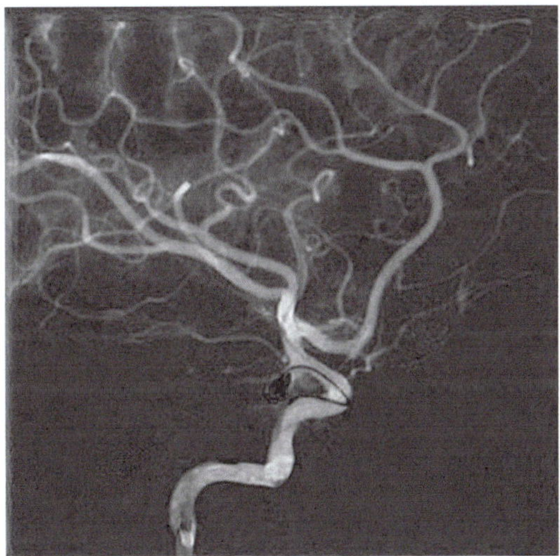

Fig. 8.9 This patient was treated by interventional embolization

providing support and access during endovascular embolization in cerebral aneurysms [87, 88]. Therefore, intraoperatively, the guiding catheter is required to be as close to or beyond the skull base as possible, especially for anterior communicating or distal aneurysms.

Choosing a good working angle is essential in initiating intracranial aneurysm embolization

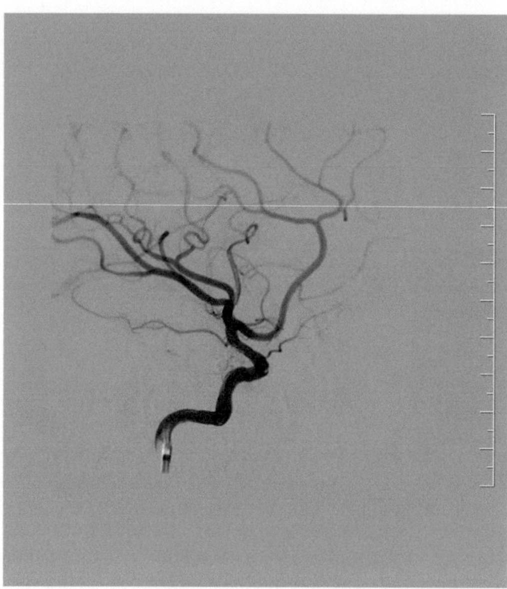

Fig. 8.10 The aneurysm was totally embolized without no residence of aneurysmal neck, the posterior communicating artery was well-protected after operation

therapy. In the embolization treatment of an aneurysm, it is crucial to avoid the herniation of the coil into the parent artery. Therefore, the intraoperative working angle should choose the projection angle of the tangential direction of the aneurysm neck. After determining the working angle, the microcatheter should be accurately shaped according to the anatomical relationship between the aneurysm and its parent artery [89, 90].

Interventional treatment techniques for intracranial aneurysms can be divided into reconstructive and non-reconstructive treatments, depending on whether the parent artery is preserved [91–93]. Non-reconstructive treatments mainly include in situ occlusion of the aneurysm body and parent artery and proximal parent artery occlusion [93, 94]. Due to the non-reconstructive treatment modality, the patients had higher ischemic complications, etc. Therefore, non-reconstructive therapy is currently only an option for some refractory aneurysms.

Reconstructive treatment techniques include coil embolization, balloon-assisted coil embolization, stent-assisted coil embolization, blood flow diversion devices, etc. [95–98] The goal of treatment is to maintain the parent artery patency while altering the intratumoral hemodynamics until the aneurysm is completely isolated from the circulatory system to eliminate the risk of bleeding. Coil embolization is the primary treatment method, and it is also the preferred treatment method for intracranial narrow neck aneurysms [16, 95]. Intracranial wide-necked aneurysms are considered unsuitable for interventional therapy in the early stage, and clipping is often used. With new interventional materials, intracranial wide-necked aneurysms can also be well cured by interventional methods [97, 99]. As a significant breakthrough in the endovascular treatment of intracranial aneurysms, the blood flow diverting device reflects the change in the treatment concept from intracranial aneurysm filling to vascular reconstruction and promotes thrombosis in aneurysms [98]. In addition, there are also blood flow disruption devices represented by WEB systems [99].

8.6 Complications

8.6.1 Complications of Surgical Treatment

Complications such as cerebral contusion, cerebral hemorrhage, or brain herniation after aneurysm surgery are caused by excessive stretching of the brain tissue during the operation [100]. The main preventive measures are to release the cerebrospinal fluid as much as possible to reduce the intracranial pressure and operate gently during the operation. Postoperative cerebral infarction may be triggered by vasospasm after SAH [101]. It can be treated by lumbar puncture or lumbar drainage of cerebrospinal fluid. Hydrocephalus may result from cerebrospinal fluid malabsorption caused by SAH blocking arachnoid granules [102]. Such complications can be treated with ventriculoperitoneal shunt. Postoperative epilepsy is caused by cortical discoloration caused by excessive lobe traction during surgery [103]. The preventive measure is to use the space where the brain tissue collapses during the operation to avoid pulling the brain lobes. Antiepileptic drugs were used during and after surgery. Postoperative aneurysm rebleeding may be caused by incomplete clipping of the aneurysm [104]. The preventive wording is to clip the aneurysm neck as completely as possible during the operation. Frail patients, elderly patients, postoperative bedridden patients, etc. can easily lead to postoperative pulmonary infection [105]. Patients should be encouraged to move early after surgery, maintain airway patency, and use antibiotics rationally. Opening the frontal sinus through tandem and sub-frontal approaches increases the chance of intracranial infection [106]. Once the frontal sinus is opened during the operation, measures such as sealing the sinus opening with bone wax should be used immediately for isolation and protection.

8.6.2 Complications of Interventional Therapy

Intraoperative aneurysm bleeding caused by microcatheter or microwire piercing the aneurysm is the most serious complication in endovascular treatment of intracranial aneurysms [107]. The main preventive measures are to place the guide catheter as close to the aneurysm as possible, to have the microcatheter tip adequately shaped, and to avoid choosing too large and hard coils. Intraoperative aneurysm embolization is not dense due to early postoperative hemorrhage after the intervention [23, 108]. The primary preventive measure is to embolize the aneurysm as tightly as possible during the operation. Thromboembolism due to vascular dissection caused by surgical procedures is the most common complication of interventional therapy [109]. The main preventive measures are standardized surgical operations to avoid damage to blood vessels. Prominence or escape of coils is also a common complication in interventional therapy due to the failure to select an appropriate auxiliary device [110, 111]. The main preventive measures are the selection of proper additional devices during treatment.

8.7 Conclusion

With the advancement of imaging technology, more and more intracranial aneurysms are discovered incidentally [7]. However, not all intracranial aneurysms require treatment [18]. Diagnosis and treatment strategies for intracranial aneurysms should be comprehensively assessed based on patient-related risk factors or aneurysm-related risks to achieve an optimal balance between the risks and benefits of surgery or follow-up [15, 35]. Clipping of intracranial aneurysms began in the 1930s, microsurgery in the 1980s, and interventional therapy in the 1990s. With the development and progress of science and technology, the safety and effectiveness of aneurysm treatment continue to improve. Interventional treatment has gradually become the mainstream technology for the treatment of intracranial aneurysms [23, 108]. However, formulating a patient's surgical plan still needs to be evaluated individually. The technique that maximizes the patient's benefit should be selected between surgical treatment and interventional therapy [2, 15, 44].

References

1. Chalouhi N, Hoh BL, Hasan D. Review of cerebral aneurysm formation, growth, and rupture. Stroke. 2013;44:3613–22. https://doi.org/10.1161/STROKEAHA.113.002390.
2. Etminan N, Rinkel GJ. Unruptured intracranial aneurysms: development, rupture and preventive management. Nat Rev Neurol. 2016;12:699–713. https://doi.org/10.1038/nrneurol.2016.150.
3. Vlak MH, Algra A, Brandenburg R, Rinkel GJ. Prevalence of unruptured intracranial aneurysms, with emphasis on sex, age, comorbidity, country, and time period: a systematic review and meta-analysis. Lancet Neurol. 2011;10:626–36. https://doi.org/10.1016/S1474-4422(11)70109-0.
4. Broderick JP, Brown RD, Sauerbeck L, Hornung R, Huston J, Woo D, Anderson C, Rouleau G, Kleindorfer D, Flaherty ML, et al. Greater rupture risk for familial as compared to sporadic unruptured intracranial aneurysms. Stroke. 2009;40:1952–7. https://doi.org/10.1161/STROKEAHA.108.542571.
5. Linn FH, Wijdicks EF, van der Graaf Y, Weerdesteyn-van Vliet FA, Bartelds AI, van Gijn J. Prospective study of sentinel headache in aneurysmal subarachnoid haemorrhage. Lancet. 1994;344:590–3.

6. Li M-H, Li Y-D, Gu B-X, Cheng Y-S, Wang W, Tan H-Q, Chen Y-C. Accurate diagnosis of small cerebral aneurysms ≤5 mm in diameter with 3.0-T MR angiography. Radiology. 2014;271:553–60. https://doi.org/10.1148/radiol.14122770.

7. Morris Z, Whiteley WN, Longstreth WT, Weber F, Lee Y-C, Tsushima Y, Alphs H, Ladd SC, Warlow C, Wardlaw JM, et al. Incidental findings on brain magnetic resonance imaging: systematic review and meta-analysis. BMJ (Clin Res Ed). 2009;339:b3016. https://doi.org/10.1136/bmj.b3016.

8. Korja M, Kaprio J. Controversies in epidemiology of intracranial aneurysms and SAH. Nat Rev Neurol. 2016;12:50–5. https://doi.org/10.1038/nrneurol.2015.228.

9. Macdonald RL, Schweizer TA. Spontaneous subarachnoid haemorrhage. Lancet. 2017;389:655–66. https://doi.org/10.1016/S0140-6736(16)30668-7.

10. Park A, Chute C, Rajpurkar P, Lou J, Ball RL, Shpanskaya K, Jabarkheel R, Kim LH, McKenna E, Tseng J, et al. Deep learning-assisted diagnosis of cerebral aneurysms using the HeadXNet model. JAMA Netw Open. 2019;2:e195600. https://doi.org/10.1001/jamanetworkopen.2019.5600.

11. Westerlaan HE, van Dijk JMC, van Dijk MJ, Jansen-van der Weide MC, de Groot JC, Groen RJM, Mooij JJA, Oudkerk M. Intracranial aneurysms in patients with subarachnoid hemorrhage: CT angiography as a primary examination tool for diagnosis—systematic review and meta-analysis. Radiology. 2011;258:134–45. https://doi.org/10.1148/radiol.10092373.

12. Kwak Y, Son W, Kim Y-S, Park J, Kang D-H. Discrepancy between MRA and DSA in identifying the shape of small intracranial aneurysms. J Neurosurg. 2020;134:1887–93. https://doi.org/10.3171/2020.4.JNS20128.

13. van Gijn J, Kerr RS, Rinkel GJE. Subarachnoid haemorrhage. Lancet. 2007;369:306–18.

14. Lawton MT, Vates GE. Subarachnoid hemorrhage. N Engl J Med. 2017;377:257–66. https://doi.org/10.1056/NEJMcp1605827.

15. Naggara ON, Lecler A, Oppenheim C, Meder J-F, Raymond J. Endovascular treatment of intracranial unruptured aneurysms: a systematic review of the literature on safety with emphasis on subgroup analyses. Radiology. 2012;263:828–35. https://doi.org/10.1148/radiol.12112114.

16. Brisman JL, Song JK, Newell DW. Cerebral aneurysms. N Engl J Med. 2006;355:928–39.

17. Krings T, Mandell DM, Kiehl T-R, Geibprasert S, Tymianski M, Alvarez H, terBrugge KG, Hans F-J. Intracranial aneurysms: from vessel wall pathology to therapeutic approach. Nat Rev Neurol. 2011;7:547–59. https://doi.org/10.1038/nrneurol.2011.136.

18. Greving JP, Wermer MJH, Brown RD, Morita A, Juvela S, Yonekura M, Ishibashi T, Torner JC, Nakayama T, Rinkel GJE, et al. Development of the PHASES score for prediction of risk of rupture of intracranial aneurysms: a pooled analysis of six prospective cohort studies. Lancet Neurol. 2014;13:59–66. https://doi.org/10.1016/S1474-4422(13)70263-1.

19. Wood AM, Kaptoge S, Butterworth AS, Willeit P, Warnakula S, Bolton T, Paige E, Paul DS, Sweeting M, Burgess S, et al. Risk thresholds for alcohol consumption: combined analysis of individual-participant data for 599 912 current drinkers in 83 prospective studies. Lancet. 2018;391:1513–23. https://doi.org/10.1016/S0140-6736(18)30134-X.

20. Wiebers DO, Whisnant JP, Huston J, Meissner I, Brown RD, Piepgras DG, Forbes GS, Thielen K, Nichols D, O'Fallon WM, et al. Unruptured intracranial aneurysms: natural history, clinical outcome, and risks of surgical and endovascular treatment. Lancet. 2003;362:103–10.

21. Sonobe M, Yamazaki T, Yonekura M, Kikuchi H. Small unruptured intracranial aneurysm verification study: SUAVe study, Japan. Stroke. 2010;41:1969–77. https://doi.org/10.1161/STROKEAHA.110.585059.

22. Yanagisawa T, Zhang H, Suzuki T, Kamio Y, Takizawa T, Morais A, Chung DY, Qin T, Murayama Y, Faber JE, et al. Sex and genetic background effects on the outcome of experimental intracranial aneurysms. Stroke. 2020;51:3083–94. https://doi.org/10.1161/STROKEAHA.120.029651.

23. Molyneux AJ, Kerr RSC, Yu L-M, Clarke M, Sneade M, Yarnold JA, Sandercock P. International subarachnoid aneurysm trial (ISAT) of neurosurgical clipping versus endovascular coiling in 2143 patients with ruptured intracranial aneurysms: a randomised comparison of effects on survival, dependency, seizures, rebleeding, subgroups, and aneurysm occlusion. Lancet. 2005;366:809–17.

24. Malhotra A, Wu X, Matouk CC, Forman HP, Gandhi D, Sanelli P. MR angiography screening and surveillance for intracranial aneurysms in autosomal dominant polycystic kidney disease: a cost-effectiveness analysis. Radiology. 2019;291:400–8. https://doi.org/10.1148/radiol.2019181399.

25. Smith MJ, Sanborn MR, Lewis DJ, Faught RWF, Vakhshori V, Stein SC. Elderly patients with intracranial aneurysms have higher quality of life after coil embolization: a decision analysis. J Neurointerv Surg. 2015;7:898–904. https://doi.org/10.1136/neurintsurg-2014-011394.

26. Morita A, Kirino T, Hashi K, Aoki N, Fukuhara S, Hashimoto N, Nakayama T, Sakai M, Teramoto A, Tominari S, et al. The natural course of unruptured cerebral aneurysms in a Japanese cohort. N Engl J Med. 2012;366:2474–82. https://doi.org/10.1056/NEJMoa1113260.

27. Fujiwara S, Fujii K, Nishio S, Matsushima T, Fukui M. Oculomotor nerve palsy in patients with cerebral aneurysms. Neurosurg Rev. 1989;12:123–32.

28. Edjlali M, Guédon A, Ben Hassen W, Boulouis G, Benzakoun J, Rodriguez-Régent C, Trystram D, Nataf F, Meder J-F, Turski P, et al. Circumferential thick enhancement at vessel wall MRI has high

specificity for intracranial aneurysm instability. Radiology. 2018;289:181–7. https://doi.org/10.1148/radiol.2018172879.

29. Fu Q, Wang Y, Zhang Y, Zhang Y, Guo X, Xu H, Yao Z, Wang M, Levitt MR, Mossa-Basha M, et al. Qualitative and quantitative wall enhancement on magnetic resonance imaging is associated with symptoms of unruptured intracranial aneurysms. Stroke. 2021;52:213–22. https://doi.org/10.1161/STROKEAHA.120.029685.

30. Backes D, Rinkel GJE, Greving JP, Velthuis BK, Murayama Y, Takao H, Ishibashi T, Igase M, ter-Brugge KG, Agid R, et al. ELAPSS score for prediction of risk of growth of unruptured intracranial aneurysms. Neurology. 2017;88:1600–6. https://doi.org/10.1212/WNL.0000000000003865.

31. Backes D, Vergouwen MDI, TielGroenestege AT, Bor ASE, Velthuis BK, Greving JP, Algra A, Wermer MJH, van Walderveen MAA, terBrugge KG, et al. PHASES score for prediction of intracranial aneurysm growth. Stroke. 2015;46:1221–6. https://doi.org/10.1161/STROKEAHA.114.008198.

32. Bijlenga P, Gondar R, Schilling S, Morel S, Hirsch S, Cuony J, Corniola M-V, Perren F, Rüfenacht D, Schaller K. PHASES score for the management of intracranial aneurysm: a cross-sectional population-based retrospective study. Stroke. 2017;48:2105–12. https://doi.org/10.1161/STROKEAHA.117.017391.

33. Rutledge C, Jonzzon S, Winkler EA, Raper D, Lawton MT, Abla AA. Small aneurysms with low PHASES scores account for Most subarachnoid hemorrhage cases. World Neurosurg. 2020;139:e580–4. https://doi.org/10.1016/j.wneu.2020.04.074.

34. Etminan N, Brown RD, Beseoglu K, Juvela S, Raymond J, Morita A, Torner JC, Derdeyn CP, Raabe A, Mocco J, et al. The unruptured intracranial aneurysm treatment score: a multidisciplinary consensus. Neurology. 2015;85:881–9. https://doi.org/10.1212/WNL.0000000000001891.

35. Tawk RG, Hasan TF, D'Souza CE, Peel JB, Freeman WD. Diagnosis and treatment of unruptured intracranial aneurysms and aneurysmal subarachnoid hemorrhage. Mayo Clin Proc. 2021;96:1970–2000. https://doi.org/10.1016/j.mayocp.2021.01.005.

36. Carpenter CR, Hussain AM, Ward MJ, Zipfel GJ, Fowler S, Pines JM, Sivilotti MLA. Spontaneous subarachnoid hemorrhage: a systematic review and meta-analysis describing the diagnostic accuracy of history, physical examination, imaging, and lumbar puncture with an exploration of test thresholds. Acad Emerg Med. 2016;23:963. https://doi.org/10.1111/acem.12984.

37. Hokari M, Shimbo D, Uchida K, Gekka M, Asaoka K, Itamoto K. Characteristics of MRI findings after subarachnoid hemorrhage and D-dimer as a predictive value for early brain injury. J Stroke Cerebrovasc Dis. 2022;31:106073. https://doi.org/10.1016/j.jstrokecerebrovasdis.2021.106073.

38. Mericle RA, Reig AS, Burry MV, Eskioglu E, Firment CS, Santra S. Endovascular surgery for proximal posterior inferior cerebellar artery aneurysms: an analysis of Glasgow outcome score by Hunt-Hess grades. Neurosurgery. 2006;58:619.

39. Frontera JA, Claassen J, Schmidt JM, Wartenberg KE, Temes R, Connolly ES, MacDonald RL, Mayer SA. Prediction of symptomatic vasospasm after subarachnoid hemorrhage: the modified fisher scale. Neurosurgery. 2006;59:21.

40. Heit JJ, Pastena GT, Nogueira RG, Yoo AJ, Leslie-Mazwi TM, Hirsch JA, Rabinov JD. Cerebral angiography for evaluation of patients with CT angiogram-negative subarachnoid hemorrhage: an 11-year experience. AJNR Am J Neuroradiol. 2016;37:297–304. https://doi.org/10.3174/ajnr.A4503.

41. Chalouhi N, Witte S, Penn DL, Soni P, Starke RM, Jabbour P, Gonzalez LF, Dumont AS, Rosenwasser R, Tjoumakaris S. Diagnostic yield of cerebral angiography in patients with computed tomography-negative, lumbar puncture-positive subarachnoid hemorrhage. Neurosurgery. 2013;73:282. https://doi.org/10.1227/01.neu.0000430291.31422.dd.

42. Catapano JS, Lang MJ, Koester SW, Wang DJ, DiDomenico JD, Fredrickson VL, Cole TS, Lee J, Lawton MT, Ducruet AF, et al. Digital subtraction cerebral angiography after negative computed tomography angiography findings in non-traumatic subarachnoid hemorrhage. J Neurointerv Surg. 2020;12:526–30. https://doi.org/10.1136/neurintsurg-2019-015375.

43. Fragata I, Canto-Moreira N, Canhão P. Comparison of cerebral perfusion in perimesencephalic subarachnoid hemorrhage and aneurysmal subarachnoid hemorrhage. Neuroradiology. 2018;60:609–16. https://doi.org/10.1007/s00234-018-1997-1.

44. Connolly ES, Rabinstein AA, Carhuapoma JR, Derdeyn CP, Dion J, Higashida RT, Hoh BL, Kirkness CJ, Naidech AM, Ogilvy CS, et al. Guidelines for the management of aneurysmal subarachnoid hemorrhage: a guideline for healthcare professionals from the American Heart Association/American Stroke Association. Stroke. 2012;43:1711–37. https://doi.org/10.1161/STR.0b013e3182587839.

45. Algra AM, Lindgren A, Vergouwen MDI, Greving JP, van der Schaaf IC, van Doormaal TPC, Rinkel GJE. Procedural clinical complications, case-fatality risks, and risk factors in endovascular and neurosurgical treatment of unruptured intracranial aneurysms: a systematic review and meta-analysis. JAMA Neurol. 2019;76:282–93. https://doi.org/10.1001/jamaneurol.2018.4165.

46. Metso TM, Metso AJ, Helenius J, Haapaniemi E, Salonen O, Porras M, Hernesniemi J, Kaste M, Tatlisumak T. Prognosis and safety of anticoagulation in intracranial artery dissections in adults. Stroke. 2007;38:1837–42.

47. Li W, Zhu W, Wang A, Zhang G, Zhang Y, Wang K, Zhang Y, Wang C, Zhang L, Zhao H, et al. Effect of adjusted antiplatelet therapy on preventing ischemic events after stenting for intracranial aneurysms.

Stroke. 2021;52:3815–25. https://doi.org/10.1161/STROKEAHA.120.032989.

48. Wan H, AlHarbi BM, Macdonald RL. Mechanisms, treatment and prevention of cellular injury and death from delayed events after aneurysmal subarachnoid hemorrhage. Expert Opin Pharmacother. 2014;15:231–43. https://doi.org/10.1517/14656566.2014.865724.

49. Fisher CM, Kistler JP, Davis JM. Relation of cerebral vasospasm to subarachnoid hemorrhage visualized by computerized tomographic scanning. Neurosurgery. 1980;6:1–9.

50. Neifert SN, Chapman EK, Martini ML, Shuman WH, Schupper AJ, Oermann EK, Mocco J, Macdonald RL. Aneurysmal subarachnoid hemorrhage: the last decade. Transl Stroke Res. 2021;12:428–46. https://doi.org/10.1007/s12975-020-00867-0.

51. Orecchia PM, Clagett GP, Youkey JR, Brigham RA, Fisher DF, Fry RF, McDonald PT, Collins GJ, Rich NM. Management of patients with symptomatic extracranial carotid artery disease and incidental intracranial berry aneurysm. J Vasc Surg. 1985;2:158–64.

52. Velly LJ, Bilotta F, Fàbregas N, Soehle M, Bruder NJ, Nathanson MH. Anaesthetic and ICU management of aneurysmal subarachnoid haemorrhage: a survey of European practice. Eur J Anaesthesiol. 2015;32:168–76. https://doi.org/10.1097/EJA.0000000000000163.

53. Harroud A, Crepeau AZ. Epilepsy and mortality after aneurysmal subarachnoid hemorrhage. Neurology. 2017;89:222–3. https://doi.org/10.1212/WNL.0000000000004125.

54. Tsunoda S, Inoue T, Ohwaki K, Akabane A, Saito N. Comparison of postoperative temporalis muscle atrophy between the muscle-preserving pterional approach and the mini-pterional approach in the treatment of unruptured intracranial aneurysms. Neurosurg Rev. 2022;45:507–15. https://doi.org/10.1007/s10143-021-01558-6.

55. Mishra S, Srivastava AK, Kumar H, Sharma BS. Reshaping the zygomatic complex: a "small step" in frontotemporal craniotomy and a "big leap" in exposure. Neurol India. 2015;63:723–6. https://doi.org/10.4103/0028-3886.166540.

56. van Furth WR, Agur AMR, Woolridge N, Cusimano MD. The orbitozygomatic approach. Neurosurgery. 2006;58:ONS103-7.

57. Fernandez-Miranda JC, Zwagerman NT, Abhinav K, Lieber S, Wang EW, Snyderman CH, Gardner PA. Cavernous sinus compartments from the endoscopic endonasal approach: anatomical considerations and surgical relevance to adenoma surgery. J Neurosurg. 2018;129:430–41. https://doi.org/10.3171/2017.2.JNS162214.

58. Klinger DR, Flores BC, Lewis JJ, Barnett SL. The treatment of cavernous sinus meningiomas: evolution of a modern approach. Neurosurg Focus. 2013;35:E8. https://doi.org/10.3171/2013.9.FOCUS13345.

59. Aversa A, Al-Mefty O. Zygomatic approach to cavernous sinus Chordoma: 2-dimensional operative video. Oper Neurosurg (Hagerstown). 2021;21:E105–6. https://doi.org/10.1093/ons/opab126.

60. Rennert RC, Brandel MG, Steinberg JA, Gonda DD, Friedman RA, Fukushima T, Day JD, Khalessi AA, Levy ML. Maturation of the anterior petrous apex: surgical relevance for performance of the middle fossa transpetrosal approach in pediatric patients. J Neurosurg. 2021:1–7. https://doi.org/10.3171/2021.3.JNS202648.

61. Lin B-J, Ju D-T, Wu Y-C, Kao H-W, Tseng K-Y, Chung T-T, Liu W-H, Hueng D-Y, Chen Y-H, Hsia C-C, et al. Endoscopic transcanal transpetrosal approach to the petroclival region: a cadaveric study with comparison to the Kawase approach. Neurosurg Rev. 2021;44:2171–9. https://doi.org/10.1007/s10143-020-01389-x.

62. Vidal CHF, Nicácio JA, Hahn Y, Caldas Neto SS, Coimbra CJ. Tentorial peeling: surgical extradural navigation to protect the temporal lobe in the focused combined transpetrosal approach. Oper Neurosurg (Hagerstown). 2020;19:589–98. https://doi.org/10.1093/ons/opaa162.

63. Kadri PAS, Essayed WIBN, Al-Mefty O. Resection of pontine Cavernoma through the anterior transpetrosal approach: 2-dimensional operative video. Oper Neurosurg (Hagerstown). 2021;21:E26–7. https://doi.org/10.1093/ons/opab103.

64. Flores BC, Boudreaux BP, Klinger DR, Mickey BE, Barnett SL. The far-lateral approach for foramen magnum meningiomas. Neurosurg Focus. 2013;35:E12. https://doi.org/10.3171/2013.10.FOCUS13332.

65. Bodon G, Kiraly K, Ruttkay T, Hirt B, Koller H. Feasibility of the far lateral suboccipital approach to the retroodontoid region. How much bone removal is truly needed? Neurospine. 2020;17:921–8. https://doi.org/10.14245/ns.2040304.152.

66. Tsunoda S, Inoue T, Naemura K, Akabane A. The efficacy of temporary clamping of V3 with a suboccipital far-lateral approach in microvascular decompression for hemifacial spasm associated with the vertebral artery. Neurosurg Rev. 2021;44:625–31. https://doi.org/10.1007/s10143-020-01262-x.

67. El Ahmadieh TY, Haider AS, Cohen-Gadol A. The far-lateral suboccipital approach to the lesions of the craniovertebral junction. World Neurosurg. 2021;155:218–28. https://doi.org/10.1016/j.wneu.2021.08.018.

68. Di G, Fang X, Hu Q, Zhou W, Jiang X. A microanatomical study of the far lateral approach. World Neurosurg. 2019;127:e932–42. https://doi.org/10.1016/j.wneu.2019.04.004.

69. Aldea S, Apra C, Chauvet D, Le Guérinel C, Bourdillon P. Interhemispheric transcallosal approach: going further based on the vascular anatomy. Neurosurg Rev. 2021;44:2831–5. https://doi.org/10.1007/s10143-021-01480-x.

70. Serra C, Türe U. The extreme anterior interhemispheric transcallosal approach for pure aqueduct tumors: surgical technique and case series. Neurosurg Rev. 2022;45:499–505. https://doi.org/10.1007/s10143-021-01555-9.

71. Pescatori L, Tropeano MP, Ciappetta P. The ipsilateral interhemispheric transprecuneal approach: microsurgical anatomy, indications, and neurosurgical applications. Neurosurg Rev. 2021;44:529–41. https://doi.org/10.1007/s10143-020-01244-z.

72. Panteli A, Güngör A, Fırat Z, Sarıtepe F, Türe H, Türe U. The posterior interhemispheric transparieto-occipital fissure approach to the atrium of the lateral ventricle: a fiber microdissection study with case series. Neurosurg Rev. 2021;45:1663. https://doi.org/10.1007/s10143-021-01693-0.

73. Aftahy AK, Barz M, Wagner A, Liesche-Starnecker F, Negwer C, Meyer B, Gempt J. The interhemispheric fissure-surgical outcome of interhemispheric approaches. Neurosurg Rev. 2021;44:2099–110. https://doi.org/10.1007/s10143-020-01372-6.

74. Bohm E, Hugosson R, Wolgast M. Carotid ligation for the treatment of carotid artery aneurysms. Pre- and peroperative studies of the cerebral blood flow with an intravenous isotope technique. Acta Neurochir (Wien). 1978;45:35–51.

75. Martinez-Perez R, Hardesty DA, Silveira-Bertazzo G, Albonette-Felicio T, Carrau RL, Prevedello DM. Safety and effectiveness of endoscopic endonasal intracranial aneurysm clipping: a systematic review. Neurosurg Rev. 2021;44:889–96. https://doi.org/10.1007/s10143-020-01316-0.

76. Meling TR, Romundstad L, Niemi G, Narum J, Eide PK, Sorteberg AG, Sorteberg WA. Adenosine-assisted clipping of intracranial aneurysms. Neurosurg Rev. 2018;41:585–92. https://doi.org/10.1007/s10143-017-0896-y.

77. Allgaier M, Neyazi B, Preim B, Saalfeld S. Distance and force visualisations for improved simulation of intracranial aneurysm clipping. Int J Comput Assist Radiol Surg. 2021;16:1297–304. https://doi.org/10.1007/s11548-021-02413-1.

78. Meling TR, Patet G. The role of EC-IC bypass in ICA blood blister aneurysms—a systematic review. Neurosurg Rev. 2021;44:905–14. https://doi.org/10.1007/s10143-020-01302-6.

79. Beitzke M, Leber KA, Deutschmann H, Gattringer T, Poltrum B, Fazekas F. Cerebrovascular complications and granuloma formation after wrapping or coating of intracranial aneurysms with cotton gauze and human fibrin adhesives: results from a single-center patient series over a 5-year period. J Neurosurg. 2013;119:1009–14. https://doi.org/10.3171/2013.6.JNS1373.

80. Germanò A, Priola S, Angileri FF, Conti A, La Torre D, Cardali S, Raffa G, Merlo L, Granata F, Longo M, et al. Long-term follow-up of ruptured intracranial aneurysms treated by microsurgical wrapping with autologous muscle. Neurosurg Rev. 2013;36:123. https://doi.org/10.1007/s10143-012-0408-z.

81. Frisoli FA, Catapano JS, Benner D, Lawton MT. Creation of a middle communicating artery with external carotid artery-radial artery graft-M2 middle cerebral artery interpositional bypass and M2 middle cerebral artery-M2 middle cerebral artery reimplantation for a recurrent middle cerebral artery aneurysm: 2-dimensional operative video. Oper Neurosurg (Hagerstown). 2020;20:E44–5. https://doi.org/10.1093/ons/opaa244.

82. Dietrich C, Hauck GH, Valvassori L, Hauck EF. Transradial access or Simmons shaped 8F guide enables delivery of flow diverters in patients with large intracranial aneurysms and type III aortic arch: technical case report. Neurosurgery. 2013;73 https://doi.org/10.1227/NEU.0b013e31827e0d67.

83. Lin L-M, Bender MT, Colby GP, Beaty NB, Jiang B, Campos JK, Huang J, Tamargo RJ, Coon AL. Use of a next-generation multi-durometer long guide sheath for triaxial access in flow diversion: experience in 95 consecutive cases. J Neurointerv Surg. 2018;10:137–42. https://doi.org/10.1136/neurintsurg-2017-013184.

84. Hassan AE, Burke EM, Monayao M, Tekle WG. Utilization of the ballast long guiding sheath for neuroendovascular procedures: institutional experience in 68 cases. Front Neurol. 2021;12:578446. https://doi.org/10.3389/fneur.2021.578446.

85. Chen SH, Peterson EC. Radial access for neurointervention: room set-up and technique for diagnostic angiography. J Neurointerv Surg. 2021;13:96. https://doi.org/10.1136/neurintsurg-2019-015692.

86. Kühn AL, Satti SR, Eden T, de Macedo Rodrigues K, Singh J, Massari F, Gounis MJ, Puri AS. Anatomic snuffbox (distal radial artery) and radial artery access for treatment of intracranial aneurysms with FDA-approved flow diverters. AJNR Am J Neuroradiol. 2021;42:487–92. https://doi.org/10.3174/ajnr.A6953.

87. Wang D, Wang Y, Su W, Wang Y, Li G, Li X. A novel approach using neuron 6F guiding catheter for the embolization of intracranial aneurysm with coiling of the parent internal carotid artery. Int J Clin Exp Med. 2015;8:1534–9.

88. Mendes Pereira V, Nicholson P, Cancelliere NM, Liu XYE, Agid R, Radovanovic I, Krings T. Feasibility of robot-assisted neuroendovascular procedures. J Neurosurg. 2021;136:992. https://doi.org/10.3171/2021.1.JNS203617.

89. Xu Y, Tian W, Wei Z, Li Y, Gao X, Li W, Dong B. Microcatheter shaping using three-dimensional printed models for intracranial aneurysm coiling. J Neurointerv Surg. 2020;12:308–10. https://doi.org/10.1136/neurintsurg-2019-015346.

90. Yamaguchi S, Ito O, Koyanagi Y, Iwaki K, Matsukado K. Microcatheter shaping using intravascular placement during intracranial aneurysm coiling. Interv Neuroradiol. 2017;23:249–54. https://doi.org/10.1177/1591019917689926.

91. Zhao K-J, Zhao R, Huang Q-H, Xu Y, Hong B, Fang Y-B, Li Q, Yang P-F, Liu J-M, Zhao W-Y. The

interaction between stent(s) implantation, PICA involvement, and immediate occlusion degree affect symptomatic intracranial spontaneous vertebral artery dissection aneurysm (sis-VADA) recurrence after reconstructive treatment with stent(s)-assisted coiling. Eur Radiol. 2014;24:2088–96. https://doi.org/10.1007/s00330-014-3225-7.

92. Cagnazzo F, Mantilla D, Rouchaud A, Brinjikji W, Lefevre PH, Dargazanli C, Gascou G, Riquelme C, Perrini P, di Carlo D, et al. Endovascular treatment of very large and Giant intracranial aneurysms: comparison between reconstructive and deconstructive techniques-a meta-analysis. AJNR Am J Neuroradiol. 2018;39:852–8. https://doi.org/10.3174/ajnr.A5591.

93. Sattur MG, Welz ME, Bendok BR, Miller JW. Balloon occlusion testing to assess retinal collateral and predict visual outcomes in the management of a fusiform intraorbital ophthalmic artery aneurysm: technical note and literature review. Oper Neurosurg (Hagerstown). 2019;16:60–6. https://doi.org/10.1093/ons/opy087.

94. Tsuji Y, Miki T, Kakita H, Sato K, Yoshida T, Shimizu F. Parent artery occlusion for treatment of a traumatic pericallosal artery aneurysm: case report and review of the literature. World Neurosurg. 2020;140:193–7. https://doi.org/10.1016/j.wneu.2020.04.186.

95. Fujimura S, Takao H, Suzuki T, Dahmani C, Ishibashi T, Mamori H, Yamamoto M, Murayama Y. Hemodynamics and coil distribution with changing coil stiffness and length in intracranial aneurysms. J Neurointerv Surg. 2018;10:797–801. https://doi.org/10.1136/neurintsurg-2017-013457.

96. Guenego A, Zerlauth J-B, Puccinelli F, Hajdu S, Rotzinger DC, Zibold F, Piechowiak EI, Mordasini P, Gralla J, Dobrocky T, et al. Balloon-assisted coil embolization and large stent delivery for cerebral aneurysms with a new generation of dual lumen balloons (Copernic 2L). J Neurointerv Surg. 2018;10:395–400. https://doi.org/10.1136/neurintsurg-2017-013218.

97. Chung J, Lim YC, Suh SH, Shim YS, Kim YB, Joo J-Y, Kim B-S, Shin YS. Stent-assisted coil embolization of ruptured wide-necked aneurysms in the acute period: incidence of and risk factors for periprocedural complications. J Neurosurg. 2014;121 https://doi.org/10.3171/2014.4.JNS131662.

98. Chua MMJ, Silveira L, Moore J, Pereira VM, Thomas AJ, Dmytriw AA. Flow diversion for treatment of intracranial aneurysms: mechanism and implications. Ann Neurol. 2019;85:793–800. https://doi.org/10.1002/ana.25484.

99. Pagano P, Paiusan L, Soize S, Pierot L. Intracranial aneurysm treatment with intrasaccular flow disruption: comparison of WEB-21 and WEB-17 systems. J Neurointerv Surg. 2021;14:904. https://doi.org/10.1136/neurintsurg-2021-017876.

100. Andrews RJ, Bringas JR. A review of brain retraction and recommendations for minimizing intraoperative brain injury. Neurosurgery. 1993;33:1052.

101. Komotar RJ, Zacharia BE, Otten ML, Mocco J, Lavine SD. Controversies in the endovascular management of cerebral vasospasm after intracranial aneurysm rupture and future directions for therapeutic approaches. Neurosurgery. 2008;62 https://doi.org/10.1227/01.neu.0000318175.05591.c3.

102. Han M-H, Won YD, Na MK, Kim CH, Kim JM, Ryu JI, Yi H-J, Cheong JH. Association between possible osteoporosis and shunt-dependent hydrocephalus after subarachnoid hemorrhage. Stroke. 2018;49:1850–8. https://doi.org/10.1161/STROKEAHA.118.021063.

103. Keränen T, Tapaninaho A, Hernesniemi J, Vapalahti M. Late epilepsy after aneurysm operations. Neurosurgery. 1985;17:897–900.

104. Sharma D. Perioperative management of aneurysmal subarachnoid hemorrhage. Anesthesiology. 2020;133:1283–305. https://doi.org/10.1097/ALN.0000000000003558.

105. Langmoen IA, Ekseth K, Hauglie-Hanssen E, Nornes H. Surgical treatment of anterior circulation aneurysms. Acta Neurochir Suppl. 1999;72:107–21.

106. Endo T, Tominaga T, Konno H, Yoshimoto T. Fatal subarachnoid hemorrhage, with brainstem and cerebellar infarction, caused by Aspergillus infection after cerebral aneurysm surgery: case report. Neurosurgery. 2002;50:1147.

107. Chang C-H, Jung Y-J, Kim J-H. Intraprocedural rupture management for intracranial aneurysm rupture during coil embolization by manual common carotid artery compression. J Clin Neurosci. 2019;62:273–6. https://doi.org/10.1016/j.jocn.2018.12.025.

108. Molyneux A, Kerr R, Stratton I, Sandercock P, Clarke M, Shrimpton J, Holman R. International Subarachnoid Aneurysm Trial (ISAT) of neurosurgical clipping versus endovascular coiling in 2143 patients with ruptured intracranial aneurysms: a randomised trial. Lancet. 2002;360:1267–74.

109. Ding D, Liu KC. Management strategies for intraprocedural coil migration during endovascular treatment of intracranial aneurysms. J Neurointerv Surg. 2014;6:428–31. https://doi.org/10.1136/neurintsurg-2013-010872.

110. Li C-H, Su X-H, Zhang B, Han Y-F, Zhang E-W, Yang L, Zhang D-L, Yang S-T, Yan Z-Q, Gao B-L. The stent-assisted coil-jailing technique facilitates efficient embolization of tiny cerebral aneurysms. Korean J Radiol. 2014;15:850–7. https://doi.org/10.3348/kjr.2014.15.6.850.

111. Gao B-L, Li M-H, Wang Y-L, Fang C. Delayed coil migration from a small wide-necked aneurysm after stent-assisted embolization: case report and literature review. Neuroradiology. 2006;48:333–7.

Incidental Cavernous Malformations

9

Meng Wang and Fuyou Guo

9.1 Introduction

Cavernous angiomas (CAs), more commonly known as "cavernomas," are low-flow vascular abnormalities of the brain composed of clusters of dilated, thin-walled capillaries filled with thrombus [1]. These lesions account for 15% of all vascular malformations and have an estimated prevalence approaching 0.6% in the general population [2]. Patients with familial CAs typically harbor multiple lesions, unlike those with a sporadic form who usually present with a single lesion [3]. CAs are typically located supratentorially; brainstem lesions account only for 8–22% of all cases.

9.2 Genetics

Up to 50% of CAs are familial and follow an autosomal dominant pattern of inheritance linked to the CCM1, CCM2, and CCM3 genes on 7q, 7p, and 3q, respectively [3–5]. In most cases, it can be a nonsense, frameshift, or splice site mutation, resulting in a non-functional protein product. In some cases, there can be a deletion or duplication of multiple exons or the entire gene [6].

9.3 Epidemiology

CAs have an incidence of <1%, an annual hemorrhage risk of up to 3%, and a rebleed risk of 4.5–23% per year [7]. They are the second most common form of intravascular malformations, after developmental venous anomaly. CAs can be presented in any age group, though it is found to be more common during the third decade of life [8]. The overall prevalence of familial CA is about 1:3300–1:3800, and the occurrence of symptomatic hereditary mutations is approximately 1:5400–1:6200 [9].

9.4 Pathology

CAs are single-layer endothelin-lined vascular spaces without intervening brain parenchymal tissue within them [10]. There is low pressure and slow flow of blood within the lesion, which results in thrombus formation, followed by its organization, and this occurs in a repetitive fashion. These features are grossly visualized as the characteristic "mulberry appearance" [11].There is insufficiency of the tight and adherens junctions of the endothelial cells, resulting in leaking and a dysfunctional blood-brain barrier [9].

M. Wang (✉) · F. Guo
Department of Neurosurgery, The First Affiliated Hospital of Zhengzhou University,
Zhengzhou, Henan Province, China

International Joint Laboratory of Nervous System Malformation, Zhengzhou, Henan Province, China

9.5 Clinical Presentation

CAs can have varied presentations depending on the location of the lesion. They can be supratentorial, which affects the cerebral cortex, and infratentorial, affecting the brainstem or the cerebellum [7]. When these lesions become symptomatic, it can have a wide array of clinical presentation that includes seizures, hemorrhage, headache, and focal neurological deficits [12]. Supratentorial lesions have been found to present more commonly with seizures, whereas infratentorial malformations present with focal neurological deficits.

9.6 Diagnosis

CA diagnosis is particularly challenging to the practicing physicians because they tend to be angiographically occult due to the slow blood flow through them. Computed tomography scans can detect lesions that are complicated by hemorrhage or calcification but lack the sensitivity and specificity to detect smaller lesions; hence, it is not the primary modality for diagnosis of these lesions. Magnetic resonance imaging (MRI) is the most sensitive and specific imaging modality for the diagnosis and follow-up of CAs [13]. Typically, the lesions appear as areas of mixed signal intensity on T1- and T2-weighted images and are surrounded by a peripheral area of hypointensity (representing a hemosiderin ring) on T2-weighted images [14]. Gradient recall echo MRI is used for the accurate detection of CA due to the characteristic hypointensity produced due to detection of hemosiderin-filled brain parenchyma [15]. Susceptibility-weighted MRI is more precise in detecting vascular malformations due to its high sensitivity to deoxyhemoglobin and iron content. This is the only imaging method that can detect capillary telangiectasias and cavernomas that are non-hemorrhagic (Fig. 9.1) [16].

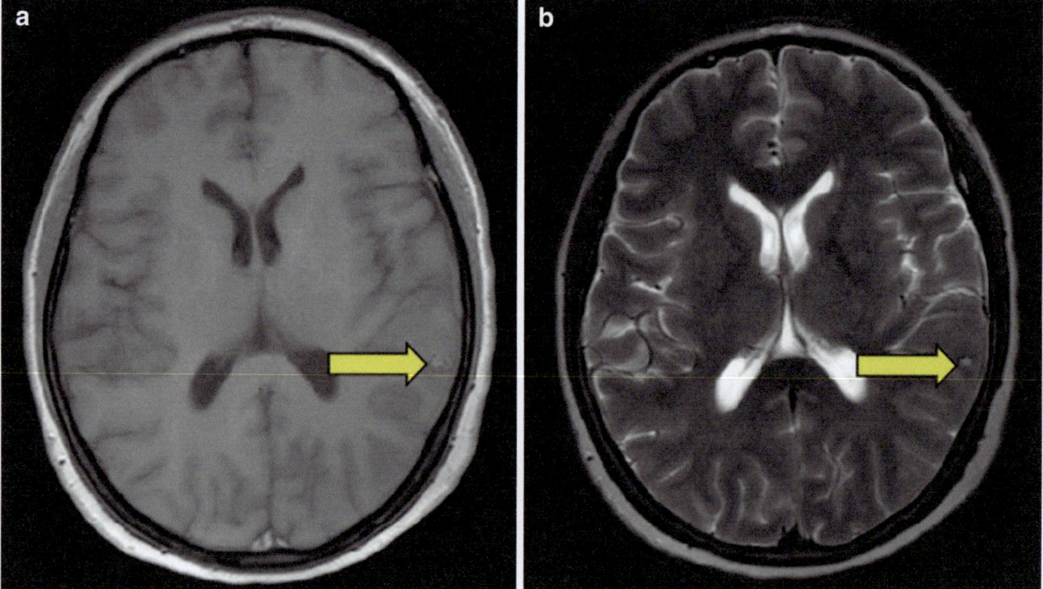

Fig. 9.1 Incidental left temporal lobe cavernous angioma in a 52-year-old woman (yellow arrows). Axial T1 (**a**), T2 (**b**), T2 FLAIR (**c**), and susceptibility-weighted magnetic resonance imaging (**d**)

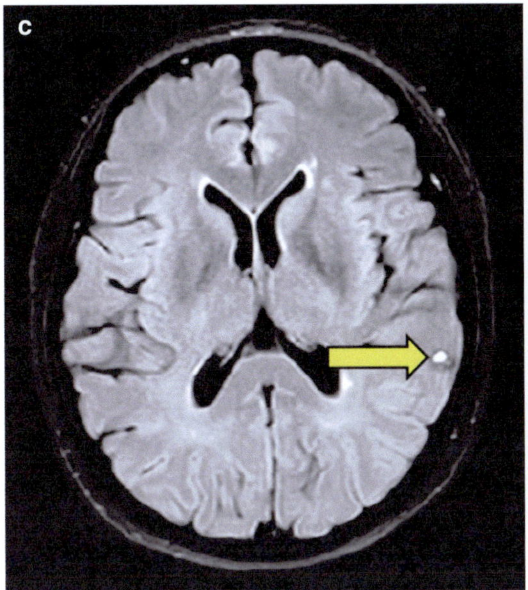 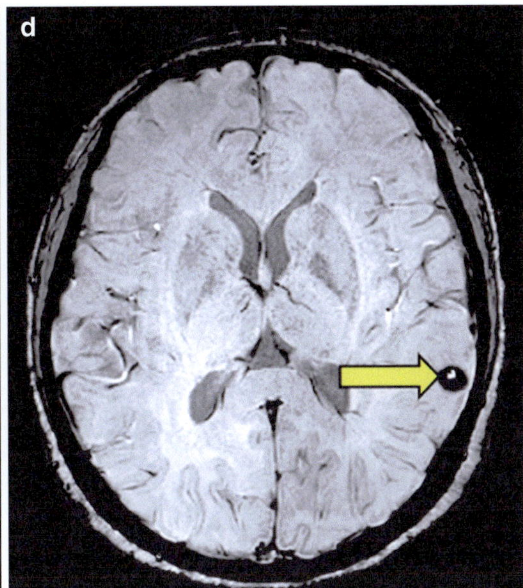

Fig. 9.1 (continued)

9.7 Natural History and Management of Incidentally Discovered Cavernous Angiomas

The annual rate of symptomatic hemorrhage from a CA ranges from 0.7% to 6% according to multiple studies and varies with a number of factors. The risk of significant bleeding is higher in patients with a prior history of hemorrhage [2]. In a study involving 122 patients with CAs, Kondziolka et al. reported an annual hemorrhage rate of 0.6% in patients with no hemorrhagic presentation versus 4.5% for patients with hemorrhagic presentation [17]. It is worth noting that the risk of rebleeding is particularly high in the 2 years following the initial hemorrhage but seems to significantly decrease thereafter. Purely incidental CAs should be managed conservatively and followed with yearly MRI. We recommend surgical management of CAs is indicated in the following situations: intractable seizures, progressive significant neurological deficit, after the first clinically significant hemorrhage in non-eloquent areas, and after the second clinically significant hemorrhage in eloquent areas including the brainstem.

9.8 Conclusion

Incidentally discovered intracranial vascular abnormalities are increasingly coming to the attention of neurosurgeons with the ubiquitous availability of high-quality, non-invasive imaging studies. CAs may be incidentally discovered on brain imaging studies. CAs are associated with their own unique natural history, and management must be tailored to the type of lesion and individual circumstances of a given patient. In this chapter, we have attempted to provide an evidence-based resource to guide neurosurgeons in the management of incidentally CAs. The quality and quantity of evidence, however, remains limited, and further studies are needed to elucidate the most appropriate management strategy in many situations.

References

1. Gault J, Sarin H, Awadallah NA, Shenkar R, Awad IA. Pathobiology of human cerebrovascular malformations: basic mechanisms and clinical relevance. Neurosurgery. 2004;55(1):1–17.
2. Chalouhi N, Dumont AS, Randazzo C, Tjoumakaris S, Gonzalez LF, Rosenwasser R, Jabbour P. Management of incidentally discovered intracranial vascular abnormalities. Neurosurg Focus. 2011;31(6):E1.
3. Laberge-le Couteulx S, Jung HH, Labauge P, Houtteville JP, Lescoat C, Cecillon M, Marechal E, Joutel A, Bach JF, Tournier-Lasserve E. Truncating mutations in CCM1, encoding KRIT1, cause hereditary cavernous angiomas. Nat Genet. 1999;23(2):189–93.
4. Bergametti F, Denier C, Labauge P, Arnoult M, Boetto S, Clanet M, Coubes P, Echenne B, Ibrahim R, Irthum B, Jacquet G, Lonjon M, Moreau JJ, Neau JP, Parker F, Tremoulet M, Tournier-Lasserve E, Société Française de Neurochirurgie. Mutations within the programmed cell death 10 gene cause cerebral cavernous malformations. Am J Hum Genet. 2005;76(1):42–51.
5. Jabbour P, Gault J, Awad IA. What genes can teach us about human cerebrovascular malformations. Clin Neurosurg. 2004;51:140–2.
6. Akers A, Al-Shahi Salman R, Awad IA, Dahlem K, Flemming K, Hart B, Kim H, Jusue-Torres I, Kondziolka D, Lee C, Morrison L, Rigamonti D, Rebeiz T, Tournier-Lasserve E, Waggoner D, Whitehead K. Synopsis of guidelines for the clinical management of cerebral cavernous malformations: consensus recommendations based on systematic literature review by the angioma alliance scientific advisory board clinical experts panel. Neurosurgery. 2017;80(5):665–80.
7. Idiculla PS, Gurala D, Philipose J, Rajdev K, Patibandla P. Cerebral cavernous malformations, developmental venous anomaly, and its coexistence: a review. Eur Neurol. 2020;83(4):360–8.
8. Dalyai RT, Ghobrial G, Awad I, Tjoumakaris S, Gonzalez LF, Dumont AS, Chalouhi N, Randazzo C, Rosenwasser R, Jabbour P. Management of incidental cavernous malformations: a review. Neurosurg Focus. 2011;31(6):E5.
9. Spiegler S, Rath M, Paperlein C, Felbor U. Cerebral cavernous malformations: an update on prevalence, molecular genetic analyses, and genetic counselling. Mol Syndromol. 2018;9(2):60–9.
10. Josephson CB, Rosenow F, Al-Shahi Salman R. Intracranial vascular malformations and epilepsy. Semin Neurol. 2015;35(3):223–34.
11. Clatterbuck RE, Eberhart CG, Crain BJ, Rigamonti D. Ultrastructural and immunocytochemical evidence that an incompetent blood-brain barrier is related to the pathophysiology of cavernous malformations. J Neurol Neurosurg Psychiatry. 2001;71(2):188–92.
12. Gross BA, Lin N, Du R, Day AL. The natural history of intracranial cavernous malformations. Neurosurg Focus. 2011;30(6):E24.
13. Rigamonti D, Johnson PC, Spetzler RF, Hadley MN, Drayer BP. Cavernous malformations and capillary telangiectasia: a spectrum within a single pathological entity. Neurosurgery. 1991;28(1):60–4.
14. Rivera PP, Willinsky RA, Porter PJ. Intracranial cavernous malformations. Neuroimaging Clin N Am. 2003;13(1):27–40.
15. de Champfleur NM, Langlois C, Ankenbrandt WJ, Le Bars E, Leroy MA, Duffau H, Bonafé A, Jaffe J, Awad IA, Labauge P. Magnetic resonance imaging evaluation of cerebral cavernous malformations with susceptibility-weighted imaging. Neurosurgery. 2011;68(3):641–8.
16. Pinker K, Stavrou I, Szomolanyi P, Hoeftberger R, Weber M, Stadlbauer A, Noebauer-Huhmann IM, Knosp E, Trattnig S. Improved preoperative evaluation of cerebral cavernomas by high-field, high-resolution susceptibility-weighted magnetic resonance imaging at 3 Tesla: comparison with standard (1.5 T) magnetic resonance imaging and correlation with histopathological findings—preliminary results. Investig Radiol. 2007;42(6):346–51.
17. Kondziolka D, Lunsford LD, Kestle JR. The natural history of cerebral cavernous malformations. J Neurosurg. 1995;83(5):820–4.

Yuchao Zuo and Fuyou Guo

10.1 Introduction

Vertebrobasilar dolichoectasia (VBD) is an uncommon disease characterized by significant expansion, elongation, and tortuosity of the vertebrobasilar arteries (Fig. 10.1a–c). Although there is no current data on the exact incidence of VBD in the general population, angiography and autopsy results suggest that the overall incidence is 0.05–0.6% [1, 2]. A Japanese study revealed that among people undergoing routine magnetic resoance imaging (MRI) and magnetic resonance angiography (MRA) examinations, the asymptomatic VBD incidence rate was 1.3% [3].

Exact etiology of VBD is unknown; however, it is observed in association with several other diseases like atherosclerosis, hypertension, collagen vascular disease, polycystic kidney disease, and sickle cell anemia [4]. An imbalance between matrix metalloproteinase and antiprotease activity within the connective tissue of arterial wall leading to aberrant vascular remodeling and defective connective tissue formation within the wall of arteries is thought to be causative mechanism in development of this disease [4]. VBD is diagnosed incidentally in most of the cases [5]. Symptomatic patients may present with vascular symptoms like episodes of transient ischemic attacks, ischemic strokes, subarachnoid hemorrhages, obstructive hydrocephalus, or with compressive symptoms related to brainstem or cranial nerve compression [5]. The natural clinical history of patients affected by VBD is unfavorable with 7.8 years of median survival [6].

Nowadays, there are no widely accepted quantitative standards for VBD diagnostic imaging. Diagnosis of VBD usually relies on assessment of the patient's vascular images by clinicians and radiologists. Dilatation can be diagnosed when, at any point, the basilar artery diameter is greater than 4.5 mm [7]. The MRA standards raised by Ubogu define extension by MRA as the length of basilar artery greater than 29.5 mm or the vertical distance from the connection of the basilar artery starting point and a bifurcation point greater than 10 mm. For vertebral arteries, if the length is greater than 23.5 mm, or at any point the vertical distance from the connection of the skull entry point and the basilar artery starting point is greater than 10 mm, it is considered extension [8].

Y. Zuo (✉) · F. Guo
Department of Neurosurgery, The First Affiliated
Hospital of Zhengzhou University,
Zhengzhou, Henan Province, China

International Joint Laboratory of Nervous System
Malformation, Zhengzhou, Henan Province, China

M. Turgut et al. (eds.), *Incidental Findings of the Nervous System*,
https://doi.org/10.1007/978-3-031-42595-0_10

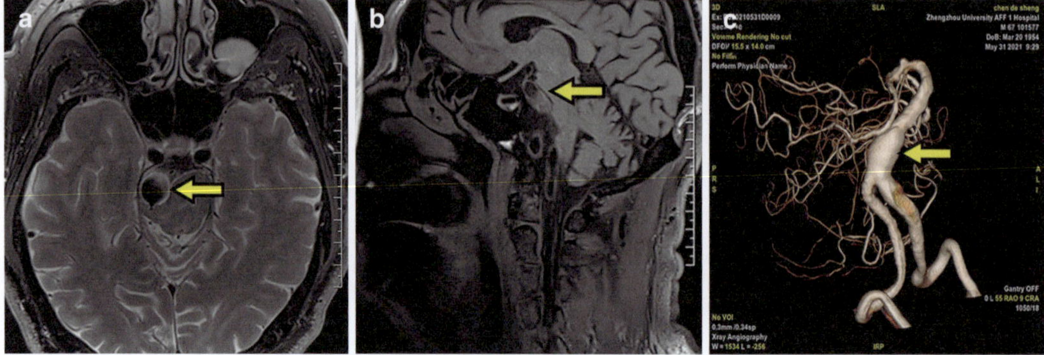

Fig. 10.1 Vertebrobasilar dolichoectasia (VBD) was incidentally found in a 68-year-old man, the typical images in view of magnetic resonance imaging (MRI) and digital subtraction angiography (DSA). (**a**) VBD showed vascular flow voids signal (yellow arrow) on T2-weighted image. (**b**) Sagittal view on T1-weighted image showed compression (yellow arrow) on the pons. (**c**) 3D-DSA showed expansion, elongation, and tortuosity of the vertebra-basilar artery (yellow arrow)

10.2 Patient Selection and Preoperative Evaluation

Preoperative evaluation including cranial computed tomography or MRI, cerebral computed tomography angiography/MRA/digital subtraction angiography (DSA), clinical presentation, associated syndromes, general status. The clinical symptoms and neuroimaging evaluation are essential factors that determine the optimal treatment planning for each patient. Surgical therapy for VBD is indicated if the patient demonstrates as follows: (1) obvious neurological deficits caused by vascular events (ischemic or hemorrhage) or hydrocephalus; (2) associated syndromes or symptoms: brainstem compression, trigeminal neuralgia, hemifacial spasm, compression of other cranial nerves, patients had previously received medical treatment for years until the treating physician determined that surgical treatment was indicated.

10.3 Surgical Principles

At present, there is no universally accepted effective treatment and surgery is associated with high morbidity and mortality. For VBD itself, there is currently no precise and effective treatment, and available treatments mainly target selected symptoms or VBD complications. Endovascular flow diverter/stent placement with or without coiling may be effective in selected patients [2].

10.4 Surgical Therapy for VBD

A variety of treatments are available to control VBD-induced drug-refractory trigeminal neuralgia and hemifacial spasm, including radiofrequency ablation, gamma-knife, percutaneous balloon compression of the trigeminal nerve, and botulinum toxin injection. However, the most effective treatment is microvascular decompression.

The patients were positioned contralaterally after general anesthesia. The dura mater was cut after retrosigmoid craniectomy and then was suspended to release the appropriate amount of cerebrospinal fluid to provide space for operation. Through arachnoid dissection and slight elevation of the cerebellum, the neurovascular conflicts located at the trigeminal nerve root entry zone were carefully observed using an operating microscope [9].

In order to decompress the trigeminal nerve by dolichoectatic artery, two different microvascular decompression techniques were used [9]: interposition technique and transposition technique. In the interposition subgroup, the author introduced the chopped Teflon felt implant into

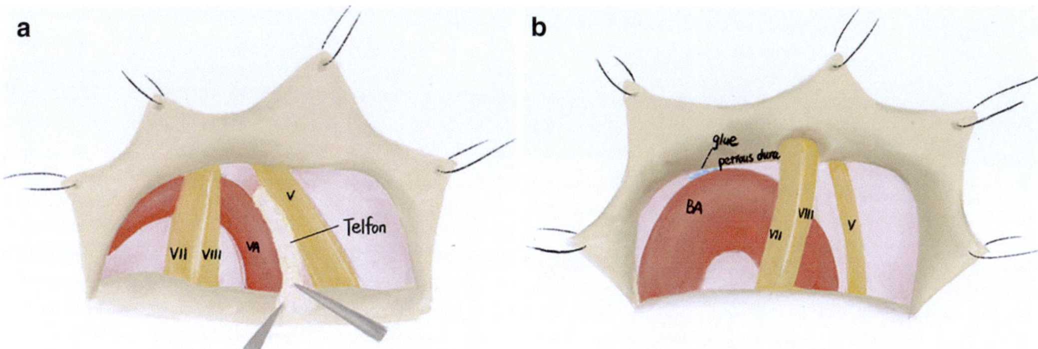

Fig. 10.2 Intraoperative pictures of intervention method and transposition method. (**a**) Intervention method: the Teflon felt was inserted between the trigeminal nerve and VA. (**b**) Transposition method: the basilar artery was fixed on the nearby petrous dura mater by using biological glue and a space was created between the trigeminal nerve and the BA. (Zhao et al. Comparison of Microvascular Decompression and Two Isocenters Gamma Knife for the Treatment of Trigeminal Neuralgia Caused by Vertebrobasilar Dolichoectasia. Front Neurol. 2021; 12: 707985)

the conflicting neurovascular area between the artery and nervous structures, thereby separating the VBD from the trigeminal nerve (Fig. 10.2a), while in the transposition subgroup, the proximal part of the vertebrobasilar artery was moved ventrally and cranially through the gap between the IX and VII–VIII nerves, and then fixed on the nearby petrous bone wall with biomedical glue (Fig. 10.2b). It is worth noting that the perforating arteries should be protected to avoid secondary damage when suspended and to avoid twisting into angles for the responsible blood vessels [10].

10.5 Endovascular Interventional Techniques

Flow diversion technology refers to the placement of stents in aneurysm-bearing arteries in order to reduce blood flow into the aneurysm and form venous stasis, which leads to gradual thrombosis and neointimal coverage, and the normal functioning of the surrounding arteries and perforating arteries is maintained.

The patient was taken to neurointerventional suite and placed under general anesthesia. A complete six-vessel cerebral DSA demonstrated severe dolichoectasia involving the left vertebral and the basilar arteries (Fig. 10.1c): Through a 6 French sheath, a 6F neuron guide catheter was used to catheterize the left vertebral artery. The patient was given 3000 units of heparin intravenous injection. A Marksman catheter (Covidien, CA) along with a Synchro 2 (Stryker, MI) standard microwire was navigated through the left dolichoectatic vertebral artery into the basilar artery [11]. Next, pipeline embolization device (PED) was deployed in a telescoping fashion starting from proximal part of the basilar artery down to the left vertebral artery, essentially reconstructing the entire length of the affected vertebrobasilar system. Six months later, a cerebral angiogram after the PED placement demonstrated good patency of the target vessels and there was thrombosis outside the PED and the cavity of VBD reduced (Fig. 10.3). The patient was continued on aspirin 100 mg and clopidogrel 75 mg daily.

The advantage of releasing of stents can reduce blood flow in the aneurysm cavity, increase forward flow, straighten tortuous vessels, and increase blood supply to branching arteries. The use of antiplatelet drugs after stent implantation can reduce thrombosis and the risk of bleeding is lower compared to using antiplatelet drugs alone.

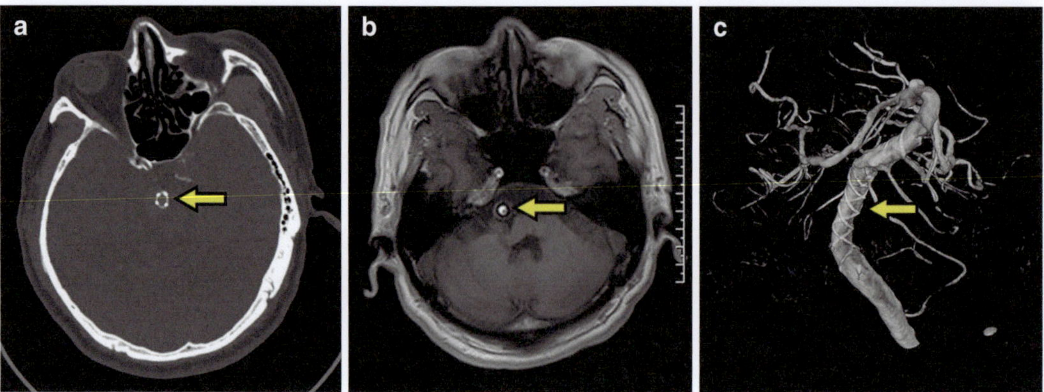

Fig. 10.3 Postoperative findings of endovascular approach. (**a**) Thrombus around the stent (yellow arrow) were shown in VBD in the axial images of computed tomography. (**b**) The cavity of the stent (yellow arrow) was shown in VBD in the axial images of MRI. (**c**) 3D-DSA showed the cavity of VBD (yellow arrow) reduced obviously

10.6 Postoperative Complications

After decompression surgery, most patients underwent pain relief, the postoperative complications mainly included hearing loss, taste hypoesthesia and wound infection, dry eyes, hearing loss, numbness, facial palsy, diplopia, and cerebrospinal fluid leakage [9].

After stent implantation, the most common complication in VBD is brain stem infarction, with an incidence rate as high as 22.2% [12], due to occlusion of the branching vessels, but excessive anticoagulation treatment may result in fatal bleeding risks. The combination of stent construction and anticoagulant therapy may lower the risk of artery rupture and bleeding compared to anticoagulant or antiplatelet therapy alone. Stent construction can reduce the cavity of VBD, thereby mitigating the mass effects of VBD, including cranial nerve compression and hydrocephalus, and thus deserves further clinical validation. The key to reducing the incidence of complications is to gradually change the hemodynamics in VBD. In light of this, staging surgery and minimizing the use of coils should be considered to optimize the surgery.

10.7 Conclusion

VBD is a complex progressive arterial disease whose pathogenesis needs further investigation. It has complex clinical manifestations, poor prognosis, and a median survival of only 7.8 years. VBD in adult likely represent an incidental finding on routine MRI. Operation for VBD was difficult, surgery should be cautious, and the surgery was used to improve the presentation of symptomatic patients and stopped the deterioration of the asymptomatic cases. Currently, there is no standard protocol for the management of VBD. However, when surgery is discussed, the surgeon should always consider his experience and institutional practice, potential operational risk as well as individual management.

References

1. Vanaclocha V, Herrera JM, Martinez-Gomez D, Rivera-Paz M, Calabuig-Bayo C, Vanaclocha L. Is there a safe and effective way to treat trigeminal neuralgia associated with vertebrobasilar dolichoectasia? Presentation of 8 cases and literature review. World Neurosurg. 2016;96:516–29.
2. Yuan YJ, Xu K, Luo Q, Yu JL. Research progress on vertebrobasilar dolichoectasia. Int J Med Sci. 2014;11(10):1039–48.
3. Ikeda K, Nakamura Y, Hirayama T, Sekine T, Nagata R, Kano O, Kawabe K, Kiyozuka T, Tamura M, Iwasaki Y. Cardiovascular risk and neuroradiological profiles in asymptomatic vertebrobasilar dolichoectasia. Cerebrovasc Dis. 2010;30(1):23–8.
4. Samim M, Goldstein A, Schindler J, Johnson MH. Multimodality imaging of vertebrobasilar dolichoectasia: clinical presentations and imaging spectrum. Radiographics. 2016;36(4):1129–46.
5. Prasad SN, Singh V, Selvamurugan V, Phadke RV. Vertebrobasilar dolichoectasia with typical radiological features. BMJ Case Rep. 2021;14(2):e239866.
6. Umana GE, Alberio N, Graziano F, Fricia M, Tomasi SO, Corbino L, Nicoletti GF, Cicero S, Scalia G. Vertebrobasilar dolichoectasia, hypoplastic third ventricle, and related biventricular hydrocephalus: case report and review of the literature. J Neurol Surg A Cent Eur Neurosurg. 2023;84(2):206–11.
7. Smoker WR, Price MJ, Keyes WD, Corbett JJ, Gentry LR. High-resolution computed tomography of the basilar artery: 1. Normal size and position. AJNR Am J Neuroradiol. 1986;7(1):55–60.
8. Ubogu EE, Zaidat OO. Vertebrobasilar dolichoectasia diagnosed by magnetic resonance angiography and risk of stroke and death: a cohort study. J Neurol Neurosurg Psychiatry. 2004;75(1):22–6.
9. Zhao Z, Chai S, Wang J, Jiang X, Nie C, Zhao H. Comparison of microvascular decompression and two Isocenters gamma knife for the treatment of trigeminal neuralgia caused by vertebrobasilar dolichoectasia. Front Neurol. 2021;12:707985.
10. Liu J, Chen Z, Feng T, Jiang B, Yuan Y, Yu Y. Biomedical glue sling technique in microvascular decompression for trigeminal neuralgia caused by atherosclerotic vertebrobasilar artery: a description of operative technique and clinical outcomes. World Neurosurg. 2019;128:e74–80.
11. Tan LA, Moftakhar R, Lopes DK. Treatment of a ruptured vertebrobasilar fusiform aneurysm using pipeline embolization device. J Cerebrovasc Endovasc Neurosurg. 2013;15(1):30–3.
12. Wu X, Xu Y, Hong B, Zhao WY, Huang QH, Liu JM. Endovascular reconstruction for treatment of vertebrobasilar dolichoectasia: long-term outcomes. AJNR Am J Neuroradiol. 2013;34(3):583–8.

Incidental Benign Developmental Venous Anomaly

11

Yan Hu and Fuyou Guo

11.1 Introduction

Developmental venous anomaly (DVA) is a congenital abnormality found in the venous circuit of the brain, which consists of a group of cerebral venous structures. Typical DVA has many dilated deep medullary veins with a "Medusa-like" or "head of jellyfish" appearance or head pulp configuration, which flow into a small number of dilated deep veins and/or superficial veins, and the arrangement of these structures forms a spider-like shape [1]. It is a rare vascular disease that can be transmitted genetically or spontaneously. However, the etiology is still unknown; some studies previously have shown that it is related to abnormal cerebral circulation and venous reflux.

The prevalence rate of DVA is approximately 0.1–0.5%, and the autopsy finding is 2.6% [2]. DVA is harmless to most patients, but in rare cases, it may be associated with cerebral hemorrhage or other neurological diseases. In general, treatment is needed only when symptoms and concomitant diseases are found. DVA can occur anywhere, usually in the form of a single lesion, most commonly in the frontal parietal lobe, with a reported range of 36–64%, while in the cerebellum, the reported range is 14–27% [2]. Previous studies have found that DVA is often accompanied with cavernous malformation (CM). According to the literature, the correlation rate between CM and DVA is that the clinical manifestations of 2–33% [3]. DVAs vary according to individual differences, and the main symptoms include headache, epilepsy, neurological dysfunction, intracranial hemorrhage, and so on. The treatment needs to be chosen according to the specific conditions of the patients. Anticoagulation therapy and surgical treatments are the main methods for DVA at present, but the effect of radiotherapy on DVA is limited.

11.2 Etiology and Epidemiology

The exact cause of DVA is not clear, but it is believed that the primitive venous drainage pattern persists due to medullary vein thrombosis during embryonic vein development. Histologically, they appear as thin and fragile veins that spread among each other in the brain parenchyma and converge into a single collecting vein, which lacks media [4]. DVA is a rare vascular disease with a prevalence rate of about 0.1–0.5%, which is more common in infants and young people. The incidence is roughly the same for men and women.

Y. Hu · F. Guo (✉)
Department of Neurosurgery, The First Affiliated Hospital of Zhengzhou University,
Zhengzhou, Henan Province, China

International Joint Laboratory of Nervous System Malformation, Zhengzhou, Henan Province, China

11.3 Classification

Based on the different modes of venous reflux, DVA can also be classified according to its relationship with other vascular abnormalities. For example, if DVA is associated with cavernous malformations, capillary hemangiomas, congenital arteriovenous malformations, etc. then it is classified as "compound DVA." In addition, it can also be classified according to different location, which is divided into supratentorial, infratentorial, brainstem DVA.

11.4 Clinical Manifestations

One study from Hon et al. is the only prospective population-based analysis of DVA, uses multiple overlapping sources of case ascertainment in a population of 5.1 million. This systematic review and prospective population-based study confirms that the presentation and clinical course of DVA are usually benign. The study also noted that 98% of DVA was found by accident, and only 2% of DVA was symptomatic and attributed to bleeding or infarction. The natural course of disease in patients with DVA shows that the risk of bleeding after the first onset of DVA is very low, ranging from 0% to 1.28% per year [5]. There may be headache, epilepsy, neurological dysfunction, intracranial hemorrhage, and other symptoms. Aoki et al. [6] reported that there was an association between DVA and venous malformations in the head and neck. Up to 20% of patients with large jugular venous malformations have DVAs. About 10% of DVA patients have CM, and their prevalence increases with age. The incidence of focal neurological disorders such as cerebral hemorrhage, focal epilepsy, and headache in patients with DVA and CM is higher.

1. Headache: headache is one of the most common symptoms of DVA, usually characterized by sudden and severe headache, often accompanied by nausea, vomiting, and other symptoms.
2. Epilepsy: DVA can cause epilepsy, but this condition is not common.
3. Neurological dysfunction: DVA may lead to neurological dysfunction, including limb weakness, sensory abnormalities.
4. Intracranial hemorrhage: with the development of DVA, they become more fragile and may rupture and lead to intracranial hemorrhage, which is a very dangerous condition.

11.5 Diagnosis of DVA

DVAs are often found incidentally on neuroimaging studies; neuroimaging examinations of DVA are the major methods for the diagnosis, including magnetic resonance imaging (MRI), computed tomography (CT), and digital subtraction angiography (DSA).

1. MRI: MRI is the capital method for the diagnosis of DVA, and MRI is the best imaging tool for detecting DVA. The typical manifestation of DVA on T1w and T2w sequences is a flow void in white matter, which passes through the cerebral cortex and may be connected with the cerebral venous system. Depending on the imaging plane, they are usually linear and/or curved or circular. It is worth noting that small DVAs may not be seen clearly in standard non-enhanced sequences [7]. DVA is characterized by low flow and low resistance hemodynamics, so it shows strong enhancement after enhancement (Fig. 11.1). The central collecting veins showed arcuate enhancement from the white matter to the connection with the dura mater or subependymal venous system. The constituent veins of DVA form a wheel-spoke appearance, and the peripheral veins gradually expand as they approach the collecting veins, which are often referred to as the "head of jellyfish" appearance (Figs. 11.2 and 11.3) [8].
2. CT: CT can also be used to diagnose DVA, but it is not as sensitive as MRI for smaller DVA diagnosis.
3. DSA: DSA is the most specific and sensitive method for the diagnosis of DVA. DSA can detect tiny DVA and accurately display its location, size, shape, and vascular supply system (Fig. 11.4) [9].

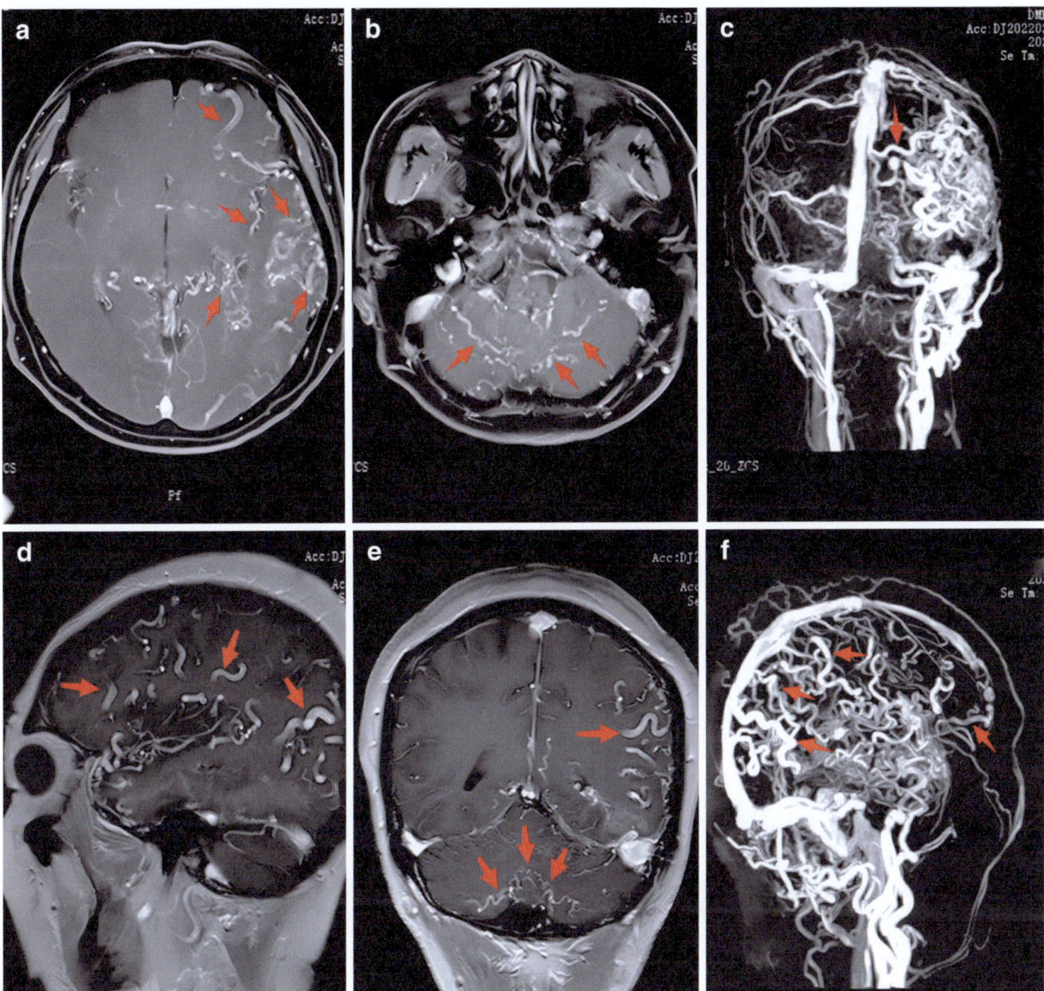

Fig. 11.1 Veins show strong enhancement after T1 enhancement (**a**, **b**, **d**, **e**). Numerous "Medusa-like" abnormal draining veins are visible in the picture, inside the brain and cerebellum (indicated by red arrows). Multiple thick veins converging into the superior sagittal sinus are visible (**c**, **f**)

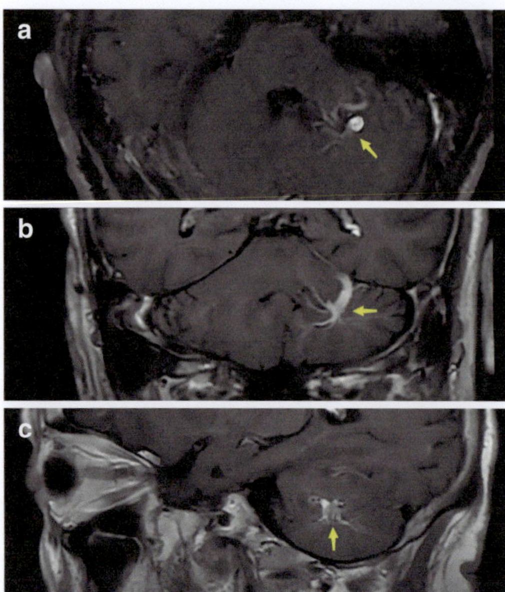

Fig. 11.2 Typical appearance in magnetic resonance imaging (MRI) resembles the "head of a jellyfish" on axial layer (**a**), coronal layer (**b**), and sagittal layer (**c**) (indicated by the yellow arrow)

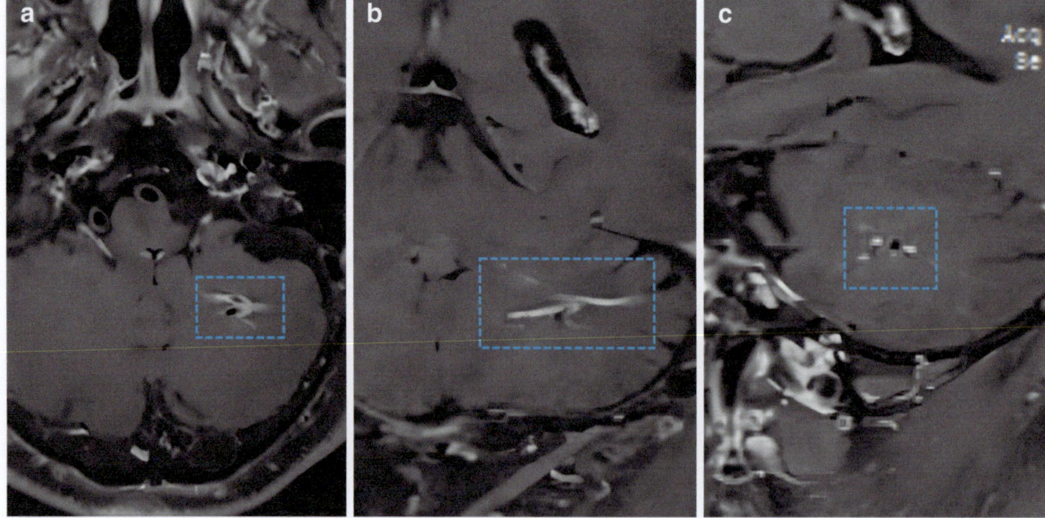

Fig. 11.3 Gadolinium-enhanced gradient-echo T1-weighted MRI showing developmental venous anomaly (DVA) (the blue rectangle) in the left cerebellar hemisphere (**a–c**). Perfusion MRI demonstrates increased values of the corresponding area (the black circle) compared with contralateral normal white matter (**d–f**). It suggests that the nature of the signal intensity abnormalities around DVAs is vasogenic edema with congestion and delayed perfusion. This may explain part of the bleeding caused by DVA

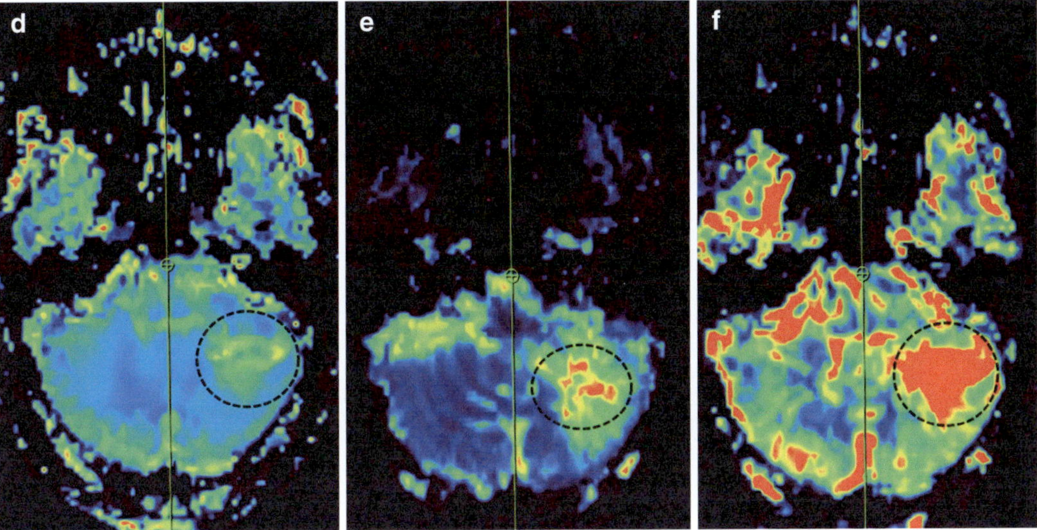

Fig. 11.3 (continued)

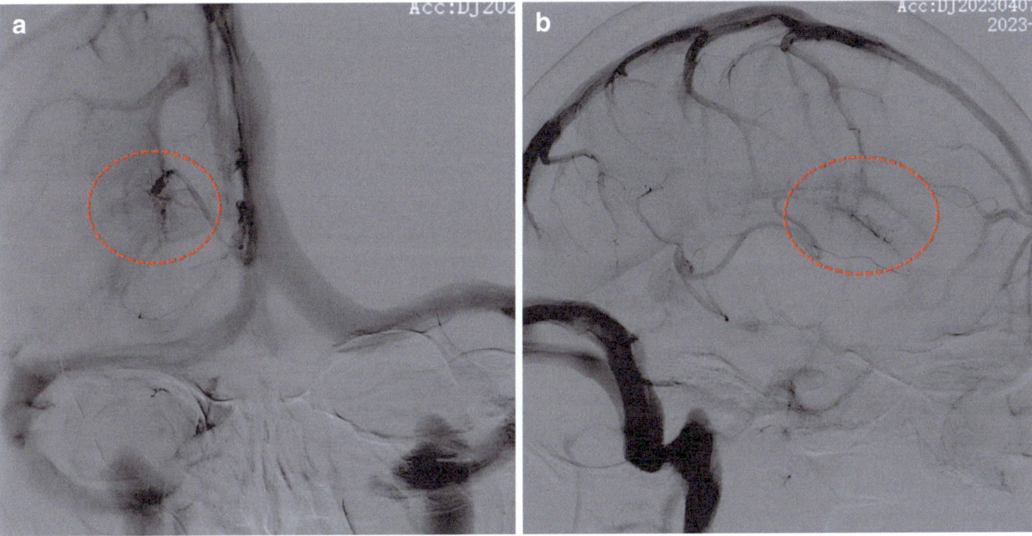

Fig. 11.4 Cerebral angiogram, lateral view depicting venous phase (**a**, **d**) revealing DVA. The lateral view depicting late venous phase (**b**, **c**) revealing DVA. DVA is best viewed in the late venous phases. The DVA (inside the red dashed line) is located superior to the cerebellar curtain and drains to the superior sagittal sinus (**a**, **b**). The DVA (inside the yellow dashed line) is located inferior to the cerebellar curtain and drains to the ethmoid sinus (**c**, **d**)

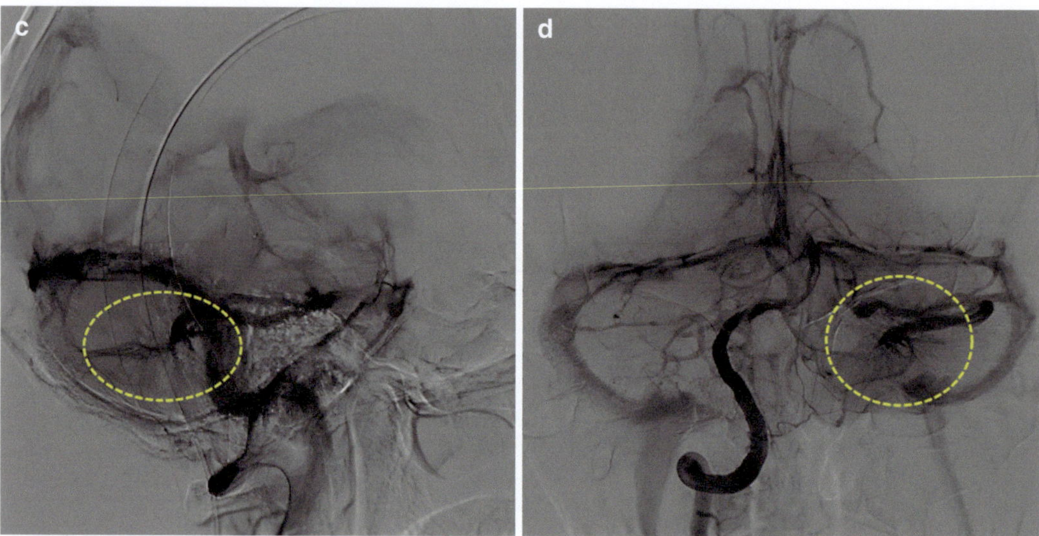

Fig. 11.4 (continued)

11.6 Management of DVA

There is no currently established consensus for DVAs. It is generally accepted that asymptomatic DVAs do not need to be treated. For symptomatic DVA caused by an increase of the inflow, the treatment of the associated arteriovenous malformation or CM by surgery, radiosurgery, or embolization is recommended regarding the high risk of rebleeding. If a draining vein thrombosis is visualized, anticoagulation should be introduced to lower the risk of rebleeding. Consequently, the diverse management should be selected based on preoperative assessment individually.

1. Anticoagulation is considered to be a first-line treatment for DVA with thrombotic symptoms, even if there is a small amount of bleeding [9]. Anticoagulant DVA is used in the treatment of thrombosis to prevent the progression of thrombosis, limit new thrombosis, and promote the recanalization of draining veins [10].

2. Surgical treatment: surgical treatment is the key method for the treatment of hemorrhagic DVA. The mode of operation can choose craniotomy or interventional operation. In the cases of severe hemorrhage and elevated intracranial pressure, intervention may be required in the form of bone flap decompression and/or removal of bleeding (Figs. 11.5 and 11.6) [11]. Interventional therapy is suitable for patients who can't be treated by craniotomy or not suitable for craniotomy. Interventional therapy includes embolization, venous balloon angioplasty, etc.

3. Radiotherapy: DVA do not respond well to gamma knife radiotherapy, have a low disappearance rate after treatment, and can cause radiation brain damage [11].

Fig. 11.5 Comparison between pre- and postcraniotomy for hemorrhage due to DVA

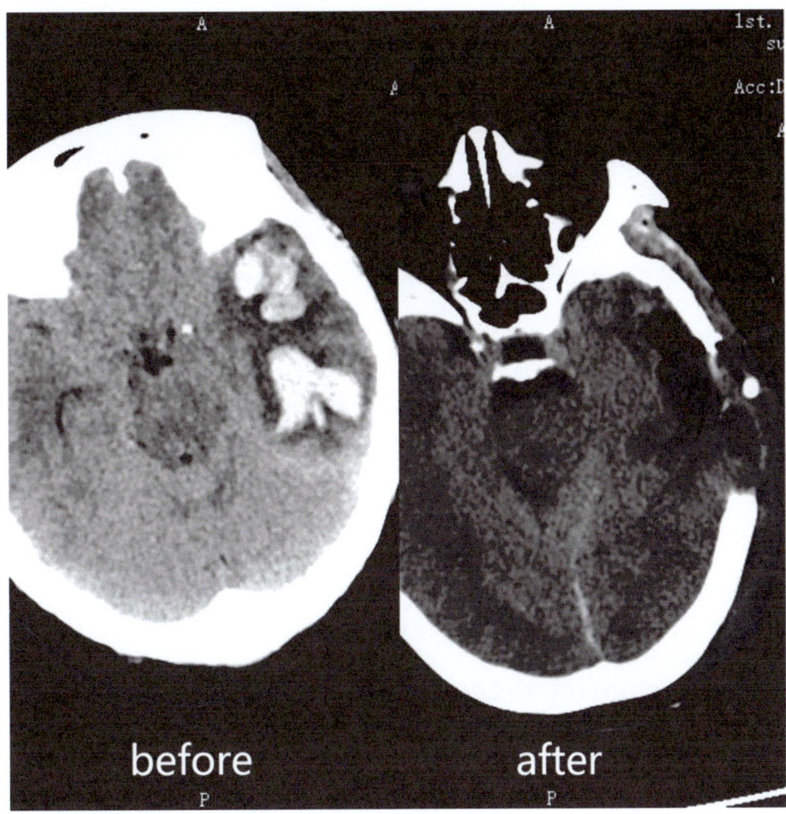

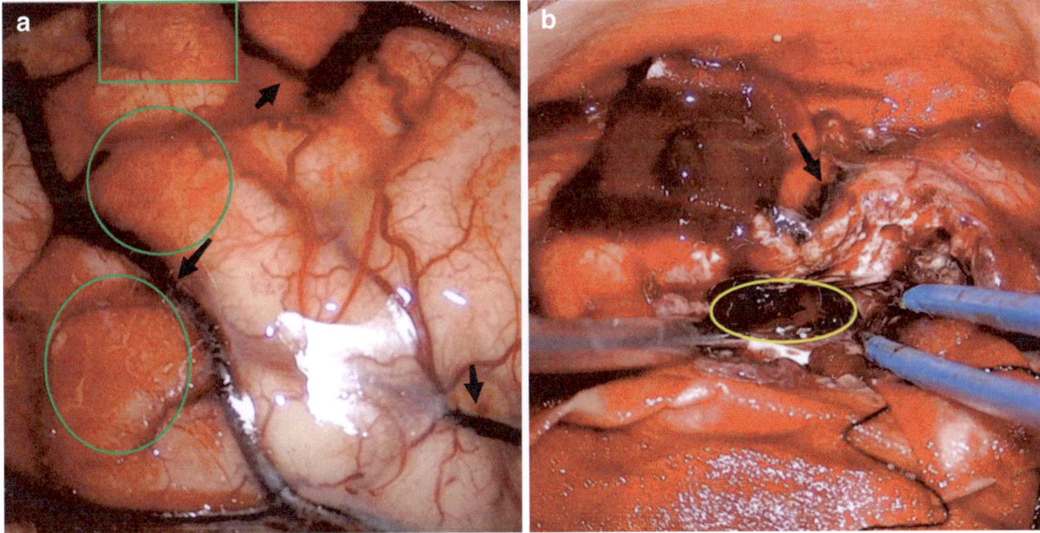

Fig. 11.6 (a) Multiple veins with thrombus can be seen in the cerebral cortex (shown by the black arrow) and capillary congestion can be seen nearby (within the green range). (b, c) Hemorrhage can be seen in the brain parenchyma (within the yellow range)

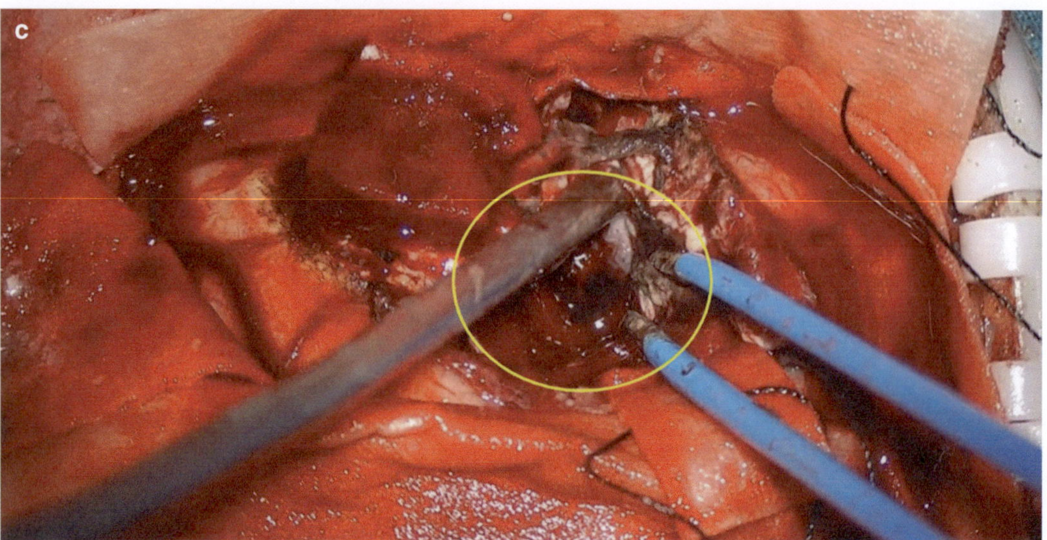

Fig. 11.6 (continued)

11.7 Postoperative Complication

In cases with cerebral hematoma or edema requiring surgical management, particular care must be taken to preserve the collecting vein of the DVA in order to avoid catastrophic venous infarction [12]. Other postoperative complications including nervous system injury, infection, and bleeding may occur following surgery.

However, in rare cases, DVA may cause cerebral hemorrhage or other neurological diseases. Therefore, timely treatment is very important for patients who have found related symptoms. Surgical treatment is the effective method for DVA at present, but attention should be paid to the prevention and treatment of postoperative complications.

11.8 Conclusion

DVA is considered to be an extreme anatomical variant of the medullary vein. It acts as a compensatory venous drainage system to drain blood from the normal brain. Because of the special vascular structure, excision of DVA may lead to the risk of regional venous congestion. It is speculated that venous congestion may induce the formation of CM, histological changes of DVAs, abnormal finding of essence, formation of varicose veins, and stenosis or blockage of collecting veins. Therefore, the evaluation of venous hyperemia perfusion study may be the key to predict the risk of symptomatic DVAs in the future. The majority of the patients with DVA have a good prognosis and do not require special treatment.

References

1. Yu T, Liu X, Lin X, Bai C, Zhao J, Zhang J, Zhang L, Wu Z, Wang S, Zhao Y, Meng G. The relation between angioarchitectural factors of developmental venous anomaly and concomitant sporadic cavernous malformation. BMC Neurol. 2016;6(1):183.
2. Narendra DP, Wang N, Erkkinen MG, Jagadeesan J, Lee TC, Zimmerman EE, Klein JP. An anomalous developmental venous anomaly. Neurology. 2014;83(11):1033–4.
3. Meng G, Bai C, Yu T, Wu Z, Liu X, Zhang J, Zhao J. The association between cerebral developmental venous anomaly and concomitant cavernous malformation: an observational study using magnetic resonance imaging. BMC Neurol. 2014;14:50.
4. Mullaguri N, Battineni A, Krishnaiah B, Migdady I, Newey CR. Developmental venous anomaly presenting with spontaneous intracerebral hemorrhage, acute ischemic stroke, and seizure. Cureus. 2019;11(8):e5412.

5. Hon JM, Bhattacharya JJ, Counsell CE, Papanastassiou V, Ritchie V, Roberts RC, Sellar RJ, Warlow CP, Al-Shahi Salman R, SIVMS Collaborators. The presentation and clinical course of intracranial developmental venous anomalies in adults: a systematic review and prospective, population-based study. Stroke. 2009;40(6):1980–5.

6. Aoki R, Srivatanakul K. Developmental venous anomaly: benign or not benign. Neurol Med Chir. 2016;56(9):534–43.

7. Marzouk O, Marzouk S, Liyanage SH, Grunwald IQ. Cerebellar developmental venous anomaly with associated cavernoma causing a hemorrhage—a rare occurrence. Radiol Case Rep. 2021;16(6):1463–8.

8. Hsu CC, Krings T. Symptomatic developmental venous anomaly: state-of-the-art review on genetics, pathophysiology, and imaging approach to diagnosis. AJNR Am J Neuroradiol. 2023;44:498. https://doi.org/10.3174/ajnr.A7829.

9. Ishigami D, Koizumi S, Miyawaki S, Hongo H, Teranishi Y, Mitsui J, Saito N. Symptomatic and stenotic developmental venous anomaly with pontine capillary telangiectasia: a case report with genetic considerations. NMC Case Rep J. 2022;9:139–44.

10. Entezami P, Boulos A, Yamamoto J, Adamo M. Paediatric presentation of intracranial haemorrhage due to thrombosis of a developmental venous anomaly. BMJ Case Rep. 2019;12(1):bcr-2018-227362.

11. Oran I, Kiroglu Y, Yurt A, Ozer FD, Acar F, Dalbasti T, Yagci B, Sirikci A, Calli C. Developmental venous anomaly (DVA) with arterial component: a rare cause of intracranial haemorrhage. Neuroradiology. 2009;51(1):25–32.

12. San Millán Ruíz D, Gailloud P. Cerebral developmental venous anomalies. Childs Nerv Syst. 2010;26(10):1395–406.

Qichang Fu and Fuyou Guo

12.1 Introduction

Intracranial large artery occlusion is mainly caused by vascular self-lesion or thromboembolism of large arteries in the neck or larger arteries at the base of the skull, which eventually leads to ischemia and hypoxia of brain tissue and presents corresponding neurological dysfunction, i.e., ischemic stroke. According to the Org10172 Trial of Acute Stroke Treatment (TOAST) typing, large artery atherosclerosis and thromboembolism are the main causes of ischemic stroke. Acute ischemic stroke is the most common type of stroke, accounting for 60%–80% of all strokes [1]. The management of acute ischemic stroke emphasizes early diagnosis, early treatment, early rehabilitation, and early prevention of recurrence.

Occlusion of large intracranial veins is mainly caused by dural sinus or cerebral vein thrombosis, resulting in cerebral ischemia and cerebral edema [2]. Intracranial venous thrombosis is a rare thrombotic disease, accounting for approximately 3.5% of ischemic cerebrovascular disease. The etiology of intracranial venous thrombosis includes mainly infectious and non-infectious factors. With the advent of antibiotics, the number of intracranial venous thrombosis with non-infectious factors as the etiology has increased year by year. The causes of non-infectious factors of intracranial venous thrombosis mainly include hormonal factors and female pregnancy and puerperium, tumors, blood and coagulation system abnormalities, systemic diseases, etc.

12.2 Patient Selection and Preoperative Evaluation

12.2.1 Selection of Patients with Intracranial Large Artery Occlusion and Preoperative Evaluation

Intracranial large artery occlusions include symptomatic or asymptomatic occlusions. Surgical or interventional treatment of patients with asymptomatic intracranial large artery occlusion remains controversial because of the low risk of stroke in this group of patients. Acute ischemic stroke due to symptomatic large artery occlusion requires aggressive intervention. The diagnosis of acute ischemic stroke includes several elements: first, acute onset of focal neurological deficit (weakness or numbness of one side of the

Q. Fu
Department of Magnetic Resonance, The First Affiliated Hospital of Zhengzhou University, Zhengzhou, Henan, China

F. Guo (✉)
Department of Neurosurgery, The First Affiliated Hospital of Zhengzhou University, Zhengzhou, China

International Joint Laboratory of Nervous System Malformation, Zhengzhou, Henan, China

face or limb, speech impairment, etc.); second, brain computed tomography (CT) or magnetic resonance imaging (MRI) to rule out hemorrhage and non-vascular causes, etc. The National Institutes of Health Stroke Scale is currently the most commonly used international scale to assess stroke severity. Although evidence-based medicine has confirmed that intravenous thrombolysis with heavy tissue-type fibrinogen activator (rt-PA) within 4.5 h of onset is the preferred treatment for acute ischemic stroke, the rate of achieving revascularization after intravenous thrombolysis in large vessel occlusive stroke is generally low, and the use of intra-arterial thrombolysis devices and revascularization devices has improved the benefit for this group of patients.

Imaging assessment of the patient's vascular condition at the early stage of the disease is important to analyze the pathogenesis of acute ischemic stroke and to initiate treatment. Imaging techniques such as MRA, CTA, or digital subtraction angiography (DSA) are effective in assessing the vascular condition of acute stroke patients. The TOAST etiology/pathogenesis staging is now widely used internationally to classify the etiology of ischemic stroke into five types: large artery atherosclerotic, cardiogenic embolic, small artery occlusive, other definite etiology, and unknown etiology. Etiological typing of acute ischemic stroke patients helps in the development of treatment plans. TOAST typing of large artery atherosclerosis and thromboembolism leading to intracranial large vessel occlusion is the main cause of ischemic stroke [3].

The goal of endovascular treatment of acute ischemic stroke is to promote recanalization of occluded large vessels and restore blood perfusion to locally ischemic brain tissue. Noncontrast computed tomography (NCCT) is clinically recognized as the routine and preferred test for acute ischemic stroke, and although it is not as sensitive for acute phase cerebral infarction, it is effective in excluding cerebral hemorrhage. Patients can significantly benefit from early recanalization therapy when the Alberta stroke program early CT score (ASPECT) score of baseline CT is >7. In contrast, patients with an ASPECT score <4 were not able to obtain clinical improvement from early revascularization. In addition, intracerebral parenchymal

hematoma is a contraindication to interventional endovascular recanalization. For brainstem and cerebellar regions where CT imaging is less sensitive, MRI imaging has a better imaging effect, with diffusion weighted image sequences being the most sensitive imaging method to show acute cerebral ischemic lesions [4].

Endovascular interventions should be performed as early as possible in patients with severe intracranial large vessel occlusions. Arterial thrombolysis is generally recommended for patients with an anterior circulation occlusion onset within 6 h and a posterior circulation onset within 24 h; or mechanical thrombolysis for patients with an anterior circulation occlusion onset within 8 h and a posterior circulation onset within 24 h. Multimodal imaging-based assessment of the ischemic semi-dark zone may widen the time window for patient treatment.

12.2.2 Selection of Patients with Large Intracranial Vein Occlusion and Preoperative Evaluation

Occlusion of large intracranial veins is mainly caused by dural sinus or cerebral vein thrombosis. Cerebral venous thrombosis (CVT) is a rare cause of stroke. It can occur at any age, and its clinical signs and symptoms are variable and non-specific, with a variety of corresponding imaging manifestations. Therefore, accurate diagnosis of cerebral venous thrombosis is difficult and treatment is often delayed. The prognosis of patients is usually good after systematic anticoagulation with drugs. For patients who do not respond well to conservative treatment, endovascular therapy may be of potential benefit.

The most common clinical manifestations in adult CVT patients are headache, optic papilledema, seizures, focal signs, and changes in consciousness. These signs and symptoms resulting from cerebral venous obstruction include non-focal syndromes due to high cranial pressure as well as focal neurological deficits due to brain parenchymal damage. Neurologic deficits vary depending on the location of the cerebral venous thrombus. 90% of patients with CVT have symptoms consistent with cranial hypertension, often combined with associated focal signs or seizures. Focal signs due to superficial venous sinus thrombosis include partial epilepsy with or without secondary aphasia, hemiparesis, and hemianopia. Deep cerebral vein thrombosis often results in an acute decrease in the level of consciousness or subacute dementia, for example. Patients with spongy sinus thrombosis are associated with corresponding ocular symptoms.

Because of the considerable challenges in the clinical diagnosis of CVT, diagnostic imaging plays an important role. Because CVT is often associated with headache and other diverse underlying clinical manifestations, NCCT of the head is usually the first imaging test. Although CT can provide diagnostic clues, it does not confirm the diagnosis of CVT the vast majority of the time; MRI can distinguish between vasogenic and cytotoxic edema, clearly show the anatomy of the venous sinuses, and detect the temporal stage of thrombosis. Therefore, if MRI is available, CT is usually not required as a starting step. noninvasive techniques such as MRI or CT can replace DSA as the gold standard for diagnosing CVT; however, DSA remains necessary when the diagnosis cannot be confirmed by noninvasive imaging [5].

12.3　Surgical Principles

12.3.1　Occlusion of Large Intracranial Arteries

The most important goal of treatment of symptomatic intracranial artery occlusion is revascularization. The value of intracranial-extracranial bypass (EC-IC bypass) as a treatment for ischemic stroke has been controversial. The results of a study by the International Randomized Trial of Extracranial/Intracranial Bypass Study Group to assess the benefit of bypass surgery in patients with symptomatic intracranial atherosclerotic stenosis showed that non-fatal and fatal strokes were more frequent and occurred earlier in the surgery group. The study led to the increasing importance of endovascular treatment techniques

after the failure of bypass as a treatment option for patients with symptomatic intracranial atherosclerosis. Within the time window, endovascular treatment of ischemic stroke due to large artery occlusion is associated with earlier treatment and better patient recovery outcomes.

The surgical plan was developed based on the patient's symptoms and preoperative imaging. Selective cannulation of the internal carotid artery or the vertebrobasilar artery is performed according to the blood supplying arteries in the cerebral ischemic area, and the patient's collateral vessel opening is understood. The specific treatment modality (arterial thrombolysis, mechanical embolization, etc.) needs to be selected individually according to the patient's condition.

12.3.2　Occlusion of Large Intracranial Veins

There is no uniform treatment protocol for intracranial venous thrombosis. Currently, treatment mostly follows the following principles: etiological treatment, cranial pressure lowering treatment and symptomatic treatment, anticoagulation and thrombolytic treatment, endovascular treatment and surgery.

12.4　Minimally Invasive Treatment of Patients with Intracranial Large Vessel Occlusion

12.4.1　Minimally Invasive Treatment of Intracranial Large Artery Occlusion

12.4.1.1　Arterial Thrombolysis

When performing arterial thrombolysis in patients with intracranial large artery occlusion, the surgical access is selected based on preoperative imaging assessment, and sex-selective thrombolysis is performed using a guiding catheter and microcatheter [6]. The microcatheter is delivered to the occluded large vessel via a microguide wire, and rt-PA or urokinase is sequentially injected into the proximal, distal, and occluded segments of the occluded vessel in order to perform contact thrombolysis. The criterion of revascularization is best achieved with the smallest dose of thrombolytic drug. After recanalization of the occluded vessel, thrombolysis should be stopped and the microcatheter withdrawn immediately. During the operation, the guidewire catheter should be handled gently to prevent secondary infarction due to dislodgement of atheromatous plaque.

12.4.1.2 Mechanical Bolt Retrieval

Mechanical intra-arterial thrombolysis has many advantages over arterial thrombolysis alone: first, it increases the contact area of thrombolytic drugs with the thrombus and improves the thrombolytic effect, thus reducing the probability of intracranial hemorrhage; second, it provides an alternative method for patients for whom anticoagulation is contraindicated, etc. Based on these advantages, mechanical thrombolysis has become an adjunct or alternative to pharmacological thrombolysis [7]. Mechanical thrombolysis is divided into the following categories: intravascular thrombolysis, intravascular aspiration, mechanical fragmentation, etc.

Endovascular thrombus removal is facilitated by applying a continuous force to the distal or proximal end of the thrombus with a thrombectomy device. The thrombus is passed through the occluded large vessel by a microguide wire in conjunction with a microcatheter to reach the distal location of the occlusion. After withdrawal of the microguide wire, the embolization device is delivered through the microcatheter to the lesion location, and when the embolization device is fully opened, the embolization device, microcatheter, and thrombus are gently pulled together to the outside of the body. (Fig. 12.1)

If a balloon-guided catheter is used, the embolization operation is performed after the balloon is filled. Intravascular thrombus aspiration works by the application of a suction technique and is suitable for fresh, not yet adherent thrombi. The use of this modality reduces the incidence of embolic events and vasospastic events. The fragmentation technique is used to break up the thrombus inside the vessel, including through balloon dilation, thus allowing for revascularization [8] (Fig. 12.2).

12.4.2 Minimally Invasive Treatment of Intracranial Large Vein Occlusion

When performing venous sinus thrombolysis for large intracranial venous occlusions due to thrombosis, the appropriate treatment is determined based on preoperative imaging assessment to define the location and extent of the venous thrombus and normal anatomic variants. The venous route is usually a 6F or 7F sheath placed in the femoral vein; occasionally, a jugular access is applied. The internal jugular vein on the side of the lesion is introduced via a guide catheter with the cephalic end placed in the jugular vein bulb [9].

Retrograde venography can clarify the extent of the distal embolism. A microguide then guides the microcatheter through the location of venous sinus occlusion under the roadmap. Intermittent imaging through the microcatheter is performed to understand the exact location of the microcatheter and the extent of the thrombus. When the microcatheter reaches the location of the venous thrombus, a thrombolytic drug such as recombinant fibrinogen activator is injected for contact thrombolysis. The drug is injected in a variety of ways, including continuous injection and pulsed

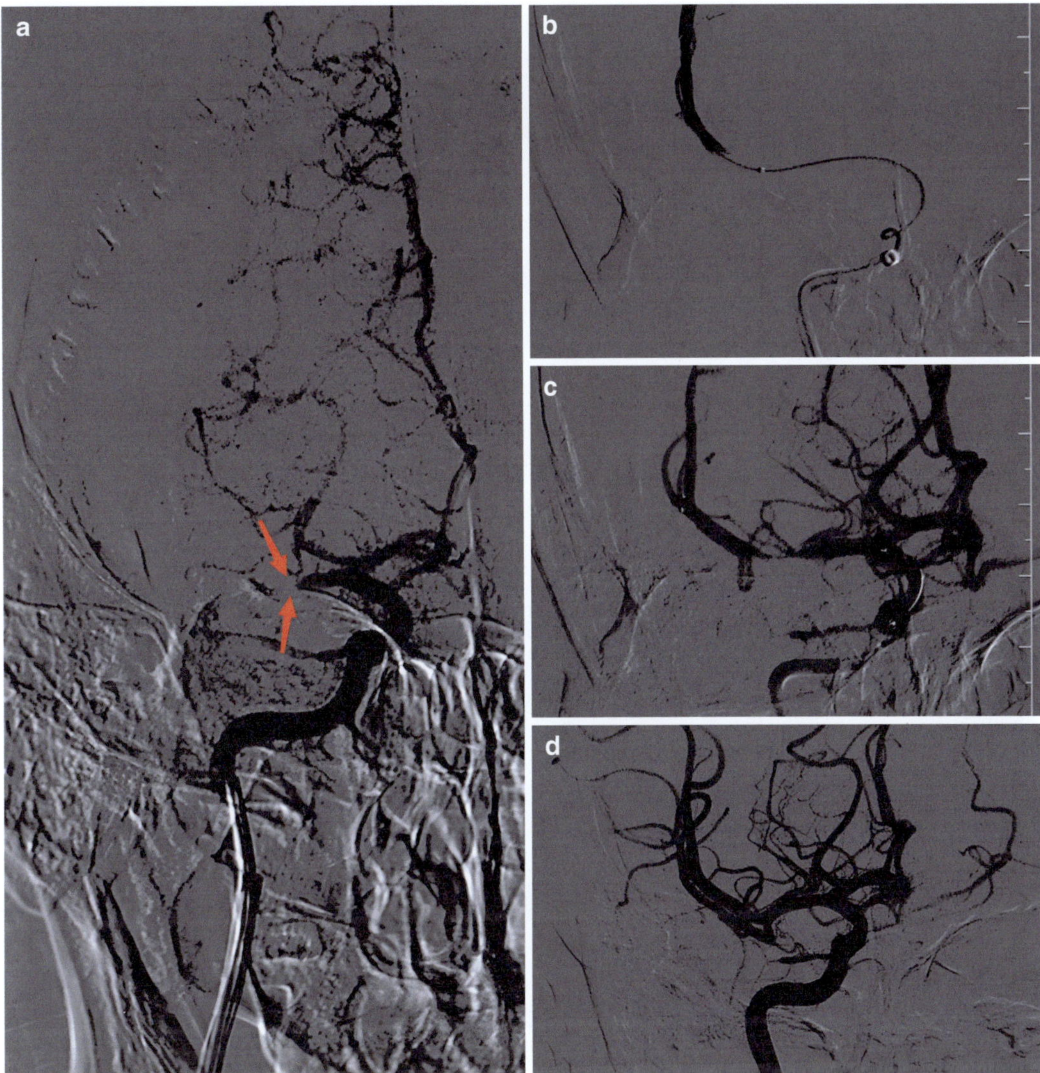

Fig. 12.1 Digital subtraction angiography (DSA) reveals middle cerebral artery occlusion (**a**) with no distal visualization. Microcatheter reaches the distal end through the area of vascular occlusion (**b**). Partial recanalization of the middle cerebral artery (**c**). Good visualization of middle cerebral artery after embolization (**d**)

injection techniques, and the dose and duration of injection vary. To accelerate thrombolysis or enhance thrombus disruption, a combination of thrombolytic drugs and mechanical fragmentation may be applied. This approach may accelerate the thrombolytic process by increasing the thrombus contact surface and improving the distribution of thrombolytic drugs within the thrombus, while also having a beneficial effect on the mechanical disruption of the thrombus [10]. Similar to the arterial aspiration technique, mechanical aspiration of venous thrombi by a suction device also allows for rapid and complete removal of venous sinus thrombi. This technique alone helps to avoid the risk of intracranial hemorrhage (Fig. 12.3).

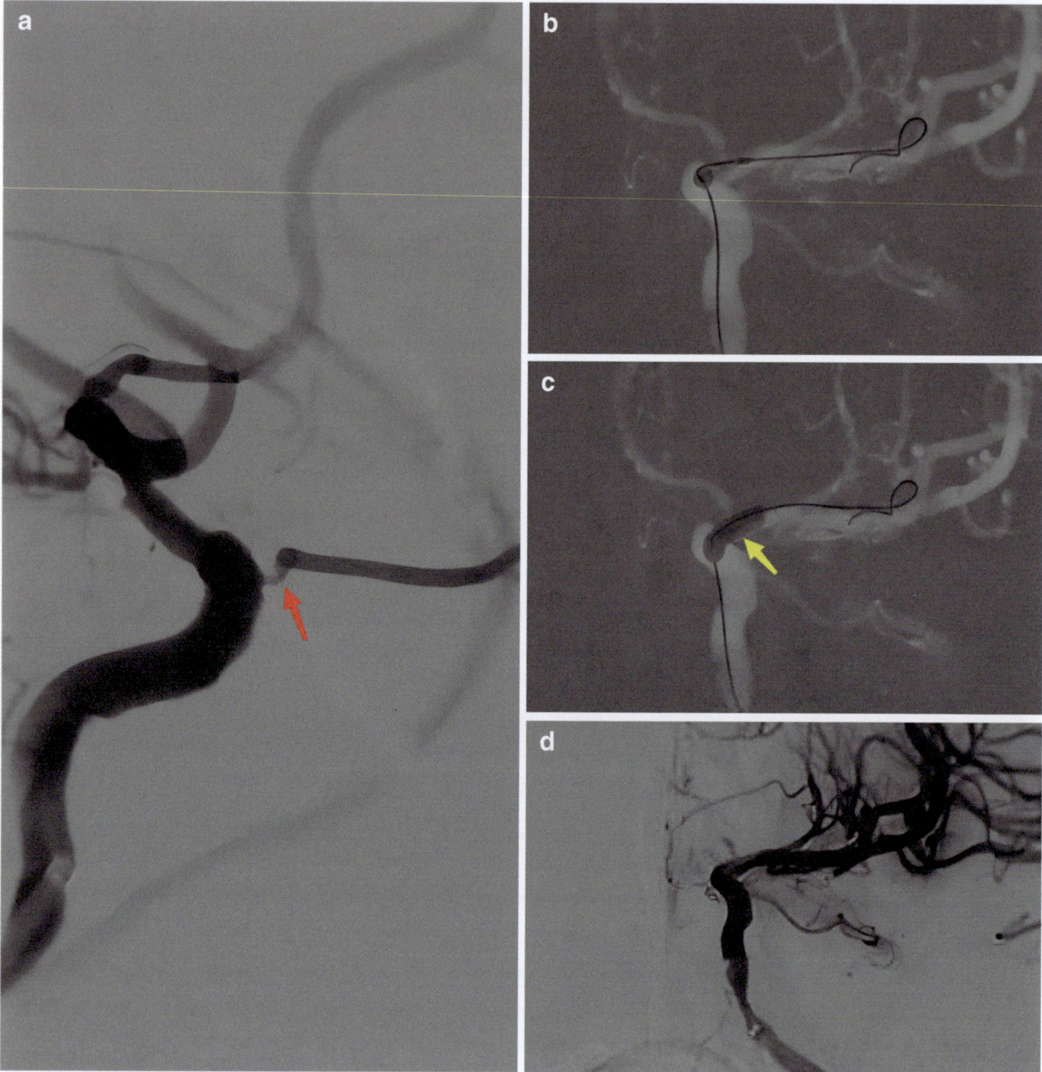

Fig. 12.2 DSA showing stenosis at the beginning of the middle cerebral artery (red arrow) (**a**). Microguide wire guides the balloon to the area of stenosis (**b**). Middle cerebral artery recanalization after intravascular balloon dilation (**c**, **d**)

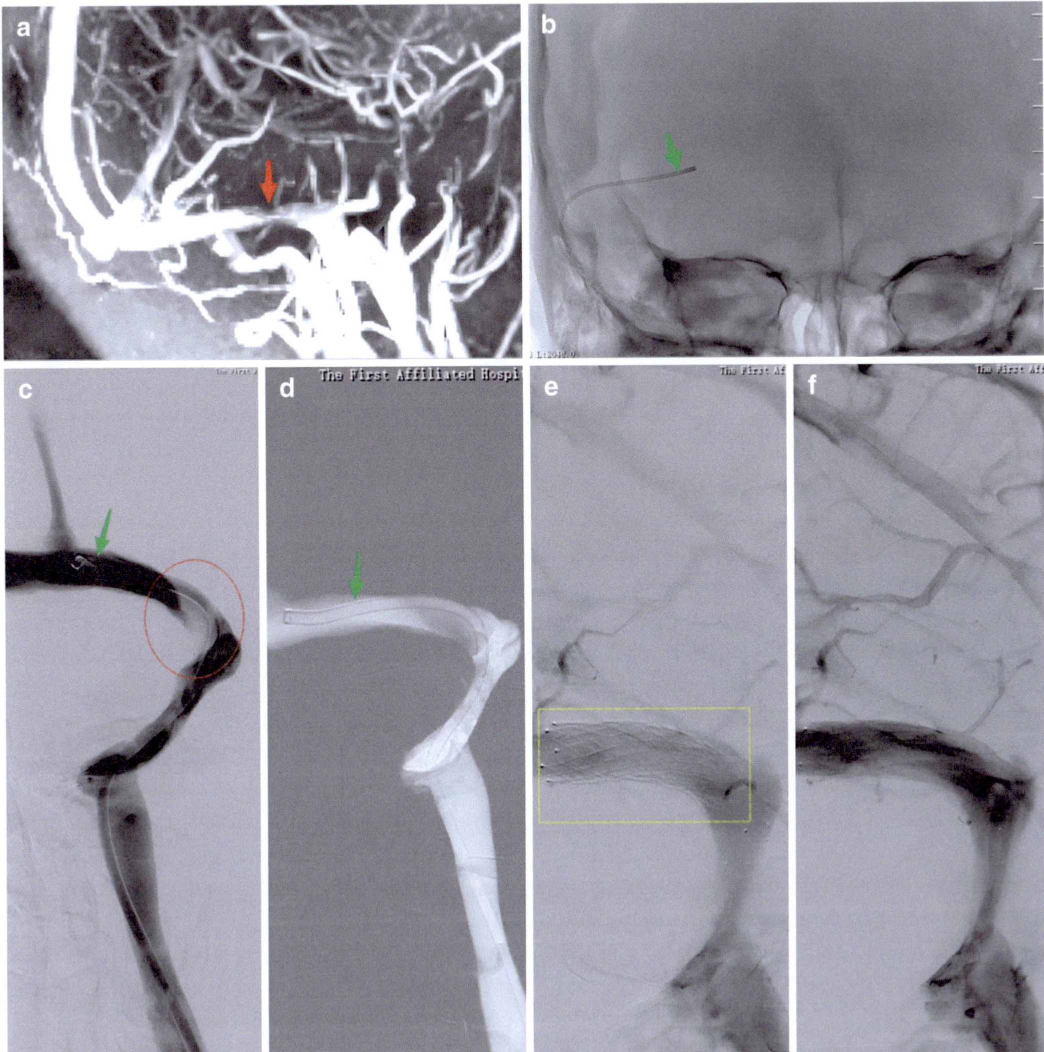

Fig. 12.3 Magnetic resonance venography showing transverse sinus stenosis (red arrow) due to thrombus (**a**). Catheter (green arrow) enters the transverse sinus to start thrombolytic therapy (**b**). Angiography after catheter passage through the stenotic area suggests partial recanalization of the transverse sinus (**c**, **d**). Release of the stent shows good filling of the transverse sinus (**e**, **f**)

12.5 Complications

12.5.1 Complications of Intracranial Large Artery Occlusion Treatment

Hemorrhagic transformation, one of the main complications of thrombolysis or endovascular therapy in acute ischemic stroke. The causes may be related to vessel wall injury, reperfusion injury, thrombolytic drug use, and combined antiplatelet and anticoagulation therapy, with bleeding occurring mostly after 36 h post-thrombolysis [11]. Strict control of indications, effective blood pressure control in the perioperative period, and reduction of the dose of thrombolytic drugs used can reduce the incidence of bleeding conversion.

Cerebral transitional perfusion injury, which refers to the reperfusion of ischemic brain tissue after recanalization of an obstructed cerebral artery, results in a significant increase in ipsilateral cerebral blood flow, leading to the occurrence of cerebral edema or even cerebral hemorrhage. Effective blood pressure control and adequate evaluation of cerebral collateral circulation during the perioperative period can reduce the incidence of hyperperfusion injury. Seizures and intracranial hemorrhage are considered to be signs of severe overperfusion injury, and anti-thrombotic therapy should be discontinued immediately once they occur.

Reocclusion, following recanalization of large intracranially occluded arteries, is a common complication of the corresponding endovascular treatment. Reocclusion is associated with worsening clinical symptoms, and early reocclusion predicts a poor long-term prognosis for reasons that may be related to thrombolytic or lipid core exposure promoting platelet aggregation after endothelial injury. Thrombolysis combined with antiplatelet therapy may reduce the incidence of reocclusion [12].

Other complications, such as vascular entrapment, stress ulcers, cardiovascular complications, puncture site injury, local hematoma formation, contrast allergy, and contrast nephropathy, have a relatively low incidence of complications.

12.5.2 Complications of Intracranial Large Vein Occlusion Treatment

The most common complication of hemorrhage conversion, during retreatment, is intracranial bleeding or bleeding from other organs after thrombolysis and anticoagulation. The cause may be excessive anticoagulation or inappropriate thrombolytic manipulation. Strict monitoring of coagulation indicators during anticoagulation and even and slow administration of appropriate doses of fibrinolytic drugs during thrombolysis can help avoid bleeding complications.

12.6 Conclusion

Advances in imaging technology have facilitated accurate and rapid diagnosis of intracranial macrovascular occlusive disease. For patients with symptomatic intracranial large vessel occlusions that do not respond well to conservative treatment, radical interventions such as endovascular therapy are becoming an important treatment option. With the innovation of endovascular thrombolytic drugs and devices, the safety and efficacy of radical interventions such as endovascular therapy have improved and have increased the benefits for patients with symptomatic intracranial macrovascular occlusions.

References

1. Elissavet E, Mitra HM, Michael A, et al. National institutes of health stroke scale zero strokes. Stroke. 2018;49:3057–9.
2. Nakase H, Heimann A, Kempski O. Local cerebral blood flow in a rat cortical vein occlusion model. J Cereb Blood Flow Metab. 1996;16(4):720–8.
3. Kohjiro N, Kei T, Yuya A, et al. ATP hydrolysis-dependent conformational changes in the extracellular domain of ABCA1 are associated with apoA-I binding. J Lipid Res. 2012;53:126–36.
4. Nguyen Thanh N, Mohamad A, Simon N, et al. Noncontrast computed tomography vs computed tomography perfusion or magnetic resonance imaging selection in late presentation of stroke with large-vessel occlusion. JAMA Neurol. 2022;79: 22–31.

5. Tetsuhiro H, Ryuzaburo K, Takanori U, et al. Difference of thrombus location between initial non-invasive vascular image and first DSA findings in mechanical thrombectomy for intracranial large vessel occlusion: post hoc analysis of the SKIP study. Neurol Med Chir (Tokyo). 2021;61:640–6.

6. Katharina F, Marius M, Moriz H, et al. Minor stroke in large vessel occlusion: a matched analysis of patients from the German Stroke Registry-Endovascular Treatment (GSR-ET) and patients from the Safe Implementation of Treatments in Stroke-International Stroke Thrombolysis Register (SITS-ISTR). Eur J Neurol. 2022;29:1619–29.

7. Baik SH, Jung C, Kim JY, et al. Local intra-arterial thrombolysis during mechanical thrombectomy for refractory large-vessel occlusion: adjunctive chemical enhancer of thrombectomy. AJNR Am J Neuroradiol. 2021;42:1986–92.

8. Yoo J, Lee SJ, Hong JH, et al. Immediate effects of first-line thrombectomy devices for intracranial atherosclerosis-related occlusion: stent retriever versus contact aspiration. BMC Neurol. 2020;20:283.

9. Farzaneh J, Gero D, Till-Karsten H, et al. Mechanical thrombectomy in cerebral venous sinus thrombosis: reports of a retrospective single-center study. J Clin Med. 2022;11:undefined.

10. Pasarikovski Christopher R, Ku Jerry C, Julia K, et al. Mechanical thrombectomy and intravascular imaging for cerebral venous sinus thrombosis: a preclinical model. J Neurosurg. 2020;135:425–30.

11. Hongzhou D, Li C, Shengli S, et al. Staged endovascular treatment for symptomatic occlusion originating from the intracranial vertebral arteries in the early non-acute stage. Front Neurol. 2021;12:673367.

12. Pierre S, Julie D, Guillaume T, et al. Thrombus length predicts lack of post-thrombolysis early recanalization in minor stroke with large vessel occlusion. Stroke. 2019;50:761–4.

Pituitary Abnormalities

13

Xueyou Liu

13.1 Introduction

Incidental pituitary abnormalities are usually detected by using sensitive brain imaging techniques, such as magnetic resonance imaging (MRI) and computed tomography scan (CT), for unrelated causes (headache, head trauma, and neurological complaints). Based on the sensitive neuroradiological imaging procedures, incidental pituitary abnormalities include pituitary incidentalomas, technical artifacts, pituitary hyperplasia, and variants of normal anatomy. Incidental pituitary abnormalities usually refer to pituitary incidentalomas in clinical practice.

Pituitary incidentalomas (rate close to 1 in 5 individuals), demonstrated only by detailed examination of pituitary gland at autopsy, were described as "subclinical adenoma" by Cosstelo as early as in 1936 [1]. In recent years, there are many reviews and original papers focus on the research of pituitary incidentalomas [2–9]. Molitch reported that the average frequency of a pituitary adenoma was 10.6% by reviewing a large number of studies [6]. Referring to the pathological diagnoses of sellar masses that performed surgery, pituitary adenomas were 91% and the none-pituitary adenomas were 9%, most

of which were craniopharyngiomas and Rathe's cleft cysts [10]. Knowing about the nature history of pituitary incidentalomas, exact evaluation and follow-up are very important for clinicians and pituitary diseases specialists to manage the patients with pituitary incidentalomas.

13.2 Nature History of Pituitary Incidentalomas

As with all pituitary lesions, micro-incidentalomas are less than 1 cm in size and macro-incidentalomas are at least 1 cm [3–5, 7, 11]. Pituitary adenomas are the most common entities in pituitary incidentalomas, accounting for 91% of all lesions [10]. Tresoldi et al.'s retrospective multicenter cohort study, over 3 years follow-up, most adenomas remained stable in size (69.5%) [9]. Macroadenomas tend to grow in time compared to microadenomas (26.8% vs. 8.3%) [9]. Pituitary incidentalomas are almost under 1 cm in size, according to Molitch's study [6], because most macro-incidentalomas compress the adjacent structures resulting in clinical manifestations, such as defect of field vision, insufficiency of hormone. However, Imran et al.'s study in Canada suggests that most pituitary incidentalomas seen in tertiary-care referral centers present as macroadenomas [4], according to Anagnostis et al.'s study [12]. In Imran et al.'s study, pituitary incidentalomas <5 mm in size at initial presenta-

X. Liu (✉)
Department of Neurosurgery, The First Affiliated Hospital of Zhengzhou University, Zhengzhou, Henan Province, China

tion, none enlarged during follow-up; in those 5–10 mm at presentation, subsequent enlargement was seen in 14%; and in those >10 mm at presentation, there was an enlargement of tumors in 25% patients ($P = 0.06$) [4]. The incidence of pituitary apoplexy was 1.1% for macroadenomas and 0.4% for microadenomas [13].

Most pituitary incidentalomas are clinically non-functioning pituitary adenomas [12, 14]. Functioning pituitary adenomas usually present with clinical symptoms of hypersecretion, such as galactorrhea amenorrhea syndrome in patients with prolactinomas, acromegaly in growth hormone (GH) secreting patients, Cushing's disease in adrenocorticotropic hormone (ACTH) secreting patients, which facilitate their diagnosis. In a 61 patients with pituitary incidentalomas cohort study, 77% were non-functioning, 18% prolactinomas, and 3% GH-secreting; and of the pituitary incidentalomas followed conservatively, 78% remained stable, 11% showed decrease, and 11% increase in size [12].

Pituitary adenomas are the most common solid (or mixed solid-cystic) lesions in the sellar regions, followed by meningiomas, craniopharyngiomas, germ cell tumors, lymphocytic hypophysitis, chordomas, and chondromas [14], which are usually distinguished by MRI and test of pituitary hormones and serum tumor markers. Cystic lesions in the sellar region need to be distinguished from a necrotic pituitary adenoma, Rathe's cleft cysts, dermoid and epidermoid cysts, and cystic craniopharyngiomas [14]. Rathke's cleft cysts should be considered, if an incidental pituitary lesion is a simple cyst without enhancement in contrast-enhanced pituitary MRI [15], and usually hyperintense on T1-weighted images [14]. In the 550 patients with pituitary incidentalomas cohort study in Japan, the MRI findings of lesions with increasing size were solid masses, while tumors of decreasing size or even sometimes cured spontaneously tended to be cystic, which were supposed to be Rathke's cleft cysts [16]. So, asymptomatic cystic pituitary incidentalomas (including Rathke's cleft cysts) should be followed up without surgical intervention [16].

13.3 Management of Pituitary Incidentalomas

13.3.1 Endocrine Evaluation

Complete pituitary and target organs' function tests are needed when patients presenting with a pituitary incidentaloma. An Endocrine Society Clinical Practice Guideline in 2011 recommend that all patients with a pituitary incidentaloma undergo clinical and laboratory evaluations for hormone hypersecretion or hypopituitarism [3]. Testing includes serum ACTH and cortisol levels for pituitary–adrenal axis, serum insulin-like growth factor-1 (IGF-1) and GH levels (oral glucose tolerance test, OGTT) for pituitary–GH axis, serum thyroid stimulating hormone (TSH) and free T4 for pituitary–thyroid axis, serum luteinizing hormone, and follicle-stimulating hormone with either testosterone in male or estradiol in female for pituitary–gonad axis, and serum prolactin levels after 1 h resting period [9, 17].

Though most of the pituitary incidentalomas are clinical none-functioning pituitary adenomas, some patients with hypersecretion incidentalomas may present subclinical symptoms (without classical signs or symptoms). If these patients with subclinical symptoms are detected early, dopamine agonists would be performed for patients with hyperprolactinemia and surgical approach would be indicated in patients with GH- or ACTH-secreting adenomas, which could reduce the long-term adverse consequences of hypersecretion [18].

Langlois et al. reviewing literatures indicate that hypopituitarism is found in 15–30% of pituitary incidentalomas, mostly in macro-incidentalomas [5], because of their compression on either the pituitary or the pituitary stalk, and the likelihood of hypopituitarism is related to the size of the pituitary incidentalomas [18]. The Endocrine Society Clinical Practice Guideline suggests that all the patients with either macro-incidentalomas or large micro-incidentalomas (diameter 6–9 mm), should be screened for hypopituitarism [3]. When clinical symptoms of hypopituitarism or hormone deficits exist, hormone replacement therapy is needed (hydrocortisone: 10–15 mg/m^2/day, levothyroxine: 1.6 µg/kg/day after hydrocortisone supplement, sex hormones and GH, and desmopressin if needed) [11, 19].

13.3.2 Radiology Evaluation

The size, composition (cystic or solid), and mass effect or invasion of pituitary lesions are important data for pituitary specialists, which can be detected by radiology. MRI and CT are the most common radiology evaluation techniques for pituitary incidentalomas. Pituitary MRI scan examination is the first choice for the diagnosis of pituitary diseases (such as pituitary microadenoma, Rathke's cleft cysts, intrasellar craniopharyngiomas, empty sella, pituitary abscess, physiologic pituitary hyperplasia, et al. in Fig. 13.1a–f) because of its soft-tissue contrast superiority [15]. While, CT scan examination plays an important role in determining the presence of calcifications relative to MRI [8], especially for the diagnosis of adamantinomatous craniopharyngiomas. Additionally, 1 mm thin slices CT scans and sagittal reconstruction images can provide detailed nasal cavity anatomy for neurosurgeon preparing for transsphenoidal surgery. Rathke's cleft cysts, described as benign pituitary diseases, are derived from remnants of the embryological Rathke's pouch [20]. Rathke's cleft cysts

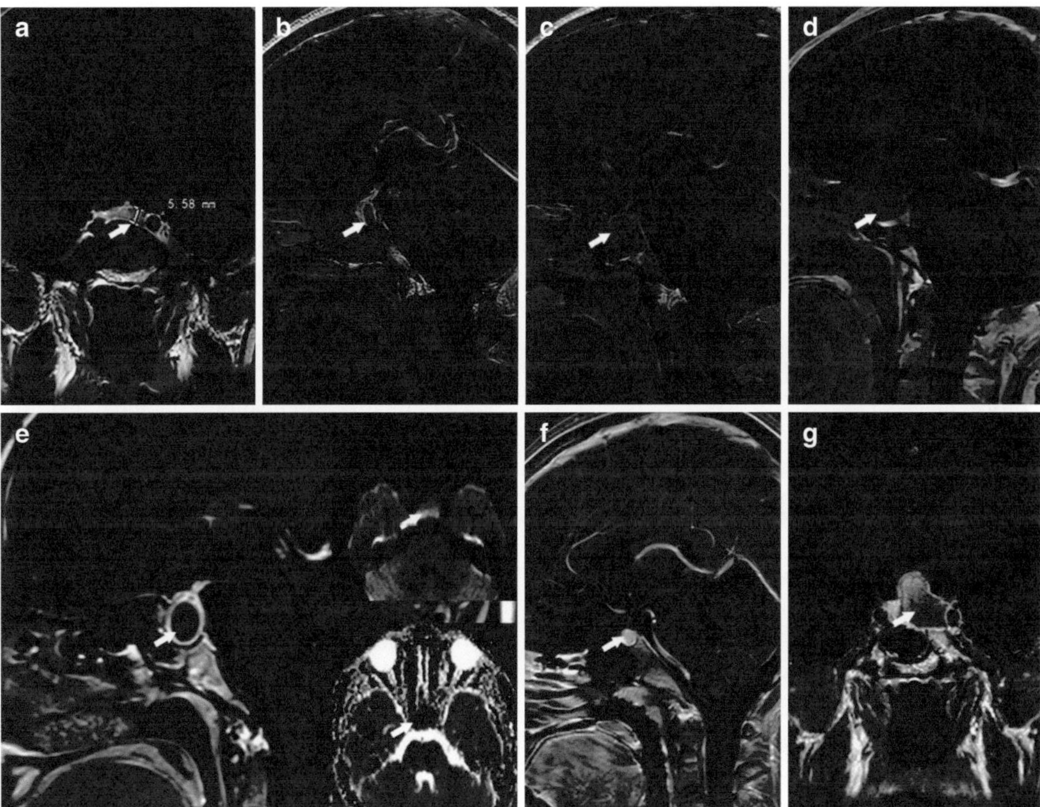

Fig. 13.1 Magnetic resonance imaging (MRI) features of pituitary incidentalomas (arrow). (**a**) Pituitary microadenoma, located at the left side of the sella, the pituitary stalk deviating toward the right; (**b**) Rathke's cleft cysts, without gadolinium enhancement of the cyst contents; (**c**) Intrasellar craniopharyngioma; (**d**) Empty sella, the subarachnoid space herniating into the sella turcica with pituitary gland flattening; (**e**) Pituitary abscess, gadolinium enhancement of the wall, and diffusion-weight MRI demonstrating increased signal intensity with a corresponding reduction in apparent diffusion coefficient; (**f**) Physiologic pituitary hyperplasia, presenting pituitary gland homogeneity on MRIs; (**g**) Pituitary apoplexy, uneven enhancement with compressed pituitary gland and optic chiasma. *(All pictures were obtained from the first Affiliated Hospital of Zhengzhou University)*

usually appear hyperintense on T2-weighted images, while different appearance (hypointense or hyperintense) on T1-weighted images depending on cyst contents, without gadolinium enhancement of the cyst contents [21]. Empty sella refers to the subarachnoid space herniating into the sella turcica with pituitary gland flattening on radiological images [22], which should be differentiated from sella arachnoid cyst. Patients with pituitary abscess usually present headache, fever, visual impairment, and hypopituitarism [23]. Pituitary abscess would be not difficult to diagnose by pituitary MRI, with gadolinium enhancement of the cyst wall, increased signal intensity on diffusion-weighted MRI, and a corresponding reduction in apparent diffusion coefficient. Physiologic pituitary hyperplasia is usually seen in pubertal girls and pregnancy women [10], presenting pituitary gland homogeneity on MRIs with or without contrast-enhancement [24].

The protocol of pituitary MRI scan should include less than 3 mm sagittal and coronal T1-weighted images with and without contrast, with a small field of view centered on the pituitary gland [15]. Besides, the anterior and posterior lobes and the stalk of pituitary should be showed in sagittal images, pituitary gland with a midline stalk between the cavernous sinuses in coronal images [15].

13.3.3 Visual Fields Evaluation

Baseline visual fields (VF) examination is recommended for all patients with a pituitary incidentaloma compressing or abutting the optic nerves or the chiasm on MRI imaging, even without visual symptoms [3]. Some patients with pituitary incidentaloma may not recognize their VF abnormalities even when visiting doctors. In Feldkamp et al.'s study, 4.5% of patients had not recognized VF defects at presentation [25]. VF follow-up is also very important. Tresoldi et al. reported that VF was stable in 71.8% of patients, worsened in 23.1%, and improved in 5.1% [9].

In a 5-year follow-up study, apoplexy developed in 9.5% of patients with clinically non-functioning pituitary incidentaloma, especially in macroadenoma [26]. Pituitary apoplexy may present as acute headache, often with panhypopituitarism and visual loss (Fig. 13.1g).

13.3.4 Treatment

The treatments of pituitary incidentalomas mainly include surgery, medical therapy, and wait-and-see (Fig. 13.2). Surgical therapy is usually recommended when there is biochemical evidence of pituitary hormone hypersecretion (except for hyperprolactinemia) or VF deficit.

According to an endocrine society clinical practice guideline for pituitary incidentaloma, absolute indications for surgical therapy include [3]:

(a) VF deficit due to the lesion compressing the chiasm or optic nerves
(b) Other visual abnormalities (such as ophthalmoplegia, diplopia) due to cavernous sinus expansion of the lesion
(c) Visual disturbance due to pituitary apoplexy
(d) Hypersecreting tumors other than prolactinomas (such as GH-, ACTH-, and TSH-secreting adenomas)

The relative indications include [3] the following:

(a) Clinically significant growth of the lesion
(b) Hypopituitarism due to the lesion
(c) A lesion close to the optic chiasm or optic nerves and with a plan for pregnancy
(d) Unremitting headache

Transsphenoidal pituitary surgery performed by an experienced team, which increases the likelihood of success of surgery for hormone hypersecreting tumors and decreases complication risk, is recommended for patients with surgical indications [3, 5]. However, the complications of surgery should not be ignored, which include loss of one or more pituitary hormones when normal before surgery, transient diabetes insipidus, cerebrospinal fluid leak, meningitis, rebleeding, visual deterioration, even mortality [27, 28].

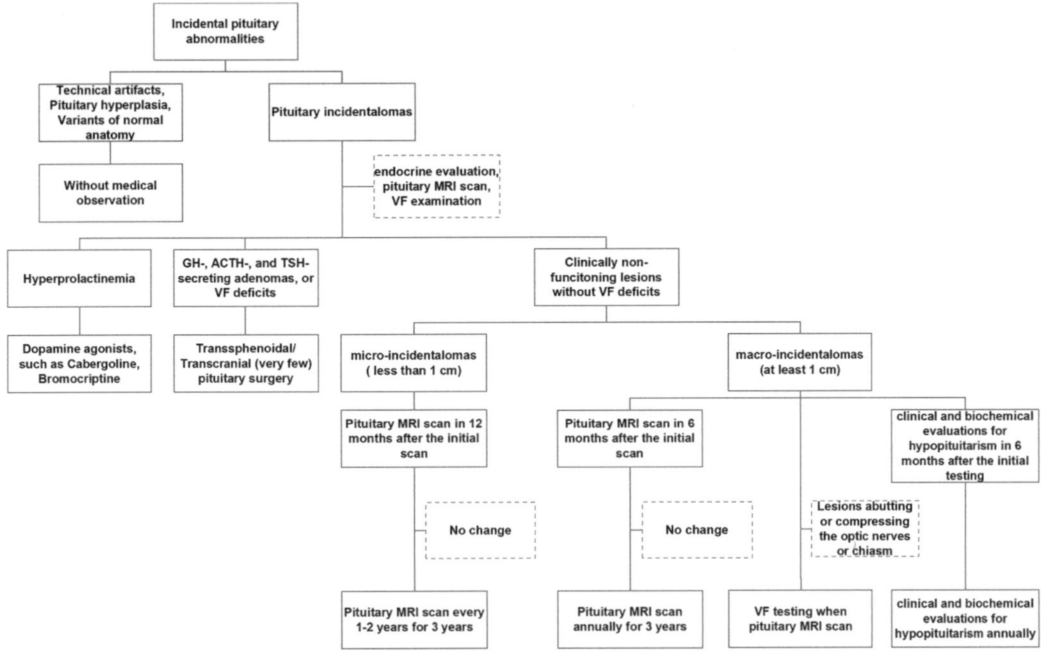

Fig. 13.2 Management flowchart of patients with incidental pituitary abnormalities

With the advances of surgery techniques (such as intraoperative MRI and intraoperative ultrasound), the proportion of gross-total resections in transsphenoidal pituitary surgery is increasing, while complications are decreasing. Hlavac et al.'s 10 years' experience with intraoperative MRI-assisted transsphenoidal pituitary surgery proved that intraoperative MRI could increase the rate of gross-total resection and improve overall outcome [29]. Intraoperative ultrasound can provide real-time feedback in transsphenoidal surgery, identifying residual tumor tissue and internal carotid artery, increasing extent of resections, and avoiding additional injury [30].

Once symptomatic prolactinoma confirmed, dopamine agonist therapy is recommended, which can lower prolactin levels, decrease tumor size, and restore gonadal function [31]. Other causes of hyperprolactinemia should be excluded, such as medication use, renal failure, hypothyroidism, and tumoral compression of the hypothalamic-pituitary stalk, before prolactinoma confirmed [3, 31]. Cabergoline is preferred to other dopamine agonists because of higher efficacy in normalizing prolactin levels and tumor shrinkage. However, patients with prolactinomas who cannot tolerate or not responsive to dopamine agonists therapy should be recommended for transsphenoidal surgery [31]. For patients with malignant prolactinomas, treatment is difficult, temozolomide therapy may be useful [31].

The majority of pituitary incidentalomas do not require surgery, managed only with wait-and-see and follow-up [2, 8, 32]. In Iglesias et al.'s study about incidental clinically non-functioning pituitary adenomas, 88.5% of lesions remained stable, 7.7% decreased, 3.8% increased [33]. In another study, tumor size increased in 10% of the microadenomas and 23% of the macroadenomas, decreased in 7% and 12% of the micro- and macroadenomas, respectively [32]. Non-surgical follow-up (including clinical assessments, MRI scan of pituitary, VF testing, and clinical and biochemical evaluations for hypopituitarism) is recommended for the patients with incidentalomas who do not meet criteria for surgery [3]. Pituitary MRI scan is recommended to repeat in 6 months after the initial scan for macro-incidentalomas and 12 months for micro-incidentalomas, and annually in macro-incidentalomas and every

1–2 years in micro-incidentalomas for the following 3 years and gradually less frequently thereafter if no changing in size [3]. VF testing should be performed in patients with incidentalomas abutting or compressing the optic nerves or chiasm when pituitary MRI scan follow-up, no need in patients whose incidentalomas are not close to the optic nerves or chiasm and without new symptoms [3]. Clinical and biochemical evaluations for hypopituitarism are recommended to repeat in 6 months after the initial testing and yearly thereafter in patients with a pituitary macro-incidentaloma. While evaluations for hypopituitarism are no need in patients with pituitary micro-incidentalomas if no changing in clinical picture, history, and MRI [3].

13.4   Conclusion

With the development and application of sensitive brain imaging techniques, more and more incidental pituitary incidentalomas are detected for unrelated causes. Surgical therapy is usually recommended for the patients with functioning pituitary adenomas (except for hyperprolactinemia) or with VF deficit. The majority of pituitary incidentalomas do not require surgery. Non-surgical follow-up (including clinical assessments, MRI scan of pituitary, VF testing, and clinical and biochemical evaluations for hypopituitarism) is recommended for the patients with incidentalomas who do not meet criteria for surgery.

References

1. Costello RT. Subclinical adenoma of the pituitary gland. Am J Pathol. 1936;12(2):205–16.
2. Boguszewski CL, de Castro Musolino NR, Kasuki L. Management of pituitary incidentaloma. Best Pract Res Clin Endocrinol Metab. 2019;33(2):101268. https://doi.org/10.1016/j.beem.2019.04.002.
3. Freda PU, Beckers AM, Katznelson L, Molitch ME, Montori VM, Post KD, et al. Pituitary incidentaloma: an endocrine society clinical practice guideline. J Clin Endocrinol Metab. 2011;96(4):894–904. https://doi.org/10.1210/jc.2010-1048.
4. Imran SA, Yip CE, Papneja N, Aldahmani K, Mohammad S, Imran F, et al. Analysis and natural history of pituitary incidentalomas. Eur J Endocrinol. 2016;175(1):1–9. https://doi.org/10.1530/EJE-16-0041.
5. Langlois F, Fleseriu M. What to do with incidentally discovered pituitary abnormalities? Med Clin North Am. 2021;105(6):1081–98. https://doi.org/10.1016/j.mcna.2021.05.015.
6. Molitch ME. Nonfunctioning pituitary tumors and pituitary incidentalomas. Endocrinol Metab Clin N Am. 2008;37(1):151–71, xi. https://doi.org/10.1016/j.ecl.2007.10.011.
7. Molitch ME. Management of incidentally found nonfunctional pituitary tumors. Neurosurg Clin N Am. 2012;23(4):543–53. https://doi.org/10.1016/j.nec.2012.06.003.
8. Sivakumar W, Chamoun R, Nguyen V, Couldwell WT. Incidental pituitary adenomas. Neurosurg Focus. 2011;31(6):E18. https://doi.org/10.3171/2011.9.FOCUS11217.
9. Tresoldi AS, Carosi G, Betella N, Del Sindaco G, Indirli R, Ferrante E, et al. Clinically nonfunctioning pituitary Incidentalomas: characteristics and natural history. Neuroendocrinology. 2020;110(7–8):595–603. https://doi.org/10.1159/000503256.
10. Freda PU, Post KD. Differential diagnosis of sellar masses. Endocrinol Metab Clin N Am. 1999;28(1):81–117, vi. https://doi.org/10.1016/s0889-8529(05)70058-x.
11. Paschou SA, Vryonidou A, Goulis DG. Pituitary incidentalomas: a guide to assessment, treatment and follow-up. Maturitas. 2016;92:143–9. https://doi.org/10.1016/j.maturitas.2016.08.006.
12. Anagnostis P, Adamidou F, Polyzos SA, Efstathiadou Z, Panagiotou A, Kita M. Pituitary incidentalomas: a single-centre experience. Int J Clin Pract. 2011;65(2):172–7. https://doi.org/10.1111/j.1742-1241.2010.02537.x.
13. Fernandez-Balsells MM, Murad MH, Barwise A, Gallegos-Orozco JF, Paul A, Lane MA, et al. Natural history of nonfunctioning pituitary adenomas and incidentalomas: a systematic review and metaanalysis. J Clin Endocrinol Metab. 2011;96(4):905–12. https://doi.org/10.1210/jc.2010-1054.
14. Vasilev V, Rostomyan L, Daly AF, Potorac I, Zacharieva S, Bonneville JF, et al. Management of endocrine disease: pituitary 'incidentaloma': neuro-radiological assessment and differential diagnosis. Eur J Endocrinol. 2016;175(4):R171–84. https://doi.org/10.1530/EJE-15-1272.
15. Hoang JK, Hoffman AR, Gonzalez RG, Wintermark M, Glenn BJ, Pandharipande PV, et al. Management of incidental pituitary findings on CT, MRI, and (18)F-fluorodeoxyglucose PET: a white paper of the ACR Incidental Findings Committee. J Am Coll Radiol. 2018;15(7):966–72. https://doi.org/10.1016/j.jacr.2018.03.037.
16. Oyama K-I, Sanno N, Tahara S, Teramoto A. Management of pituitary incidentalomas: according to a survey of pituitary incidentalomas in Japan.

Semin Ultrasound CT and MRI. 2005;26(1):47–50. https://doi.org/10.1053/j.sult.2004.10.001.

17. Fleseriu M, Hashim IA, Karavitaki N, Melmed S, Murad MH, Salvatori R, et al. Hormonal replacement in hypopituitarism in adults: an endocrine society clinical practice guideline. J Clin Endocrinol Metab. 2016;101(11):3888–921. https://doi.org/10.1210/jc.2016-2118.

18. Lania A, Beck-Peccoz P. Pituitary incidentalomas. Best Pract Res Clin Endocrinol Metab. 2012;26(4):395–403. https://doi.org/10.1016/j.beem.2011.10.009.

19. Higham CE, Johannsson G, Shalet SM Hypopituitarism. Lancet. 2016;388(10058):2403–15. https://doi.org/10.1016/S0140-6736(16)30053-8.

20. Voelker JL, Campbell RL, Muller J. Clinical, radiographic, and pathological features of symptomatic Rathke's cleft cysts. J Neurosurg. 1991;74(4):535–44. https://doi.org/10.3171/jns.1991.74.4.0535.

21. Han SJ, Rolston JD, Jahangiri A, Aghi MK. Rathke's cleft cysts: review of natural history and surgical outcomes. J Neuro-Oncol. 2014;117(2):197–203. https://doi.org/10.1007/s11060-013-1272-6.

22. Mehla S, Chua AL, Grosberg B, Evans RW. Primary Empty Sella. Headache. 2020;60(10):2522–5. https://doi.org/10.1111/head.13987.

23. Aranda F, Garcia R, Guarda FJ, Nilo F, Cruz JP, Callejas C, et al. Rathke's cleft cyst infections and pituitary abscesses: case series and review of the literature. Pituitary. 2021;24(3):374–83. https://doi.org/10.1007/s11102-020-01115-2.

24. Chanson P, Daujat F, Young J, Bellucci A, Kujas M, Doyon D, et al. Normal pituitary hypertrophy as a frequent cause of pituitary incidentaloma: a follow-up study. J Clin Endocrinol Metab. 2001;86(7):3009–15. https://doi.org/10.1210/jcem.86.7.7649.

25. Feldkamp J, Santen R, Harms E, Aulich A, Modder U, Scherbaum WA. Incidentally discovered pituitary lesions: high frequency of macroadenomas and hormone-secreting adenomas - results of a prospective study. Clin Endocrinol. 1999;51(1):109–13. https://doi.org/10.1046/j.1365-2265.1999.00748.x.

26. Arita K, Tominaga A, Sugiyama K, Eguchi K, Iida K, Sumida M, et al. Natural course of incidentally found nonfunctioning pituitary adenoma, with special reference to pituitary apoplexy during follow-up examination. J Neurosurg. 2006;104(6):884–91. https://doi.org/10.3171/jns.2006.104.6.884.

27. Mortini P, Losa M, Barzaghi R, Boari N, Giovanelli M. Results of transsphenoidal surgery in a large series of patients with pituitary adenoma. Neurosurgery. 2005;56(6):1222–33.; discussion 1233. https://doi.org/10.1227/01.neu.0000159647.64275.9d.

28. Nomikos P, Ladar C, Fahlbusch R, Buchfelder M. Impact of primary surgery on pituitary function in patients with non-functioning pituitary adenomas—a study on 721 patients. Acta Neurochir. 2004;146(1):27–35. https://doi.org/10.1007/s00701-003-0174-3.

29. Hlavac M, Knoll A, Mayer B, Braun M, Karpel-Massler G, Etzrodt-Walter G, et al. Ten years' experience with intraoperative MRI-assisted transsphenoidal pituitary surgery. Neurosurg Focus. 2020;48(6):E14. https://doi.org/10.3171/2020.3.FOCUS2072.

30. Marcus HJ, Vercauteren T, Ourselin S, Dorward NL. Intraoperative ultrasound in patients undergoing transsphenoidal surgery for pituitary adenoma: systematic review [corrected]. World Neurosurg. 2017;106:680–5. https://doi.org/10.1016/j.wneu.2017.07.054.

31. Melmed S, Casanueva FF, Hoffman AR, Kleinberg DL, Montori VM, Schlechte JA, et al. Diagnosis and treatment of hyperprolactinemia: an Endocrine Society clinical practice guideline. J Clin Endocrinol Metab. 2011;96(2):273–88. https://doi.org/10.1210/jc.2010-1692.

32. Huang W, Molitch ME. Management of nonfunctioning pituitary adenomas (NFAs): observation. Pituitary. 2018;21(2):162–7. https://doi.org/10.1007/s11102-017-0856-0.

33. Iglesias P, Arcano K, Trivino V, Garcia-Sancho P, Diez JJ, Villabona C, et al. Prevalence, clinical features, and natural history of incidental clinically non-functioning pituitary adenomas. Horm Metab Res. 2017;49(9):654–9. https://doi.org/10.1055/s-0043-115645.

Pineal Cyst

14

Mehmet Turgut, Menekşe Aygün,
and Steffen Fleck

14.1 Anatomy of Pineal Gland

The pineal gland is a neuroendocrine gland geometrically located at the midpoint of the intracranial cavity and contributes to the regulation of biological rhythm [1–3]. It is the corpus callosum at the top, the cerebellum at the bottom, the galena vein and the quadrigeminal cistern at the back, and the third ventricle and the thalamus at the anterior [1, 4–10]. The pineal gland has a vascular supply by the medial posterior choroidal artery from the posterior cerebral artery. Also bilateral choroidal, pericallosal artery, superior cerebellar artery, and quadrigeminal artery anastomoses also contribute to its nutrition. Venous drainage is provided by the vein of galena [11, 12]. Although the gland is small, it is the second bloodiest organ in the body [13].

M. Turgut (✉)
Department of Neurosurgery, Aydın Adnan Menderes
University Faculty of Medicine, Efeler, Aydın, Turkey

Department of Histology and Embryology, Aydın
Adnan Menderes University Health Sciences
Institute, Efeler, Aydın, Turkey

M. Aygün
Department of Neurosurgery, Aydın Adnan Menderes
University Faculty of Medicine, Efeler, Aydın, Turkey

S. Fleck
Neurochirurgische Gemeinschaftspraxis Greifswald,
Greifswald, Germany
e-mail: sfleck@uni-greifswald.de

14.2 Histology of Pineal Gland

The mammalian pineal gland has both "peripheral innervation," i.e., sympathetic and parasympathetic nerve fibers, and "central innervation," i.e., those arising from the central nervous system [6]. Histologically, the structure of the gland composed of two types of cells, pinealocytes and astrocytes. Pinealocytes form 95% of parenchymal cells in a lobular manner. Astrocytes also surround these cells. The lobules formed by pinealocytes are separated from each other by septa, and there are connective tissue cells in the structure of these septa. They also form vascular structures, although epithelial cells are few in number [6, 14–17]. It has been reported that calcification of the gland increases with age, although it has been encountered in children in western countries [7, 18].

14.3 Pathology of Pineal Gland

Pineal gland tumors constitute less than 1% of all intracranial tumors [19]. It is more common in child age-group than adults and is malignant at a rate of 60% [20]. The presence of many cell types in the structure of the gland allows the development of different tumor types [15–17]. Pineal region tumors can be evaluated in four groups as germ cell tumors, pineal parenchymal tumors, pineal interstitial cell tumors, and cysts [21]. In this chapter, we will consider pineal cysts from pineal region lesions.

14.4 Pineal Cyst

Pineal cysts, which is the most common lesion of the pineal gland, has been reported to be more than 10% in magnetic resonance imaging (MRI) examinations that were taken for other reasons [4, 19, 22–28]. In autopsy series, incidence of *pineal cyst was reported to be up to 40%* [29]. Pineal cysts are benign and mostly asymptomatic [27, 29–32]. Although it can be seen at any age starting from the fetal period; it is mostly seen between the ages of 21 and 30 and its frequency decreases with age [27, 32]. The incidence in women is higher than in men and it is also more common in women when they are symptomatic [28, 33].

Histologically, pineal cyst wall consists of 3 distinct layers: an inner glial, middle pineal, and outer fibrous connective tissue including the collagen fibers [16, 21]. The glial layer is the inner layer of glial tissue with/without hemosiderin, and the middle pineal layer is pineal parenchymal tissue which may contain calcium deposits, called incidental "pineal gland calcification" [16]. Collagen layer is the outermost thin layer of leptomeningeal fibrous tissue in the pineal gland [33, 34]. When we look at its etiology, there is no clear information; various theories have been put forward. During brain development, the diverticula forms the cavum pineale, which forms the pineal gland. Disturbances in this process may cause the cavum epiphysis not to close completely and a middle cavity to form [34].

(i) According to some researchers, pineal cysts may arise from ischemic degeneration of the glial layer or from necrotic epiphyseal parenchyma [35, 36]. The above-mentioned theories can explain the etiopathogenesis of cysts smaller than 1 cm.

(ii) There are also those who suggest that larger cysts are developed owing to fusion of several small epiphyseal cysts, but this theory is considered unlikely since the size increase in the cysts is not much.

(iii) After the cyst was resected, when it was examined under a microscope, hemosiderin deposits were observed in its structure and it was suggested as a different theory that the cysts were formed secondary to bleeding [23, 33, 35–37].

(iv) When Klein and L. Rubinstein examined that the incidence of pineal cysts is higher in women and especially during puberty, and its incidence prevalence decreases with age; This suggests that cyst development is hormone dependent [28, 36].

14.5 Clinical Symptoms

The most frequent presenting symptom encountered in individuals with pineal cysts in the brain is headache [9, 28]. It is widely believed that giant pineal cysts can lead to headache-inducing hydrocephalus, although some researchers suggest that the mechanisms that cause headaches in individuals are not always associated with the mass effect. The fact that many patients with pineal cysts that show compression on the quadrigeminal lamina on MRI are asymptomatic supports this view [38].

In the study of Seifert et al., the fact that none of the patients had hydrocephalus and the size of the pineal cyst did not differ between patients with and without complaint of headache, suggesting a possible role for abnormal production of melatonin, instead of its mass effect, in the etiology of headache. Less frequently, ataxia, motor and sensory disorders, mental and emotional disorders, seizure, circadian rhythm disorders, and nausea/emesis, visual disturbances resulting from tectal compression may be seen in patients [5, 9, 19, 33, 35, 39, 40]. In recent years, secondary parkinsonism is also seen as a symptom related to pineal cyst [41].

Impairment in the secretion of the hormone melatonin by the pineal gland can lead to irregular melatonin production, resulting in hormonal imbalance. Less frequently, various endocrine dysfunction findings, such as precocious puberty, hypogonadism, and diabetes insipidus, have been reported in patients with pineal cyst [42].

14.6 Pineal Cyst and Apoplexy

A rare but serious condition in epiphyseal cysts is bleeding within the pineal gland, called pineal apoplexy. It is not necessarily symptomatic, but a large proportion of hemorrhagic lesions of the pineal gland become to pineal apoplexy [26]. As a rule, apoplexy is symptomatic and patients present with severe symptoms and this condition is associated with acute obstructive hydrocephalus. Even patients of pineal cyst can experience sudden death [43]. It is rare in the pediatric population. The youngest case described so far is a 10-year-old girl when we searched the literature [44].

The most common symptoms in pineal cyst apoplexy are most common headache, eye movement disorder or visual impairment, nausea/vomiting, transient loss of consciousness, and postural tone disorder [45]. A fluid-liquid level is seen on MRI, representing the stratification of blood products associated with acute bleeding, known as hallmark of pineal cyst apoplexy [46]. It has been reported that this radiological finding was observed in almost all of patients with pineal cyst apoplexy [34, 46–49].

14.7 Radiological Features

14.7.1 Computed Tomography (CT)

Pineal cysts may appear circular on computed tomography (CT) with a thin capsule and hypodense compared to the cerebrospinal fluid (CSF) (Fig. 14.1). Hyperdense areas on CT usually reflect hemorrhage or capsular calcification [35, 40]. 25–33% of cysts contain thin ring-shaped calcifications along the walls of the pineal cysts [50, 51]. Radiologically, the contents of pineal cysts are homogeneous or heterogeneous, and these cystic lesions are unilocular or polycystic [24]. Some small epiphyseal cysts cannot be detected on CT and MRI is required. Unfortunately, the similar density of CSF and pineal cyst contents makes it difficult to detect cysts on CT [35].

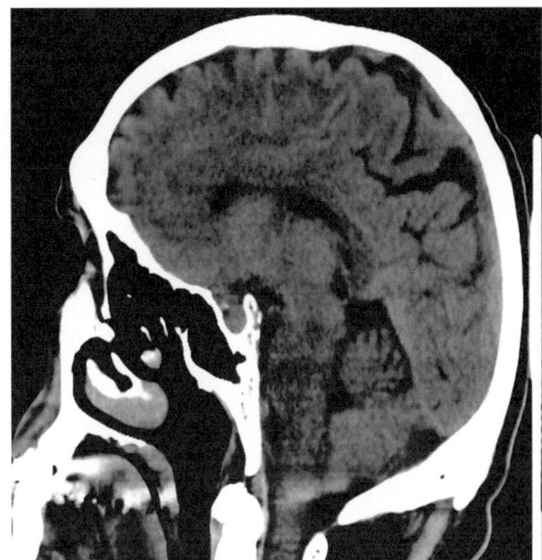

Fig. 14.1 A 64-year-old male patient with pineal cyst, sagittal section computed tomography study

14.7.2 Magnetic Resonance Imaging (MRI)

On MRI, pineal cysts are well-circumscribed, oval cystic lesions [26, 32, 52]. Pineal cysts generally have signaling properties similar to CSF, due to their lipid or protein content [50, 51]. In T1-weighted imaging; hypointense compared to white matter and according to CSF, it is either isointense or diffusely hyperintense [37] (Figs. 14.2 and 14.3). The cyst wall is slightly hypointense or isointense compared to the adjacent brain tissue [53].

In T2-weighted imaging, mixtures of pineal cysts are homogeneous and they are isointense/hyperintense according to CSF (Figs. 14.4, 14.5, 14.6, 14.7, 14.8). The thickness of a cyst wall is typically 2 mm or less [22, 26, 40]. In contrast imaging, roughly 60% of pineal cysts have contrast enhancement as a result of absence of the blood–brain barrier in the cyst wall and this fine contrast rim (<2 mm) appears extremely intense [34] (Fig. 14.9). In FLAIR imaging, because the pineal cyst content is not suppressed, it typically appears slightly hyperintense compared to CSF [25, 26] (Figs. 14.10, 14.11, 14.12).

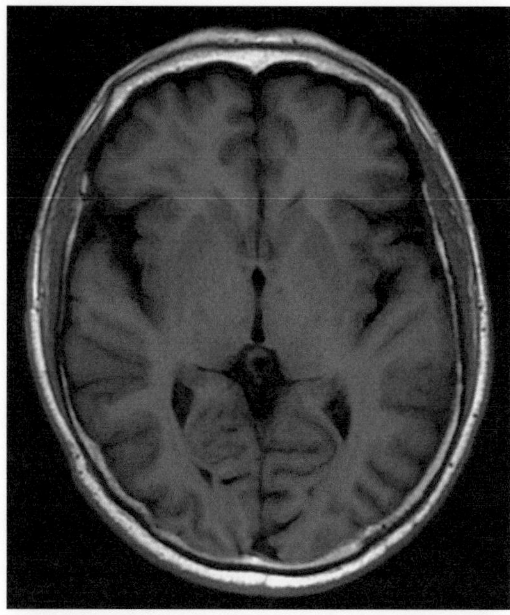

Fig. 14.2 A 64-year-old male patient (same patient in Fig. 14.1); axial section T1-weighted magnetic resonance imaging (MRI)

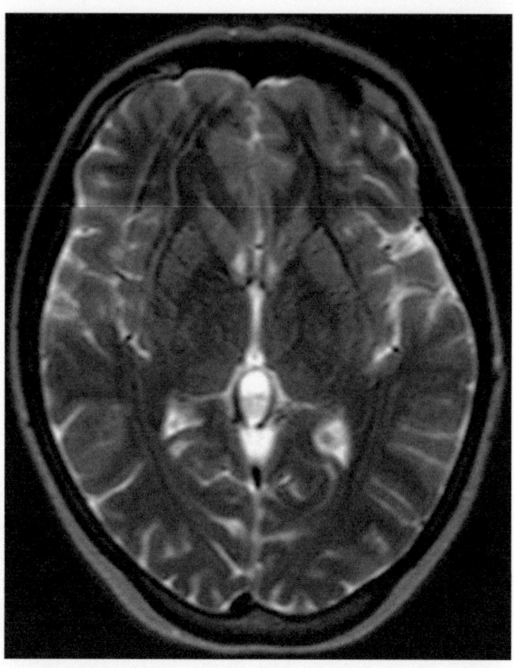

Fig. 14.4 A 21-year-old female patient; axial section T2-weighted MRI

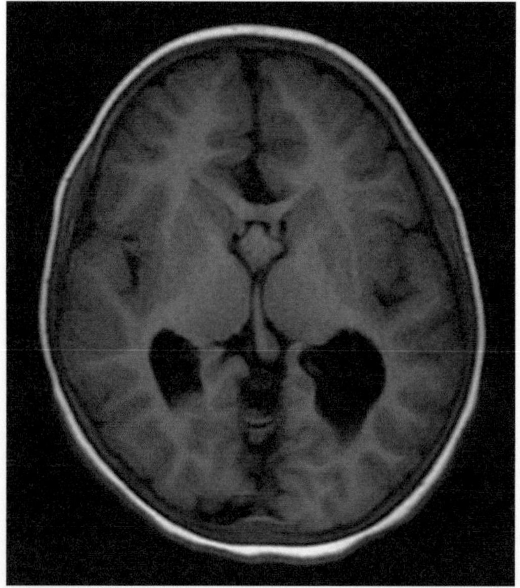

Fig. 14.3 A 9-year-old female patient with small pineal cyst, axial section T1-weighted MRI

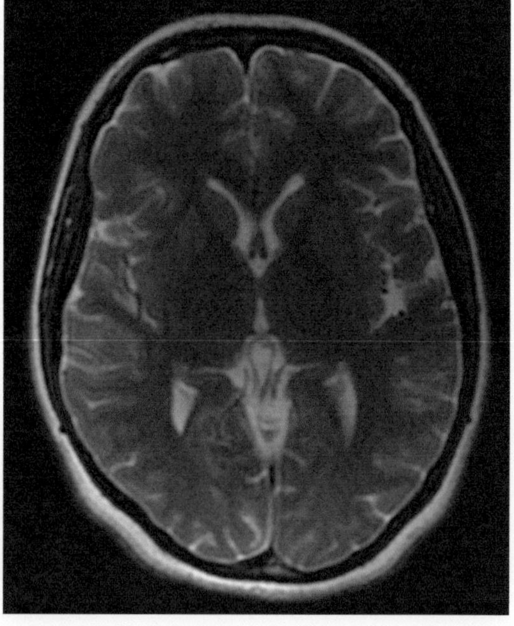

Fig. 14.5 A 28-year-old female patient; axial section T2-weighted MRI

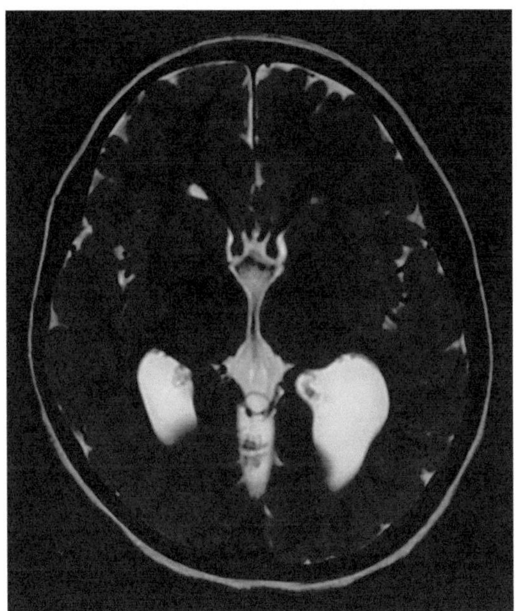

Fig. 14.6 A 9-year-old female patient (same patient in Fig. 14.3); axial section T2-weighted MRI

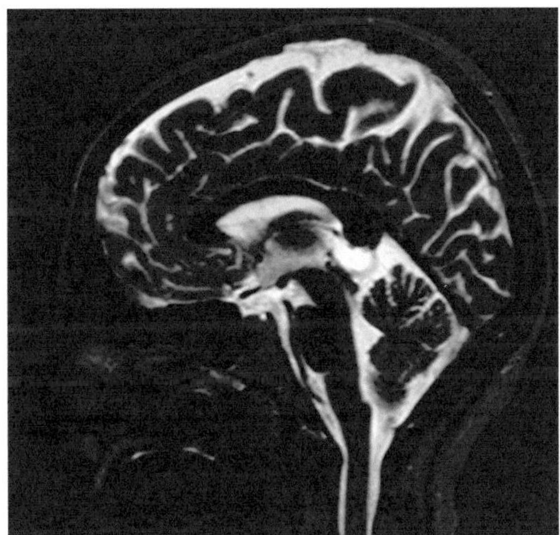

Fig. 14.7 A 21-year-old female patient (same patient in Fig. 14.4); sagittal section T2-weighted MRI

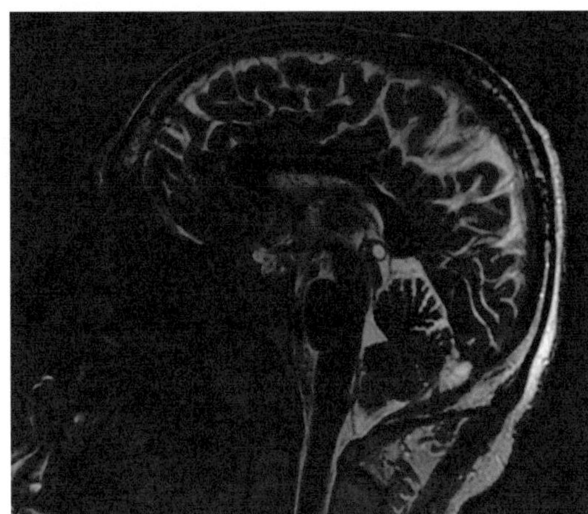

Fig. 14.8 A 64-year-old male patient (same patient in Figs. 14.1 and 14.2); mid-sagittal section T2-weighted MRI

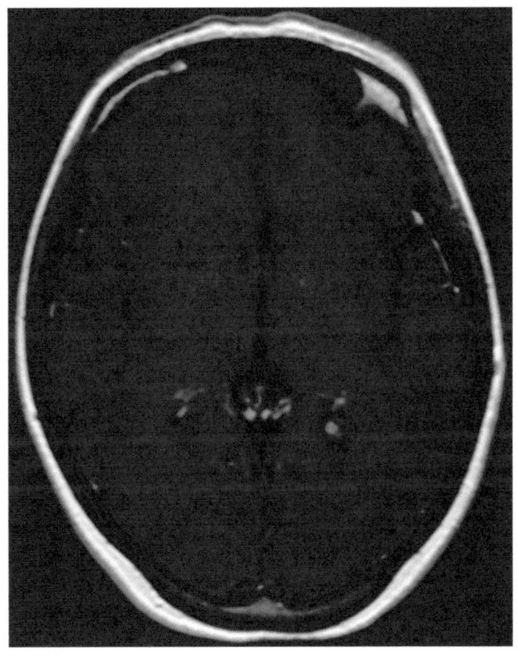

Fig. 14.9 A 21-year-old female patient (same patient in Figs. 14.4 and 14.7); axial section MRI following contrast material administration

14.7.3 Transcranial Sonography

Transcranial sonography (TCS) study is an ultrasound-based, non-invasive imaging technique that can produce black and white two-dimension (2D) planar images. First time, Harrer et al. demonstrated the feasibility of TCS as a radiological option in the diagnosis and follow-up of young patients with incidental asymptomatic pineal cysts [54]. In another study, the reliability of TCS was confirmed by Budisic et al. [55, 56]. They concluded that TCS is a cost-effective and reliable alternative radiological study in the follow-up of individuals with pineal cysts [55, 56].

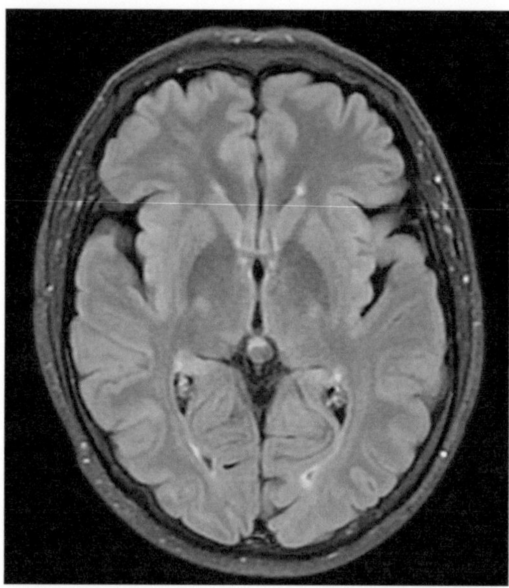

Fig. 14.10 A 64-year-old male patient (same patient in Figs. 14.1, 14.2 and 14.8); axial section FLAIR MRI

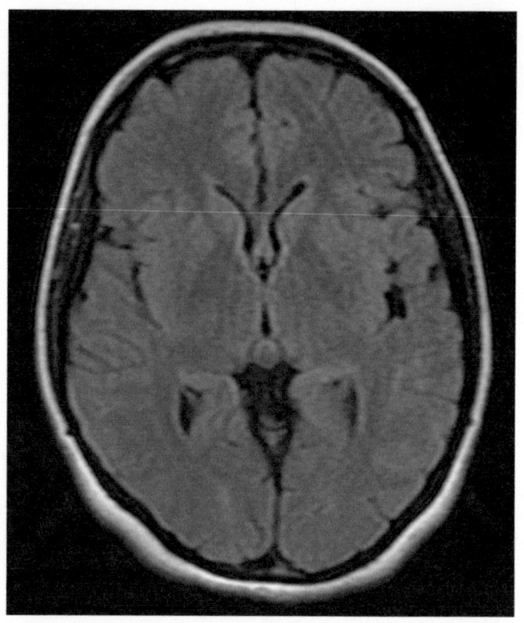

Fig. 14.12 A 28-year-old female patient (same patient in Fig. 14.5); axial section FLAIR MRI

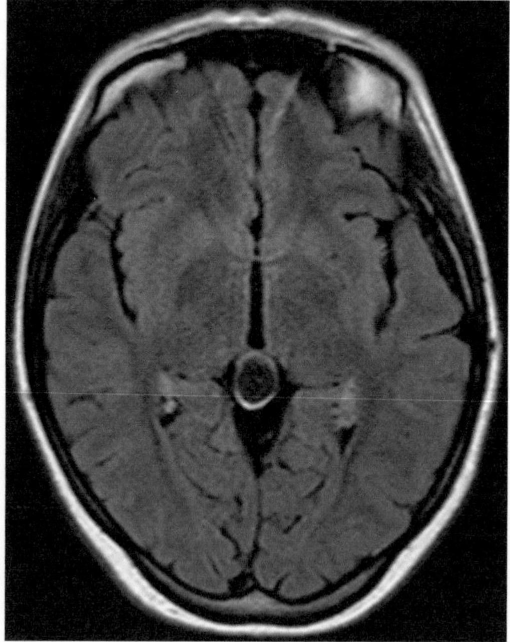

Fig. 14.11 A 21-year-old female patient (same patient in Figs. 14.4, 14.7 and 14.9); axial section FLAIR MRI

14.8 Treatment

As a rule, in symptomatic patients of in pineal cysts with consecutive obstructive hydrocephalus due to aqueductal stenosis, the surgery is clearly indicated [31]. Historically, first in 1914 in St. Petersburg, the microsurgical removal of a symptomatic pineal cyst was carried out by Pussep, the founder of Russian neurosurgery and head of the world's first Neurosurgery Department [2, 31, 57]. Pussep used an infratentorial supracerebellar approach to remove the cyst. This approach is still the most commonly used [31, 35, 36, 57–62].

Even today, scientific knowledge regarding surgical treatment of patients with pineal cysts without hydrocephalus is still limited. There might be an indication in very selected patients. In patients with pineal cysts presenting with clinical symptoms such as headache, nausea, and vision problems, other etiologies should be considered. The most obvious explanation of causing these symptoms is an intermittent occlusion of the aqueduct leading to repeated intracranial hypertension. The primary treatment method in symptomatic pineal cysts is microsurgical resection via supracerebellar-infratentorial approach [31]. Exact preoperative planning (e.g., regarding position and venous anatomy) is mandatory. Second, the occipital transtentorial approach is used. Transient homonymous hemianopsia and convulsive syndrome are complications that can be seen in this approach [58]. In case of wide ventricles, endoscopic transventricular fenestration might be an option.

Nowadays, stereotactic cyst fenestration can be used as an alternative to open surgery. Stereotactic aspiration, a minimal invasive procedure, may provide elimination of the mass effect, in spite of risk of bleeding or recurrence. In the stereotactic aspiration method, usually no histological sample is taken and the aspirated fluid is analyzed and analyzed. Hence the potential to miss a completely cystic neoplasm. It has been reported that a long-term follow-up is mandatory if stereotactic aspiration is used as a treatment method [63].

14.9 Conclusion

Pineal cysts are the most common observed lesions of the pineal gland, and their etiology is not known exactly. Clinically, they usually present with headache ataxia, motor and sensory disorders, mental and emotional disorders, epilepsy, circadian rhythm disorders, and secondary parkinsonism. Radiologically, MRI, CT, and TCS are used to visualize these lesions. Cases with obstructive hydrocephalus due to aqueductal stenosis may require surgical resection of the cyst, while minimally invasive methods such as endoscopic transventricular resection in hydrocephalic patients and stereotactic aspiration are alternative approaches for these lesions.

References

1. Lombardi G, Poliani PL, Manara R, Berhouma M, Minniti G, Tabouret E, Razis E, Cerretti G, Zagonel V, Weller M, Idbaih A. Diagnosis and treatment of pineal region tumors in adults: a EURACAN overview. Cancers (Basel). 2022;14(15):3646.
2. Shoja MM, Hoepfner LD, Agutter PS, Singh R, Tubbs RS. History of the pineal gland. Childs Nerv Syst. 2016;32(4):583–6.
3. Turgut M, Ozkaya B. Pineal region tumors: pathological features and surgical approaches (in Turkish). Archive. 2001;10:100–18.
4. Bosnjak J, Budisic M, Azman D, Strineka M, Crnjakovic M, Demarin V. Pineal gland cysts–an overview. Acta Clin Croat. 2009;48(3):355–8.
5. Majovsky M, Benes V. Natural course of pineal cysts-a radiographic study. Chin Neurosurg J. 2018;4:33.
6. Møller M. Fine structure of the pinealopetal innervation of the mammalian pineal gland. Microsc Res Tech. 1992;21(3):188–204.
7. Patel S, Rahmani B, Gandhi J, Seyam O, Joshi G, Reid I, Smith NL, Waltzer WC, Khan SA. Revisiting the pineal gland: a review of calcification, masses, precocious puberty, and melatonin functions. Int J Neurosci. 2020;130(5):464–75.
8. Rhoton AL Jr, Yamamoto I, Peaca DA. Microsurgery of the third ventricle. Part 2. Operative approaches. Neurosurgery. 1981;8:357.
9. Seifert CL, Woeller A, Valet M, Zimmer C, Berthele A, Tölle T, Sprenger T. Headaches and pineal cyst: a case-control study. Headache. 2008;48:448–52.
10. Simon E, Afif A, M'Baye M, Mertens P. Anatomy of the pineal region applied to its surgical approach. Neurochirurgie. 2015;61(2–3):70–6.
11. Kappers AJ. The mammalian pineal gland, a survey. Acta Neurochir. 1976;34:109–49.
12. Quest DQ, Kleragia E. Microsurgical anatomy of the pineal region. Neurosurgery. 1980;6:385–90.
13. Reiter RJ. The mammalian pineal gland: structure and function. Am J Anat. 1981;162:287–313.
14. Cho ZH, Choi SH, Chi JG, Kim YB. Classification of the venous architecture of the pineal gland by 7T MRI. J Neuroradiol. 2011;38(4):238–41.
15. Erlich SS, Apuzzo KLJ. The pineal gland: anatomy, physiology and clinical significance. J Neurosurg. 1985;63:321–41.
16. Fawcett DW, Jenesh RP. Pineal gland. In: Bloom M, Fawcett DW, editors. Concise histology. New York: Chapman & Hall International Thomson Publishing; 1977. p. 164.
17. King AS, McLelland J. Birds. Their structure and function. London: Bailliere Tindall; 1984.
18. Turgut AT, Karakaş HM, Ozsunar Y, Altın L, Ceken K, Alıcıoğlu B, Sönmez I, Alparslan A, Yürümez B, Celik T, Kazak E, Geyik PÖ, Koşar U. Age-related

changes in the incidence of pineal gland calcification in Turkey: a prospective multicenter CT study. Pathophysiology. 2008;15(1):41–8.

19. Engel U, Gottschalk S, Niehaus L, Lehmann R, May C, Vogel S, Jänisch W. Cystic lesions of the pineal region-MRI and pathology. Neuroradiology. 2000;42:399–402.

20. Herrmann HD, Winkler D, Westphal M. Treatment of tumors of the pineal region and posterior part of the third ventricle. Acta Neurochir. 1992;116:137–46.

21. Kumar P, Tatke M, Sharma A, Singh D. Histological analysis of lesions of the pineal region: a retrospective study of 12 years. Pathol Res Pract. 2006;202:85–92.

22. Di Costanzo A, Tedeschi G, Di Salle F, Golia F, Morrone R, Bonavita V. Pineal cysts: an incidental MRI finding? J Neurol Neurosurg Psychiatry. 1993;56:207–8.

23. Fleege MA, Miller GM, Fletcher GP, Fain JS, Scheithauer BW. Benign glial cysts of the pineal gland: unusual imaging characteristics with histologic correlation. AJNR Am J Neuroradiol. 1994;15(1):161–6.

24. Jinkins JR, Xiong L, Reiter RJ. The midline pineal «eye»: MR and CT characteristics of the pineal gland with and without benign cyst formation. J Pineal Res. 1995;19(2):64–71.

25. Korogi Y, Takahashi M, Ushio Y. MRI of pineal region tumors. J Neuro-Oncol. 2001;54(3):251–61.

26. Mamourian AC, Towfighi J. Pineal cysts: MR imaging. AJNR Am J Neuroradiol. 1986;7(6):1081–6.

27. Pu Y, Mahankali S, Hou J, Li J, Lancaster JL, Gao JH, Appelbaum DE, Fox PT. High prevalence of pineal cysts in healthy adults demonstrated by high-resolution, noncontrast brain MR imaging. AJNR Am J Neuroradiol. 2007;28(9):1706–9.

28. Sawamura Y, Ikeda J, Ozawa M, Minoshima Y, Saito H, Abe H. Magnetic resonance images reveal a high incidence of asymptomatic pineal cysts in young women. Neurosurgery. 1995;37:11–5.

29. Hasegawa A, Ohtsubo K, Mori W. Pineal gland in old age; quantitative and qualitative morphological study of 168 human autopsy cases. Brain Res. 1987;409:343–9.

30. Nolte I, Brockmann MA, Gerigk L, Groden C, Scharf J. TrueFISP imaging of the pineal gland: more cysts and more abnormalities. Clin Neurol Neurosurg. 2010;112(3):204–8.

31. Kennedy BC, Bruce JN. Surgical approaches to the pineal region. Neurosurg Clin N Am. 2011;22(3):367–80. viii

32. Mandera M, Marcol W, Bierzynska-Macyszyn G, Kluczewska E. Pineal cysts in childhood. Childs Nerv Syst. 2003;19:750–5.

33. Mena H, Armonda RA, Ribas JL, Ondra SL, Rushing EJ. Nonneoplastic pineal cyst: a clinicopathologic study of twenty-one cases. Ann Diagn Pathol. 1997;1:11–8.

34. Osborn AG, Preece MT. Intracranial cysts: radiologic-pathologic correlation and imaging approach. Radiology. 2006;239:650–64.

35. Fain JS, Tomlinson FH, Scheithauer BW, Parisi JE, Fletcher GP, Kelly PJ, Miller GM. Symptomatic glial cysts of the pineal gland. J Neurosurg. 1994;80:454–60.

36. Klein P, Rubinstein LJ. Benign symptomatic glial cysts of the pineal gland: a report of seven cases and review of the literature. J Neurol Neurosurg Psychiatry. 1989;52:991–5.

37. Al-Holou WN, Garton HJL, Muraszko KM, Ibrahim M, Maher CO. Prevalence of pineal cysts in children and young adults. Clinical article. J Neurosurg Pediatr. 2009;4:230–6.

38. Molina-Martinez FJ, Jimenez-Martinez MC, Vives-Pastor B. Some questions provoked by a chronic headache (with mixed migraine and cluster headache features) in a woman with a pineal cyst. Answers from a literature review. Cephalalgia. 2010;30:1031–40.

39. Fleck S, Damaty AE, Lange I, Matthes M, Rafaee EE, Marx S, Baldauf J, Schroeder HWS. Pineal cysts without hydrocephalus: microsurgical resection via an infratentorial-supracerebellar approach-surgical strategies, complications, and their avoidance. Neurosurg Rev. 2022;45(5):3327–37.

40. Tamaki N, Shirataki K, Lin TK, Masumura M, Katayama S, Matsumoto S. Cysts of the pineal gland. A new clinical entity to be distinguished from tumors of the pineal region. Childs Nerv Syst. 1989;5: 172–6.

41. Morgan JT, Scumpia AJ, Webster TM, Mittler MA, Edelman M, Schneider SJ. Resting tremor secondary to a pineal cyst: case report and review of the literature. Pediatr Neurosurg. 2008;44:234–8.

42. Smirniotopoulos JG, Rushing EJ, Mena H. Pineal region masses: differential diagnosis. Radiographics. 1992;12:577–96.

43. Richardson JK, Hirsch CS. Sudden, unexpected death due to "pineal apoplexy". Am J Forensic Med Pathol. 1986;7:64–8.

44. Majeed K, Enam SA. Recurrent pineal apoplexy in a child. Neurology. 2007;69:112–4.

45. Patel AJ, Fuller GN, Wildrick DM, Sawaya R. Pineal cyst apoplexy: case report and review of the literature. Neurosurgery. 2005;57(5):E1066; discussion E1066.

46. Koenigsberg RA, Faro S, Marino R, Turz A, Goldman W. Imaging of pineal apoplexy. Clin Imaging. 1996;20:91–4.

47. Musolino A, Cambria S, Rizzo G, Cambria M. Symptomatic cysts of the pineal gland: stereotactic diagnosis and treatment of two cases and review of the literature. Neurosurgery. 1993;32:315–20.

48. Swaroop GR, Whittle IR. Pineal apoplexy: an occurrence with no diagnostic clinicopathological features. Br J Neurosurg. 1998;12:274–6.

49. Turtz AR, Hughes WB, Goldman HW. Endoscopic treatment of a symptomatic pineal cyst: technical case report. Neurosurgery. 1995;37:1013–4.

50. Gaillard F, Jones J. Masses of the pineal region: clinical presentation and radiographic features. Postgrad Med J. 2010;86(1020):597–607.

51. Peres MFP, Zukerman E, Porto PP, Brandt RA. Headaches and pineal cyst: a (more than) coincidental relationship? Headache. 2004;44: 929–30.

52. Pastel DA, Mamourian AC, Duhaime AC. Internal structure in pineal cysts on high-resolution magnetic resonance imaging: not a sign of malignancy. J Neurosurg Pediatr. 2009;4(1):81–4.
53. Fakhran S, Escott EJ. Pineocytoma mimicking a pineal cyst on imaging: true diagnostic dilemma or a case of incomplete imaging? AJNR Am J Neuroradiol. 2008;29(1):159–63.
54. Harrer JU, Klötzsch C, Oertel MF, Möller-Hartmann W. Sonographic detection and follow up of an atypical pineal cyst: a comparison with magnetic resonance imaging. Case report. J Neurosurg. 2005;103(3):564–6.
55. Budisic M, Bosnjak J, Lovrencic-Huzjan A, Mikula I, Bedek D, Demarin V. Pineal gland cyst evaluated by transcranial sonography. Eur J Neurol. 2008;15:229–33.
56. Budisic M, Bosnjak J, Lovrencic-Huzjan A, Strineka M, Bene R, Azman D, Bedek D, Trkanjec Z, Demarin V. Transcranial sonography in the evaluation of pineal lesions: two-year follow up study. Acta Clin Croat. 2008;47:205–10.
57. Kalani MY, Wilson DA, Koechlin NO, Abuhusain HJ, Dlouhy BJ, Gunawardena MP, Nozue-Okada K, Teo C. Pineal cyst resection in the absence of ventriculomegaly or Parinaud's syndrome: clinical outcomes and implications for patient selection. J Neurosurg. 2015;123(2):352–6.
58. Berhoumaa M, Nia H, Delabara V, Tahhana N, Memou S, Mottolesea C. Update on the management of pineal cysts: case series and a review of the literature. Neurochirurgie. 2015;61(2–3):201–7.
59. Maurer PK, Ecklund J, Parisi JE, Ondra S. Symptomatic pineal cyst: case report. Neurosurgery. 1990;27:451–345.
60. Michielsen G, Benoit Y, Baert E, Meire F, Caemaert J. Symptomatic pineal cysts: clinical manifestations and management. Acta Neurochir. 2002;144:233–42.
61. Oeckler R, Feiden W. Benign symptomatic lesions of the pineal gland. Report of seven cases treated surgically. Acta Neurochir. 1991;108:40–4.
62. Sarikaya-Seiwert S, Turowski B, Hänggi D, Sela G, Han S, Steiger JB, Stummer W. Symptomatic intracystic hemorrhage in pineal cysts. J Neurosurg Pediatr. 2009;4
63. Steven DA, Gregory JM, McClarty BM. A choroid plexus papilloma arising from an incidental pineal cyst. AJNR Am J Neuroradiol. 1996;17:939–42.

Chiari Malformation

15

Mehmet Turgut, Ahmet Kürşat Kara,
and R. Shane Tubbs

15.1 Introduction

Chiari malformation (CM) was defined by Hans Chiari in 1891. It is accepted as a congenital anomaly of the craniovertebral junction. Symptoms occur because the cerebellar tonsils are herniated downwards from the foramen magnum, disrupting the dynamics of free flow at the craniovertebral junction and compressing neurological structures. The prevalence of CMs is less than 1% in the United States [1]. CM type 1 is more common and preponderantly affects females [2]. Its incidence is higher in the pediatric population [3].

Clinically, CM can progress asymptomatically or present with neurological symptoms such as headache, ataxia, dysphagia, sleep apnea, and sudden death. The herniation degree of tonsilla cerebelli shows a correlation with the symptoms [4]. The gold standard for diagnosis is sagittal plane magnetic resonance imaging (MRI). Downward displacement of the excess foreman magnum is diagnostic for CM type 1. In Fig. 15.1, a 71-year-old man was diagnosed with CM but had no symptoms. Tonsillar displacement up to 2 mm asymptomatically is considered normal [5]. Although tonsil involvement is usually bilateral and unilateral, tonsillar herniation is also seen.

M. Turgut (✉)
Department of Neurosurgery, Aydın Adnan Menderes University Faculty of Medicine, Efeler, Aydın, Turkey

Department of Histology and Embryology, Aydın Adnan Menderes University Health Sciences Institute, Efeler, Aydın, Turkey

A. K. Kara
Department of Neurosurgery, Aydın Adnan Menderes University Faculty of Medicine, Efeler, Aydın, Turkey

R. S. Tubbs
Department of Neurosurgery, Tulane University School of Medicine, New Orleans, LA, USA

Department of Structural and Cell Biology, Tulane University School of Medicine, New Orleans, LA, USA

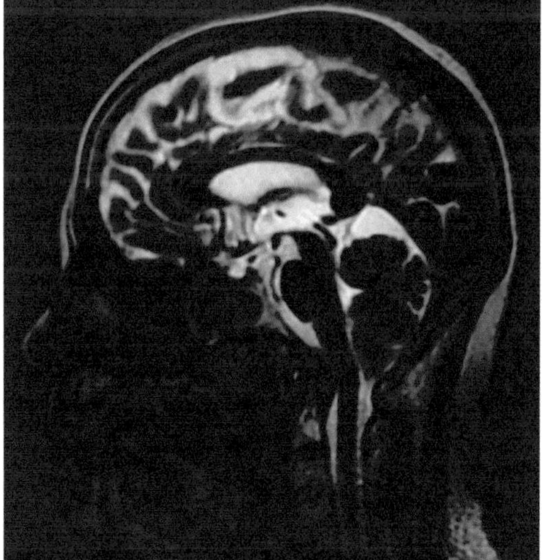

Fig. 15.1 A 71-year-old female patient was diagnosed with Chiari malformation (CM) type 1. The cerebellar tonsils herniated downward from the foramen magnum

Syrinx forms because cerebrospinal fluid (CSF) flow is disrupted at the craniovertebral junction and circulation in the subarachnoid space is impaired. Characteristically, there is a small posterior fossa and downward displacement of the brainstem in patients with CM type 2. This malformation is accompanied by spinal dysraphism in almost every case, and symptoms such as dysphagia, stridor, apnea, and motor weakness are attributable to brainstem compression [6].

15.2 Definition and Classification

The Chiari classification used today is the one proposed by Hans Chiari at the end of the nineteenth century. It distinguishes four types. Chiari created this classification on the basis of autopsy studies. CM type 1 is downward displacement of the tonsilla cerebelli of the cerebellum of 5 mm or more. However, the brain stem is not displaced downwards, and no neural tube defect is observed. Syrinx can accompany CM type 1.

A neural tube defect accompanies almost every case of CM type 2. The defect is usually a myelomeningocele. The brain stem is displaced caudally. Hydrocephalus is common in these patients. Ventriculoperitoneal (VP) shunting surgery or third ventriculostomy is required.

CM type 3 is very rare, and it is likely to be fatal. The brain stem and cerebellum migrate out of the posterior fossa. CM type 3.5 was defined as a new and very rare type. In CM type 3.5, an occipitocervical encephalocele communicates with the stomach [7].

CM type 4 is hindbrain hypoplasia [8]. However, there is misunderstanding about CM type 4 and misuse of the term [9]. Comparisons were made with different pathologies involving the posterior fossa. This is the classification defined by Hans Chiari.

New classifications were subsequently determined for patients who did not fully fit these four types but did fit the definition of CM. Two of these were named CM type 0 and type 1.5. In CM type 0, the cerebellar tonsils show less than 5 mm caudal displacement, but there is a crowded appearance and syrinx formation. CM type 1.5 appears to be halfway between types 1 and 2. There is no neural tube defect, as in in type 2I, but there is downward displacement of the brain stem. Figure 15.2 shows MRI of a patient followed up with a diagnosis of CM type 1.5.

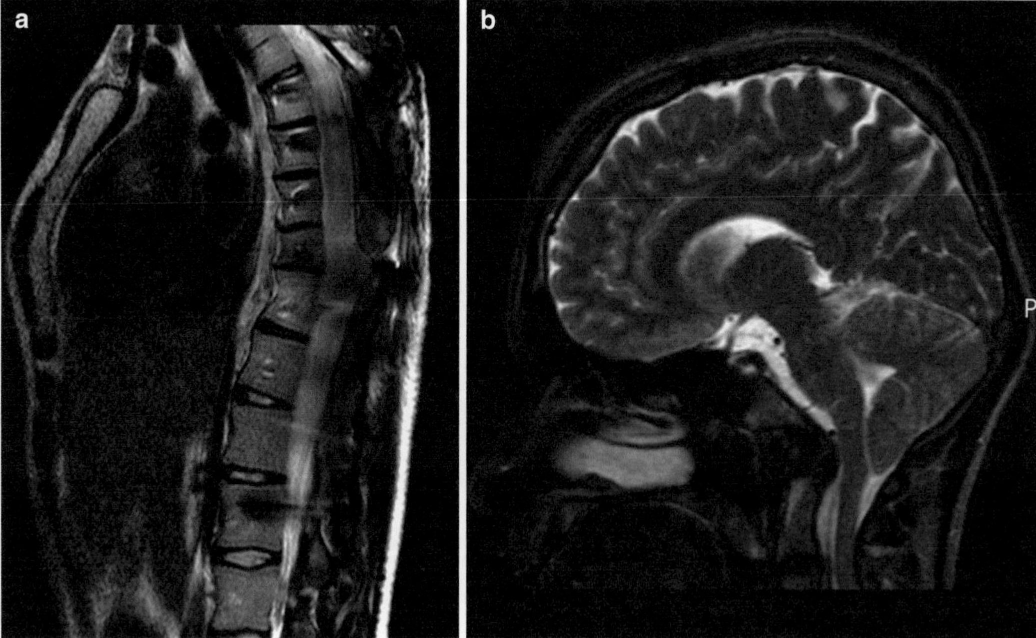

Fig. 15.2 A 17-year-old male patient with diagnosis of CM type 1.5

Complex CM is characterized by bone and soft tissue abnormalities. The brainstem is herniated downward from the foramen magnum. Complex CM can be accompanied by medullary kink, occipitalization of the atlas, syringomyelia, basilar invagination, and retroflexed odontoid process [10]. Recently, a case of suboccipital decompressive craniectomy for "complex CM" associated with necrotizing encephalopathy caused by H1N1 viral infection has been reported by senior author this chapter [11].

Downward herniation of the occipital lobe along the foramen magnum was classed as CM type 5. This is a very rare condition [12].

15.3 Epidemiology

Although CM is now more commonly diagnosed because of the widespread use of MRI, its incidence is around 0.01% in symptomatic patients. Radiologically, it is around 1%. The population incidence of tonsillar ectopia is 3.5% [13]. The occurrence of symptoms is correlated with the extent of tonsillar herniation. However, individual anatomical variations affect the symptoms.

The etiology of CM is multifactorial; both environmental and genetic factors are involved. Some studies show that familial factors affect its incidence. There is a case report of monozygotic twins with CM type I but different degrees of tonsillar herniation [14]. The cohort study by Milhorat et al. supports this [15]. However, CM can be seen together with Ehlers Danlos, Marfan, and Klippel Feil syndromes [16].

Genetic factors in the etiology of CM have been investigated, but no particular gene has been identified. However, the hla-a9 gene is common among patients with CM [17]. CM is more common in women. Elster found that 62% of his study participants were women [18]. The onset and symptoms of the disease, and its prevalence, differ among ethnic groups [19, 20]. CM can

develop because of birth trauma and can also be caused by trauma in adults [21]. Increased intracranial pressure can cause it [22]. However, a VP shunt helps in the regression of tonsillar herniation in cases with hydrocephalus. Considering the incidence of CM, more cases are needed for epidemiological information.

15.4 Radiological Diagnosis

Radiological examinations are the gold standard for the diagnosis and surgical planning of CM. In CM type 1, there is a small posterior fossa, tonsillar herniation, deterioration of CSF flow dynamics, and compression of neural structures at the level of the tonsillar herniation [23]. These characteristics explain the symptoms. There is crowding at the level of the foramen magnum. Syringomyelia is observed in the spinal cord [24]. Sagittal plane MRI reveals the presence and extent of herniation of tonsilla cerebelli. In MRI examination, the sections should not be thicker than 3 mm for accurate evaluation. Radiologically, downward displacement of the cerebellar tonsils of 5 mm or more is diagnostic [25].

It is important to determine whether neural structures are under pressure in the foramen magnum. A mass effect at the foramen magnum level from various other causes will give symptoms similar to CM [26]. Therefore, other pathologies that can cause a mass effect in this region should be included in the differential diagnosis. Hydrocephalus, resulting from fourth ventricular compression, can be seen with cranial MRI. At the same time there is downward displacement of the brain stem. In Fig. 15.3, a 21-year-old patient had all the clinical signs of CM type 2.

In CM type 2, the spinal defect and related CSF leakage can result in intracranial hypotension [4]. In CM type 3, structures in the posterior fossa herniate out of the defect [27].

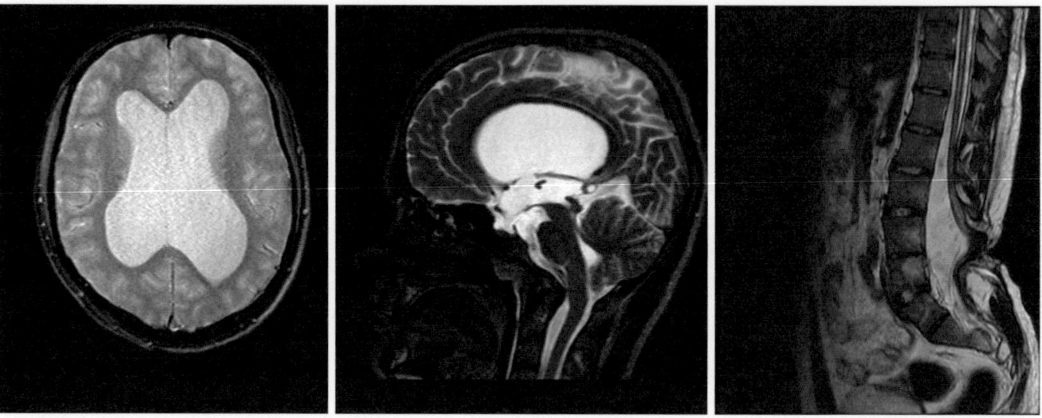

Fig. 15.3 A 21-year-old male patient was diagnosed with CM type 2. Myelomeningocele and hydrocephalus accompany the malformation

15.5 Pathophysiology

Despite research on the pathophysiology of CM, it has not been clarified. Since it is a group of diseases of different types, the pathophysiology of each type needs to be explained separately. For example, CMs types 1 and 2 have very different characteristics and components. Therefore, the symptoms and mechanisms of their manifestation are also different. While tonsillar herniation is prominent in CM type 1, downward displacement of the brain stem and brain stem compression predominate in type 2. The symptoms are therefore different.

Langhans proposed a mechanism of syringomyelia formation hypothesis and pathological tonsillar ectopia in 1881. Syringomyelia was thought to form because of the obstruction at the level of the foramen magnum [28]. Gardner tried to explain the mechanism: While the central canal remains open in the obex, the exit foramen of the fourth ventricle is closed [29]. The CSF in the fourth ventricle continues to force the central canal as it is the only outlet. This cavity pressure, pulsation, and continuity in the central canal are thought to cause syringomyelia. Figure 15.4 shows syringomyelia extending through the entire thoracic passage. However, this hypothesis does not fully explain the pathophysiology; it does not explain why CM may develop secondary to trauma or teth-

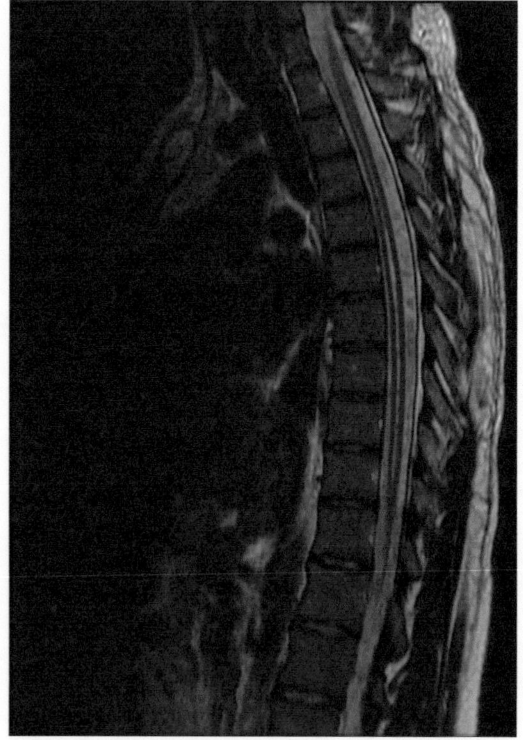

Fig. 15.4 Thoracic syringomyelia

ered cord [30]. Goel proposed that atlantoaxial instability causes syringomyelia and CM [31]. CM is thought to be caused by the difference in cranial and spinal pressure before the tonsilla cerebelli of the cerebellum and brain stem are fully developed [32].

The anatomy of the posterior fossa in the pathophysiology of CM has been studied to elucidate the etiology [33]. Milhorat showed that patients with CM had a smaller posterior cranial fossa than the control group [34]. MRI is valuable for measuring the posterior fossa [35]. CM type 2 is associated with spina bifida [21].

The incidence of hydrocephalus is 4–18% in cases of CM. Tubbs et al. found that 10% of their 500 CM patients had hydrocephalus [36]. The formation of hydrocephalus is explained by blocking the drainage of the fourth ventricle [37]. However, CM is thought to occur secondary to hydrocephalus [38]. Spinal defects, hyperostosis, and bone mineral diseases are also thought to be involved in the pathophysiology [39].

15.6 Clinical Findings

CM type 1 presents with different clinical features. The extent of tonsillar herniation and compression of neural tissues in the foramen magnum affect the presentation [40]. Although it can be asymptomatic, patients with CM type I can experience double or blurred vision, tinnitus, and hearing impairment [41]. Clinical findings can include nystagmus, loss of gag reflex, hoarseness, and tongue atrophy [42]. In some patients, suboccipital headache is the only symptom [3]. Symptoms begin to appear in early childhood, appearing in the 20 s in adults. CM can manifest itself with cranial nerve involvement [43]. The effects can include tonsillar herniation, cranial nerve traction, and brain stem compression due to impaired CSF circulation. CM type 1 can be accompanied by syndromic conditions such as Pierre Robin syndrome [44].

The Valsalva Maneuver especially provokes suboccipital headache [45], usually lasting for a short time and tending to recur during the day [4]. Headache occurs in almost all patients. Visual and balance disturbances occur because of brain stem compression. Although nystagmus is seen in these patients, it has been reported with different incidences in different series, up to 70% [25]. Swallowing difficulties, dizziness, and syncope also occur as a result of brain stem compression. Sudden death in CM has been presented in case reports [46].

CM type 2 presents with caudal elongation and migration of the cerebellar vermis [47]. A neural tube defect, myelomeningocele or encephalocele, is present in almost every patient. Hydrocephalus is common in this patient group, and VP shunting is needed [48]. In these patients, bulging in the fontanelles and separation of the cranial sutures can present with hydrocephalus.

CM type 3 is extremely rare. It results from external herniation of posterior fossa structures owing to a bone defect in the occipital region [25]. Clinically, it presents with myelomeningocele, tethered cord, and hydrocephalus.

15.7 Treatment

There are surgical and conservative options for treating CM. Patient selection for surgery is a controversial issue [49]. Since there is no primary cause in most patients, decompression surgery is performed rather than etiological treatment. If the etiology is known, treatment for it can be planned; for example, in CM associated with craniosynostosis. However, even in this case, the primary question of craniosynostosis surgery or decompressive surgery is controversial [50].

While radiological imaging is the gold standard for diagnosing CM, the clinic is more important for selecting patients for surgical treatment [2]. Surgery is recommended for patients with significant symptoms in CM type 1 and also for patients with syringomyelia formation to stop its progression [19]. Although the extent of tonsillar herniation correlates with the severity of symptoms, we cannot decide on the indication for surgery only by looking at its extent. One study showed tonsillar herniation of more than 5 mm with a prevalence of 0.9% with no symptoms [51]. There is no indication for surgical treatment in that patient group.

Surgical treatment involves suboccipital decompression and VP shunting. The accompanying myelomeningocele and hydrocephalus in CM type 2 are part of the treatment management [26]. Decompressive surgery should be combined with VP shunting surgery and a treatment plan for myelomeningocele. As an alternative to VP shunting, third ventriculostomy is preferred in suitable cases. A VP shunt has a high rate of complications such as shunt infection and shut failure in these patients [52].

15.8 Prognosis

The prognosis in CM is very variable and the factors affecting it are still not fully known. Since the pathophysiology of the disease is not completely clear, its natural course is also unknown. Which patients will be followed conservatively and which will be operated on is still controversial. The presence of syringomyelia, nystagmus, and ataxia indicates a poor prognosis [53]. The prognosis is better for patients with a small posterior fossa [54], and for patients with cerebellar syndrome and brain stem syndrome [17]. Patients with only headache respond well to conservative treatment, but the prognosis is poor for patients with ataxia and cranial nerve signs [55]. Even patients who benefit rapidly after surgery can return to the clinic with a condition like that before surgery, or even worse [56].

In a study of patients with CM type 1, the clinical improvement was 69.6% after surgery [57]. In a patient population without syringomyelia, clinical improvement was around 80% [58]. In a clinical series, the rate of benefit from surgical treatment in CM Type 2 was 60% [59]. Some argue that surgical treatment in CM type 2 does not benefit the patient but even causes clinical worsening [60]. Hindbrain compression, which causes neurological symptoms, is a surgical indication and benefits from surgery [61].

15.9 Conclusion

CM is a rare pathology with different subtypes. Each subtype has different clinical features and diagnostic criteria. There is a large spectrum of clinical manifestations from asymptomatic to sudden death. MRI is the gold standard for diagnosis of CM. CM is a clinical condition that was frequently overlooked before the widespread use of imaging methods. In recent years, these imaging methods

have increased the rate of diagnosis, especially for asymptomatic patients. Treatment is not recommended for patients who show no symptoms, but the patient should be followed up. Incidental detection of CM has also increased.

References

1. Vernooij MW, Ikram MA, Tanghe HL, et al. Incidental findings on brain MRI in the general population. N Engl J Med. 2007;357(18):1821–8. https://doi.org/10.1056/NEJMoa070972.
2. Arnautovic A, Splavski B, Boop FA, Arnautovic KI. Pediatric and adult Chiari malformation Type I surgical series 1965-2013: a review of demographics, operative treatment, and outcomes. J Neurosurg Pediatr. 2015;15(2):161–77. https://doi.org/10.3171/2014.10.PEDS14295.
3. Taylor FR, Larkins MV. Headache and Chiari I malformation: clinical presentation, diagnosis, and controversies in management. Curr Pain Headache Rep. 2002;6(4):331–7. https://doi.org/10.1007/s11916-002-0056-z.
4. Milhorat TH. Cerebrospinal fluid physiology. In: Milhorat TH, editor. Hydrocephalus and the cerebrospinal fluid. Baltimore: Williams & Wilkins; 1972. p. 1–41.
5. Barkovich AJ, Wippold FJ, Sherman JL, Citrin CM. Significance of cerebellar tonsillar position on MR. AJNR Am J Neuroradiol. 1986;7(5):795–9.
6. Paul KS, Lye RH, Strang FA, Dutton J. Arnold-Chiari malformation. Review of 71 cases. J Neurosurg. 1983;58(2):183–7. https://doi.org/10.3171/jns.1983.58.2.0183.
7. Fisahn C, Shoja MM, Turgut M, Oskouian RJ, Oakes WJ, Tubbs RS. The Chiari 3.5 malformation: a review of the only reported case. Childs Nerv Syst. 2016;32(12):2317–9. https://doi.org/10.1007/s00381-016-3255-3.
8. Semple DA, McClure JH. Arnold-chiari malformation in pregnancy. Anaesthesia. 1996;51(6):580–2. https://doi.org/10.1111/j.1365-2044.1996.tb12570.x.
9. Tubbs RS, Turgut M. Defining the Chiari malformations: past and newer classifications. In: Tubbs RS, Turgut M, Oakes WJ, editors. The Chiari malformations. Springer Nature Switzerland AG; 2020. p. 21–39.
10. Brockmeyer DL, Spader HS. Complex Chiari malformations in children: diagnosis and management. Neurosurg Clin N Am. 2015;26(4):555–60. https://doi.org/10.1016/j.nec.2015.06.002.
11. Turgut M, Sağıroğlu S. Suboccipital decompressive craniectomy in a case of complex Chiari malformation complicated with influenza a (H1N1) necrotizing encephalopathy. Childs Nerv Syst. 2020;36(7):1335–6. https://doi.org/10.1007/s00381-020-04659-7.

12. Tubbs RS, Muhleman M, Loukas M, Oakes WJ. A new form of herniation: the Chiari V malformation. Childs Nerv Syst. 2012;28(2):305–7. https://doi.org/10.1007/s00381-011-1616-5.
13. Cavender RK, Schmidt JH 3rd. Tonsillar ectopia and Chiari malformations: monozygotic triplets. Case report. J Neurosurg. 1995;82(3):497–500. https://doi.org/10.3171/jns.1995.82.3.0497.
14. Turgut M. Chiari type I malformation in two monozygotic twins. Br J Neurosurg. 2001;15(3):279–80. https://doi.org/10.1080/026886901750353773.
15. Speer MC, Enterline DS, Mehltretter L, et al. Review article: Chiari type I malformation with or without syringomyelia: prevalence and genetics. J Genet Couns. 2003;12(4):297–311. https://doi.org/10.1023/A:1023948921381.
16. Braca J, Hornyak M, Murali R. Hemifacial spasm in a patient with Marfan syndrome and Chiari I malformation. Case report. J Neurosurg. 2005;103(3):552–4. https://doi.org/10.3171/jns.2005.103.3.0552.
17. Newman PK, Wentzel J, Foster JB. HLA and syringomyelia. J Neuroimmunol. 1982;3(1):23–6. https://doi.org/10.1016/0165-5728(82)90015-7.
18. Elster AD, Chen MY. Chiari I malformations: clinical and radiologic reappraisal. Radiology. 1992;183(2):347–53. https://doi.org/10.1148/radiology.183.2.1561334.
19. Guo F, Turgut M. Precise management of Chiari malformation with Type I. Front Surg. 2022;9:850879. Published 2022 Mar 28. https://doi.org/10.3389/fsurg.2022.850879.
20. Krucoff MO, Cook S, Adogwa O, et al. Racial, socioeconomic, and gender disparities in the presentation, treatment, and outcomes of adult Chiari I malformations. World Neurosurg. 2017;97:431–7. https://doi.org/10.1016/j.wneu.2016.10.026.
21. McLone DG, Knepper PA. The cause of Chiari II malformation: a unified theory. Pediatr Neurosci. 1989;15(1):1–12. https://doi.org/10.1159/000120432.
22. Yadav YR, Parihar V, Sinha M. Lumbar peritoneal shunt. Neurol India. 2010;58(2):179–84. https://doi.org/10.4103/0028-3886.63778.
23. Banerji NK, Millar JH. Chiari malformation presenting in adult life. Its relationship to syringomyelia. Brain. 1974;97(1):157–68. https://doi.org/10.1093/brain/97.1.157.
24. Pillay PK, Awad IA, Little JR, Hahn JF. Symptomatic Chiari malformation in adults: a new classification based on magnetic resonance imaging with clinical and prognostic significance. Neurosurgery. 1991;28(5):639–45.
25. Ciaramitaro P, Ferraris M, Massaro F, Garbossa D. Clinical diagnosis-part I: what is really caused by Chiari I. Childs Nerv Syst. 2019;35(10):1673–9. https://doi.org/10.1007/s00381-019-04206-z.
26. Tachibana S, Harada K, Abe T, Yamada H, Yokota A. Syringomyelia secondary to tonsillar herniation caused by posterior fossa tumors. Surg Neurol. 1995;43(5):470–7. https://doi.org/10.1016/0090-3019(95)80092-u.
27. Chiari H. Ueber Veranderungen des Kleinhirns in folge von Hydrocephalie des Grosshirns. Dtsch Med Wochenschr. 1891;17:1172–5.
28. Tubbs RS, Turgut M, Oakes WJ. A history of the Chiari malformations. In: Tubbs RS, Turgut M, Oakes WJ, editors. The Chiari malformations. Springer Nature Switzerland AG; 2020. p. 3–20.
29. Gardner WJ, Goodall RJ. The surgical treatment of Arnold-Chiari malformation in adults; an explanation of its mechanism and importance of encephalography in diagnosis. J Neurosurg. 1950;7(3):199–206. https://doi.org/10.3171/jns.1950.7.3.0199.
30. Moscote-Salazar LR, Zabaleta-Churio N, Alcala-Cerra G, et al. Symptomatic Chiari malformation with syringomyelia after severe traumatic brain injury: case report. Bull Emerg Trauma. 2016;4(1):58–61.
31. Goel A. Is atlantoaxial instability the cause of Chiari malformation? Outcome analysis of 65 patients treated by atlantoaxial fixation. J Neurosurg Spine. 2015;22(2):116–27. https://doi.org/10.3171/2014.10.SPINE14176.
32. Tubbs RS, Turgut M, Oakes WJ. Conclusions. In: Tubbs RS, Turgut M, Oakes WJ, editors. The Chiari malformations. Springer Nature Switzerland AG; 2020. p. 611–3.
33. Nishikawa M, Sakamoto H, Hakuba A, Nakanishi N, Inoue Y. Pathogenesis of Chiari malformation: a morphometric study of the posterior cranial fossa. J Neurosurg. 1997;86(1):40–7. https://doi.org/10.3171/jns.1997.86.1.0040.
34. Milhorat TH, Nishikawa M, Kula RW, Dlugacz YD. Mechanisms of cerebellar tonsil herniation in patients with Chiari malformations as guide to clinical management. Acta Neurochir. 2010;152(7):1117–27. https://doi.org/10.1007/s00701-010-0636-3.
35. Acer N, Turgut M, Yılmaz S, Güler HS. Measurement of the volume of the posterior cranial fossa using MRI. In: Tubbs RS, Turgut M, Oakes WJ, editors. The chiari malformations. Springer Nature Switzerland AG; 2020. p. 329–39.
36. Tubbs RS, McGirt MJ, Oakes WJ. Surgical experience in 130 pediatric patients with Chiari I malformations. J Neurosurg. 2003;99(2):291–6. https://doi.org/10.3171/jns.2003.99.2.0291.
37. Williams H. A unifying hypothesis for hydrocephalus, Chiari malformation, syringomyelia, anencephaly and spina bifida. Cerebrospinal Fluid Res. 2008;5:7. Published 2008 Apr 11. https://doi.org/10.1186/1743-8454-5-7.
38. Di Rocco C, Frassanito P, Massimi L, Peraio S. Hydrocephalus and Chiari type I malformation. Childs Nerv Syst. 2011;27(10):1653–64. https://doi.org/10.1007/s00381-011-1545-3.
39. Albert L Jr, Hirschfeld A. Acquired Chiari malformation secondary to hyperostosis of the skull: a case report and literature review. Surg Neurol. 2009;72(2):157–61. https://doi.org/10.1016/j.surneu.2008.02.030.

40. Pascual J, Oterino A, Berciano J. Headache in type I Chiari malformation. Neurology. 1992;42(8):1519–21. https://doi.org/10.1212/wnl.42.8.1519.

41. Milhorat TH, Chou MW, Trinidad EM, et al. Chiari I malformation redefined: clinical and radiographic findings for 364 symptomatic patients. Neurosurgery. 1999;44(5):1005–17. https://doi.org/10.1097/00006123-199905000-00042.

42. Goodwin D, Halvorson AR. Chiari I malformation presenting as downbeat nystagmus: clinical presentation, diagnosis, and management. Optometry. 2012;83(2):80–6. Published 2012 Feb 15

43. Dahdaleh NS, Menezes AH. Incomplete lateral medullary syndrome in a patient with Chiari malformation Type I presenting with combined trigeminal and vagal nerve dysfunction. J Neurosurg Pediatr. 2008;2(4):250–3. https://doi.org/10.3171/PED.2008.2.10.250.

44. Turgut M. Pierre-Robin syndrome associated with Chiari type I malformation. Childs Nerv Syst. 2004;20(1):3–7. https://doi.org/10.1007/s00381-003-0830-1.

45. Martins HA, Ribas VR, Lima MD, et al. Headache precipitated by Valsalva maneuvers in patients with congenital Chiari I malformation. Arq Neuropsiquiatr. 2010;68(3):406–9. https://doi.org/10.1590/s0004-282x2010000300015.

46. Martinot A, Hue V, Leclerc F, Vallee L, Closset M, Pruvo JP. Sudden death revealing Chiari type 1 malformation in two children. Intensive Care Med. 1993;19(2):73–4. https://doi.org/10.1007/BF01708364.

47. Tubbs RS, Oakes WJ. Treatment and management of the Chiari II malformation: an evidence-based review of the literature. Childs Nerv Syst. 2004;20(6):375–81. https://doi.org/10.1007/s00381-004-0969-4.

48. McLone DG, Dias MS. The Chiari II malformation: cause and impact. Childs Nerv Syst. 2003;19(7–8):540–50. https://doi.org/10.1007/s00381-003-0792-3.

49. Strahle J, Muraszko KM, Kapurch J, Bapuraj JR, Garton HJ, Maher CO. Natural history of Chiari malformation type I following decision for conservative treatment. J Neurosurg Pediatr. 2011;8(2):214–21. https://doi.org/10.3171/2011.5.PEDS1122.

50. Turgut M, Tubbs RS. Chiari I malformation and craniosynostosis. In: Tubbs RS, Turgut M, Oakes WJ, editors. The Chiari Malformations. Springer Nature Switzerland AG; 2020. p. 239–59.

51. Wu YW, Chin CT, Chan KM, Barkovich AJ, Ferriero DM. Pediatric Chiari I malformations: do clinical and radiologic features correlate? Neurology. 1999;53(6):1271–6. https://doi.org/10.1212/wnl.53.6.1271.

52. Jenkinson MD, Campbell S, Hayhurst C, et al. Cognitive and functional outcome in spina bifida-Chiari II malformation. Childs Nerv Syst. 2011;27(6):967–74. https://doi.org/10.1007/s00381-010-1368-7.

53. Dyste GN, Menezes AH, VanGilder JC. Symptomatic Chiari malformations. An analysis of presentation, management, and long-term outcome. J Neurosurg. 1989;71(2):159–68. https://doi.org/10.3171/jns.1989.71.2.0159.

54. Badie B, Mendoza D, Batzdorf U. Posterior fossa volume and response to suboccipital decompression in patients with Chiari I malformation. Neurosurgery. 1995;37(2):214–8. https://doi.org/10.1227/00006123-199508000-00004.

55. Killeen A, Roguski M, Chavez A, Heilman C, Hwang S. Non-operative outcomes in Chiari I malformation patients. J Clin Neurosci. 2015;22(1):133–8. https://doi.org/10.1016/j.jocn.2014.06.008.

56. Kalb S, Perez-Orribo L, Mahan M, Theodore N, Nakaji P, Bristol RE. Evaluation of operative procedures for symptomatic outcome after decompression surgery for Chiari type I malformation. J Clin Neurosci. 2012;19(9):1268–72. https://doi.org/10.1016/j.jocn.2012.01.025.

57. Giammattei L, Messerer M, Daniel RT, Aghakhani N, Parker F. Long-term outcome of surgical treatment of Chiari malformation without syringomyelia. J Neurosurg Sci. 2020;64(4):364–8. https://doi.org/10.23736/S0390-5616.17.04063-2.

58. Akbari SH, Limbrick DD Jr, Kim DH, et al. Surgical management of symptomatic Chiari II malformation in infants and children. Childs Nerv Syst. 2013;29(7):1143–54. https://doi.org/10.1007/s00381-013-2040-9.

59. Cameron AH. The Arnold-Chiari and other neuroanatomical malformations associated with spina bifida. J Pathol Bacteriol. 1957;73:195–211.

60. Salman MS. Posterior fossa decompression and the cerebellum in Chiari type II malformation: a preliminary MRI study. Childs Nerv Syst. 2011;27(3):457–62. https://doi.org/10.1007/s00381-010-1359-8.

61. Pollack IF, Pang D, Albright AL, Krieger D. Outcome following hindbrain decompression of symptomatic Chiari malformations in children previously treated with myelomeningocele closure and shunts. J Neurosurg. 1992;77(6):881–8. https://doi.org/10.3171/jns.1992.77.6.0881.

Agenesis of Corpus Callosum

Arad Iranmehr, Sara Hanaei,
and Ahmet Tuncay Turgut

16.1 Introduction

Agenesis of the corpus callosum (ACC) is the total or partial loss of at least one of the components of corpus callosum (CC) since birth, resulting in a shorter anterior to posterior length of this structure. A hypoplastic CC is one that is thinner than normal yet has a normal anterior to posterior extent [1]. Tractography studies using diffusion tensor imaging enhanced our knowledge of how the CC connects to the brain in healthy subjects, and how these connections are disrupted or redirected in patients with ACC. The known sigmoid bundles, which connect the frontal cortex to the contralateral occipitoparietal cortex asymmetrically, are of special interest. Sigmoid bundles have been observed in individuals with incomplete ACC and may reflect a pathologic neural plasticity not previously connected with the well-

A. Iranmehr
Department of Neurosurgery, Sina Hospital, Tehran University of Medical Sciences (TUMS), Tehran, Iran

S. Hanaei (✉)
Department of Neurosurgery, Imam Khomeini Hospital Complex (IKHC), Tehran University of Medical Sciences (TUMS), Tehran, Iran

Universal Scientific Education and Research Network (USERN), Tehran, Iran

Borderless Research, Advancement and Innovation in Neuroscience Network (BRAINet), Tehran, Iran

A. T. Turgut
Department of Radiology, Faculty of Medicine, Ankara Medipol University, Ankara, Turkey

documented longitudinal bundles of Probst [2, 3]. The processes behind this apparent adaptability of interhemispheric connectivity in individuals with incomplete ACC remain to be seen whether such types of heterotopic connections are compensating or detrimental.

16.2 Embryology

Early forebrain patterning and the eventual creation of the commissural plate, which is where all forebrain commissures travel, are dependent on midline-located FGF8 expression. Midline-located FGF8 expression is essential for initial forebrain segmentation and later growth in the commissural plate, which is where all forebrain commissures flow. Molecularly, the commissural plate may be divided into four different anatomical sub-structures, each defined by patterning molecules in the midline that presumably function downstream of FGF8 signaling. Each forebrain commissure corresponds to distinct anatomical sub-structures. The CC flows through an EMX1 and NFIA-expressing domain; the hippocampus commissure (HC) navigates via NFIA, ZIC2, and SIX3-expressing domains; and the anterior commissure (AC) flows by a SIX3-expressing domain in the septum [4].

The human commissural plate divides to the massa commissuralis, which contains the CC and HC, and the area septalis, which contains the AC [5]. For many years, it was assumed that the

M. Turgut et al. (eds.), *Incidental Findings of the Nervous System*,
https://doi.org/10.1007/978-3-031-42595-0_16

human CC developed from anterior to posterior, with the first callosal axons crossing the midline at the anterior genu, while rostrum-related pathways were added later. However, neuroimaging investigations have recently revealed that the axons primarily cross the commissural plate in the hippocampus primordium, with the following bidirectional connections [6, 7].While midline crossing of neocortical neurons in both mice and humans is followed by the crossing of pioneering axons from the cingulate cortex, callosal neurons come from layers 2/3, 5, and 6 of the neocortex. Pioneering axons start crossing the midline during weeks 13 and 14; anterior portions begin to develop by weeks 14 and 15, while posterior sections grow between weeks 18 and 19 [4, 5]. Because of the obvious delay in the formation of the posterior and anterior callosal components, it was assumed that early callosal disruption results in complete ACC, while later developmental perturbations cause partial agenesis limited to the posterior part of CC and rostrum. However, recent evidence suggests that connections are formed in two distinct locations: the AC and the HC. The HC's posterior shift, as well as the related callosal splenium, occurs from early frontal brain enlargement, while the anterior CC grows. As a result, it has been proposed that the lack of the posterior section of the CC in partial ACC is usually caused by unsuccessful dorsoventral growth of the splenium [4, 6]. The ultimate morphology of the CC completes by 20 weeks, while axonal development continues approximately 2 months following birth, after which molecular- and activity-dependent axonal trimming takes over [8]. While the quantity of callosal fibers is essentially fixed at birth, structural alterations occur throughout postnatal development, with the most pronounced modifications occurring throughout childhood and adolescence [9, 10].

16.3 Pathophysiology

The CC is the biggest white matter tract in the human brain, with around 200–300 million axons connecting the left and right cerebral hemispheres: it accounts for roughly 2–3% of all cortex fibers. It makes up one of the five major cerebral commissures (bundles of neurons which traverse the midline of the cerebral cortex), together with the anterior, posterior, hippocampal, and habenular commissures. The CC is specific to placental mammals and is considered to have an important role in cognition in humans [4, 11]. Its main task is to improve cognition and neurological function by coordinating and transferring information across the two cerebral hemispheres [6, 12]. Various genetic factors, prenatal infections, and maternal alcohol consumption may disrupt the fetal development of this structure [13]. Genetic changes linked to axon guidance, ciliary formation, cell adhesion, proliferation, differentiation, and migration are the most common causes of ACC. Probst bundles are a prominent indicator of aberrant commissure development. These bundles are groups of neurons that are aligned longitudinally rather than transversely. As a result, they can't do the task of linking the two hemispheres. Imaging and morphometric approaches reveal a range of callosal developmental abnormalities, from thinning to full agenesis. Complete ACC is defined as the loss of all portions of CC, in contrast to the lack of partial elements. This deformity could be an independent defect, or it may be part of a syndrome including other neurological disorders [13–15]. The prevalence of ACC in the general population differs based on the source and is likely understated owing to the condition's silent nature. The typical incidence range is 1:5000 to 1:4000 [16], although greater incidence (0.2–0.7%) has also been reported in different investigations [17, 18]. This impairment can be found in as many as 1–3% of people with poor neurodevelopment [19, 20]. The genetic origin of 30% to 45% of ACC patients has been identified, with roughly 10% having chromosome-related abnormalities and the other 20–35% having single-gene alterations. Although the identification of total ACC is not in dispute, the specific definitions of partial ACC are up for debate, making it impossible to compare the incidence of the two. Typically, the inclusion of hypoplastic CC cases as incomplete ACC is the cause of contention [14, 20].

16.4   Radiological Manifestations

Ultrasonography (US) sometimes fails to identify less dramatic cases of incomplete ACC or callosal hypoplasia [21, 22]. As a result, in instances where suspected ACC and accompanying anomalies were not found by US, prenatal magnetic resonance imaging (MRI) maintains the recommended imaging modality for inspection of the CC. This is especially crucial for providing early advice to parents, since other brain abnormalities detected by MRI may indicate broader neurode-velopmental issues associated with more severe neurological disabilities [23]. Computed tomography and MRI of the brain reveal parallel running lateral ventricles with complete ACC, and dilatation of the occipital horns of lateral ventricles (Figs. 16.1 and 16.2). Two characteristic imaging findings of MRI of the brain are as follows: [1] radial arrangement of the gyri outward in a radial pattern from the ventricle itself due to absence of the CC and everted cingulate gyrus in the midsagittal image giving "sunray appearance" (Figs. 16.1, 16.2 and 16.3); [2] widely spaced lat-

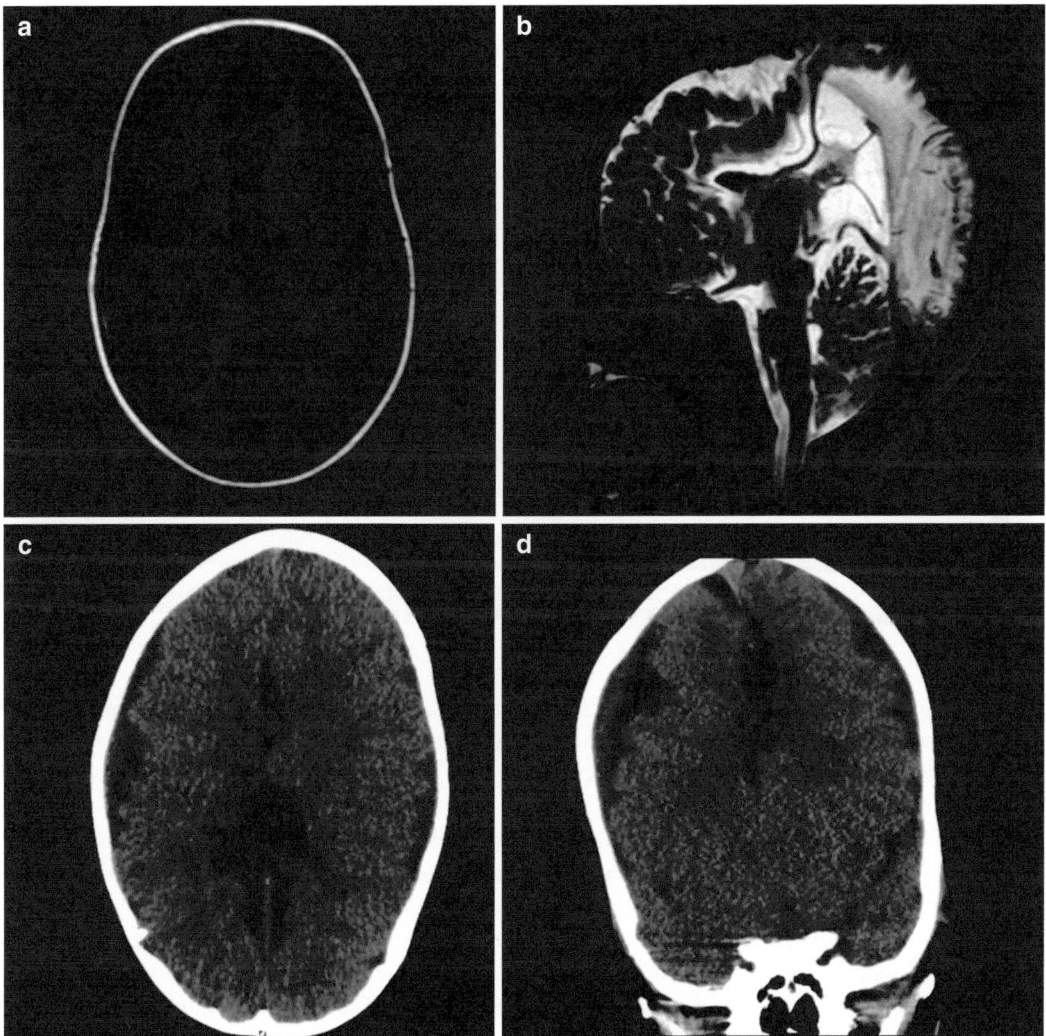

Fig. 16.1 T1-weighted axial (**a**) and T2-weighted (**b**) sagittal brain magnetic resonance imaging (MRI) and as axial (**c**) and coronal (**d**) brain CT images showing com-plete agenesis of the corpus callosum (ACC) in a 7-year-old child with history of gross developmental delay and minor intelligence issue (Courtesy of Dr. M Turgut)

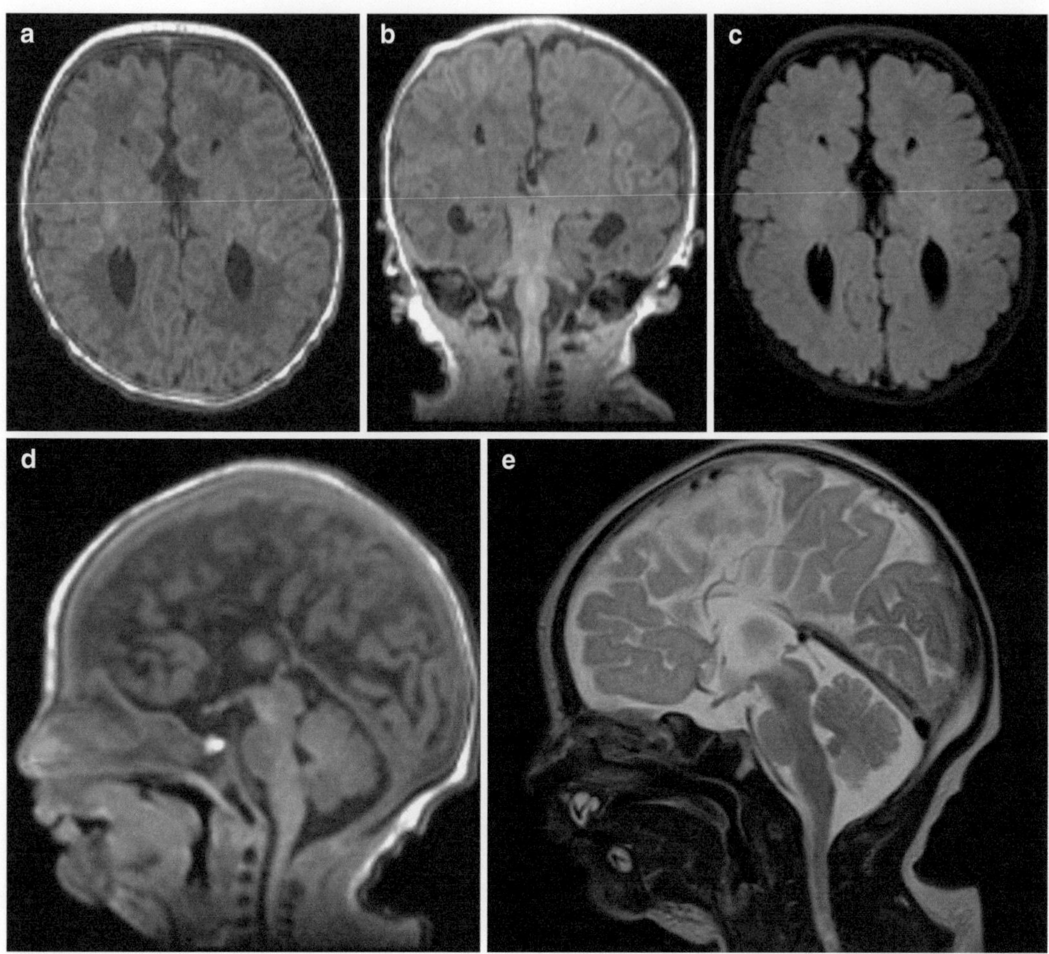

Fig. 16.2 Complete ACC was detected on brain MRI of a 2-month-old male child with respiratory distress, generalized tonic-clonic seizures, and delayed milestones. Axial (**a**) and coronal (**b**) T1-weighted and FLAIR (**c**) sequences show diagnostic "race car sign," while midsagittal T1- (**d**) and T2- (**e**) weighted sequences demonstrate frontal microgyri and elevation of the third ventricle, suggesting ACC (Courtesy of Dr. Y Türk)

eral ventricles due to ACC with intervening Probst bundles giving "race car sign" (Fig. 16.2); and [3] widely spaced lateral ventricles in the coronal image giving a characteristic the "**moose head appearance**" of the ventricles (also known as the Viking helmet, **steer-horn**, **Texas longhorn**, **buffalo horn**, or trident-shaped appearance or **Poseidon ventricles**) [23] (Fig. 16.3). Tractography with diffusion weighted image is a more accurate clinical estimation method that gives a visual picture of the brain's white matter corticospinal networks. In neuroimaging investigations, colpocephaly is common in the affected

population. A characteristic imaging indication of this developmental anomaly is a *"race car sign,"* which is generated by ventriculomegaly and the lack of CC with adjacent Probst bundles. In the absence of CC, the neural fibers expand parallel rather than perpendicular to the interhemispheric fissure. They, along with the previously described dilated lateral ventricles, produce the picture of a racing vehicle. The higher fractions of Probst bundles are associated with more adaptation and better social outcomes [19, 24]. The septum pellucidum is a structure positioned as the medial wall of the lateral ventricles. Although an aberrant

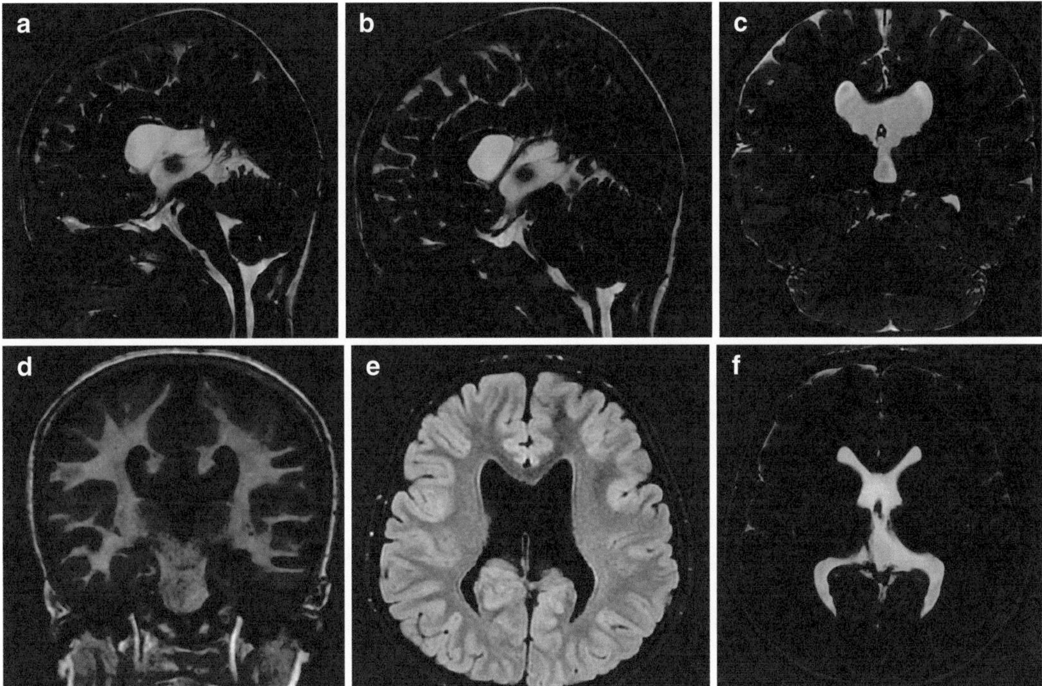

Fig. 16.3 Partial ACC was found on brain MRI of an 11-year-old girl with mental disability and antiepileptic therapy with a diagnosis of epilepsy. Sagittal (**a, b**) and coronal (**c**) T2-weighted as well as coronal T1- (**d**) axial T1- (**e**) and T2- (**f**) weighted sequences show "sunray appearance," dilated high-riding third ventricle and the "**moose head,** viking helmet, **steer-horn**, **Texas long-horn, buffalo horn appearance**" of the ventricles. Note that the cingulate gyrus is everted into narrowed and elongated frontal horns (Courtesy of Dr. S Oktay)

septum pellucidum (ASP) is not found in every patient with partial ACC, it might be a possible sign of this developmental abnormality due to the common occurrence of ventriculomegaly. When acquiring high contrast imaging of the brain in the midsagittal location is challenging, like prenatal screening, indirect indications such as ASP could be beneficial. This symptom was present in 52% of isolated partial ACC patients [25–27]. It was found that callosal dysmorphism was related to a decrease in length and an increase in width of ASP [28]. In some affected individuals, either the hippocampus or AC could be absent. As a result, every commissure defect observed on prenatal US should be evaluated by MRI, since it may be associated with ACC. MRIs could reveal variations in normal brain sulci patterns in isolated ACC which is distinguishable after first trimester of pregnancy. These changes are distinct from those seen in the developing fetal cortex [25, 29, 30].

16.5 Clinical Manifestations

One of the most common cerebral anomalies is agenesis of the CC, the biggest white matter tract in the brain. Patients with this condition are presented with a variety of symptoms, with some significantly affected, while others may be unaware of the abnormality since it has no impact on their regular function. Because only symptomatic patients are documented, the prevalence of ACC may be underestimated [4]. As previously stated, the neurodevelopmental prognosis of ACC patients might vary significantly. The extent of the symptoms varies depending upon if the ACC is complete or incomplete, if it is a single instance of ACC, or if it is linked with other anomalies [19, 31]. It must be mentioned that age has a significant effect on the patient's presentation. Even if the person previously had normal intellect and neuropsychological development, the end of childhood and beginning of adolescence might be the moment when complaints begin to appear, particularly in the case of isolated ACC. During this time, the CC's growth and myelination are completed, making the compensatory potential of other cerebral commissures inadequate for normal function. Based on discussed facts, each person with asymptomatic ACC needs a scheduled follow-up plan [32]. The CC links both brain hemispheres, allowing for higher cognitive functions as well as emotional and social behavior. These skills are compromised in autistic people. Some signs of ACC and autism spectrum disorder (ASD) are identical, such as issues with communication and social skills, affective prosody, abstract reasoning, and emotional and behavioral disorders [33]. It prompted scientists to investigate the link between CC alterations and autistic spectrum diseases. The majority of studies did reveal the presence of agenesis or the thinning of CC in autistic individuals. The average thickness of CC in autistic people was 15% smaller than in the control group [34]. While 76.04% of infants were prenatally identified with isolated complete ACC had normal neuro-development, developmental delay, and retardation in attaining milestones are often observed by caregivers of children with ACC. Extra-callosal anomalies raise the likelihood of additional issues, such as speech delay or epilepsy [31]. In people with ACC, muscular tone can be normal or abnormal, hypotonia or hypertonia. Axial hypotonia has been observed in the case of CC thinning. Appendicular hypertonia is also reported on these patients. A similar disparity exists in terms of head size. Patients have been documented to have microcephaly or macro-cephaly. Porencephaly, on the other hand, has been found in the ACC population. Fetuses with isolated anomalies are more likely to have chromosomal abnormalities [35–37]. ACC can lead to changes in the osmoregulatory system. While ACC with hyponatremia will be an incredibly unusual association, such instances have lately been documented [35].

16.6 Prognosis

Even among children with similar neuroanatomic profiles, neurodevelopmental outcome for individuals with callosal abnormalities can be highly different, and there is frequently overlap in neu-ropsychological performance between patients with complete ACC and those with partial ACC [38]. The most prevalent symptoms identified in people with ACC include delays in motor and cognitive skills, seizures, and social and linguistic abnormalities; also, ACC has been associated with the incidence of, attention deficit hyperactivity disorder and schizophrenia. Yet, pediatric series have a significant bias since only symptomatic cases have been identified and included [31, 39]. Although advances in prenatal imaging methods have increased the diagnosis rate of ACC, antenatal counseling when a fetus is identified with this defect remains difficult [39]. According to recent findings, the neurodevelopmental prognosis could be classified into three categories: normal, borderline/moderate, and severe. The neurodevelopmental assessment in affected patients should contain motor control, sensory status, visual control, epilepsy, language, coordination, and cognitive status. Neurodevelopmental outcome was reported to be normal in 71.42% of patients with an isolated partial ACC in recent meta-analysis. In these children, the incidences of borderline/moderate and severe neurodevelopmental outcomes were 14.92% and 12.52%, respectively. 11.74% of the patients had impaired fine motor skills, and 16.11% of these children had epilepsy. Impairment in language was observed in 17.25% of the patients, whereas cognitive status was impacted in 17.25% of the cases. Lastly, abnormal coordination occurred in 11.74% of the patients [31]. Fetuses with isolated callosal agenesis (complete ACC or partial ACC) are predisposed to chromosomal abnormalities. Even if traditional karyotyping is normal, there is a substantial probability of genetic defects being found only with chromosomal micro-array analysis. In fetuses with complete ACC and partial ACC, the likelihood of related malformations identified solely at fetal MRI is around 8% and 12%, respectively, but accompanying abnormalities discovered following the birth are possible in about 5% of fetuses with complete ACC and 14% of those with partial ACC [4, 31].

16.7 Conclusion

Patients with ACC may either be asymptomatic or present with a variety of symptoms. In this regard, some may be significantly affected, while others may even be unaware of the abnormality since it has no impact on their regular function. The extent of the symptoms varies depending upon if the ACC is complete or incomplete and whether it is accompanied by other anomalies. Prenatal MRI enables visualization of the CC, in instances where suspected ACC and accompanying anomalies were not found by US. This is especially crucial for prenatal counseling, since other brain abnormalities detected by MRI may be consistent with broader neurodevelopmental issues associated with more severe neurological disabilities.

References

 1. Santo S, et al. Counseling in fetal medicine: agenesis of the corpus callosum. Ultrasound Obstetr Gynecol. 2012;40:513–21. https://doi.org/10.1002/uog.12315.
 2. Wahl M, et al. Variability of homotopic and heterotopic callosal connectivity in partial agenesis of the corpus callosum: a 3T diffusion tensor imaging and Q-ball tractography study. AJNR Am J Neuroradiol. 2009;30:282–9. https://doi.org/10.3174/ajnr.A1361.
 3. Tovar-Moll F, et al. Neuroplasticity in human callosal dysgenesis: a diffusion tensor imaging study. Cerebral Cortex New York NY 1991. 2007;17:531–41. https://doi.org/10.1093/cercor/bhj178.
 4. Edwards TJ, Sherr EH, Barkovich AJ, Richards LJ. Clinical, genetic and imaging findings identify new causes for corpus callosum development syndromes. Brain. 2014;137:1579–613. https://doi.org/10.1093/brain/awt358.
 5. Rakic P, Yakovlev PI. Development of the corpus callosum and cavum septi in man. J Comp Neurol. 1968;132:45–72. https://doi.org/10.1002/cne.901320103.
 6. Paul LK. Developmental malformation of the corpus callosum: a review of typical callosal development and examples of developmental disorders with callosal involvement. J Neurodev Disord. 2011;3:3–27. https://doi.org/10.1007/s11689-010-9059-y.
 7. Barkovich AJ, Lyon G, Evrard P. Formation, maturation, and disorders of white matter. AJNR Am J Neuroradiol. 1992;13:447–61.
 8. Innocenti GM, Price DJ. Exuberance in the development of cortical networks. Nat Rev Neurosci. 2005;6:955–65. https://doi.org/10.1038/nrn1790.
 9. Garel C, et al. Biometry of the corpus callosum in children: MR imaging reference data. AJNR Am J Neuroradiol. 2011;32:1436–43. https://doi.org/10.3174/ajnr.A2542.
10. Luders E, Thompson PM, Toga AW. The development of the corpus callosum in the healthy human brain. J Neurosci. 2010;30:10985–90. https://doi.org/10.1523/jneurosci.5122-09.2010.
11. Bartha-Doering L, et al. Effect of corpus callosum agenesis on the language network in children and adolescents. Brain Struct Funct. 2021;226:701–13. https://doi.org/10.1007/s00429-020-02203-6.
12. Hinkley LB, et al. The role of corpus callosum development in functional connectivity and cognitive processing. PLoS One. 2012;7:e39804. https://doi.org/10.1371/journal.pone.0039804.
13. Hong M, Krauss RS. Ethanol itself is a holoprosencephaly-inducing teratogen. PLoS One. 2017;12:e0176440. https://doi.org/10.1371/journal.pone.0176440.
14. Hofman J, Hutny M, Sztuba K, Paprocka J. Corpus callosum agenesis: an insight into the etiology and Spectrum of symptoms. Brain Sci. 2020;10 https://doi.org/10.3390/brainsci10090625.
15. Neal JB, Filippi CG, Mayeux R. Morphometric variability of neuroimaging features in children with agenesis of the corpus callosum. BMC Neurol. 2015;15:116. https://doi.org/10.1186/s12883-015-0382-5.
16. Chadie A, et al. Neurodevelopmental outcome in prenatally diagnosed isolated agenesis of the corpus callosum. Acta Paediatrica (Oslo, Norway: 1992). 2008;97:420–4. https://doi.org/10.1111/j.1651-2227.2008.00688.x.
17. Weise J, et al. Analyses of pathological cranial ultrasound findings in neonates that fall outside recent indication guidelines: results of a population-based birth cohort: survey of neonates in Pomerania (SNiP-study). BMC Pediatr. 2019;19:476. https://doi.org/10.1186/s12887-019-1843-6.
18. Sefidbakht S, Dehghani S, Safari M, Vafaei H, Kasraeian M. Fetal central nervous system anomalies detected by magnetic resonance imaging: a two-year experience. Iran J Pediatr. 2016;26:e4589. https://doi.org/10.5812/ijp.4589.
19. Al-Hashim AH, Blaser S, Raybaud C, MacGregor D. Corpus callosum abnormalities: neuroradiological and clinical correlations. Dev Med Child

Neurol. 2016;58:475–84. https://doi.org/10.1111/dmcn.12978.

20. Jouan L, et al. Exome sequencing identifies recessive CDK5RAP2 variants in patients with isolated agenesis of corpus callosum. Eur J Human Genet EJHG. 2016;24:607–10. https://doi.org/10.1038/ejhg.2015.156.

21. Ghi T, et al. Prenatal diagnosis and outcome of partial agenesis and hypoplasia of the corpus callosum. Ultrasound Obstetr Gynecol. 2010;35:35–41. https://doi.org/10.1002/uog.7489.

22. Paladini D, Pastore G, Cavallaro A, Massaro M, Nappi C. Agenesis of the fetal corpus callosum: sonographic signs change with advancing gestational age. Ultrasound Obstetr Gynecol. 2013;42:687–90. https://doi.org/10.1002/uog.12506.

23. Tang PH, et al. Agenesis of the corpus callosum: an MR imaging analysis of associated abnormalities in the fetus. AJNR Am J Neuroradiol. 2009;30:257–63. https://doi.org/10.3174/ajnr.A1331.

24. Agarwal DK, Patel SM, Krishnan P. Classical imaging in callosal agenesis. J Pediatr Neurosci. 2018;13:118–9. https://doi.org/10.4103/jpn.jpn_150_17.

25. Griffiths PD, et al. Anatomical subgroup analysis of the MERIDIAN cohort: failed commissuration. Ultrasound Obstetr Gynecol. 2017;50:753–60. https://doi.org/10.1002/uog.17502.

26. Shen O, et al. Abnormal shape of the cavum septi pellucidi: an indirect sign of partial agenesis of the corpus callosum. Ultrasound Obstetr Gynecol. 2015;46:595–9. https://doi.org/10.1002/uog.14776.

27. Ben M'Barek I, et al. Antenatal diagnosis of absence of septum pellucidum. Clin Case Reports. 2020;8:498–503. https://doi.org/10.1002/ccr3.2666.

28. Karl K, Esser T, Heling KS, Chaoui R. Cavum septi pellucidi (CSP) ratio: a marker for partial agenesis of the fetal corpus callosum. Ultrasound Obstetr Gynecol. 2017;50:336–41. https://doi.org/10.1002/uog.17409.

29. Cesaretti C, et al. Variability of forebrain commissures in Callosal agenesis: a prenatal MR imaging study. AJNR Am J Neuroradiol. 2016;37:521–7. https://doi.org/10.3174/ajnr.A4570.

30. Tarui T, et al. Disorganized patterns of Sulcal position in fetal brains with agenesis of corpus callosum. Cerebral Cortex (New York, N.Y. : 1991). 2018;28:3192–203. https://doi.org/10.1093/cercor/bhx191.

31. D'Antonio F, et al. Outcomes associated with isolated agenesis of the corpus callosum: a meta-analysis. Pediatrics. 2016;138 https://doi.org/10.1542/peds.2016-0445.

32. Guadarrama-Ortiz P, Choreño-Parra JA, de la Rosa-Arredondo T. Isolated agenesis of the corpus callosum and normal general intelligence development during postnatal life: a case report and review of the literature. J Med Case Rep. 2020;14:28. https://doi.org/10.1186/s13256-020-2359-2.

33. Patra S, Naik S, Jha M. Corpus callosum agenesis: neuroanatomical model of autism Spectrum disorder? Indian J Psychol Med. 2019;41:284–6. https://doi.org/10.4103/ijpsym.ijpsym_281_18.

34. Wegiel J, et al. Partial agenesis and hypoplasia of the corpus callosum in idiopathic autism. J Neuropathol Exp Neurol. 2017;76:225–37. https://doi.org/10.1093/jnen/nlx003.

35. Silveira MAD, et al. Chronic hyponatremia due to the syndrome of inappropriate Antidiuresis (SIAD) in an adult woman with corpus callosum agenesis (CCA). Am J Case Reports. 2018;19:1345–9. https://doi.org/10.12659/ajcr.911810.

36. Cohen JS, et al. Further evidence that de novo missense and truncating variants in ZBTB18 cause intellectual disability with variable features. Clin Genet. 2017;91:697–707. https://doi.org/10.1111/cge.12861.

37. Volodarsky M, et al. CDC174, a novel component of the exon junction complex whose mutation underlies a syndrome of hypotonia and psychomotor developmental delay. Hum Mol Genet. 2015;24:6485–91. https://doi.org/10.1093/hmg/ddv357.

38. Palmer EE, Mowat D. Agenesis of the corpus callosum: a clinical approach to diagnosis. Am J Med Genet C Semin Med Genet. 2014;166c:184–97. https://doi.org/10.1002/ajmg.c.31405.

39. Siffredi V, Anderson V, Leventer RJ, Spencer-Smith MM. Neuropsychological profile of agenesis of the corpus callosum: a systematic review. Dev Neuropsychol. 2013;38:36–57. https://doi.org/10.1080/87565641.2012.721421.

Dattatraya Muzumdar and Sarvender Rai

17.1 Introduction and Definition

Dandy–Walker complex (DWC) is a malformative association of the central nervous system. Dandy–Walker variant (DWV) is a less severe form of the spectrum of Dandy–Walker malformation (DWM) [1–5]. The distinction between other congenital posterior fossa cyst can be sometimes difficult and may have diagnostic and therapeutic challenges. The exact etiology of the DWM or its variant is still unknown. The association of congenital anomalies and hydrocephalus has an impact on the developmental outcome [4, 6]. Hence it is important to diagnose with relative certainty and differentiate DWV from other malformations of the posterior fossa early in the prenatal period to allow for proper counselling and management of the posterior fossa cyst.

17.2 Clinical Symptomatology

DWV is defined by classic DWM findings but with limited vermin hypoplasia. Due to the variant being less severe, patients may present with milder symptoms and the malformation may be found incidentally later in life [4, 7–9]. There are no two people in the universe who have experienced similar experiences in the symptomatology. Many patients have lived their entire life without being aware that they have had it. Dandy–Walker syndrome (DWS) or its variant has been noted in babies who have died from unknown causes but seemingly healthy at full term. They lead a happy and healthy life with adaptable social integration. A review of 12 cases of incidental DWM discovery found preserved communication between the fourth ventricular cyst and surrounding basal cisterns which may allow DWM to remain asymptomatic in these patients [4]. In these patients, watchful waiting without specific treatment may be indicated if they remain asymptomatic. The isolated DWV abnormality has the highest incidence of survival, and there are reported cases of people who have had DWV their entire lives without any symptoms. Patients with DWV are more likely to present in adulthood than in infancy or childhood [4]. Any child presenting with macrocephaly or congenital anomaly associated with normal neurology should undergo magnetic resonance imaging (MRI) to rule out DWV and other associated congenital anomalies. Any family with special genetic history needs evaluation.

D. Muzumdar (✉) · S. Rai
Department of Neurosurgery, Seth G S Medical
College and King Edward VII Memorial Hospital,
Parel, Mumbai, India

17.3 Embryology, Development, and Association of Congenital Anomalies

The cerebellar vermis completes its development from superior to inferior at about 17 ± 18 weeks' gestation [10]. However, it is not uncommon to find the cerebellar vermis being incompletely formed at 15 ± 16 weeks. Consequently, DWV should not be diagnosed too early in the course. In two fetuses, after 18 weeks of gestation with findings of DWV, they were reported to be normal on later (USG) and at birth [11–14].

17.4 Association with Other Congenital Anomalies

The association of DWV with other congenital anomalies, radiographic abnormalities, incidence of hydrocephalus, and developmental outcomes is largely limited to case reports. Various USG studies have demonstrated that associated anomalies occur in between 47% and 80% of fetuses with DWV and between 46% and 86% of those with DWM [13, 15, 16]. Aberrations in the CNS, gastrointestinal, genitourinary, craniofacial, and musculoskeletal systems are also associated with DWV. It is also associated with the various syndromes including Pierre Robin sequence, Smith–Lemli–Opitz syndrome, and Senior–Loken syndrome, Menkes syndrome (kinky-hair disease), Coffin–Siris syndrome, and Ehlers–Danlos syndrome, as well as neurocutaneous melanosis [4, 5, 16–18]. The DWV may be associated with X-linked inheritance, as suggested by an ultrasound evaluation of a pedigree of 5 fetuses with isolated DWV, in whom only the males were affected [6, 7, 17, 19]. Other studies have suggested a correlation with autosomal recessive inheritance, as was observed in a case of 2 siblings with concomitant diagnoses of DWV and spastic hereditary paraplegia [8, 19]. Chromosomal abnormalities were also observed with defects on chromosomes 9, 11, 13, and 8. A full spectrum of the Dandy–Walker com-plex (DWC), also referred to as Dandy-Walker spectrum or Dandy-Walker continuum, can occur in Coffin–Siris syndrome [18]. DWV may result from a more specific local insult to the developing cerebellum, with little effect on the roof of the fourth ventricle. The presence of other anomalies, such as Meckel–Gruber syndrome or severe chromosomal anomalies, is related to a poor prognosis.

In summary, both DWM cyst and DWV are commonly associated with a high incidence of other anomalies and karyotypic abnormalities. The presence of other anomalies is associated with worst prognosis but not uniformly fatal. Isolated DWV has the chance of having the best prognosis.

17.5 Etiology and Diagnosis

DWC comprises of four different types, viz. DWM, DWV, mega cisterna magna, and posterior fossa arachnoid cyst. DWM is defined by agenesis or hypoplastic cerebellar vermis, cystic dilatation of the fourth ventricle, and a large posterior fossa [2, 4, 5, 13, 20]. A DWV is characterized by vermis hypoplasia, cystic dilatation of the fourth ventricle, and a normal posterior fossa. A mega cisterna magna presents with a large posterior fossa, normal vermis, and fourth ventricle. A posterior fossa arachnoid cyst can produce enlargement of the posterior fossa and the upward displacement of the tentorium who can be appreciated by the high position of the torcula and of the sinuses. It may be difficult to appreciate the differences between them unless one looks at the MRI sequences closely. It is thought that all these variations represent a continuum of developmental abnormalities in a spectrum which is collectively called as DWC.

The DWV, as defined by Raybaud (1982), differs in that the vermis is typically less hypoplastic, the posterior fossa is less enlarged, the brainstem is not compressed, and the fourth ventricle is enlarged. In 1976, Harwood-Nash and Fitz described an addition to this spectrum, the

DWV [21]. This diagnosis is manifested by variable vermian hypoplasia, a normal-sized posterior fossa, and a cystic lesion that demonstrates open communication with the fourth ventricle. Specific size criteria to denote a normal-sized posterior fossa and vermian hypoplasia are not established in the literature. Rather, DWV is a diagnosis often made according to the expertise of individual neuroradiologists.

The overall prevalence of DWM was 6.79 per 100,000 births (95% CI 5.79–7.96) with 39.2% livebirths, 4.3% fetal deaths from 20 weeks gestational age, and 56.5% terminations of pregnancy after prenatal diagnosis of fetal anomaly at any gestation [8]. The prevalence of DWV was 2.08 per 100,000 (95% CI 1.39–3.13). The overall prevalence of DWM and DWV was 8.85 per 100,000 (95%CI: 7.43–10.54). A significantly higher proportion of trisomy 13 (Patau's syndrome) was observed in DWV (10.5%) than in DWM (4.1%) [8]. The exact etiology of the DWM is unknown and is believed to be a combination of environmental and genetic factors. It is a manifestation of abnormal development of the rhombencephalon with incomplete formation of the vermis or due to a defect within the tela choroidea which leads to cystic dilation of the fourth ventricle [10, 12, 15]. It is believed that DWV develops along the same embryological pathway since it has a comparable appearance to DWM. Definitive diagnosis of DWM or DWV depends on neuroimaging as most of the clinical signs are not conclusive [2, 4, 7, 22]. In the neuroradiological literature, a distinction is often made between DWM and DWV; the latter term is applied if the posterior fossa is not enlarged, the hypoplasia of the cerebellar vermis is less pronounced, or both [5, 6, 8, 23]. The introduction of modern imaging techniques, specifically MRI, has radically changed the evaluation of symptoms related to the posterior fossa. MRI usually is performed for detailed evaluation of DWM lesions and complications [6, 14, 20]. Sometimes, DWM and DWV cases show many similarities that a clear-cut distinction is difficult. There was no significant difference in the spectrum of associated anomalies and postnatal prognosis between DWM and DWV cases.

Some degree of vermian dysgenesis can be found in cases with mega cisterna magna [12, 13, 15]. These fetuses typically have the fewest posterior fossa abnormalities, usually limited to isolated enlargement of the cisterna magna. The cerebellar vermis is intact, and there is a variably enlarged posterior fossa volume [1]. An association with chromosomal abnormalities, especially with trisomy-18 has been reported, and fetal karyotyping has been suggested for cases of mega cisterna magna [24].

Vermian defects may be over- or underdiagnosed on prenatal USG examination, and the distinction between DWV and other abnormalities of the posterior fossa is difficult [11–13, 15]. If USG is incorrectly performed, it is relatively easy to create the appearance of a DWV malformation. On the basis of available evidence it is believed that antenatal USG allows a definitive diagnosis of only the severe anatomic varieties of the DWC, those characterized by both a large posterior fossa cystic mass and a wide defect in the cerebellar vermis, referred to as classic DWM. It is difficult to solve prenatally the doubt of either a mega cisterna magna or a small inferior defect of the vermis as in DWV and this can only be resolved by postnatal imaging studies. Distinction between DWV and mega cisterna magna in the fetus is difficult as definitive criteria have not been firmly established. The former condition should be suspected when a thin communication is found between the fourth ventricle and the cisterna magna, the latter when the cisterna magna has a depth greater than 10 mm [13]. The prenatal differentiation between DWV and mega cisterna magna should be made with caution, especially in the early second trimester because the relatively large fourth ventricle and the incompletely formed inferior cerebellar vermis may give a false impression of vermian defect and a follow-up scan at 18 weeks or later is recommended.

17.6 Ventriculomegaly, Hydrocephalus, and Radiographic Findings

The finding of ventriculomegaly and hydrocephalus in patients with the DWV has not been clearly ascertained. By comparison, a 55–96% rate of hydrocephalus has been observed in patients with DWM [1, 2, 5, 17]. Based on prenatal USG studies, it has been estimated that ventriculomegaly will occur in 24–27% of patients with DWV and approximately half required treatment with cerebrospinal fluid (CSF) diversion [6, 11–13, 15, 20]. The only factor that significantly predicted the need for a shunt was the presence of ventriculomegaly. Other radiographic features observed such as agenesis of the corpus callosum, gyral abnormalities, and cortical atrophy were comparable to those described in the literature for DWM [1, 2, 5, 17]. Notably, no occipital encephaloceles were observed. Ghane et al. report a one and a half year old female child who had absence of obvious external congenital malformation, had brachycephaly instead of occipital prominence, had microcephaly instead of macrocephaly which were suggestive of milder spectrum of DWM, i.e., DWV [25]. But contrary to the above-examination findings, child had severe neurological impairment involving white and gray matter manifesting as significant motor delay and seizures. The definitive diagnosis, though an incidental finding was due to advanced neuroimaging techniques like MRI.

17.7 Neuropathology

The gross anatomical examination of the brain demonstrated only mild neurodevelopmental anomalies [26]. It revealed cystic dilatation of the fourth ventricle combined with mild vermian hypoplasia, confirming the clinical diagnosis of DWV. In most cases, the foramina of Magendie and Luschka were open. The microscopic examination showed significant morphological alterations of neurons and dendrites including focal dilatation of dendrites in temporal lobe, notable reduction of dendritic spines in the cerebral cortex, poverty of dendritic arborization in the cerebellum, and neurofibrillary alterations in the temporal lobe. In the hippocampus, the most prominent finding is the tortuous configuration of the apical dendrites of the pyramidal neurons. The degenerative changes are milder in the occipital cortex. These alterations are possibly caused by hydrocephalus which could present even after 10 years survival from CSF diversion treatment [26]. This substantiates that neuronal damage caused by long exposure to increased intracranial pressure may not be possible to be reversed in its entirety. Hence, early diagnosis and treatment with shunt are crucial for the prognosis of the malformation.

17.8 Developmental Status

The reported developmental outcomes in patients with DWV tend to be more encouraging. In a study with a small follow-up period of only 6 weeks, USG analysis showed that 7 of 13 patients in whom the DWV was diagnosed exhibited normal development [13]. In another retrospective USG analysis with a longer follow-up study ranging from 4 months to 4 years, 9 of 11 surviving infants were developing normally, and that in 75% of those no associated extracranial USG anomaly was identified [15]. The sensitivity of prenatal MRI imaging found 77% of infants were developmentally normal and 3 exhibited only mild motor delay, with a confirmed postnatal diagnosis of DWV [9, 22]. Hence it is generally understood that isolated DWV is associated with a good outcome. The presence of other neurological anomalies or syndromes appears to increase the association with developmental delay (Figs. 17.1, 17.2, 17.3, 17.4).

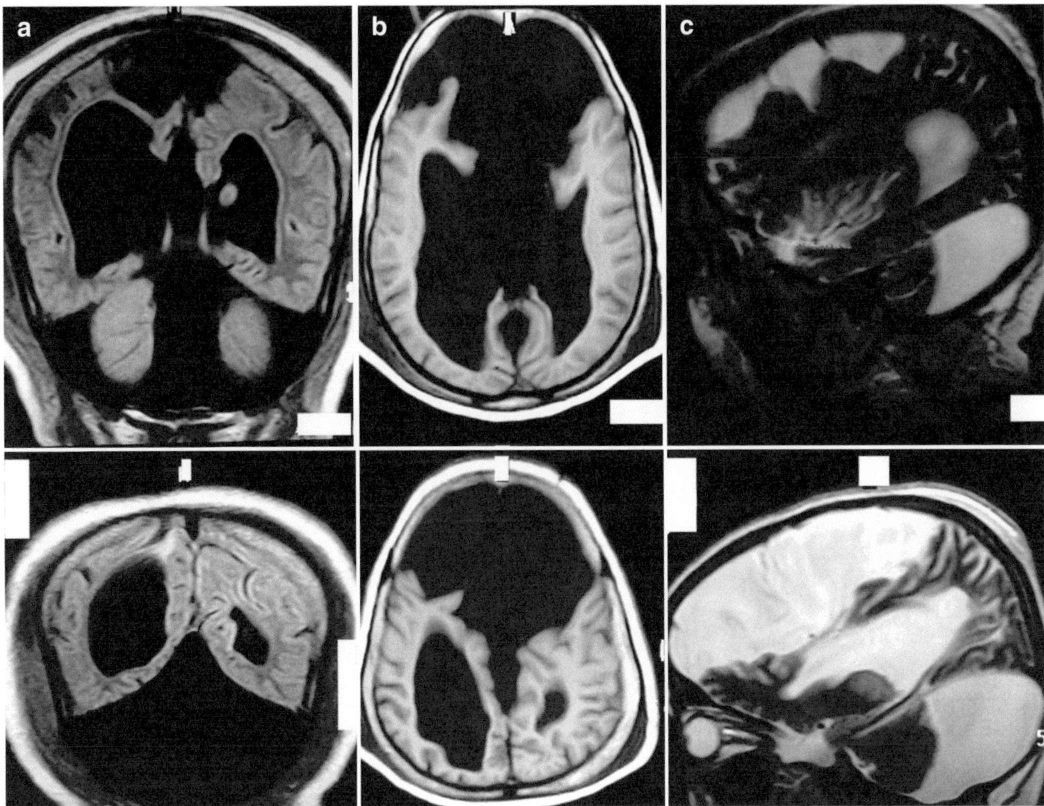

Fig. 17.1 Dandy–Walker variant (DWV) associated with holoprosencephaly and lip schizencephaly in a 8-month-old child. (**a**) Coronal view. (**b**) Axial view. (**c**) Sagittal view

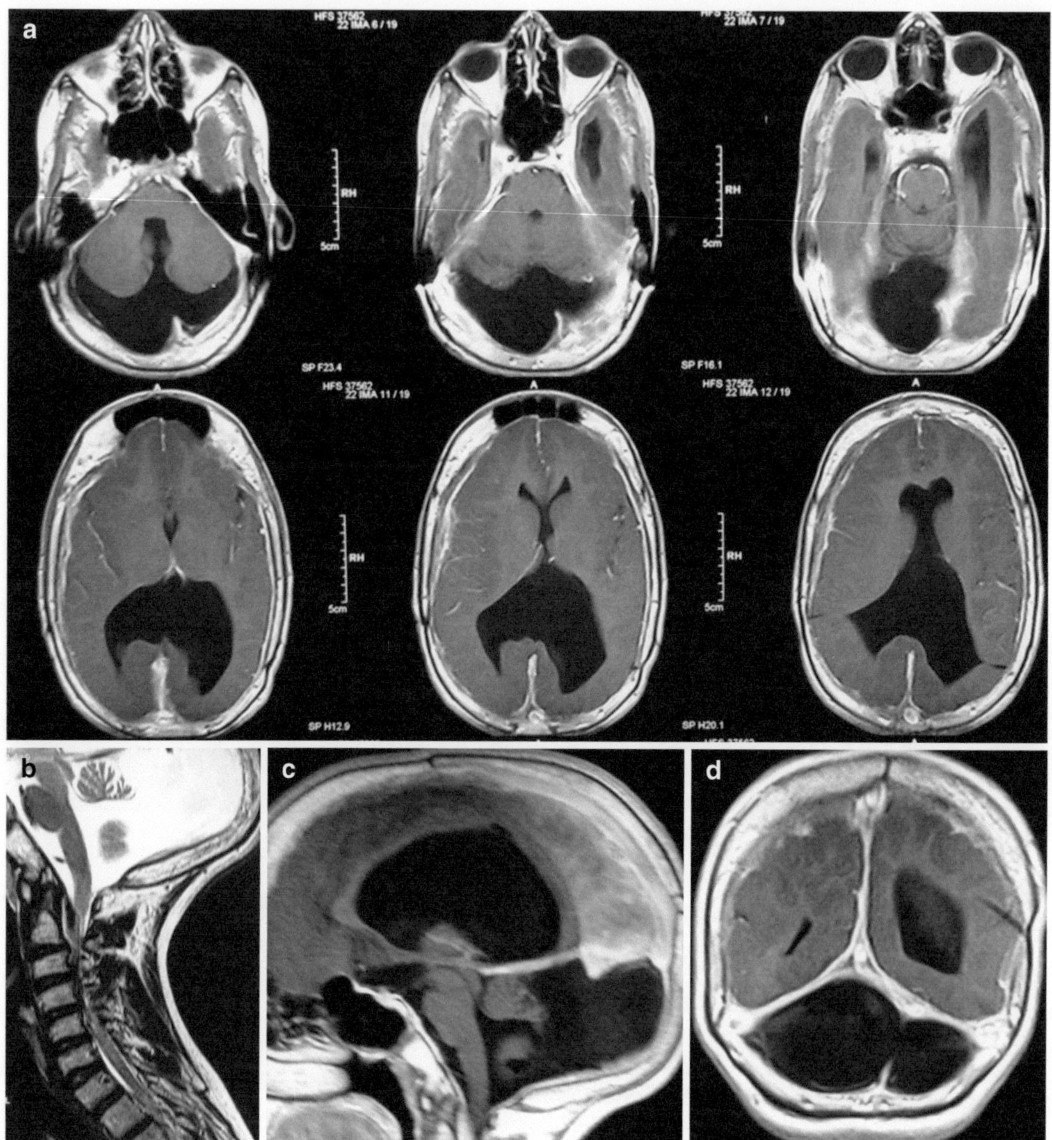

Fig. 17.2 DWV associated with C2-C5 compressive degenerative spondylotic myelopathy in a 58-year-old male patient.. (**a**) Axial view. (**b**) Sagittal view showing the posterior fossa cyst along with C2 to C5 cord compression. (**c**) Sagittal view of the posterior fossa cyst and vermin hypoplasia. (**d**) Coronal view

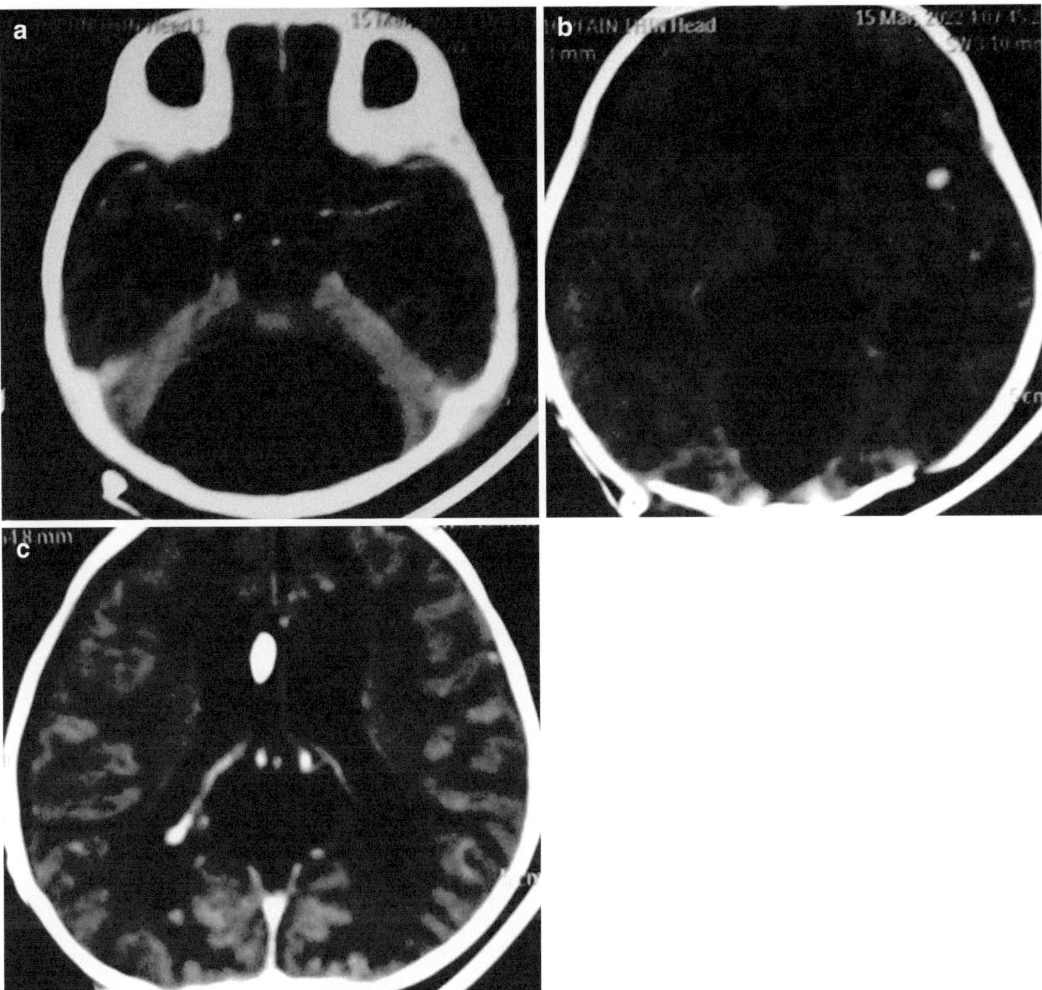

Fig. 17.3 Magnetic resonance imaging brain showing large posterior fossa cyst but normal posterior fossa volume and associated hydrocephalus in a 3-month-old child. (**a**) Axial view at level of cyst. (**b**) Axial view at level of the tentorial notch. (**c**) Axial view showing shunt in situ

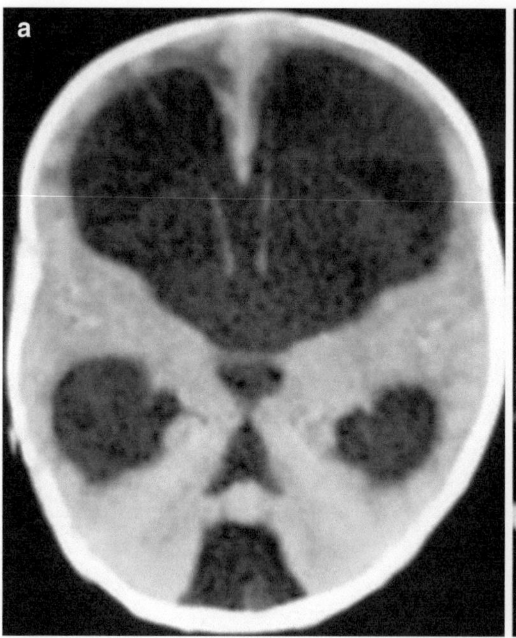

Fig. 17.4 Computed tomography brain showing Dandy–Walker complex showing mega cistern magna in a 3 month old child. . (**a**) Axial view. (**b**) Partial vermian hypoplasia. Communication of the mega cisterna magna with fourth ventricle and hydrocephalus

17.9 Medicolegal Considerations

In today's era, failure to diagnose DWC and hydrocephaly in a neonate or a child can have serious medicolegal implications apart from the neurological complications. DWM misunderstood or diagnosed as mega cisterna magna or arachnoid cyst can be cause of morbidity or mortality [4–6]. In a recent study, Carroll et al. [12] reported the correlation between antenatal sonographic diagnosis and pathologic findings in fetal brain abnormalities. The most common disparity they found was in cases with presumed DW or DWV. Hence, the potential discrepancy in findings between ultrasound and autopsy should be explained to patients who are considering termination of pregnancy.

17.10 Asymptomatic Dandy–Walker Syndrome

Asymptomatic DWM can be found incidentally with unrelated diseases [3–5, 27]. Absence of associated fatal congenital anomalies increases life expectancy in such cases. Presentation at extremes of age signifies the fact that some valve-like mechanism exist between outlet of foramen of Luschka and Magendie of fourth ventricle and membranous wall of posterior fossa cyst with surrounding subarachnoid spaces. Although reports are available where cases had been surgically treated at extreme old age but it seems impractical to treat such cases without overt manifestations of DWS and interfere in natural mechanism which had led them to live their life normally till date. Cases with good CSF communication of posterior fossa cyst with surrounding CSF space may remain asymptomatic throughout their life and only regular follow-up is needed.

17.11 Surgical Management

The DWV is a continuum of the DWC (Figs. 17.1, 17.2, 17.3, 17.4). The boundaries between DWM, DWV, mega cisterna magna, Blake's pouch cyst are indistinct and are not of any significance in the management of DWC associated hydrocephalus [4, 6, 27, 28]. Each may be associated with hydrocephalus, the common pathology being anomalous fourth ventricle/posterior fossa CSF outflow. In majority of infants below 12 months of age, endoscopic ventriculostomy (ETV) and choroid plexus cauterization is successful while in children more than 1–2 years of age, ETV alone is sufficient in most cases [4, 6, 27, 28]. Aqueductal obstruction is infrequently seen in infants at time of presentation, however secondary aqueductal obstruction can be seen following shunting of lateral ventricle [4, 6, 27, 28]. Hence endoscopic third ventriculostomy is strongly advised as a primary modality of treatment.

17.12 Conclusion

DWV is a distinct entity which needs to be differentiated from DWM. A normal-sized posterior fossa and mild vermian hypoplasia are the differentiating features. It is a milder form of the DWC. There are no rigid objective measurement for its diagnosis although it remains a frequent source of referrals for neurosurgeons. It has a developmental pathway similar to DWM. Ventriculomegaly appears to be much commoner than hydrocephalus. It can also be associated with other extracranial malformations, chromosomal abnormalities, and syndromes. Hence a close follow-up of these patients is essential to determine the possible need for CSF diversion. The developmental outcome seems to be good in patients with isolated DWV and uncertain when associated congenital anomalies are prominent.

References

1. Asai A, Hoffman HJ, Hendrick EB, Humphreys RP. Dandy-Walker syndrome: experience at the hospital for sick children, Toronto. Pediatr Neurosci. 1989;15:66–73.
2. Hirsch JF, Pierre-Kahn A, Renier D, Sainte-Rose C, Hoppe- Hirsch E. The Dandy-Walker malformation. A review of 40 cases. J Neurosurg. 1984;61:515–22.
3. Hochberg E, Niles E. An incidental finding of Dandy-Walker malformation. JAAPA. 2021;34(1):22–4.
4. Jha VC, Kumar R, Srivastav AK, Mehrotra A, Sahu RN. A case series of 12 patients with incidental asymptomatic Dandy-Walker syndrome and management. Childs Nerv Syst. 2012;28(6):861–7.
5. Osenbach RK, Menezes AH. Diagnosis and management of the Dandy-Walker malformation: 30 years of experience. Pediatr Neurosurg. 1992;18:179–89.
6. Sasaki-Adams D, Elbabaa SK, Jewells V, Carter L, Campbell JW, Ritter AM. The Dandy-Walker variant: a case series of 24 pediatric patients and evaluation of associated anomalies, incidence of hydrocephalus, and developmental outcomes. J Neurosurg Pediatr. 2008;2(3):194–9.
7. Jurcă MC, Kozma K, Petcheşi CD, Bembea M, Pop OL, MuŢiu G, et al. Anatomic variants in Dandy-Walker complex. Romanian J Morphol Embryol. 2017;58(3):1051–5.
8. Santoro M, Coi A, Barišić I, Garne E, Addor MC, Bergman JEH, et al. Epidemiology of Dandy-Walker malformation in Europe: a EUROCAT population-based registry study. Neuroepidemiology. 2019;53(3–4):169–79.
9. Sinha P, Tarwani J, Kumar P, Garg A. Dandy-Walker variant with schizophrenia: comorbidity or cerebellar cognitive affective syndrome? Indian J Psychol Med. 2017;39(2):188–90.
10. Bromley B, Nadel AS, Pauker S, Estroff JA, Benacerraf BR. Closure of the cerebellar vermis: evaluation with second trimester US. Radiology. 1994;193(3):761 3.
11. Alam A, Chander BN, Bhatia M. Dandy-Walker variant: prenatal diagnosis by ultrasonography. Med J Armed Forces India. 2004;60(3):287–9.
12. Carrol SGM, Porter H, Abdel-Fattah S, Kyle PM, Soothil PW. Correlation of prenatal ultra- sound diagnosis and pathologic findings in fetal brain abnormalities. Ultrasound Obstet Gynecol. 2000;16:149–53.
13. Ecker JL, Shipp TD, Bromley B, Benacerraf B. The sonographic diagnosis of Dandy-Walker and Dandy-Walker variant: associated findings and outcomes. Prenat Diagn. 2000;20(4):328–32.
14. Has R, Ermiş H, Yüksel A, Ibrahimoğlu L, Yildirim A, Sezer HD, et al. Dandy-Walker malformation: a review of 78 cases diagnosed by prenatal sonography. Fetal Diagn Ther. 2004;19(4):342–7.
15. Estroff JA, Scott MR, Benacerraf BR. Dandy-Walker variant: prenatal sonographic features and clinical outcome. Radiology. 1992;185:755–8.

16. Gross PL, Kays JL, Shura RD. Neuropsychological function in a case of Dandy-Walker variant in a 68-year-old veteran. Appl Neuropsychol Adult. 2016;23(1):70–4.

17. Golden JA, Rorke LB, Bruce DA. Dandy-Walker syndrome and associated anomalies. Pediatr Neurosci. 1987;13:38–44.

18. Imai T, Hattori H, Miyazaki M, Higuchi Y, Adachi S, Nakahata T. Dandy-Walker variant in coffin-Siris syndrome. Am J Med Genet. 2001;100(2):152–5.

19. Tadakamadla J, Kumar S, Mamatha GP. Dandy-Walker malformation: an incidental finding. Indian J Hum Genet. 2010;16(1):33–5.

20. Warf BC, Dewan M, Mugamba J. Management of Dandy-Walker complex-associated infant hydrocephalus by combined endoscopic third ventriculostomy and choroid plexus cauterization. J Neurosurg Pediatr. 2011;8(4):377–83.

21. Harwood-Nash DC, Fitz CR. Neuroradiology in infants and children. St. Louis: Mosby; 1976. p. 1014–9.

22. Limperopoulos C, Robertson RL, Estroff JA, Barnewolf C, Levine D, Bassan H, et al. Diagnosis of inferior vermian hypoplasia by fetal magnetic resonance imaging: potential pitfalls and neuro-8developmental outcome. Am J Obstet Gynecol. 2006;194:1070–6.

23. Shinde RS, Dhungat PP, Kulkarni JS, Bhoge DP, Joshi RS, Bedekar AA. Incidental presentation of Dandy Walker variant in 66 year male patient. J Assoc Physicians India. 2021;69(4):11–2.

24. Lavanya T, Cohen M, Gandhi SV, Farrell T, Whitby EH. A case of a Dandy-Walker variant: the importance of a multidisciplinary team approach using complementary techniques to obtain accurate diagnostic information. Br J Radiol. 2008;81(970):e242–5.

25. Ghane VR, Patra KC, Meshram N, Chauhan A, Kalbhande A, Wankhede S. Dandy Walker variant mimicking as cerebral palsy with severe neurological impairment. Int J Res Med Sci. 2014;2:1191–3.

26. Mytilinaios DG, Tsamis KI, Njau SN, Polyzoides K, Baloyannis SJ. Neuropathological findings in Dandy Walker variant. Dev Neurorehabil. 2010;13(1):64–7.

27. Garg A, Suri A, Chandra PS, Kumar R, Sharma BS, Mahapatra AK. Endoscopic third ventriculostomy: 5 years' experience at the All India Institute of Medical Sciences. Pediatr Neurosurg. 2009;45:1–5.

28. Mohanty A, Biswas A, Satish S, Praharaj SS, Sastry KV. Treatment options for Dandy-Walker malformation. J Neurosurg. 2006;105(5 Suppl):348–56.

Subdural Hematoma

18

Mehmet Turgut, Sinan Sağıroğlu, and Ali Akhaddar

18.1 Introduction

Since acute subdural hematoma (aSDH) is a pathology that is frequently diagnosed post-traumatic in emergency services, data on its frequency cannot be determined exactly and it varies between countries [1]. The incidence of non-traumatic aSDH cases is thought to be 3–5% [2]. Coombs et al. [3] in their literature review on non-traumatic aSDH screened 193 cases and stated that there was only a small number of cases reported in the current literature. 171 of the cases were over 40 years old and predominantly male. Arterial (61.5%), idiopathic (10.8%), coagulopathy (10.1%), oncologic (5.4%), spontaneous intracranial hypotension (5.4%), cocaine abuse (2.0%), arteriovenous malformation (1.4%) and arachnoid cyst, spontaneous occlusion of the Circle of Willis, brittle bone disease, meningioma, lifting heavy objects (0.07% each) are reported. Symptoms begin with gradually worsening severe headache and may evolve into symptoms of raised intracranial pressure (ICP) such as abducens palsy [3]

In epidemiological studies on chronic subdural hematoma (cSDH), incidence has been reported as 1.72–20.6 per 100.000, although it increases with the elderly [4–7]. The leading risk factors are advanced age, male gender, trauma/fall, anticoagulant/antiaggregant use, diabetes mellitus, alcohol abuse, epilepsy, and cardiovascular disease [1, 3, 6–9]. In cSDH, unlike aSDH, there is a process that spreads over time [1, 6]. In young patients, it often presents with a headache not accompanied by a neurological deficit [5, 9]. Common causes of admission are headache, gait disturbance, limb weakness and paralysis, altered mental status (delirium, confusional state, drowsiness, or coma), speech impairment, and epilepsy [5, 9, 10].

In the pediatric population, the most common cause of subdural hematoma (SDH) is shaken baby syndrome with a rate of 21/100.000 [11]. Caretaker abuse is most likely associated with retinal hemorrhages and additional physical injuries [12]. Other causes have been reported as trauma, surgical complications, fetal SDH, traumatic birth, aneurysm, arachnoid cyst (AC), hematological diseases causing coagulopathy, glutaric aciduria, galactosemia, and hypernatre-

M. Turgut (✉)
Department of Neurosurgery, Aydın Adnan Menderes University Faculty of Medicine, Efeler, Aydın, Turkey

Department of Histology and Embryology, Aydın Adnan Menderes University Health Sciences Institute, Efeler, Aydın, Turkey

S. Sağıroğlu
Department of Neurosurgery, Aydın Adnan Menderes University Faculty of Medicine, Efeler, Aydın, Turkey

A. Akhaddar
Department of Neurosurgery, Avicenne Military Hospital of Marrakech, Mohammed V University in Rabat, Rabat, Morocco

mia [12]. There are few cases of idiopathic SDH in teenagers [2, 13, 14]. The authors suggest that spontaneous intracranial hypotension could be the etiology after the Valsalva maneuver [14].

SDH can have a range of symptoms that include headache, confusion, memory loss, difficulty speaking, weakness gait imbalance, and even coma [10]. However, it is also possible for a SDH to be present without any of these symptoms, or symptoms may have been relieved and forgotten at admission [14–16]. This is more likely to occur in cases where the hematoma is small or develops slowly over time. In this section, we will focus on rare cases in which intracranial SDH can be detected incidentally on radiological studies taken for patients with unrelated clinical presentations, apart from the causes of SDH that are frequently mentioned in the literature and that come to mind immediately today.

18.2 Subdural Hematoma in Adult Population

The main reason for the development of aSDH is trauma, and depending on the study, the incidence is 5–25% after severe head trauma [1]. Epidemiologic studies found around 24% of aSDH to be spontaneous, the rest is primarily of traumatic origin [1, 17]. Spontaneous SDHs generally have an underlying cause [2]. Very few cases were reported with negative work-up for underlying disease and considered idiopathic [2, 3, 14] (Fig. 18.1).

18.2.1 Idiopathic Subdural Hematoma

A few cases were reported in the literature with idiopathic aSDH or cSDH [2, 3, 14]. All of the cases were previously healthy, with no documented vascular malformation, coagulopathy, drug abuse, or oncologic etiology. Common factors in these cases are young age, a profession in which physical actions equivalent to the Valsalva maneuver are highly likely routine [2, 3, 14, 18, 19]. Four of these patients, also engage in vigorous physical activity [2, 3, 18]. Some papers reported the use of nonsteroidal anti-inflammatory drugs which may cause enlargement of SDH by hindering platelet function [3, 18, 19]. SDH specimens containing large blasts of atypical lymphoid proliferation or myeloid process may be seen [3].

Illicit drugs have been reported with SDH in literature such as cocaine and methamphetamine abuse [20, 21]. Both drugs are sympathomimetic

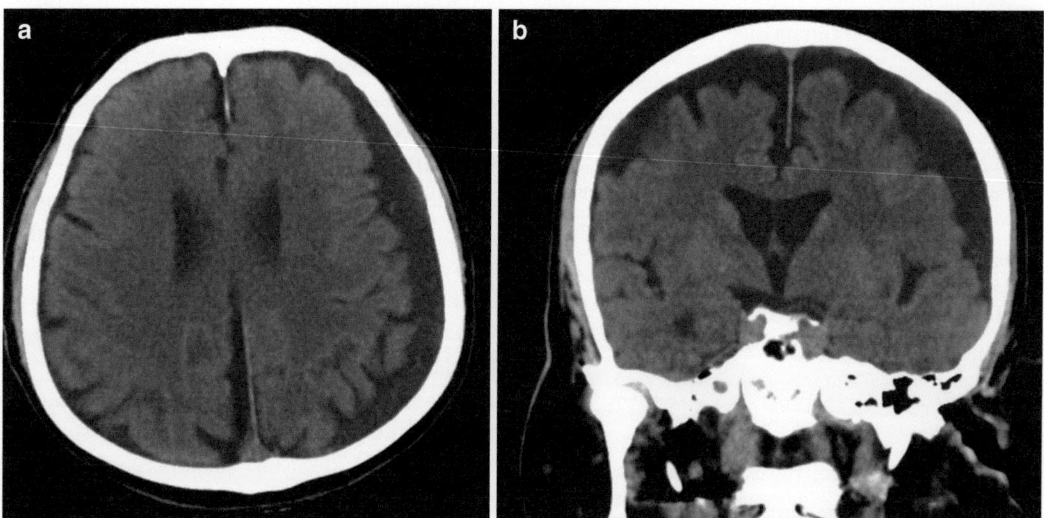

Fig. 18.1 Axial (**a**) and coronal (**b**) computed tomography (CT) images of a case of chronic subdural hematoma (cSDH) of an asymptomatic patient

and hypothesized to cause hypertensive SDH. High altitude may cause SDH in unaccustomed individuals [22, 23]. Increased cerebral blood flow and as a consequence, increased venous pressure might explain the pathogenicity of SDH [24, 25]. While reasons are unknown, momentary intracranial hypertension or hypotension, increased venous pressure, submaximal dynamic exercise, Valsalva maneuver, or dehydration are suggested mechanisms for the tearing of bridging veins [14, 18, 19, 25].

18.2.2 Arterial Hemorrhages and Vascular Malformations

Rupture of the cortical artery is the leading etiology in spontaneous aSDH [3]. Multiple studies found male predominance for arterial aSDH [26, 27]. Patients refer to their sudden severe headache as "the worst headache ever," similar to the thunderclap headache of subarachnoid hematoma [28]. There are several theories of which artery may rupture without trauma. One theory is that arterial twigs arising from cortical artery or attachment of these twigs to the arachnoid, which is thought to be the result of a previous microhemorrhage, is a structural weakness and flimsy to pressure difference, such as hypertension and sudden movement [27–32]. This theory is supported by direct intraoperative and autopsy observation of defects in the cortical cerebral wall [27, 29, 32, 33]. Hypertension is the main risk factor for these hematomas, especially combined with alcoholism [26, 27, 29, 30, 34]. The most common anatomic location of rupture is arteries at or near the Sylvian fissure [27, 29, 34] (Fig. 18.2).

Aneurysm, arteriovenous malformation (AVM), dural arteriovenous fistula (dAVF), and moyamoya disease are rare conditions accompanied by aSDH [35–42]. A ruptured aneurysm may present with SDH with an incidence of 2–5.8%, while pure aSDH is a rare finding [3, 33, 35, 39, 43]. Cortical arterial aneurysms are likely to result in aSDH but few reports are available, while other locations such as internal carotid artery (ICA), posterior communicating artery (PCoA), ICA-PCoA bifurcation, anterior cerebral artery (ACA),

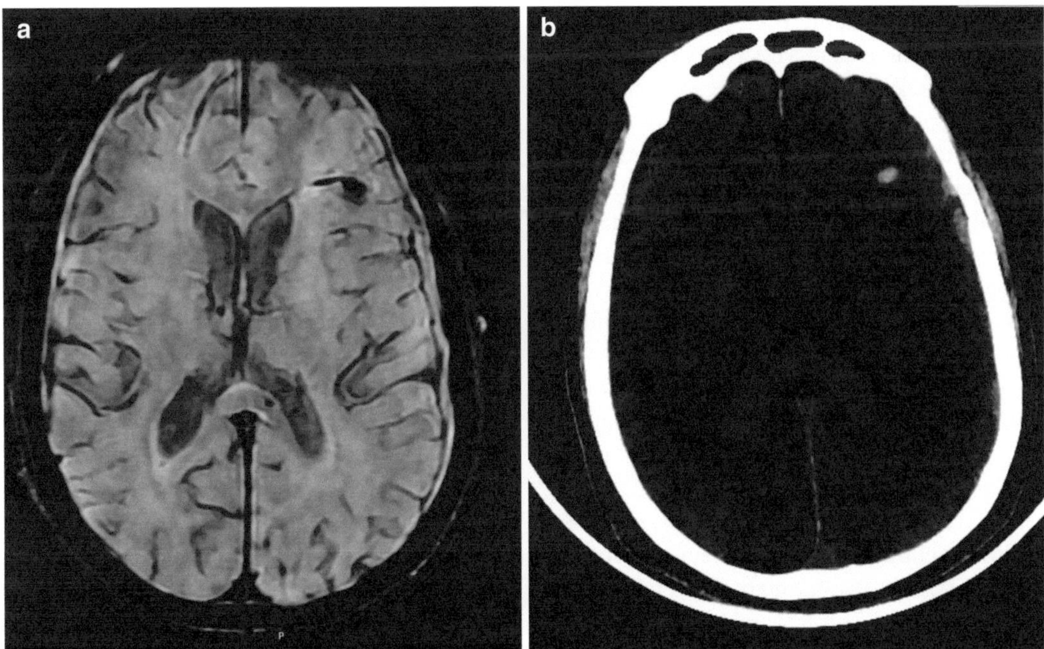

Fig. 18.2 A vascular malformation accompanied with a subacute subdural hematoma. Axial susceptibility weighted imaging sequence magnetic resonance imaging (**a**) and CT (**b**) images

anterior communicating artery (ACoA), middle cerebral artery (MCA) reported frequently [36, 39, 42–44]. High blood pressure during aneurysm rupture, especially in the setting of previous self-contained bleeds causing arachnoid adhesions, may lead to arachnoid rupture, resulting in aSDH [39, 42, 43, 45]. A recent study suggests that previous unremembered microtraumas may cause rupture and self-limiting hemorrhage in the distal part of cortical arteries of Sylvian fissure, which develop into pseudoaneurysms. A second minor trauma or hypertension may cause aSDH [46].

Mycotic aneurysm incidence is 2.5–4.5% among all aneurysms [47]. Infective endocarditis is a known risk factor [47–50]. While extremely rare, aSDH secondary to mycotic aneurysms of distal MCA had been reported. The infective SDH mechanism is explained with distal eventual localization of the mobile vegetation, causing cortical aneurysm, or arterial rupture without the evidence of an aneurysm [47–50]. Dural AVF is extremely rare to present with acute or chronic SDH and may be responsible for unexplained recurrent cSDH [38, 40, 41]. Dural AVF resulting from a middle meningeal artery (MMA) has been most frequently associated with SDH [41]. One explanation is bleeding from the venous part of dAVF originating from MMA may lead to cSDH [38]. Another recent study suggests that local venous pressure is amplified with arterial pressure due to the shunt, which may cause rupture of dural veins, resulting in SDH [40]. Endovascular embolization may be a sufficient treatment for such cases [38, 41]. AVM is another extremely rare cause of SDH [37, 42]. Adhesions of AVM to the arachnoid and strain of the arachnoid are thought to cause SDH [37, 51].

Moyamoya disease is an unusual condition in individuals with stenosis of supraclinoidal ICA and in those with collateral circulation [52]. While extremely rare to present with SDH, and with a variety of vascular malformations of moyamoya, rupture of an occult aneurysm or moyamoya vessel itself, high cerebral venous pressure, rupture or transdural anastomoses [52–54]. On the other hand, cerebral venous thromboses (CVTs) account for 0.5–1% of all strokes, which are known to result in intracranial hyper-

tension, brain edema, venous infarction, and SAH, and may rarely present with SDH [55–57]. One explanation is venous hypertension may rupture dural veins, similar to dAVF [25, 40, 58].

Today, it is strongly suggested to take an angiogram in non-traumatic aSDH, if the neurological status of the patient can tolerate the time delay, to rule out underlying vascular malformations as it may change the surgical approach and survival of the patient [29, 33, 34, 37–39, 42, 45, 53, 59]. The initial angiogram may be negative for microaneurysms [36]. As an endnote, arterial ruptures may mimic saccular aneurysms in digital subtraction angiography through extravasation of contrast into SDH, especially in settings of anti-aggregation or antiplatelet drugs [27, 29, 30, 33, 34].

18.2.3 Oncologic Etiology

Shekarchizadeh et al. [44] reported that acute SDH due to neoplastic disease has an incidence of 7.8% of all spontaneous SDHs. Various primary intracranial tumors and metastatic tumors with dural involvement have been documented to present with SDH [44, 60]. While 20% of dural metastases are clinically silent, about 41% percent of dural involvement is also accompanied by SDH. Dural metastases may be an extension of skull metastases with an incidence of 57%, primarily lung, prostate, breast carcinomas, and Ewing sarcoma [60–64]. Hematogenous spread with 43% incidence, associated with advanced stages and with lung involvement [60, 62]. Another type of dural spread is from brain parenchyma, mostly seen in nonocular malignant melanoma [62] Sporadic cases of SDH as an accidental finding of malignancy have been reported [61, 65, 66] (Fig. 18.3).

Hematologic malignancies have a high incidence of 31% for SDH [67]. Acute myeloid leukemia (AML), lymphoma, acute promyelocytic leukemia(APL), and acute lymphocytic leukemia (ALL) may present with SDH [67–69]. Repeated lumbar punctures for intrathecal therapy, especially with coagulopathic cases may be the culprit [68, 69]. Various hematological oncologies

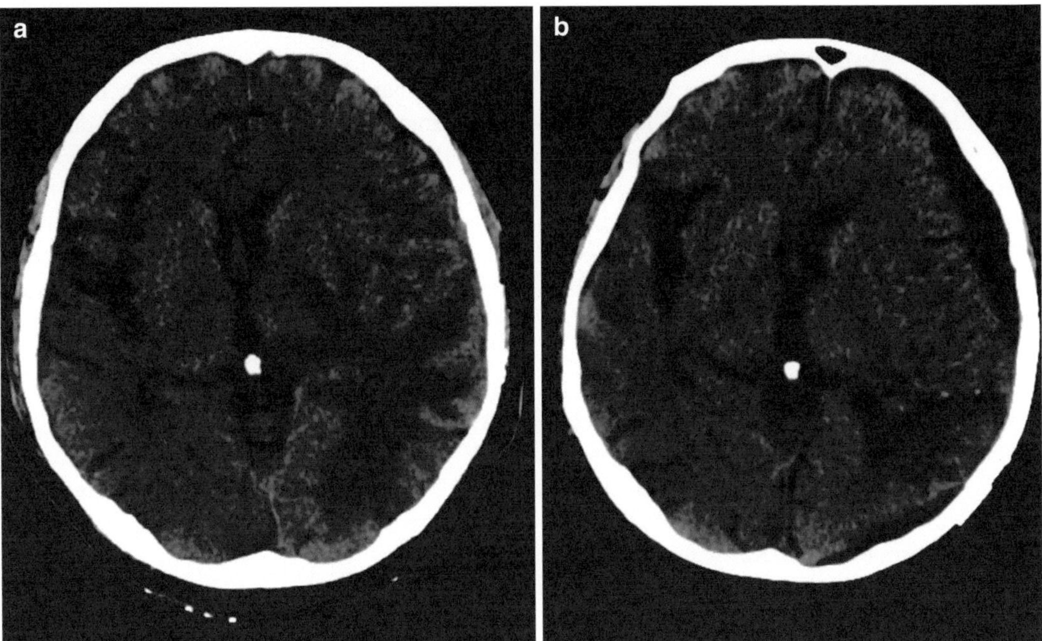

Fig. 18.3 The images show development of cSDH in a patient with glioblastoma multiforme over a 10-month period, with the pre-operative CT image (**a**) and the post-operative CT image (**b**)

such as chronic lymphocytic leukemia (CLL), and chronic myeloid leukemia (CML), have been suggested SDH as an initial finding of the underlying disease [70, 71]. Meningiomas are the most frequent primary tumor of the brain with an extremely rare presentation with SDH [72, 73]. Hematoma pathogenesis is unclear whether primary tumoral bleeding, vascular insult due to lesion mass, or secreted pro-angiogenic factors are the primary mechanisms [72, 73]. As a rule, SDH with surrounding membrane should be examined histopathologically if malignancy is suspected in patients such as elder patients, a history of weight loss, accompanied thrombocytopenia, or unexplained recurrence [64, 71, 74].

18.2.4 Spontaneaous İntracranial Hypotension

Spontaneous intracranial hypotension is an entity presenting with postural headache and low opening lumbar puncture pressure [75, 76]. Annual incidence is 5 in 100.000 per year [77]. Cases reported in the literature suggest spontaneous intracranial hypotension (SIH) associated with aSDH has an incidence of 5–10 and favors young and middle-aged with good neurological outcomes if treated promptly [3, 76]. Ferrante et al. [78] found the incidence of SDH with SIH was 16% and 97% of these were bilateral SDH. Hypotension may be idiopathic, as a result of cerebrospinal fluid (CSF) leak, or possibly postexertional to resistance exercise [19]. CSF leak may be spontaneous, or due to possibly trivial trauma, invasive procedures, or connective tissue diseases like Marfan's syndrome or Ehler–Danlos syndrome [68, 75, 78, 79]. Gadolinium-enhanced brain MRI and myelography of the central nervous system are recommended to differentiate [75, 80].

In this context, the critical point that the physician should pay attention to is whether the patient has a CSF leak because the treatment method is determined accordingly [75, 76]. SIH should come to mind in unexplained, bilateral SDH in middle-aged and young patients [78, 81, 82]. Without treatment of underlying CSF leakage, hematoma evacuation can lead to hematoma recurrence and even rapid deterioration after surgery [76, 78, 82].

18.2.5 Anticoagulants, Antiaggregants, and Coagulopathy

SDH may be the incidental finding of an underlying coagulopathy, which is mostly seen in the elderly, with a relatively high mortality rate [3, 59]. Thrombocytopenia may cause aSDH or cSDH in all age-groups [59, 83–85]. Several oncologic cases, with thrombocytopenia, have also been reported to result in SDH [65, 66, 74]. Liver cirrhosis also may lead to coagulopathy and increase the risk of SDH development [86].

Many infective pathogens are known to cause thrombocytopenia or coagulopathy with a variety of mechanisms. Kleib et al. [87] described a case of aSDH caused by coagulopathy due to Crimean-Congo hemorrhagic fever. Raj et al. [88] reported incidental SDH discovered in the setting of thrombocytopenia in a patient with malaria. Sandouno et al. [89] reported an interesting case of systemic lupus erythematosus (SLE) with the initial finding of aSDH. Jokonya et al. [90] reported human immunodeficiency virus (HIV) with cSDH in young patients. The authors propose coagulopathy due to retroviral infection as the culprit, while stating that dampened liver function via pathogen or antivirals may also cause coagulation factor deficiencies or dehydration that may result in cSDH.

cSDH with idiopathic thrombocytopenic purpura (ITP) may benefit from medical treatment without surgery if initial symptoms were mild, as restoring platelet function leads to the remission of hematoma [83–85]. Coagulation factor deficiencies such as factor I (fibrinogen), II, V, VII, VIII (hemophilia A), IX (Hemophilia B), X, XI, XII, von Willebrand disease have been proposed to create a predisposition to SDH [86, 89, 91–95]. Coagulopathy is associated with worse initial symptoms and poor outcomes in SDH [59].

Liver cirrhosis is a systemic disease with hindered factor synthesis, with a risk of 1–2% development of intracerebral hemorrhage [86, 96]. Hemophilia-related intracranial hematoma occurs at all ages but tends to favor the pediatric population [95]. Warfarin, which is a vitamin K antagonist, has a higher incidence of non-traumatic SDH, compared to traumatic cases [4, 17]. The use of warfarin may lead to an arterial rupture in hypertensive patients or due to minor trauma, making it more significant risk factor when compared to antiplatelet aggregation agents [4, 29].

Anticoagulant and antiaggregant treatment somewhat increase the incidence of cSDH, yet figures might be overestimated [4, 17, 59]. Antiplatelet therapy, commonly used in stroke patients and coronary diseases, is also a risk factor for SDH development and expansion [29, 59]. Anticoagulants have been shown to increase the mortality of SDH in hemodialysis patients [97]. Heparinization is a known risk factor and has a high incidence of SDH development, especially in patients undergoing routine hemodialysis [59, 97].

18.3 Subdural Hematoma in Pediatric Population

SDH is a rare condition in the young population, and the incidence of SDH in infants is increased compared to the rest of the pediatric population and is found to be 16.5/100.000 [11, 98]. However, it is not easy to diagnose in young children and infants. While it may be asymptomatic in newborns, it may present with clinical symptoms such as convulsions, apnea, and bradycardia [99, 100]. Infants and young children may have general symptoms such as fatigue, irritability, nausea, lethargy, and confusion [11, 101, 102].

18.3.1 Labor, Benign External Hydrocephalus, and Macrocephaly

Vaginal labor, whether traumatic or atraumatic, has been a known risk factor for perinatal intracranial hemorrhages [99, 103]. Compression during labor, tearing of falx or tentorium, and tearing of bridging veins are thought to result in SDH [104]. Blood products envelop the dural capillary bed, which is the primary CSF evacuation mechanism (minor CSF pathway) until the latter half of the first age [102, 105]. This hindrance of the minor

CSF pathway leads to hygroma formation, which leads to macrocephaly [102, 106]. This mechanism may be vice versa, rebleeding of stretched bridging veins due to hygroma resulting in recurrence of SDH [106, 107]. Thus, SHD may be an incidental finding of macrocephaly [106, 108].

While these mechanisms may explain SDH without a history of trauma, child abuse called shaken baby syndrome (SBS) should always be kept in mind. Occipital or infratentorial location of the SDH is a common sign of asymptomatic SDH. Likewise, the prognosis of incidental SDH is benign, and spontaneous resolution is expected by 2–3 years of age [99, 103, 109, 110].

18.3.2 Fetal Subdural Hematoma

There are limited reports on the suspected fetal origin of SDH, while it has 32% mortality [111]. One of the key features of this entity is the lack of apparent trauma or difficulty of birth, as almost all fetal SDH newborns are delivered with cesarean section [112–114]. The reports of vaginal birth with documented intrauterine SDH are scarce [115, 116]. Some reports document intrauterine intracranial hemorrhage and an increase in head circumference [114, 116]. Suspected etiology for in utero SDHs are maternal injury, bleeding disorders, and intracranial vascular malformations, yes most of the time prepartum history and postnatal evaluations fail to document such findings [113, 116, 117]. These reports show that however rare, routine intrauterine ultrasound evaluation may find incidental hydrocephalus which is revealed postnatally accompanying SDH [113, 116, 117]. Prenatal US features are intracranial echogenicity (42%), enlarged lateral ventricles (38%), presence of an intracranial mass (31), macrocephaly, (24%), displacement of falx cerebri from the midline (20%), intracranial fluid-filled collection (11%), reversed diastolic flow in MCA(11%) [111]. In such suspicious findings, fetal MRI could be considered may prove useful for revealing underlying pathology [115]. A multidisciplinary approach and swift response to minimize neurological sequelae to such cases are advised.

18.3.3 Arachnoid Cysts

AC is considered to be one of the most common intracranial masses with an incidence of 1% [118]. The annual risk for hemorrhage in the middle cranial fossa is thought to be below 0.1% [119]. AC is a known source of headaches in children, and gradual worsening may be the clue for hemorrhage [75, 120]. Hemorrhage may be spontaneous or after minor head trauma [120]. One of the theorized mechanisms is AC wall which is less compliant and this may cause to the rupture of bridging veins or unsupported veins around the AC wall, leading to SDH [121]. One of the alternative explanations is a one-way valve mechanism of CSF flow into AC or secretions of the AC wall itself may cause increased cyst pressure and rupture of the vascular AC wall [121, 122].

AC is a common entity and is mostly an incidental finding in children with headaches, with a benign outcome. Physicians should keep in mind AC is a predisposing factor for SDH development, especially after minor trauma. When patients who followed up with AC come with an advanced headache, control imaging should not be delayed.

18.3.4 Vascular Malformations

Fetal vascular malformations such as AVM, and aneurysms are well-researched and common causes of intracranial hemorrhage in the pediatric population [123]. Although aneurysms, dAVFs, and AVMs are known etiology of SDH in adults, vascular malformations seem rarely a cause of SDH in the pediatric population [3, 45]. Only a handful of cases with SDH had an aneurysmal origin [117, 124, 125]. AVMs in children are the main cause of spontaneous intracranial hemorrhage, and SDH is mostly reported to be a component of complex intraparenchymal-subarachnoid-SDH seen in AVM rupture [123, 126]. Development of aSDH is accepted to be the rupture of arterialized bridging vein from an AVM [126]. There is one pediatric case of SDH developed after AVF embolization. The authors commend rapid deflation of giant malformation may be the culprit [127]. CVT has a prevalence of 0.67 per 100.000 among the pediatric population [128]. While the rare occurrence of CVT with SDH limits the number of cases, recent reports postulate previous SDH with mass effect is the reason for the development of CVT in infants, not vice versa [129, 130].

18.3.5 Hematologic Diseases and Coagulation Disorders

The factors affecting the coagulation pathway are on a wide spectrum and it is difficult to follow all diseases up to date. One of the well-reported conditions is SDH in the setting of hemophilia, both type A (factor VIII) and B (factor IX). Hemophilia is reported to have a central nervous system bleeding rate of 7.5%, and the incidence increases to 85.2% in the severe forms. SDH accounts for 19–29.8% of intracranial hematomas in hemophilia patients [95, 131]. Trauma accounts for 54.3% of SDH in hemophilia [95].

Hemophilia is a serious risk factor for an intracranial hematoma in general, carrier women should have genetic counseling. The delivery method should be decided accordingly by a multidisciplinary approach. And prophylaxis should start as soon as possible to avoid further complications [132]. Other factor deficiencies seldom reported with intracranial hematomas such as fibrinogen (factor I), factor VII, X, XIII, and von Willebrand factor [92–94, 131]. Accompanying hemorrhages such as muscular or retinal hematomas makes it difficult to differentiate unknown coagulopathy or nonaccidental trauma such as SBS [92, 94]. Idiopathic thrombocytic purpura is a very common hematologic condition in children and an extremely rare cause of intracerebral hematoma, approximately 1–10/1.000.000 [133]. Only a few cases were reported in the pediatric population with SDH [134–136].

Various types of leukemia may present with SDH as a first sign, and lack of abuse history and repeated infections may be the clue for neoplastic disease in children [137]. These hematological cancer types are acute lymphocytic leukemia (ALL), acute myeloid leukemia (AML), juvenile myelomonocytic leukemia, acute monocytic leukemia, and other variants [17, 137–142]. In earlier studies, ALL is found to be predisposing to cSDH, and the authors claimed morphological studies did not support lumber puncture as a cause [142]. Initial hemorrhage mechanism is due to intradural bleeding secondary to thrombocytopenia. Meningeal spread of leukemia is thought to be a prominent factor in sustaining SDH [139, 142].

18.3.6 Metabolic Disorders

Glutaric aciduria type 1 (GA1) is a rare metabolic disorder with an incidence of 20–30% of subdural hematoma development [143]. Microcephalic macrocephaly is the initial sign of the disease most of the time [144]. A recent review of GA1 with SDH found that 40% of the cases were related to trauma [145]. The probable pathogenesis of SDH is thought to be the rupture of bridging veins due to cerebral atrophy [144–147]. Another very rare disease, D-2-hydoxyglutaric aciduria type 1 has been diagnosed after incidental SDH, which was initially suspected to be abuse due to retinal hemorrhages and bilateral SDH [148]. In a clinical investigation of 9 infants with neuronal ceroid lipofuscinosis (NCL), 4 of 9 patients had incidental SDH without additional symptoms. NCL causes progressive brain atrophy, which is associated with stretching and tearing of the bridging veins [149]. Menkes disease is a disease of copper absorption and transport abnormality, characterized by seizures, developmental delay, and kinky hair [150–152]. This rare disease is another example of neurodegeneration and atrophy, resulting in stretching of the bridging veins [146, 150–152]. Lastly, SDH alone does not provide evidence for abuse or a genetic disorder [146]. A variety of genetic diseases rarely causes SDH, except for GA1, and may provide a challenge for physicians because of similarities with non-incidental trauma. Herewith, we compiled known cases to keep in mind the probability of underlying genetic origin.

18.4 Conclusion

SDH is one of the most common diseases a neurosurgeon encounters during practice. Acute forms usually result from trauma and chronic forms are seen mostly in the elderly after minor head trauma, which every neurosurgeon is accustomed to. Non-traumatic SDH is an overlooked entity, while incidence is around 24% for aSDHs. If an aSDH is suspected to be of arterial origin, craniotomy should cover the Sylvian fissure, which is the most probable origin of the hematoma. Underlying pathologies such as aneurysms, AVM, dAVF, and moyamoya disease require additional pre-operative planning and may require advanced surgical techniques compared to regular aSDH or cSDH operations. While rare in the pediatric population, vascular anomalies may also play a role in SDH development. Mycotic aneurysms have a chance to resolve with anti-biotherapy alone, and surgery can be reserved for cases with mass effects or deterioration. cSDH associated with dAVFs and with CSF leak may cause unexplained recurrence and the patient may go through several cranial surgeries to no avail. Additional evaluation of the patients such as an angiogram or enhanced MR myelography should come to mind in such cases. Bilateral unexplained SDH in middle-aged and young patients might be the clue for SIH. SDH may be a sign of a primary intracranial tumor, metastasis of cancer, or hematologic oncology.

Pre-operative evaluation of blood work-up should be carefully examined because several hematologic malignancies cause SDH, which may be the initial finding of the underlying disease. If there is a suspicion of oncological etiology, hematoma and surrounding membranes should be examined histopathologically. Various infections, factor deficiencies, liver cirrhosis, autoimmune diseases, anticoagulants, and anti-aggregant drugs have been reported with SDH. A comprehensive history of the patient should be taken carefully, and a hematologic work-up including bleeding time and hematology consult for additional tests are advised. In pediatric patients, hematologic diseases such as hemophilia, factor deficiencies, ITP, or malignancies may be accompanied by SDH. The neurosurgeon must be scrupulous with pediatric cases, as the majority of SDH is caused by abuse, which is accompanied by retinal hemorrhages and additional physical injuries. There are several diseases in the differential diagnosis of SBS. Fetal screening with ultrasound might find suspicious findings, and further investigation with MRI may be considered for revealing underlying pathology. A multidisciplinary approach, planning of delivery, and early intervention may minimize neurological sequelae. Vaginal labor itself may change the cranial vault due to compression, which may result in asymptomatic SDH, and have a benign outcome. Macrocephaly is a subject for research on SDH in newborns and infants.

Today, the most common genetic diseases are included in newborn screening. However, screening tests vary from one country to another, physicians should also keep in mind rare diseases may present initially with SDH. AC is a common intracranial mass that is mostly found as an incidental finding. The neurosurgeon may come upon the new onset of headache in followed-up patients with AC. SDH in the setting of AC should come to mind and control imaging is advised. In this chapter, the goal is to inform the neurosurgeon of the incidental appearance of SDH in literature. Proper diagnosis of the underlying disease is crucial for appropriate treatment, and benefit of the patient.

References

1. Miljković A, Milisavljević F, Bogdanović I, Pajić S. Epidemiology and prognostic factors in patients with subdural hematoma. Facta Univ Ser Med Biol. 2021;22:49.
2. Arnold PM, Christiano LD, Klemp JA, Anderson KK. Nontraumatic spontaneous acute subdural hematoma in identical teenage twins 1 year apart. Pediatr Emerg Care. 2011;27:649–51.
3. Coombs JB, Coombs BL, Chin EJ. Acute spontaneous subdural hematoma in a middle-aged adult: case report and review of the literature. J Emerg Med. 2014;47:e63–8.
4. Aspegren OP, Åstrand R, Lundgren MI, Romner B. Anticoagulation therapy a risk factor for the

development of chronic subdural hematoma. Clin Neurol Neurosurg. 2013;115:981–4.

5. Kolias AG, Chari A, Santarius T, Hutchinson PJ. Chronic subdural haematoma: modern management and emerging therapies. Nat Rev Neurol. 2014;10:570–8.

6. Mekaj AY, Morina AA, Mekaj YH, et al. Surgical treatment of 137 cases with chronic subdural hematoma at the university clinical center of Kosovo during the period 2008-2012. J Neurosci Rural Pract. 2015;6:186–90.

7. Yang W, Huang J. Chronic subdural hematoma: epidemiology and natural history. Neurosurg Clin N Am. 2017;28:205–10.

8. Baechli H, Nordmann A, Bucher HC, Gratzl O. Demographics and prevalent risk factors of chronic subdural haematoma: results of a large single-center cohort study. Neurosurg Rev. 2004;27:263.

9. Mori K, Maeda M. Surgical treatment of chronic subdural hematoma in 500 consecutive cases: clinical characteristics, surgical outcome, complications, and recurrence rate. Neurol Med Chir (Tokyo). 2001;41:371–81.

10. Turgut M, Akhaddar A, Hall WA, Turgut AT. Subdural hematoma: past to present to future management. Springer Nature; 2021.

11. Jayawant S, Rawlinson A, Gibbon F, et al. Subdural haemorrhages in infants: population based study. BMJ. 1998;317:4.

12. Kemp AM. Investigating subdural haemorrhage in infants. Arch Dis Child. 2002;86:98–102.

13. Kulah A, Taşdemir N, Fiskeci C. Acute spontaneous subdural hematoma in a teenager. Childs Nerv Syst. 1992;8:343–6.

14. Wang HS, Kim SW, Kim SH. Spontaneous chronic subdural hematoma in an adolescent girl. J Korean Neurosurg Soc. 2013;53:201.

15. Ban SP, Hwang G, Byoun HS, et al. Middle meningeal artery embolization for chronic subdural hematoma. Radiology. 2018;286:992–9.

16. Soleman J, Nocera F, Mariani L. The conservative and pharmacological management of chronic subdural haematoma. Swiss Med Wkly. 2017;147:w14398.

17. Lindvall P, Koskinen L-OD. Anticoagulants and antiplatelet agents and the risk of development and recurrence of chronic subdural haematomas. J Clin Neurosci. 2009;16:1287–90.

18. Brennan PM, Fuller E, Shanmuganathan M, et al. Spontaneous subdural haematoma in a healthy young male. Case Rep. 2011;2011:bcr0120113694.

19. Dickerman RD, Morgan J. Pathogenesis of subdural hematoma in healthy athletes: postexertional intracranial hypotension? Acta Neurochir. 2005;147:349–50.

20. Nguyen A, Reed L, Daly SR, et al. Spontaneous atraumatic subdural hematoma related to methamphetamine use. Cureus. 2021;13:e18383. https://doi.org/10.7759/cureus.18383.

21. Saleh T, Badshah A, Afzal K. Spontaneous acute subdural hematoma secondary to cocaine abuse. South Med J. 2010;103:714–5.

22. Ganau L, Prisco L, Ganau M. High altitude induced bilateral non-traumatic subdural hematoma. Aviat Space Environ Med. 2012;83:899–901.

23. Ilbasmis S. High altitude induced subdural hematoma. Aviat Space Environ Med. 2013;84:260.

24. Lu H, Wang X-B, Tang Y. Subdural hematoma associated with high altitude. Chin Med J. 2015;128:407–8.

25. Missori P, Domenicucci M, Sassun TE, et al. Alterations in the intracranial venous sinuses in spontaneous nontraumatic chronic subdural hematomas. J Clin Neurosci. 2013;20:389–93.

26. Koç RK, Paşaoğlu A, Kurtsoy A, et al. Acute spontaneous subdural hematoma of arterial origin: a report of five cases. Surg Neurol. 1997;47:9–11.

27. Tokoro K, Nakajima F, Yamataki A. Acute spontaneous subdural hematoma of arterial origin. Surg Neurol. 1988;29:159–63.

28. McDermott M, Fleming JF, Vanderlinden RG, Tucker WS. Spontaneous arterial subdural hematoma. Neurosurgery. 1984;14:13–8.

29. Abecassis ZA, Nistal DA, Abecassis IJ, et al. Ghost aneurysms in acute subdural hematomas: a report of two cases. World Neurosurg. 2020;139:e159–65.

30. Arai H. Acute hypertensive subdural hematoma from arterial rupture shortly after the onset of cerebral subcortical hemorrhage: leakage of contrast medium during angiography. Stroke. 1983;14:281–5.

31. Drake CG. Subdural haematoma from arterial rupture. J Neurosurg. 1961;18:597–601.

32. Vance BM. Ruptures of surface blood vessels on cerebral hemispheres as a cause of subdural hemorrhage. AMA Arch Surg. 1950;61:992–1006.

33. Sung SK, Kim SH, Son DW, Lee SW. Acute spontaneous subdural hematoma of arterial origin. J Korean Neurosurg Soc. 2012;51:91.

34. Yasui T, Komiyama M, Kishi H, et al. Angiographic extravasation of contrast medium in acute "spontaneous" subdural hematoma. Surg Neurol. 1995;43:61–7.

35. Avis SP. Nontraumatic acute subdural hematoma. A case report and review of the literature. Am J Forensic Med Pathol. 1993;14:130–4.

36. Awaji K, Inokuchi R, Ikeda R, Haisa T. Nontraumatic pure acute subdural hematoma caused by a ruptured cortical middle cerebral artery aneurysm: case report and literature review. NMC Case Rep J. 2016;3:63–6.

37. Choi HJ, Lee JI, Nam KH, Ko JK. Acute spontaneous subdural hematoma due to rupture of a tiny cortical arteriovenous malformation. J Korean Neurosurg Soc. 2015;58:547.

38. Kim E. Refractory spontaneous chronic subdural hematoma: a rare presentation of an intracranial arteriovenous fistula. J Cerebrovasc Endovasc Neurosurg. 2016;18:373.

39. Koerbel A, Ernemann U, Freudenstein D. Acute subdural haematoma without subarachnoid haemor-

rhage caused by rupture of an internal carotid artery bifurcation aneurysm: case report and review of literature. Br J Radiol. 2005;78:646–50.

40. Lebeau J, Moïse M, Bonnet P, et al. The dural vascular plexus in subdural hematoma: illustration through a case of dural arteriovenous fistula. Surg Neurol Int. 2022;13:212.

41. Li G, Zhang Y, Zhao J, et al. Isolated subdural hematoma secondary to Dural arteriovenous fistula: a case report and literature review. BMC Neurol. 2019;19:43.

42. Rengachary SS, Szymanski DC. Subdural hematomas of arterial origin. Neurosurgery. 1981;8:166–72.

43. Ohkuma H, Shimamura N, Fujita S, Suzuki S. Acute subdural hematoma caused by aneurysmal rupture: incidence and clinical features. Cerebrovasc Dis. 2003;16:171–3.

44. Shekarchizadeh A, Masih S, Reza P, Seif B. Acute subdural hematoma and subarachnoid hemorrhage caused by ruptured cortical artery aneurysm: case report and review of literature. Adv Biomed Res. 2017;6:46.

45. Gao X, Yue F, Zhang F, et al. Acute non-traumatic subdural hematoma induced by intracranial aneurysm rupture: a case report and systematic review of the literature. Medicine (Baltimore). 2020;99:e21434.

46. Yanagawa T, Yamashita K, Harada Y, et al. Location of hemorrhage with nontraumatic acute subdural hematoma due to ruptured microaneurysm. Surg Neurol Int. 2021;12:401.

47. Lee S, Park H-S, Choi J-H, Huh J-T. Ruptured mycotic aneurysm of the distal middle cerebral artery manifesting as subacute subdural hematoma. J Cerebrovasc Endovasc Neurosurg. 2013;15:235.

48. Boukobza M, Duval X, Laissy J-P. Mycotic intracranial aneurysms rupture presenting as pure acute subdural hematoma in infectious endocarditis. Report of 2 cases and review of the literature. J Clin Neurosci. 2019;62:222–5.

49. Geisenberger D, Huppertz LM, Büchsel M, et al. Non-traumatic subdural hematoma secondary to septic brain embolism: a rare cause of unexpected death in a drug addict suffering from undiagnosed bacterial endocarditis. Forensic Sci Int. 2015;257:e1–5.

50. Peters PJ, Harrison T, Lennox JL. A dangerous dilemma: management of infectious intracranial aneurysms complicating endocarditis. Lancet Infect Dis. 2006;6:742–8.

51. Pozzati E, Tognetti F, Gaist G. Chronic subdural haematoma from cerebral arteriovenous malformation. Min Minim Invasive Neurosurg. 1986;29:61–2.

52. Vijayasaradhi M, Prasad VB. Moyamoya disease presenting as bilateral acute subdural hematomas without deficits. Asian J Neurosurg. 2017;12:228–31.

53. Oppenheim JS, Gennuso R, Sacher M, Hollis P. Acute atraumatic subdural hematoma associated with moyamoya disease in an African-American. Neurosurgery. 1991;28:616–8.

54. Takeuchi S, Nawashiro H, Uozumi Y, et al. Chronic subdural hematoma associated with moyamoya disease. Asian J Neurosurg. 2014;9:165.

55. Alharshan R, Qureshi HU, AlHada A, et al. Cerebral venous sinus thrombosis manifesting as a recurrent spontaneous subdural hematoma: a case report. Int J Surg Case Rep. 2020;67:223–6.

56. Bansal H, Chaudhary A, Mahajan A, Paul B. Acute subdural hematoma secondary to cerebral venous sinus thrombosis: case report and review of literature. Asian J Neurosurg. 2016;11:177.

57. Ramesh R, Hazeena P, Javed TP, Venkatasubramanian S. Isolated cortical vein thrombus presenting with subdural hematoma. Ann Indian Acad Neurol. 2020;23:566–7.

58. Akins P, Axelrod Y, Ji C, et al. Cerebral venous sinus thrombosis complicated by subdural hematomas: case series and literature review. Surg Neurol Int. 2013;4:85.

59. Depreitere B, Van Calenbergh F, van Loon J. A clinical comparison of non-traumatic acute subdural haematomas either related to coagulopathy or of arterial origin without coagulopathy. Acta Neurochir. 2003;145:541–6.

60. Laigle-Donadey F, Taillibert S, Mokhtari K, et al. Dural metastases. J Neuro-Oncol. 2005;75:57–61.

61. Chye C-L, Lin K-H, Ou C-H, et al. Acute spontaneous subdural hematoma caused by skull metastasis of hepatocellular carcinoma: case report. BMC Surg. 2015;15:60.

62. Kleinschmidt-DeMasters BK. Dural metastases. A retrospective surgical and autopsy series. Arch Pathol Lab Med. 2001;125:880–7.

63. Sugawara A, Miura S, Suda Y, et al. Chronic subdural hematoma secondary to metastasis of adenocarcinoma of the dura mater and skull—a case report. Gan No Rinsho Jpn J Cancer Clin. 1986;32:190–5.

64. Zheng JX, Tan TK, Kumar DS, et al. Subdural haematoma due to dural metastases from bronchogenic carcinoma in a previously well patient: an unusual cause of non-traumatic recurrent intracranial haematomata. Singap Med J. 2011;52:e66–9.

65. Ichimura S, Ichimura S, Horiguchi T, et al. Nontraumatic acute subdural hematoma associated with the myelodysplastic/myeloproliferative neoplasms. J Neurosci Rural Pract. 2012;03:98–9.

66. Kitano A, Yamamoto K, Nagao T, et al. Successful treatment with drainage of hematoma and chemotherapy in a case of Burkitt leukemia presenting with subdural hematoma. Rinsho Ketsueki. 2005;46:278–80.

67. Chen C-Y, Tai C-H, Cheng A, et al. Intracranial hemorrhage in adult patients with hematological malignancies. BMC Med. 2012;10:97.

68. Chia XX, Bazargan A. Subdural hemorrhage—a serious complication post-intrathecal chemotherapy. A case report and review of literature. Clin Case Rep. 2015;3:57–9.

69. Jourdan E, Dombret H, Glaisner S, et al. Unexpected high incidence of intracranial subdural haematoma during intensive chemotherapy for acute myeloid leukaemia with a monoblastic component. Br J Haematol. 1995;89:527–30.

70. Abdulhamid MM, Li YM, Hall WA. Spontaneous acute subdural hematoma as the initial manifestation of chronic myeloid leukemia. J Neuro-Oncol. 2011;101:513–6.

71. Bromberg JE, Vandertop WP, Jansen GH. Recurrent subdural haematoma as the primary and sole manifestation of chronic lymphocytic leukaemia. Br J Neurosurg. 1998;12:373–6.

72. Matos D, Pereira R. Meningioma-related subacute subdural hematoma: a case report. Surg Neurol Int. 2020;11:264.

73. Mezzacappa FM, Chen J, Punsoni M, et al. Acute, nontraumatic subdural hemorrhage as a presentation of meningioma: a report of two cases and literature review. Interdiscip Neurosurg. 2022;28:101518.

74. George K, Ellis M, Fehlings M, et al. Metastatic coagulopathic subdural hematoma: a dismal prognosis. Surg Neurol Int. 2012;3:60.

75. Hou K, Li CG, Zhang Y, Zhu BX. The surgical treatment of three young chronic subdural hematoma patients with different causes. J Korean Neurosurg Soc. 2014;55:218.

76. de Noronha RJ. Subdural haematoma: a potentially serious consequence of spontaneous intracranial hypotension. J Neurol Neurosurg Psychiatry. 2003;74:752–5.

77. Schievink WI. Spontaneous spinal cerebrospinal fluid leaks and intracranial hypotension. JAMA. 2006;295:2286–96.

78. Ferrante E, Rubino F, Beretta F, et al. Treatment and outcome of subdural hematoma in patients with spontaneous intracranial hypotension: a report of 35 cases. Acta Neurol Belg. 2018;118:61–70.

79. Dangra V, Bharucha N, Sharma Y, Deopujari C. An interesting case of headache. Ann Indian Acad Neurol. 2011;14:130.

80. Chazen JL, Talbott JF, Lantos JE, Dillon WP. MR Myelography for identification of spinal CSF leak in spontaneous intracranial hypotension. Am J Neuroradiol. 2014;35:2007–12.

81. Kim HJ, Lee JW, Lee E, et al. Incidence of spinal CSF leakage on CT myelography in patients with nontraumatic intracranial subdural hematoma. Diagnostics. 2021;11:2278.

82. Kim J-H, Kim JH, Kwon TH, Chotai S. Brain herniation induced by drainage of subdural hematoma in spontaneous intracranial hypotension. Asian J Neurosurg. 2013;8:112.

83. Patnaik A, Mishra S, Senapati S, Pattajoshi A. Management of chronic subdural haematoma in a case of idiopathic thrombocytopenic purpura. J Surg Tech Case Rep. 2012;4:132.

84. Seçkin H, Kazanci A, Yigitkanli K, et al. Chronic subdural hematoma in patients with idiopathic thrombocytopenic purpura: a case report and review of the literature. Surg Neurol. 2006;66:411–4.

85. Takase H, Tatezuki J, Ikegaya N, et al. Therapeutic suggestions for chronic subdural hematoma associated with idiopathic thrombocytopenic purpura: a case report and literature review. NMC Case Rep J. 2014;2:118–22.

86. Ahmad S, Ali H, Ikram S, et al. Spontaneous bilateral subdural hematomas in a patient with cryptogenic liver cirrhosis. Cureus. 2021;13:e16100.

87. Kleib AS, Salihy SM, Ghaber SM, et al. Crimean-Congo hemorrhagic fever with acute subdural hematoma, Mauritania, 2012. Emerg Infect Dis. 2016;22:1305–6.

88. Mallela AR, Hariprasad S, Koya R, et al. Spontaneous subdural haemorrhage: a rare association with plasmodium vivax malaria. J Clin Diagn Res JCDR. 2016;10:OD05–6.

89. Sandouno TM, Bachir H, Alaoui HB, et al. Acute spontaneous subdural hematoma as an inaugural presentation of systemic lupus erythematosus with acquired factor XIII deficiency: a case report. Pan Afr Med J. 2021;39:207.

90. Jokonya L, Musara A, Cakana A, KazadiKN K. Spontaneous chronic subdural hematomas in human immunodeficiency virus-infected patients with normal platelet count and no appreciable brain atrophy: two case reports and review of literature. Surg Neurol Int. 2016;7:437.

91. Agrawal D, Mahapatra AK. Spontaneous subdural hematoma in a young adult with hemophilia. Neurol India. 2003;51:114–5.

92. Senturk S, Guzel E, Hasanefendioglu Bayrak A, et al. Factor X deficiency presenting with bilateral chronic subdural hematoma. Pediatr Neurosurg. 2010;46:54–7.

93. de Sousa C, Clark T, Bradshaw A. Antenatally diagnosed subdural haemorrhage in congenital factor X deficiency. Arch Dis Child. 1988;63:1168–70.

94. Stray-Pedersen A, Omland S, Nedregaard B, et al. An infant with subdural hematoma and retinal hemorrhages: does von Willebrand disease explain the findings? Forensic Sci Med Pathol. 2011;7:37–41.

95. de Tezanos PM, Fernandez J, Perez Bianco PR. Update of 156 episodes of central nervous system bleeding in hemophiliacs. Haemostasis. 1992;22:259–67.

96. Lai C-H, Cheng P-Y, Chen Y-Y. Liver cirrhosis and risk of intracerebral hemorrhage: a 9-year follow-up study. Stroke. 2011;42:2615–7.

97. Fayed A, Tarek A, Refaat MI, et al. Retrospective analysis of nontraumatic subdural hematoma incidence and outcomes in Egyptian patients with end-stage renal disease on hemodialysis. Ren Fail. 2021;43:1322–8.

98. Högberg U, Andersson J, Squier W, et al. Epidemiology of subdural haemorrhage during infancy: a population-based register study. PLoS One. 2018;13:e0206340.

99. Looney CB, Smith JK, Merck LH, et al. Intracranial hemorrhage in asymptomatic neonates: prevalence on MR images and relationship to obstetric and neonatal risk factors. Radiology. 2007;242:535–41.

100. Palmer TW, Donn SM. Symptomatic subarachnoid hemorrhage in the term newborn. J Perinatol Off J Calif Perinat Assoc. 1991;11:112–6.

101. Gerstl L, Badura K, Heinen F, et al. Childhood haemorrhagic stroke: a 7-year single-centre experience. Arch Dis Child. 2019;104:1198–202.

102. Zahl SM, Wester K, Gabaeff S. Examining perinatal subdural haematoma as an aetiology of extra-axial hygroma and chronic subdural haematoma. Acta Paediatr. 2020;109:659–66.

103. Rooks VJ, Eaton JP, Ruess L, et al. Prevalence and evolution of intracranial hemorrhage in asymptomatic term infants. Am J Neuroradiol. 2008;29:1082–9.

104. Huang AH, Robertson RL. Spontaneous superficial parenchymal and leptomeningeal hemorrhage in term neonates. AJNR Am J Neuroradiol. 2004;25:469–75.

105. Oi S, Di Rocco C. Proposal of "evolution theory in cerebrospinal fluid dynamics" and minor pathway hydrocephalus in developing immature brain. Childs Nerv Syst. 2006;22:662–9.

106. Ravid S, Maytal J. External hydrocephalus: a probable cause for subdural hematoma in infancy. Pediatr Neurol. 2003;28:139–41.

107. Caré MM. Macrocephaly and subdural collections. Pediatr Radiol. 2021;51:891–7.

108. Azais M, Echenne B. Idiopathic pericerebral swelling (external hydrocephalus) of infants. Ann Pediatr (Paris). 1992;39:550–8.

109. Lee HC, Chong S, Lee JY, et al. Benign extracerebral fluid collection complicated by subdural hematoma and fluid collection: clinical characteristics and management. Childs Nerv Syst. 2018;34:235–45.

110. Mori K, Sakamoto T, Nishimura K, Fujiwara K. Subarachnoid fluid collection in infants complicated by subdural hematoma. Childs Nerv Syst ChNS Off J Int Soc Pediatr Neurosurg. 1993;9:282–4.

111. Cheung KW, Tan LN, Seto MTY, et al. Prenatal diagnosis, management, and outcome of fetal subdural haematoma: a case report and systematic review. Fetal Diagn Ther. 2019;46:285–95.

112. Copley PC, Dean B, Davidson AL, et al. Spontaneous subdural haematoma in a neonate requiring urgent surgical evacuation. Acta Neurochir. 2021;163:1743–9.

113. MacDonald JT, Weitz R, Sher PK. Intrauterine chronic subdural hematoma. Arch Neurol. 1977;34:777–8.

114. Powers CJ, Fuchs HE, George TM. Chronic subdural hematoma of the neonate: report of two cases and literature review. Pediatr Neurosurg. 2007;43:25–8.

115. Diaz A, Taha S, Vinikoff L, et al. Chronic subdural hematoma in utero. Case report with literature review. Neurochirurgie. 1998;44:124–6.

116. Nogueira GJ. Chronic subdural hematoma in utero: report of a case with survival after treatment. Childs Nerv Syst. 1992;8:462–4.

117. Sohda S, Hamada H, Takanami Y, Kubo T. Prenatal diagnosis of fetal subdural haematomas. BJOG Int J Obstet Gynaecol. 1996;103:89–90.

118. Cincu R, Agrawal A, Eiras J. Intracranial arachnoid cysts: current concepts and treatment alternatives. Clin Neurol Neurosurg. 2007;109:837–43.

119. Parsch CS, Krauss J, Hofmann E, et al. Arachnoid cysts associated with subdural hematomas and hygromas: analysis of 16 cases, long-term follow-up, and review of the literature. Neurosurgery. 1997;40:483–90.

120. Liu Z, Xu P, Li Q, et al. Arachnoid cysts with subdural hematoma or intracystic hemorrhage in children. Pediatr Emerg Care. 2014;30:345–51.

121. Page A, Paxton RM, Mohan D. A reappraisal of the relationship between arachnoid cysts of the middle fossa and chronic subdural haematoma. J Neurol Neurosurg Psychiatry. 1987;50:1001–7.

122. Santamarta D, Aguas J, Ferrer E. The natural history of arachnoid cysts: endoscopic and cine-mode MRI evidence of a slit-valve mechanism. Min Minim Invasive Neurosurg. 1995;38:133–7.

123. Ciochon UM, Bindslev JBB, Hoei-Hansen CE, et al. Causes and risk factors of pediatric spontaneous intracranial hemorrhage—a systematic. Review. 2022;12

124. Strigini FAL, Nardini V, Carmignani A, Valleriani AM. Second-trimester diagnosis of intracranial vascular anomalies in a fetus with subdural hemorrhage: fetal intracranial vascular anomalies. Prenat Diagn. 2004;24:31–4.

125. Vapalahti PM, Schugk P, Tarkkanen L, af Björkesten G. Intracranial arterial aneurysm in a three-month-old infant: case report. J Neurosurg. 1969;30:169–71.

126. Oikawa A, Aoki N, Sakai T. Arteriovenous malformation presenting as acute subdural haematoma. Neurol Res. 1993;15:353–5.

127. Ye Z, Hao J, Zhang L, Lv X. Development of bilateral subdural hematoma after endovascular embolization of a dural sinus malformation. Childs Nerv Syst. 2022;38:211–5.

128. deVeber G, Andrew M, Adams C, et al. Cerebral sinovenous thrombosis in children. N Engl J Med. 2001;345:417–23.

129. McLean LA, Frasier LD, Hedlund GL. Does intracranial venous thrombosis cause subdural hemorrhage in the pediatric population? Am J Neuroradiol. 2012;33:1281–4.

130. Vaslow DF. Chronic subdural hemorrhage predisposes to development of cerebral venous thrombosis and associated retinal hemorrhages and subdural rebleeds in infants. Neuroradiol J. 2022;35:53–66.

131. Patiroglu T, Ozdemir MA, Unal E, et al. Intracranial hemorrhage in children with congenital factor deficiencies. Childs Nerv Syst. 2011;27:1963–6.

132. Zanon E, Pasca S. Intracranial haemorrhage in children and adults with haemophilia A and B: a literature review of the last 20 years. Blood Transfus Trasfus Sangue. 2019;17:378–84.

133. Butros LJ, Bussel JB. Intracranial hemorrhage in immune thrombocytopenic purpura: a retrospective analysis. J Pediatr Hematol Oncol. 2003;25:660–4.

134. González B, Fodor P, Schuh W. Use of intravenous gamma globulin in idiopathic thrombocytopenic purpura in children. Rev Chil Pediatr. 1984;55:417–9.

135. Kolluri VR, Reddy DR, Reddy PK, et al. Subdural hematoma secondary to immune thrombocytopenic purpura: case report. Neurosurgery. 1986;19:635–6.

136. Panicker JN, Pavithran K, Thomas M. Management of subdural hematoma in immune thrombocytopenic purpura: report of seven patients and a literature review. Clin Neurol Neurosurg. 2009;111:189–92.

137. Lambert WA, DiGiuseppe JA, Lara-Ospina T, et al. Juvenile myelomonocytic leukemia presenting in an infant with a subdural hematoma. Childs Nerv Syst. 2021;37:2075–9.

138. Basmaci M, Hasturk AE. Chronic subdural hematoma in a child with acute myeloid leukemia after leukocytosis. Indian J Crit Care Med. 2012;16:222–4.

139. Bean SC, Ladisch S. Chorea associated with a subdural hematoma in a child with leukemia. J Pediatr. 1977;90:255–6.

140. Lin C-H, Hung G-Y, Chang C-Y, Chien J-C. Subdural hemorrhage in a child with acute promyelocytic leukemia presenting as subtle headache. J Chin Med Assoc. 2005;68:437–40.

141. Mashiyama S, Fukawa O, Mitani S, et al. Chronic subdural hematoma associated with malignancy: report of three cases. No Shinkei Geka. 2000;28:173–8.

142. Pitner SE, Johnson WW. Chronic subdural hematoma in childhood acute leukemia. Cancer. 1973;32:185–90.

143. Hoffmann G, Athanassopoulos S, Burlina A, et al. Clinical course, early diagnosis, treatment, and prevention of disease in Glutaryl-CoA dehydrogenase deficiency. Neuropediatrics. 1996;27:115–23.

144. Strauss KA, Puffenberger EG, Robinson DL, Morton DH. Type I glutaric aciduria, part 1: natural history of 77 patients. Am J Med Genet. 2003;121C:38–52.

145. Vester MEM, Bilo RAC, Karst WA, et al. Subdural hematomas: glutaric aciduria type 1 or abusive head trauma? A systematic review. Forensic Sci Med Pathol. 2015;11:405–15.

146. Shur NE, Summerlin ML, McIntosh BJ, et al. Genetic causes of fractures and subdural hematomas: fact versus fiction. Pediatr Radiol. 2021;51:1029–43.

147. Woelfle J, Kreft B, Emons D, Haverkamp F. Subdural hemorrhage as an initial sign of glutaric aciduria type 1: a diagnostic pitfall. Pediatr Radiol. 1996;26:779–81.

148. Perales-Clemente E, Hewitt AL, Studinski AL, et al. Bilateral subdural hematomas and retinal hemorrhages mimicking nonaccidental trauma in a patient with D-2-hydroxyglutaric aciduria. JIMD Rep. 2021;58:21–8.

149. Levin SW, Baker EH, Gropman A, et al. Subdural fluid collections in patients with infantile neuronal ceroid lipofuscinosis. Arch Neurol. 2009;66:1567.

150. Johnsen DE, Coleman L, Poe L. MR of progressive neurodegenerative change in treated Menkes' kinky hair disease. Neuroradiology. 1991;33:181–2.

151. Nassogne M-C, Sharrard M, Hertz-Pannier L, et al. Massive subdural haematomas in Menkes disease mimicking shaken baby syndrome. Childs Nerv Syst. 2002;18:729–31.

152. Tayal A, Elwadhi A, Sharma S, Patra B. An unusual presentation of Menkes disease masquerading as a Leukodystrophy with macrocephaly. J Pediatr Neurosci. 2020;15:57–9.

Asymptomatic Craniofacial Fibrous Dysplasia

Ashutosh Kumar, Ashish Sharma,
and Sanjay Behari

19.1 Introduction

Fibrous dysplasia (FD) is a benign bone tumor that manifests as a broad clinical spectrum. The spectrum ranges from an isolated asymptomatic lesion diagnosed incidentally, to a trivial lesion with minimal symptoms, to the presence of severe disease that may involve the whole of the skeletal system. FD is one of the component of the clinical triad of McCune–Albright syndrome (MAS), with others being café-au-lait skin macules and precocious puberty [1]. It occurs from a gain of function mutation in the GNAS gene, which encodes the α-subunit of the G_s signaling protein. The resultant alteration of intrinsic GTPase activity of $G_s\alpha$ leads to persistent stimulation of adenylyl cyclase and dysregulated production of cAMP and downstream signaling [2, 3].

The clinical features and the management depend largely on the location and distribution of the lesions. It most commonly involves the craniofacial skeleton, known as craniofacial FD (CFD), while the skull base is the most commonly affected site in CFD [4]. The bony lesions may present in isolation or in combination with the extraskeletal disease [5]. Depending upon the number of bones involved, it may be monostotic (one bone) or polyostotic (multiple bones). No extraskeletal manifestations should be present. MAS is diagnosed if extraskeletal are present with or without FD [6]. This chapter deals with the management of asymptomatic CFD.

19.2 Clinical Presentation

The typical clinical presentation of CFD is a gradual, painless swelling leading to facial asymmetry. A significant number of CFD patients are diagnosed incidentally who are completely asymptomatic for the disease [7]. Becelli et al. reported that 36.3% ($n = 24$) of their patients had an insidious onset of the disease, lacked evident symptomatology, and the diagnosis was fortuitous [8]. Most of these patients have lesions detected on imaging done following trauma or in dental radiographs [9]. Mostly, these patients have monostotic CFD. The lesions are either too small to cause any noticeable cosmetic deformity or lie in cryptic areas like the skull base with no compression of neurological structures. Due to the high importance of location, these lesions are classified based on the anatomical zones of the skull (Table 19.1) [10, 11].

A. Kumar · A. Sharma · S. Behari (✉)
Department of Neurosurgery, Sanjay Gandhi
Postgraduate Institute of Medical Sciences,
Lucknow, India

Table 19.1 Classification of craniofacial fibrous dysplasia (CFD) based on skull zones involved and managerial implications

Zones	Bones involved		Management
Zone 1	Frontal, orbital, nasal, ethmoid, zygoma, and upper maxilla		• Most conspicuous regions • Complete excision and reconstruction in most cases
Zone 2	Parietal, parts of occipital area, and lateral cranial base of the temporal bone.		• Covered with hair (less cosmetic problem) • Both conservative and radical excision are viable options
Zone 3	Central cranial base, petrous, mastoid, pterygoid, and sphenoid bones		• Difficult to access • If asymptomatic— conservatively managed
Zone 4	4a	Maxillary alveolar bone	• Teeth bearing area • Conservative resection and recontouring
	4b	Mandible	

Evaluation of asymptomatic CFD must include:

1. Further evaluation for the presence of any other skeletal disease (monostotic/polyostotic).
2. Presence of extra-skeletal manifestation.

19.2.1 Skeletal Survey

The skeletal survey to find other cryptic FD lesions encompasses three arms. Firstly, clinical history and examination including a prior history of fracture, bone pain, and minor joint deformities. Secondly, biochemical tests for bone pathology like alkaline phosphatase (ALP), renal profile, bicarbonate, albumin adjusted serum calcium, phosphates, 25OH-Vit D, and parathyroid hormone (PTH) should be carried out. Finally, a radiological survey involving whole body imaging with bone scintigraphy, whole body magnetic resonance imaging (MRI), computed tomography (CT) of the suspected areas, and low dose 2D/3D radiography may be carried out.

19.2.2 Extraskeletal Manifestation Evaluation

The extraskeletal manifestations include endocrine abnormalities and dermatological lesions (café-au-lait macules). Patients need to be tested for ovarian, testicular, thyroid, adrenal, and pituitary hormones.

The monostotic forms never progress to polyostotic FD or MAS. Also, these lesions do not undergo spontaneous resolution. They have a myriad of manifestations ranging from a quiescent lesion (with stable with no growth), to a non-aggressive (slow growing) or aggressive (rapid growth and may be associated with pain, neurological compression, pathological fractures, or undergoing malignant transformation) lesion. The former two are mostly diagnosed incidentally and remain asymptomatic [12]. These features of CFD have critical implications in the expectant management of the incidental asymptomatic CFDs.

19.3 Radiological Diagnosis

The detection of an asymptomatic CFD is a radiological diagnostic challenge. The radiological differential diagnoses of such lesions are broad and myriad (Table 19.2). CT study is currently regarded as the investigation for choice, with a characteristic sign of "ground glass appearance" and bone expansion (Fig. 19.1). It appears homogenously grayish due to the presence of woven bone components with a variable amount of mineralization. Due to age-related variations in the pathological progression of the disease, the radiological picture varies considerably. In children less than 2 years of age, the lesion often appears heterogeneous with a lack of classic ground glass appearance. In older patients, the lesions become denser and more sclerotic [13, 14].

The diagnosis of CFD based on MRI findings is challenging due to the high variability of the signals on the T2 and contrast-enhanced imaging (Fig. 19.1) [15]. The lesions appear hypointense in both T1 and T2 sequences in most cases, with a variable degree of contrast enhancement with gadolinium. The combined use of CT scan and contrast-enhanced MRI could differentiate this entity from other lesions and may also help to characterize most cases of CFD [16].

Table 19.2 Radiological differential diagnoses of monostotic craniofacial fibrous dysplasia (CFD) include:

Pathologies mimicking CFD on radiological imaging	Intra-osseous meningioma
	Ossifying fibroma
	Fibro-osseous lesion
	Cherubism
	Aseptic mandibular osteitis (SAPHO syndrome)
	Central giant cell granuloma
	Aneurysmal bone cyst
	Giant cell tumor
	Langerhans cell histiocytosis
	Paget's disease of bone

Technetium 99 m-methyl diphosphonate bone scan is used to detect the extent of the disease by identifying the metabolically active lesions. After the establishment of the initial diagnosis, these scans are not recommended during the follow-up visit of the patient. These lesions also show 18-F-fluorodeoxyglucose uptake on positron emission tomography/CT mimicking malignant lesions and metastasis [17]. The lesion may not be detected if it is small. Their detection may also be difficult in patients less than 5 years of age.

19.4 Management

Most asymptomatic monostotic CFD cases can be managed conservatively with the expectant follow-up [6]. Serial imaging is done to confirm that the lesion is biologically inactive and insignificant to cause any neurological deficit. Even in symptomatic cases, the surgical indications are limited and restricted to addressing the functional

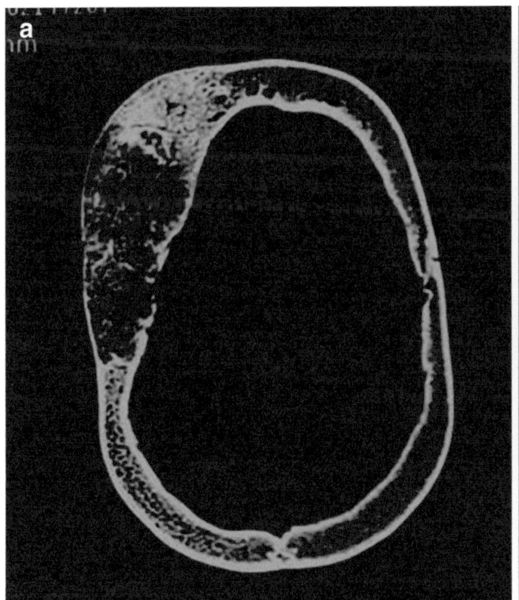
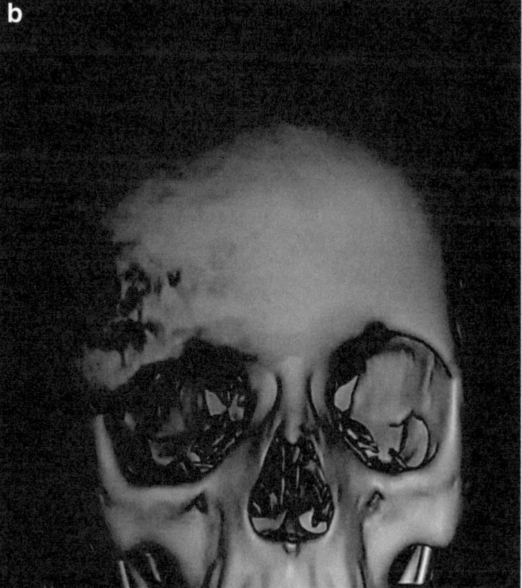

Fig. 19.1 A 20-year-old girl presented with minor facial asymmetry due to craniofacial fibrous dysplasia (CFD) involving the right frontal bone. The plain CT head (**a**) showed a ground glass appearance of the CFD lesion involving the right frontal bone. The (**b**) 3D reconstruction of the CT showed the extent of boney involvement of the frontal bone, especially the orbital roof causing facial asymmetry. Due to unacceptable cosmesis, the patient opted for surgical intervention

impairment, such as compressive neuropathies, otic canal obstruction, severe malocclusion, symptomatic cranial base deformities, and lesions causing a profound cosmetic problem.

The majority of the patients incidentally diagnosed on CT, with the presence of the ground glass appearance on imaging, can be managed conservatively with no need for confirmation with a biopsy. A biopsy is indicated when the radiological features are atypical, especially in the case of monostotic lesions. Lesions that have a minimal risk of neurological deficit or deformity can be observed, depending upon the location, age of the patient, type of CFD, and patient's view towards surgery.

Optic nerve encasement is common with CFD, and it is usually asymptomatic. Visual deterioration is reported in less than 5% of the cases. These cases are managed conservatively with periodic imaging to assess the progression of the disease. In asymptomatic patients with optic nerve compression, surgical decompression (complete or partial) is not recommended due to the high risk of optic nerve injury [18]. Similarly, patients with CFD involving temporal bone develop mild hearing loss, which is mostly conductive. It results from the fixation of the ossicles within the epitympanum and is less common due to the narrowing of the external auditory meatus. Most of these cases are managed conservatively [19].

While managing a patient conservatively, a follow-up regimen is essential to confirm the non-progression of the lesion or the occurrence of a new lesion, neurological deficit, or a change in the character of an existing lesion. The frequency depends upon the extent of the disease and the risk of complications. The baseline and periodic CT scan of the head should be performed in children, usually every 2 years (or less frequently based on the localization and the severity of the disease). While in adults, the follow-up scan is usually performed every 5 years (or earlier if there is an onset of any new clinical finding). A hearing assessment should be done on a yearly basis in skull base lesions. The onset of night pain, visHal loss, or hearing deterioration, or the presence of new neurological deficits sug-

gest disease progression. There may be a co-existing aneurysmal bone cyst, or rarely there may be a malignant transformation of the lesion. Such changes in the behavior of the lesions warrant urgent imaging with or without subsequent biopsy for confirmation [20, 21].

Lifestyle modification for optimum bone health is an essential component of CFD management. Appropriate calcium and Vit D3 supplements with cessation of alcohol and smoking should be promoted. Concurrent management of endocrinopathies and other extraskeletal manifestations should be done under the guidance of a multidisciplinary team involving physicians and surgeons of respective specialties. Incidentally diagnosed asymptomatic CFD with no extensive disease and extraskeletal problems does not require treatment with bisphosphonates. An important component of managing such a disease is to make the patient aware of the non-hereditary and benign nature of the disease. Thus, with regular follow-up and interval imaging, most cases of asymptomatic CFD can be managed conservatively.

References

1. McCune D. Osteitis fibrosa cystica: the case of a nine year old girl who also exhibits precocious puberty, multiple pigmentation of the skin and hyperthyroidism. Am J Child. 1936;52:743–4.
2. Weinstein LS, Shenker A, Gejman PV, Merino MJ, Friedman E, Spiegel AM. Activating mutations of the stimulatory G protein in the McCune–Albright syndrome. N Engl J Med. 1991;325:1688–95.
3. Landis CA, Masters SB, Spada A, Pace AM, Bourne HR, Vallar L. GTPase inhibiting mutations activate the α chain of Gs and stimulate adenylyl cyclase in human pituitary tumours. Nature. 1989;340:692–6.
4. Kelly M, Brillante B, Collins M. Pain in fibrous dysplasia of bone: age-related changes and the anatomical distribution of skeletal lesions. Osteoporos Int. 2008;19:57–63.
5. Boyce AM, Florenzano P, de Castro LF, Collins MT. Fibrous dysplasia/McCune-Albright syndrome. GeneReviews®[Internet]; 2019.
6. Javaid MK, Boyce A, Appelman-Dijkstra N, Ong J, Defabianis P, Offiah A, et al. Best practice management guidelines for fibrous dysplasia/McCune-Albright syndrome: a consensus statement from the FD/MAS international consortium. Orphanet J Rare Dis. 2019;14:139.

7. Freyschmidt J, Ostertag H, Jundt G. Fibröse dysplasie (FD). Knochentumoren Klin Radiol Pathol 3rd Ed Berl Heidelb Ger Springer 2010;762–801.
8. Becelli R, Perugini M, Cerulli G, Carboni A, Renzi G. Surgical treatment of fibrous dysplasia of the cranio-maxillo-facial area. Review of the literature and personal experience from 1984 to 1999. Minerva Stomatol. 2002(51):293–300.
9. Burke A, Collins MT, Boyce AM. Fibrous dysplasia of bone: craniofacial and dental implications. Oral Dis. 2017;23:697–708.
10. Chen Y-R, Noordhoff MS. Treatment of craniomaxillofacial fibrous dysplasia: how early and how extensive? Plast Reconstr Surg. 1990;86:835–42.
11. Ricalde P, Horswell BB. Craniofacial fibrous dysplasia of the fronto-orbital region: a case series and literature review. J Oral Maxillofac Surg. 2001;59:157–67.
12. Lee J, FitzGibbon E, Chen Y, Kim H, Lustig L, Akintoye SO, et al. Clinical guidelines for the management of craniofacial fibrous dysplasia. Springer; 2012. p. 1–19.
13. Leet AI, Collins MT. Current approach to fibrous dysplasia of bone and McCune–Albright syndrome. J Child Orthop. 2007;1:3–17.
14. Kuznetsov SA, Cherman N, Riminucci M, Collins MT, Robey PG, Bianco P. Age-dependent demise of GNAS-mutated skeletal stem cells and "normalization" of fibrous dysplasia of bone. J Bone Miner Res. 2008;23:1731–40.
15. Kinnunen A-R, Sironen R, Sipola P. Magnetic resonance imaging characteristics in patients with histopathologically proven fibrous dysplasia-a systematic review. Skelet Radiol. 2020;49:837–45.
16. Cappabianca S, Colella G, Russo A, Pezzullo M, Reginelli A, Iaselli F, et al. Maxillofacial fibrous dysplasia: personal experience with gadolinium enhanced magnetic resonance imaging. Radiol Med (Torino). 2008;113:1198–210.
17. Kushchayeva YS, Kushchayev SV, Glushko TY, Tella SH, Teytelboym OM, Collins MT, et al. Fibrous dysplasia for radiologists: beyond ground glass bone matrix. Insights Imaging. 2018;9:1035–56.
18. Amit M, Collins MT, FitzGibbon EJ, Butman JA, Fliss DM, Gil Z. Surgery versus watchful waiting in patients with craniofacial fibrous dysplasia: a meta-analysis. J Neurol Surg Part B Skull Base. 2012;73:A002.
19. Boyce AM, Brewer C, DeKlotz TR, Zalewski CK, King KA, Collins MT, et al. Association of hearing loss and otologic outcomes with fibrous dysplasia. JAMA Otolaryngol Neck Surg. 2018;144:102–7.
20. Attri G, Maurya VP, Srivastava AK, Behari S, Bhaisora KS, Sardhara J, et al. Calvarial lesions: a tertiary centre's experience over fifteen years. Neurol India. 2021;69(3):650–58. https://doi.org/10.4103/0028-3886.319236.
21. Singh AK, Srivastava AK, Sardhara J, Bhaisora KS, Das KK, Mehrotra A, et al. Skull base bony lesions: Management nuances; a retrospective analysis from a Tertiary Care Centre. Asian J Neurosurg. 2017;12(3):506–13. https://doi.org/10.4103/1793-5482.185068.

Incidental Lacunar and Cortical Infarcts

20

Harsh Deora and Dwarakanath Srinivas

20.1 Introduction

"Lacune" was first used as a term in 1838 by Dechambre to describe "softenings in subcortical regions of the brain" found on autopsy. While the etiology was unclear at that time the possible causes included encephalitis, a late phase of a small hemorrhage, or ischemic necrosis. "Marche a petits pas de Dejerine" was a clinical syndrome associated with multiple lacunes, characterized by sudden hemiplegia with good recovery, a characteristic gait with small steps, pseudobulbar palsy, and dementia and was first described by Marie in 1901. Later in the 1960s, after pathological examinations, Fischer generated the so-called lacunar hypothesis, which suggested that lacunes are due to a chronic vasculopathy related to systemic hypertension, cause a variety of defined clinical syndromes, and imply a generally good prognosis (Figs. 20.1, 20.2, 20.3).

Lacunar infarcts were thus defined as small (2–15 mm in diameter) noncortical infarcts caused by occlusion of a single penetrating branch of a large cerebral artery. These branches arise at acute angles from the large arteries of the circle of Willis, the stem of the middle cerebral artery (MCA), or the basilar artery. Although this definition implies that pathological confirmation is necessary, diag-nosis in vivo may be made in the setting of appropriate clinical syndromes and radiological tests. Silent lacunar infarcts are covert cerebral ischemic lesions that are detected on brain imaging of individuals presenting with non-specific or atypical neurological symptoms without the classical features of an acute stroke. Not all small deep infarcts are lacunar, and the diagnosis of lacunar infarction also requires the exclusion of other etiologies of ischemic stroke. Neuroimaging studies in the acute phase (<10 days from stroke onset) have used 20 mm (instead of 15 mm) as the upper size limit for lacunes since some volume reduction is expected over time and all the pathological studies were done on chronic strokes.

The introduction of modern radiology like computed tomography (CT) and magnetic resonance imaging (MRI) has led to a debate on the lacunar theory. While many detractors have pointed out the lack of embolic phenomenon in most of these cases, proponents point to the difference among the strokes caused by emboli and others. This has further been complicated by the description of white matter rarefactions termed as "Leukoaraiosis" as first described by Hachinski et al. [1]. Leukoaraiosis has been linked to age, hypertension, arteriosclerosis, cigarette smoking, and glucose intolerance which are the same factors considered responsible for Lacunar infarcts. Overtime these infarcts tend to grow due to either chronic apoptosis induced by ischemia or repeated embolic episodes.

H. Deora · D. Srinivas (✉)
Department of Neurosurgery, National Institute of
Mental Health and Neurosciences, Bangalore, India

"

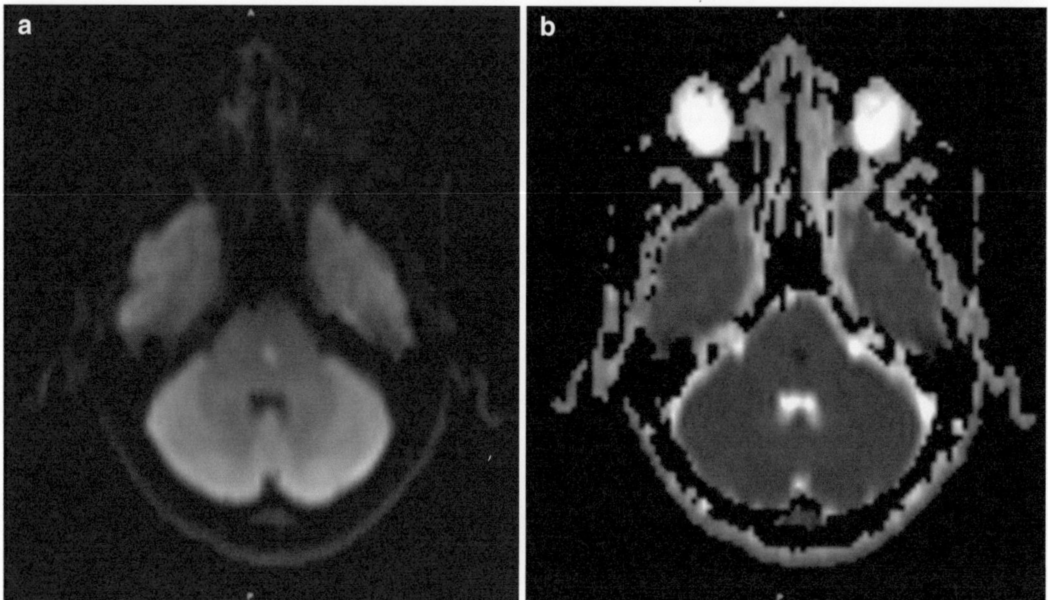

Fig. 20.1 (**a**, **b**) Axial section of diffusion-weighted (DWI) and apparent diffusion coefficient (ADC) on a magnetic resonance imaging (MRI) showing a silent/incidental acute lacunar infarct of the pons in a case of intracranial hypotension. Increased DWI signal in ischemic brain tissue is observed within a few minutes after arterial occlusion and progresses through a stereotypic sequence of ADC reduction, followed by a subsequent increase, pseudo-normalization, and, finally, permanent elevation

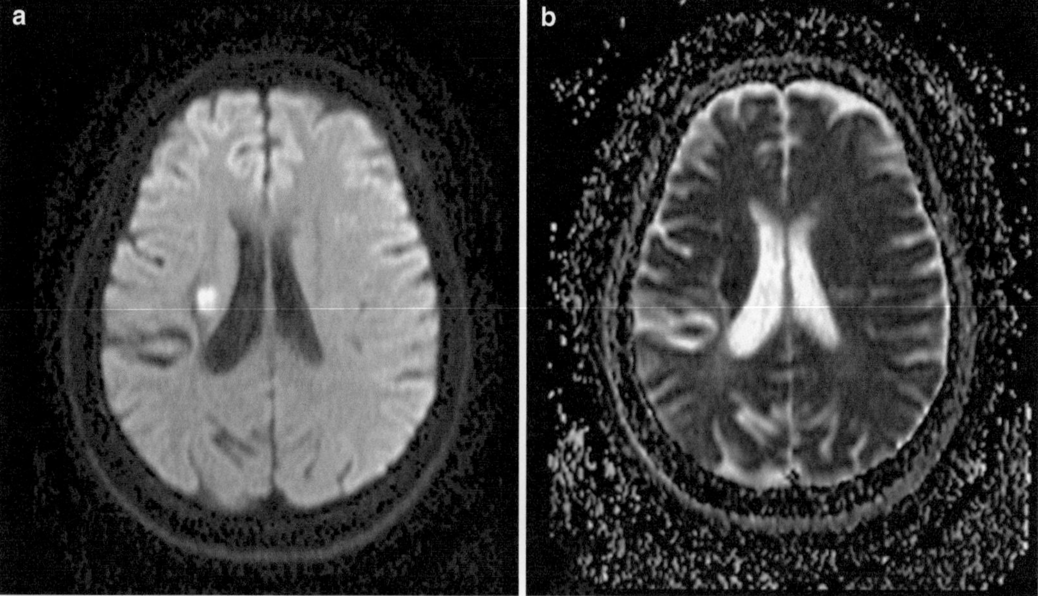

Fig. 20.2 (**a**, **b**) Axial section of diffusion-weighted and apparent diffusion coefficient sequences on a MRI showing a silent/incidental acute lacunar infarct of the corona radiata

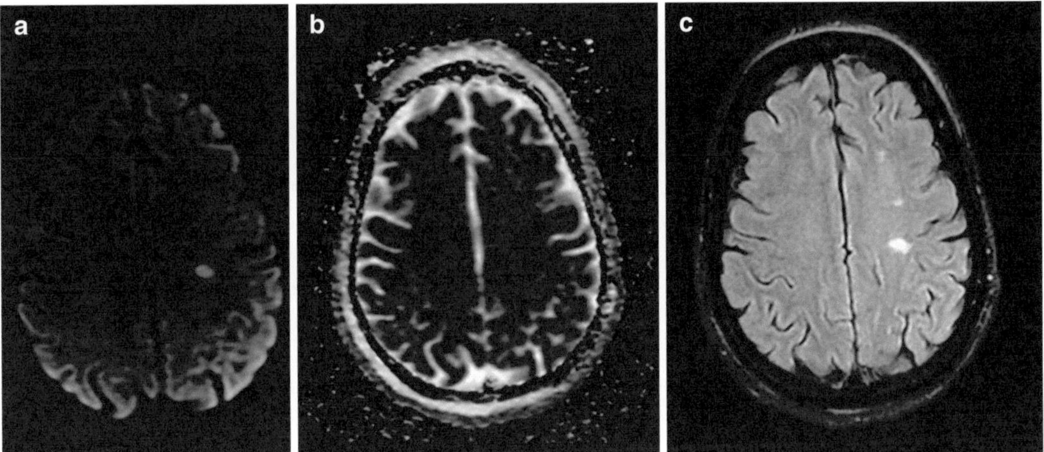

Fig. 20.3 (a–c) Axial section of diffusion-weighted and apparent diffusion coefficient and fluid-attenuated and inversion recovery (FLAIR) sequences on a MRI showing a silent/incidental acute lacunar infarct of the post central gyrus with additional old lacunar infarcts seen on FLAIR

Incidental infarcts have increased since the advent of diffusion-weighted imaging (DWI) which has a unique contrast property and a relatively short acquisition time. This imaging technique has been incorporated into many routine brain MRI protocols, including, among others, protocols for strokes, headaches, seizures, and tumors. Currently, around 10% of all silent infarcts are cortical in nature while the rest are lacunar [2–16].

20.1.1 Relevant Vascular Anatomy

Lacunar infarcts occur in the basal ganglia (putamen, globus pallidus, caudate), thalamus, subcortical white matter (internal capsule and corona radiata), and pons. These locations correspond to vascular territories of the lenticulostriate branches from the anterior and middle
cerebral arteries, the recurrent artery of Heubner from the anterior cerebral artery, the anterior choroidal artery from the distal internal carotid artery, thalamo-perforator branches from the posterior cerebral artery, and paramedian branches from the basilar artery. These small branches originate directly from large arteries, making them particularly vulnerable to the effects of hypertension, probably explaining this peculiar distribution.

20.2 Etiology of Silent Infarcts

One interesting observation from a systematic review of 19 cohort studies with 5864 cases was that cases with lacunar strokes have a higher risk of having a repeat lacunar stroke than a non-lacunar stroke recurrence. This gives credence to the theory that these types of strokes have a distinct pathophysiology.

20.2.1 Hypertension

Majority of the cases of lacunar infarcts are caused by hypertensive microangiopathy. Hypertension leads to arteriolar wall thickening and narrowing of the lumen of the small penetrating arteries due to arteriolosclerosis and related pathologies including lipohyalinosis, fibrinoid necrosis, and segmental arterial disorganization, sometimes accompanied by microaneurysm formation. Another observation that has strengthened the hypertensive microangiopathy theory is the reduction in the incidence and natural history of lacunar strokes with antihypertensive therapy.

20.2.2 Atherosclerosis

Microatheroma or branch atheromatous disease is also a major contributor of these strokes with the origin being from the middle cerebral artery or the vertebrobasilar artery. Serial sections of the basilar artery in lacunar stroke cases have proven the same.

20.2.3 Embolism

This hypothesis has been supported by cases of lacunar infarcts in cases of cardiac sources of emboli and in post angiography cases of cardiac and arch of aorta. Also the presence of simultaneous multiple infracts on DWI imaging in acute or sub-acute phase supports this hypothesis.

20.2.4 Blood–Brain Barrier Disruption

Arteriolar and capillary endothelial failure can lead to small vessel disease, lacunar stroke, and white matter lesions. Blood products extravasate in the perivascular area and can lead to edema and further damage to the vessel wall, neurons, and glia.

20.3 Epidemiology and Associations of Incidental Infarcts

Lacunar infarcts can account for 15–26 percent of ischemic stroke and in a hospital-based study over 4 years in which 16,2026 consecutive MRI images of asymptomatic individuals were viewed, the incidence of incidental infarcts was 0.37%. Interestingly, all of these cases had some vascular risk factors which are detailed below.

20.3.1 Hypertension and Diabetes

Hypertension and diabetes mellitus are associated with an increased risk of lacunar stroke. Lacunar stroke incidence rates are higher in Black Americans due to a higher incidence of risk factors such as diabetes and hypertension. The rates of hypertension and current smoking were found to be significantly increased in patients with lacunar infarcts compared with other stroke subtypes. Other studies have also found a difference in the incidence of risk factors between patients with lacunar stroke and those with other stroke subtypes. In the Stroke Data Bank, patients with lacunar stroke had fewer previous transient ischemic attacks (TIAs) and strokes than those with large vessel atherosclerotic infarction and, compared with patients who had cardioembolic strokes, those with lacunar infarcts more frequently had hypertension and diabetes.

20.3.2 Genetic Factors

The incidence of hereditary small vessel ischemic stroke is estimated to be 16–25 percent [3, 4]. A pooled analysis of individual patient data and genome-wide association studies reported 12 loci that were associated with lacunar stroke. Five of these loci were directly associated with lacunar stroke, and seven were associated jointly with lacunar stroke and white matter hyperintensities, including two loci (COL4A2 and HTRA1) that are linked to monogenic small vessel stroke [5].

- Cerebral autosomal dominant arteriopathy with subcortical infarcts and leukoencephalopathy (CADASIL). This is probably the most common monogenic cause of cerebral small vessel disease.
- Familial cerebral amyloid angiopathy (CAA) is an important cause of primary lobar intracerebral hemorrhage in older adults. It is characterized by the deposition of congophilic material in small- to medium-sized blood vessels of the brain and leptomeninges.
- Autosomal dominant retinal vasculopathy with cerebral leukoencephalopathy and systemic manifestations (RVCL-S), which is due to pathogenic variants in the TREX1 gene.

The major clinical manifestations are retinopathy, focal neurological symptoms including ischemic events, and cognitive impairment.

- Cerebral autosomal recessive arteriopathy with subcortical infarcts and leukoencephalopathy (CARASIL) due to HTRA1 pathogenic variants.
- Cathepsin A-related arteriopathy with strokes and leukoencephalopathy (CARASAL), an autosomal dominant, adult-onset disorder caused by a pathogenic variant in the CTSA gene.

20.4 Presentation

While most of lacunar infarcts are _silent or asymptomatic_, some do present with classical syndromes (Table 20.1).

While other strokes have the maximum symptoms at onset and evolve rapidly, lacunar stroke evolve over time and the symptoms typically worsen after hospital admission. Cases may present with multitude of symptoms (Table 20.2), and these should be kept in mind.

The lack of symptoms in most cases must be explained, especially in incidental cases. Lesion location and lesion size are undoubtedly the most important factors determining whether the patient becomes symptomatic. In previous studies, it has been pointed out that subcortical infarcts are not associated with obvious symptoms and are silent simply because they occur in clinically ineloquent regions of the brain. The right hemispheric preponderance may also support this hypothesis.

Table 20.2 Other presentations of lacunar stroke in symptomatic cases

Modified pure motor hemiparesis with motor aphasia
Pure motor hemiparesis sparing face
Mesencephalo-thalamic syndrome
Thalamic dementia
Pure motor hemiparesis with horizontal gaze palsy
Pure motor hemiparesis with crossed third-nerve palsy (Weber syndrome)
Pure motor hemiparesis with crossed sixth-nerve palsy
Pure motor hemiparesis with confusion
Cerebellar ataxia with crossed third-nerve palsy (Claude syndrome)
Hemiballismus
Lower basilar branch syndrome—dizziness, diplopia, gaze palsy, dysarthria, cerebellar ataxia, trigeminal numbness
Lateral medullary syndrome
Lateral pontomedullary syndrome
Locked-in syndrome (bilateral pure motor hemiparesis)
Pure dysarthria
Acute dystonia of thalamic origin
Lacunar state

Table 20.1 Classic lacunar stroke presentations in symptomatic cases

Lacunar syndrome	Location	Clinical findings	Positive predictive value
Pure motor hemiparesis (45–57%)	Internal capsule, corona radiata, basal pons, medial medulla	Unilateral paralysis of face, arm, and leg, no sensory signs, dysarthria, and dysphagia may be present	52–85%
Pure sensory syndrome (7–18%)	Thalamus, pontine tegmentum, corona radiata	Unilateral numbness of face, arm, and leg without motor deficit	95–100%
Ataxic hemiparesis (3–18%)	Internal capsule-corona radiata, basal pons, thalamus	Unilateral weakness and limb ataxia	59–95%
Sensorimotor syndrome (15–20%)	Thalamocapsular, maybe basal pons or lateral medulla	Hemiparesis or hemiplegia of face, arm, and leg with ipsilateral sensory impairment	51–87%
Dysarthria-clumsy hand syndrome (2–6%)	Basal pons, internal capsule, corona radiata	Unilateral facial weakness, dysarthria, and dysphagia, with mild hand weakness and clumsiness	About 96%

20.5 Evaluation of Lacunar Infarcts

20.5.1 Computed Tomography

Non-contrast CT is the initial imaging modality for most patients presenting with an acute stroke. CT has, however, low sensitivity for detecting small acute infarcts such as lacunes (30–44%). This goes even lower when we consider the sensitivity of CT for lacunes in the hyperacute phase (<6 h). Hence most lacunar infarcts seen on CT are frequently chronic and incidental. CT also is limited in identifying posterior fossa infarcts and in defining the degree of cortical extension in subcortical infarcts.

20.5.2 Magnetic Resonance Imaging

Standard brain MRI protocols that include conventional T1-weighted, T2-weighted, fluid-attenuated inversion recovery (FLAIR), and T2*-weighted gradient-recalled echo (GRE) sequences along with DWI can reliably diagnose both acute ischemic stroke and acute hemorrhagic stroke in emergency settings. Incidental or symptomatic lacunar infarcts are visualized as focal lesions characterized by decreased T1-weighted and increased T2-weighted signal intensity. Conventional MRI has a higher sensitivity and specificity than CT.

20.5.3 Diffusion-Weighted Imaging

DWI is a fast MRI technique that demonstrates a hyperintense signal whenever there is an area of restricted water diffusion, as occurs during acute ischemia. DWI has the advantages of higher sensitivity for acute lesions than T2-weighted MRI or FLAIR. It can differentiate between acute and chronic lacunar infarcts and identify multiple acute infarcts potentially linked to embolic sources or even incidental ones. However, symptoms association is important as DWI may overestimate acute/clinically relevant infarcts by 25% especially when multiple subcortical infarcts of various ages are present. The size of acute lacunar infarction is overestimated on DWI by approximately 40 percent when compared with final infarct size at 30 days or more after stroke onset on conventional MRI (T2 or FLAIR sequences) and CT.

20.5.4 Other Studies

Genetic screening for pathogenic variants in NOTCH3 is appropriate if there is suspicion for CADASIL, as suggested by a family history of stroke and dementia, absence of hypertension, or known vascular risk factors.

20.6 Differential Diagnosis of Incidental Infarcts

Since most of lesions are incidentally diagnosed on imaging especially magnetic resonance imaging and are seen in the white matter, they are also called white matter lesions/hyperintensities/changes. Less commonly they are also referred to as unidentified bright objects, a term which is now used to refer to focal areas of high signal intensity seen in children with neurofibromatosis 1. Nonetheless, a broad differential for incidental infarcts include the following:

1. Arteriolosclerosis or age-related and vascular risk factor-related small vessel disease: e.g., Binswanger disease
2. Cerebral amyloid angiopathy (sporadic or hereditary)
3. Inherited/genetic small vessel diseases other than cerebral amyloid angiopathy, such as
    (a) CADASIL
    (b) CARASIL
    (c) MELAS
    (d) Fabry disease
    (e) Retinal vasculopathy with cerebral leukoencephalopathy
    (f) COL4A1 brain small vessel disease
4. Inflammatory and immunologically mediated small vessel diseases (CNS vasculitis)
5. Venous collagenosis

6. Other small vessel diseases, such as
   (a) Post-radiation angiopathy
   (b) Non-amyloid microvessel degeneration in Alzheimer's disease

20.7 Management

20.7.1 Incidental/Silent Lacunar Strokes

Incidental presence of these lesions and the association with vascular risk factors [2] begets prevention of further such lesions (secondary prevention). Risk factor management, including blood pressure control, antiplatelet and statin therapy, and lifestyle modification is the cornerstone of management. The risk/benefit of antiplatelet therapy has not been adequately studied for patients with incidental lacunar infarcts. After the acute phase of stroke (when permissive hypertension is often employed), antihypertensive therapy should be resumed in previously treated, neurologically stable patients with known hypertension for prevention of recurrent stroke and other vascular events. In addition, antihypertensive therapy should be started in previously untreated or incidental cases who have an established blood pressure that is above goal. Once the acute phase of TIA and ischemic stroke (i.e., >21 days) is over, and in the absence of an indication for oral anticoagulation, long-term single-agent antiplatelet therapy for secondary stroke prevention should be continued with aspirin, clopidogrel, or aspirin-extended-release dipyridamole. Long-term dual antiplatelet therapy with aspirin and clopidogrel is not recommended. Patients with ischemic stroke, all of whom are at high risk for recurrent cerebrovascular and cardiovascular events, should receive high-intensity statin therapy. Lifestyle modifications to reduce the risk of stroke include smoking cessation, limited alcohol consumption, weight control, regular aerobic physical activity, salt restriction, and a Mediterranean diet.

The efficacy of aspirin and other antiplatelet agents for preventing second strokes and mortality has been illustrated for patients with non-cardioembolic ischemic stroke in general. A 2015 meta-analysis identified two trials that evaluated antiplatelets versus placebo and reported outcomes in the subgroup of patients with lacunar stroke; in the pooled analysis, treatment with any single antiplatelet agent was associated with a significant reduction in ischemic stroke recurrence (relative risk 0.48, 95% CI 0.30–0.78) [6]. Despite early enthusiasm, results from the SPS3 trial suggest that the long-term use of combined antiplatelet therapy with aspirin plus clopidogrel is harmful to patients with lacunar stroke because it leads to an increased risk of hemorrhage and death but does not reduce the risk of recurrent stroke [7]. Therefore, it should not be employed for secondary prevention in this population in the absence of proven indications [8–14].

20.7.2 Acute Management of Symptomatic Stroke

Reperfusion therapy for any stroke has well-established guidelines (Table 20.3) [15]. In short, intravenous alteplase improves functional outcome in ischemic stroke within 4.5 h of onset or in select cases outside the window which show a perfusion-diffusion mismatch. However, this may not apply to most cases of lacunar stroke cases. Aspirin alone or in combination should be given within 24 h of any acute stroke.

20.7.3 Prognosis of Silent/Incidental Infarcts

Most incidental strokes remain asymptomatic and whether the same can lead to further strokes remains to established. In cases who are symptomatic, lacunar strokes have a better outcome than other strokes. Only cases with worse motor symptoms at onset have a poorer outcome. Secondary prevention has been shown to be effective and should be the primary goal in incidental cases.

Table 20.3 Eligibility criteria for reperfusion in acute symptomatic stroke (adapted from AHA 2018 guidelines) [15]

Inclusion criteria
Clinical diagnosis of ischemic stroke causing measurable neurologic deficit
Onset of symptoms <4.5 h before beginning treatment; if the exact time of stroke onset is not known, it is defined as the last time the patient was known to be normal or at neurologic baseline
Age ≥18 years
Exclusion criteria
Patient history
Ischemic stroke or severe head trauma in the previous 3 months
Previous intracranial hemorrhage
Intra-axial intracranial neoplasm
Gastrointestinal malignancy
Gastrointestinal hemorrhage in the previous 21 days
Intracranial or intraspinal surgery within the prior 3 months
Clinical
Symptoms suggestive of subarachnoid hemorrhage
Persistent blood pressure elevation (systolic ≥185 mmHg or diastolic ≥110 mmHg)
Active internal bleeding
Presentation consistent with infective endocarditis
Stroke known or suspected to be associated with aortic arch dissection
Acute bleeding diathesis, including but not limited to conditions defined under "hematologic"
Hematologic
Platelet count <100,000/mm^3
Current anticoagulant use with an INR >1.7 or PT >15 s or aPTT>40 s
Therapeutic doses of low molecular weight heparin received within 24 h (e.g., to treat VTE and ACS); this exclusion does not apply to prophylactic doses (e.g., to prevent VTE)
Current use (i.e., last dose within 48 h in a patient with normal renal function) of a direct thrombin inhibitor or direct factor Xa inhibitor with evidence of anticoagulant effect by laboratory tests such as aPTT, INR, ECT, TT, or appropriate factor Xa activity assays
Head CT
Evidence of hemorrhage
Extensive regions of obvious hypodensity consistent with irreversible injury
Warnings
Only minor and isolated neurologic signs or rapidly improving symptoms
Serum glucose <50 mg/dL (<2.8 mmol/L)◊
Serious trauma in the previous 14 days§
Major surgery in the previous 14 days¥
History of gastrointestinal bleeding (remote) or genitourinary bleeding‡
Seizure at the onset of stroke with postictal neurologic impairments†
Pregnancy
Arterial puncture at a noncompressible site in the previous 7 days
Large (≥10 mm), untreated, unruptured intracranial aneurysm
Untreated intracranial vascular malformation
Additional warnings for treatment from 3 to 4.5 h from symptom onset
Age >80 years
Oral anticoagulant use regardless of INR
Severe stroke (NIHSS score >25)
Combination of both previous ischemic stroke and diabetes mellitus

20.7.4 Long-Term Outcomes After Silent Infarcts

In a study done primarily on the Asian population, among all silent lacunar and cortical infarct cases, about 4 in 10 had a recurrent stroke and about 1 in 10 died by 5 years consistent with event rates for symptomatic infarcts [16]. While the risks of a recurrent stroke at 5 years did not differ by age, sex, and area, the all-cause mortality rates were higher in men, in rural areas, and in those aged over 65 years. The 5-year risks of all-cause mortality for silent infarcts in this study were comparable with those in cases with a hospital diagnosis of TIA or minor stroke (10.6% risk of all-cause mortality) in Western countries. Overall, most studies place the risk of recurrent stroke around 4.6% per year.

Long-term functional decline like dementia has received much less attention than survivorship or recurrent stroke. Crude measures such as the ability to activities of daily living have been recently replaced by the International classification of functioning as adopted by the WHO. Lacunar strokes, however, tend to have a better functional outcome as compared to other cortical strokes. Cognitive decline is another major long-term result of these infarcts which may only be subjective, e.g., reduced speed of mental processing. Dementia rates vary from 11% a 2–3 years to 15% at 9 years in various studies.

Progression of asymptomatic lesions is another area of concern which has not been studied adequately. Studies concluded that new silent infarcts develop at twice the rate of symptomatic ones and at an average of 3 years since the index infarcts 50% of all cases of silent infarcts will have progression of leukoaraiosis [17].

20.7.5 Conclusion

Lacunar infarcts are small (0.2–15 mm in diameter) noncortical infarcts caused by occlusion of a single penetrating branch of a large cerebral artery. These branches arise at acute angles from the large arteries of the circle of Willis, the stem of the middle cerebral artery, and the basilar artery. Most lacunes occur in the basal ganglia (putamen, globus pallidus, caudate), thalamus, subcortical white matter (internal capsule and corona radiata), and pons. They account for 15–26% of ischemic strokes and are associated with systemic hypertension. Other likely risk factors include diabetes mellitus and possibly smoking. As a general rule, lacunar syndromes lack findings such as aphasia, agnosia, neglect, apraxia, or hemianopsia. Monoplegia, stupor, coma, loss of consciousness, and seizures also are typically absent. Radiologic diagnosis of lacunar infarction relies upon finding a small noncortical infarct on computed tomography or magnetic resonance imaging whose location is consistent with the clinical lacunar syndrome defined by history and examination. Secondary prevention, most patients with ischemic stroke or TIA should be treated with risk factor management, including blood pressure control, antiplatelet and statin therapy, and lifestyle modification. Lacunar strokes have a better prognosis than cortical ones, and their incidental presence may be associated with vascular risk factors which beget prevention of symptomatic strokes.

References

1. Hachinski VC, Potter P, Merskey H. Leukoaraiosis. Arch Neurol. 1987;44:21–3.
2. Yamada K, Nagakane Y, Sasajima H, Nakagawa M, Mineura K, Masunami T, Akazawa K, Nishimura T. Incidental acute infarcts identified on diffusion-weighted images: a university hospital-based study. AJNR Am J Neuroradiol. 2008;29(5):937–40. https://doi.org/10.3174/ajnr.A1028. Epub 2008 Mar 5.
3. Bevan S, Traylor M, Adib-Samii P, et al. Genetic heritability of ischemic stroke and the contribution of previously reported candidate gene and genome wide associations. Stroke. 2012;43:3161.
4. Traylor M, Bevan S, Baron JC, et al. Genetic architecture of lacunar stroke. Stroke. 2015;46:2407.
5. Traylor M, Persyn E, Tomppo L, et al. Genetic basis of lacunar stroke: a pooled analysis of individual patient data and genome-wide association studies. Lancet Neurol. 2021;20:351.
6. Kwok CS, Shoamanesh A, Copley HC, et al. Efficacy of antiplatelet therapy in secondary prevention following lacunar stroke: pooled analysis of randomized trials. Stroke. 2015;46:1014.

7. SPS3 Investigators, Benavente OR, Hart RG, et al. Effects of clopidogrel added to aspirin in patients with recent lacunar stroke. N Engl J Med. 2012;367:817.

8. Low molecular weight heparinoid, ORG 10172 (danaparoid), and outcome after acute ischemic stroke: a randomized controlled trial. The publications Committee for the Trial of ORG 10172 in acute stroke treatment (TOAST) investigators. JAMA. 1998;279:1265.

9. Ganesh A, Gutnikov SA, Rothwell PM, Oxford Vascular Study. Late functional improvement after lacunar stroke: a population-based study. J Neurol Neurosurg Psychiatry. 2018;89:1301.

10. Hart RG, Pearce LA, Bakheet MF, et al. Predictors of stroke recurrence in patients with recent lacunar stroke and response to interventions according to risk status: secondary prevention of small subcortical strokes trial. J Stroke Cerebrovasc Dis. 2014; 23:618.

11. Shoamanesh A, Pearce LA, Bazan C, et al. Microbleeds in the secondary prevention of small subcortical strokes trial: stroke, mortality, and treatment interactions. Ann Neurol. 2017;82:196.

12. Samuelsson M, Söderfeldt B, Olsson GB. Functional outcome in patients with lacunar infarction. Stroke. 1996;27:842.

13. Deora H, Rao KVLN, Somanna S, Srinivas D, Shukla DP, Bhat DI. Surgically managed pediatric intracranial aneurysms: how different are they from adult intracranial aneurysms? Pediatr Neurosurg. 2017;52(5): 313–7. https://doi.org/10.1159/000477815. Epub 2017 Aug 29.

14. Kumar K, Das KK, Singh S, Khatri D, Deora H, Singh J, Bhaisora K, Srivastava AK, Jaiswal AK, Behari S. Vascular offenders in trigeminal neuralgia: a unified classification and assessment of the outcome of microvascular decompression. World Neurosurg. 2019;127:e366–75. https://doi.org/10.1016/j. wneu.2019.03.128. Epub 2019 Mar 21.

15. Powers WJ, Rabinstein AA, Ackerson T, Adeoye OM, Bambakidis NC, Becker K, Biller J, Brown M, Demaerschalk BM, Hoh B, Jauch EC, Kidwell CS, Leslie-Mazwi TM, Ovbiagele B, Scott PA, Sheth KN, Southerland AM, Summers DV, Tirschwell DL. Guidelines for the early management of patients with acute ischemic stroke: 2019 Update to the 2018 guidelines for the early Management of Acute Ischemic Stroke: a guideline for healthcare professionals from the American Heart Association/American Stroke Association. Stroke. 2019;50(12):e344–418. https://doi.org/10.1161/STR.0000000000000211. Epub 2019 Oct 30. Erratum in: stroke. 2019 Dec;50(12):e440–e441.

16. Hao Z, Chen Y, Wright N, Qin H, Turnbull I, Guo Y, Kartsonaki C, Sansome S, PeiPei YC, Gu Q, Hu J, Lv J, Li L, Liu M, Wang Y, Clarke R, Chen Z. Natural history of silent lacunar infarction: 10-year follow-up of a community-based prospective study of 0.5 million Chinese adults. Lancet Reg Health West Pac. 2021;17:100309. https://doi.org/10.1016/j. lanwpc.2021.100309.

17. Norrving B. Long-term prognosis after lacunar infarction. Lancet Neurol. 2003;2(4):238–45. https://doi. org/10.1016/s1474-4422(03)00352-1.

Incidental Findings in Intracranial Lipoma

21

Fuyou Guo

21.1 Introduction

Intracranial lipomas are rare congenital malformations, accounting for less than 1% of all intracranial lesions [1]. They are benign lesions, which are usually found by physical examination or other diseases progress asymptomatically, however, epilepsy, headache, behavioral disorders, and cranial nerve paralysis may be observed. The prevailing proportion of cases tend to be involved in the midline location such as the area around the corpus callosum and quadrigeminal cisterns, and majority of patients demonstrated no symptom [2]. The onset of these symptoms is generally believed to be due to the neurodevelopmental abnormalities that often accompany them. Intracranial lipomas are easy to diagnose and usually have typical computerized cranial tomography (CT) and magnetic resonance imaging (MRI) findings.

Surgical treatment may result in high morbidity and mortality due to the highly vascular nature of intracranial lipomas' and their severe adhesion with surrounding tissue [3].Surgical intervention of intracranial lipomas is not usually considered necessary in the most of patients unless which caused obstructive hydrocephalus or requiring management of coexisting conditions.

21.2 Representative Imagings of Intracranial Lipomas

According to report by Truwit and Barcovich [4] in 44 intracranial lipomas, interhemispheric lipomas were the most common, which accounting for 45% of all cases. The remainder of the lesions were clustered in the quadrigeminal/superior cerebellar (25%), suprasellar/interpeduncular (14%), cerebellopontine angle (9%), and Sylvian (5%) cisterns. The detailed distributions of intracranial lipomas were analyzed in Table 21.1 based on Türk O' description [5], which is the largest series of 163 cases with intracranial lipomas recently. In addition, 55% of the lesions were associated with brain malformations of varying degrees. The representative figures of diverse intracranial lipomas were demonstrated as following (all pictures were obtained from the first affiliated hospital of Zhengzhou University) (Figs. 21.1, 21.2, 21.3, 21.4, 21.5).

F. Guo (✉)
Department of Neurosurgery, First Affiliated Hospital of Zhengzhou University,
Zhengzhou, Henan Province, China

International Joint Laboratory of Nervous System Malformations, First Affiliated Hospital of Zhengzhou University,
Zhengzhou, Henan Province, China

Table 21.1 Anatomic distribution of intracranial lipomas

	N	%
Quadrigeminal cistern	36	22.09
Interhemispheric cistern	20	12.27
Corpus callosum and pericallosal region	19	11.66
Lateral ventricle	11	6.75
Supracerebellar cistern	10	6.13
Crista galli	10	6.13
Perimesencephalic cistern	7	4.29
Cerebellopontine angle	7	4.29
Cerebellar vermis and its neighbor	6	3.68
Ambient cistern	6	3.68
Hypothalamus-chiasmatic cistern-suprasellar cistern	5	3.07
Third ventricle	5	3.07
Interpeduncular cistern	4	2.45
Tectum-perirectal region	4	2.45
Silvian aqueduct	2	1.23
Pericerebellar cistern	2	1.23
Temporal lobe and convexity of the temporal lobe	2	1.23
Prepontine cistern	2	1.23
Cerebellomedullary cistern	1	0.61
Parietal lobe	1	0.61
Pineal region	1	0.61
Fourth ventricle	1	0.61
Silvian cistern	1	0.61
Total	163	

The content of this table was obtained from Türk O, et al. Ideggyogy Sz. 2019, 72:89–92.

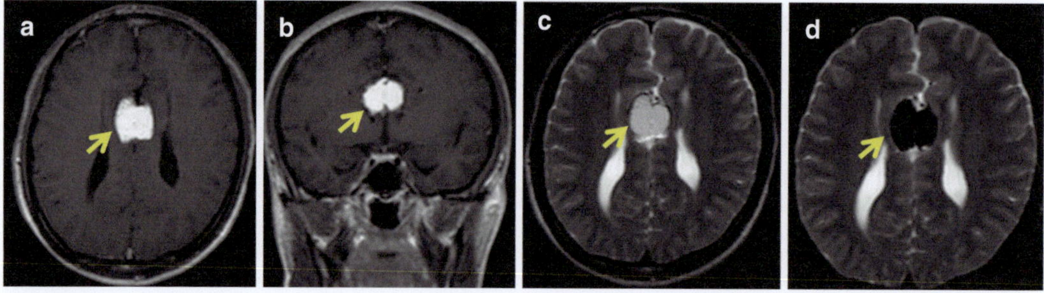

Fig. 21.1 (a–d) One male aged 36 years was admitted with accidental headache for 6 months. Axial and coronal magnetic resonance imaging (MRI) showing a hyperintense mass located deep in pericallosal area on T1-weighted image (a, b), axial T2-weighted image also showing high signal intensity involved in corpus callosum (c), MRI sequences on T2-weighted suppress signal from fat display fat-containing tissues and lesions. (d) Yellow arrow indicating the lesion

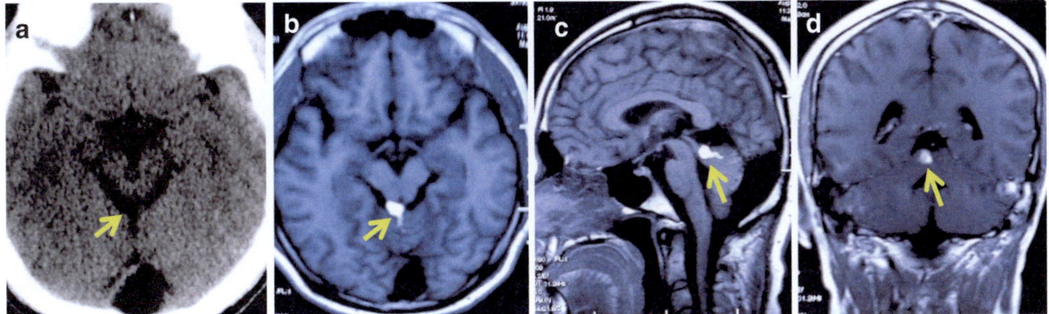

Fig. 21.2 (**a–d**) Male patient aged 34 years was admitted with dizziness for 3 days, computed tomography (CT) scan showing low density on right quadrigeminal cistern (**a**). Axial, sagittal, and coronal T1-weighted MRI showing high signal intensity located in right quadrigeminal cistern on MRI, respectively (**b–d**). Additionally, arachnoid cyst of cerebellomedullary cistern was observed in this case. Yellow arrow indicating the lesion

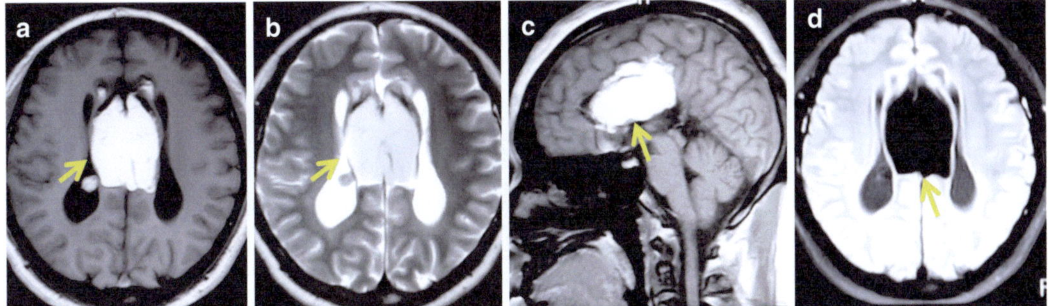

Fig. 21.3 (**a–d**) A 34-year-old male was admitted with one-month of fatigue and intermittent headache. Axial MRI showing a hyperintense mass located deep in corpus callosum area on T1-weighted and T2-weighted image, respectively (**a, b**), sagittal T1-weighted image also showing high signal intensity involved in corpus callosum area (**c**), MRI sequences suppress signal from fat display fat-containing tissues and lesions (**d**). Yellow arrow indicating the lesion. MRI also showed the absence of corpus callosum, bilateral ventricular triangle area, and bilateral cingulate gyrus. Yellow arrow indicating the lesion

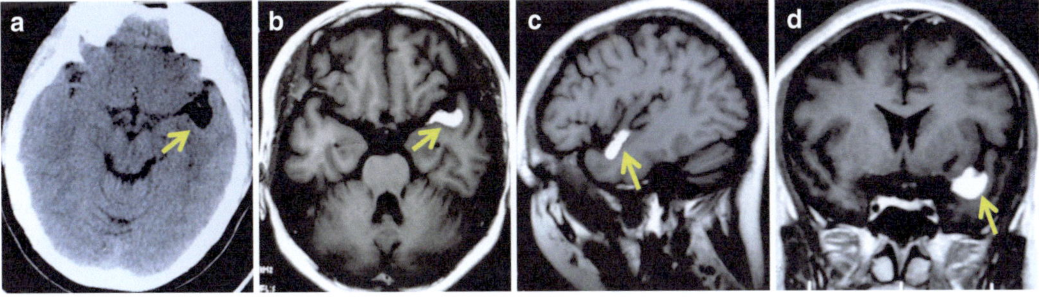

Fig. 21.4 (**a–d**) A 32-year-old female patient was admitted with intracranial lesion due to routine physical examination. No symptom was occurred in this patient. Axial noncontrast-enhanced CT scan revealing a low-density mass in the left sylvian fissure. Axial, sagittal, and coronal T1-weighted MRI showing high signal intensity located in left sylvian fissure on MRI, respectively (**b–d**). Yellow arrow indicating the lesion, due to no obvious symptoms, the patient was closely observed instead of surgical treatment

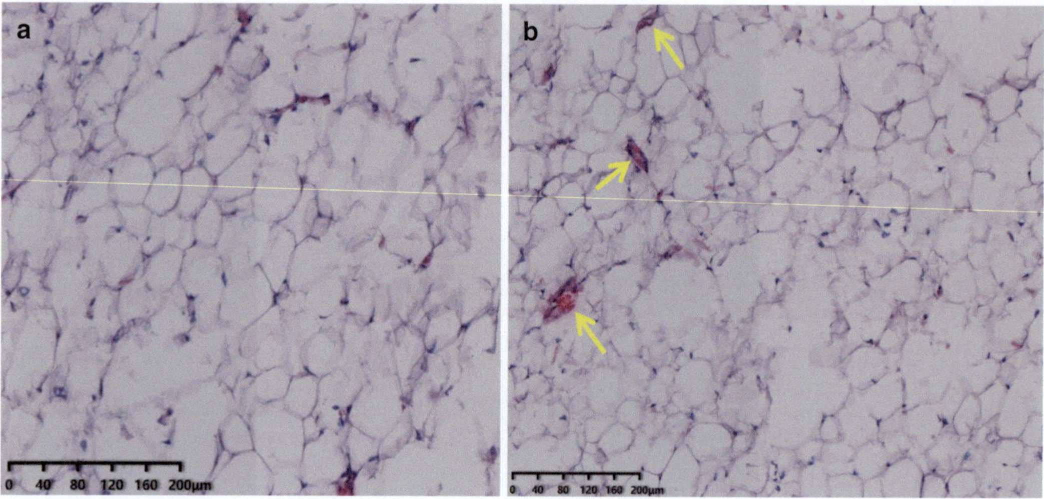

Fig. 21.5 (**a–b**) Hematoxylin and eosin staining revealed adipose tissue from the sample of resection (**a**, ×20). Adipose tissue scatter blood vessels were noted (**b**, ×10, yellow arrow indicate)

21.3 Epidemiology and Clinical Features

Intracranial lipomas are uncommon congenital lesions resulting from abnormal persistence and maldifferentiation of the meninx primitiva during the development of the subarachnoid cisterns [6]. Majority of intracranial lipomas are usually observed incidentally on brain imaging performed for another reason. *There are several striking features in clinical manifestation regarding intracranial lipomas:*

1. Most lipomas are located at or near the midline—typically in the pericallosal cistern and quadrigeminal/superior cerebellar [4].
2. More than half of all intracranial lipomas are associated with brain malformations. Agenesis or dysgenesis of the corpus callosum is the most frequently associated brain anomaly. Others include the absence of the septum pellucidum, cranium bifidum, spina bifida, encephalocele, myelomeningocele, hypoplasia of the vermis, and malformation of the cortex [3].
3. The clinical symptoms are non-specific and depend on their location, headache is the most common symptom of intracranial lipomas and up for 67.48% of all cases with intracranial lipomas, the initial symptoms at admission were found in Table 21.2 [5].
4. Primary symptoms are also including vertigo, mental retardation, dyskinesia, vomiting, dizziness, hearing impairment, and so on. Approximately 80% of cerebellopontine angle lipomas had dizziness, ataxia, and progressive hearing loss About 50% of lipomas in the corpus callosum area had headache, seizure, mental disorder, mental disorder, behavior change, and dementia, while about 50% of lipomas in the sylvian fissure had seizure and paresis. The incidence of focal symptoms in the quadruplex cistern and circumferential cistern was about 20%, and hydrocephalus could be seen in a few patients [7, 8].
5. Intracranial lipomas are often managed conservatively, and attempts for total resection are associated with high mortality.

Table 21.2 Initial symptoms of the patients with intracranial lipomas

	N	%
Headache	110	67.48
Vertigo	25	15.34
Incidental finding while head trauma diagnostics	9	5.52
Epilepsy	4	2.45
Syncope	4	2.45
Dementia	3	1.84
Facial paralysis	3	1.84
Speech impairment	3	1.84
Defect of vision	2	1.23
Ataxia	2	1.23
Incidental finding while tumor screening	2	1.23

The content of this table was obtained from Türk O, et al. Ideggyogy Sz. 2019, 72:89–92 [5].

21.4 Histology and Pathology

On histologic examination, intracranial lipomas, similar to mature fat cells elsewhere, may have anaplastic cartilaginous, bony and osseous components, but are rare in the cerebellopontine angle region. Large lipomas have a thickening fibrous capsule around the margin, the latter or its, and calcification of the adjacent cerebral parenchyma. Blood vessels and nerves run in the tumor body, do not invade the surrounding, meninges, and nerve structures, biological behavior is similar to malformation. Therefore, most authors now believe that intracranial lipoma is neither a teratoma nor a true tumor, but a congenital malformation with long-term abnormalities of the protomeninges, frequently present, poorly differentiated, and poorly formed. Specimen following postoperation showed a yellow and tan tissue mass that was soft and pliable but fibrous and not easily fragmented. Hematoxylin and eosin staining revealed adipose tissue surrounded by a fibrous capsule. Blood vessels and a focal aggregate of melanocytes on microscopic examination were also observed [9].

There are various theories as to the mechanism of the disease, and the main ones are the following: (1) the presence of ectopic fat in the embryo; (2) deposition of fat metabolites; (3) pial adipocyte hyperplasia; (4) allosteric fat cells; (5) fatty interchanges in connective tissue or soft, meningeal tissue; (6) the fat of the neural embryo is stunted; (7) fat degeneration of the gelatinous tissue. Primary meningeal hypoplasia during the development of subarachnoid cisterns is actually the most accredited theory [4, 10].

21.5 Imaging Characteristics and Differential Diagnosis

The clinical diagnosis of intracranial lipoma mainly depends on imaging. At present, CT and MRI are the two most commonly used imaging methods in clinic. Intracranial lipomas generally have specific imaging findings. On CT, lipomas demarcate areas of marked hypodensity that do not show enhancement after administration of intravenous contrast. They usually have a CT density of between -50 UH and -100 UH. Calcification is often present in interhemispheric lipomas—usually within the fibrous capsule surrounding the lesion. MRI shows a homogeneous, hyperintense mass on T1-weighted images which is hypointense with fat suppression, hyperintense on T2-weighted images. In addition, lipomas may be confused with subacute hemorrhage due to imaging similarities. Fat-saturation can help refine this diagnosis, since subacute hemorrhage is not suppressed by fat-saturation [11].

Lipoma is easy to be diagnosed preoperatively and postoperatively because of its typical imaging and pathological features. Clinically, lipomas can be distinguished from teratomas, craniopharyngiomas, dermoid cysts, and epidermoid cyst [10]. Dermoid cyst and teratoma were located in the posterior third ventricle and the inferior frontal lobe. The density and MRI signal intensity were not uniform. The epidermoid cyst was frequently located in the cerebellopontine angle, the parahypophyseal area or the fourth ventricle, and the CT value was lower than that of cerebrospinal fluid (CSF). Bursa of craniopharyngioma is sometimes fat-dense, but its location is mostly in the saddle [12–14].

21.6 Surgical Therapy for Intracranial Lipoma

The essential principles toward intracranial lipomas should be conservatively management. Biopsy may be considered when the diagnosis is in doubt. When surgery is considered to be absolutely necessary, it should be limited to partial removal. Because the risks of surgical intervention far outweigh the potential benefits, aggressively total removal of intracranial lipoma is technically hazardous because of the dense adhesion of lipoma to surrounding structures and almost invariably result in severe neural injury. In addition, surgical resection should be considered in epileptic patients who fail to respond to the medical treatment. The epileptic seizures which have been reported in about 50% of patients are not likely to be relieved by surgery [15].

Surgical therapy for intracranial lipoma is indicated in two following situations: (1) The lesion progressively increased in size with resulting compression of surrounding structures and develop new neurological deficits; (2) symptoms of increased intracranial pressure caused by obstructive hydrocephalus located in the midline lipoma. However, in view of the high incidence of postoperative cranial nerve deficits after surgery for intracranial lipoma. It is wise to adopt the partial microsurgical decompression if the lesion is highly suspective of intracranial lipomas. Of course, patients subjected to obstructive hydrocephalus can be treated by CSF diversion procedure rather than resection.

For the treatment of intracranial lipoma, it is generally believed that radical surgical treatment should not be advocated for two main reasons. First, intracranial lipomas usually attach to the surrounding dense blood vessels or nerve tissue, especially the cranial nerves, making surgery difficult and extremely dangerous. Secondly, intracranial lipoma is a benign congenital malformation with slow growth. Based on the report of Yilmaz MB [16], the mean follow-up period was 17.2 months (range 3–36 months) for 12 cases with intracranial lipomas and no patient showed progression.

The space occupying effect of intracranial lipoma is weak and not easy to break. Therefore, the first choice for the accidental discovery of asymptomatic lipoma may be closely follow-up without surgical intervention. The non-specific symptoms and signs presented by the patient may not be caused by the lipoma itself, but may be attributable to concurrent malformations such as callosum hypoplasia or multiple sclerosis [17]. If the symptom is obvious caused by obstructive hydrocephalus secondary to lipoma, ventriculoperitoneal shunt operation should be performed as soon as possible.

The primary objective of the remove operation should be to meticulously relieve the pressure on the adjacent tissue, rather than to seek total resection of the lipoma. Up to now, surgery for symptomatic intracranial lipoma was frequently described as exceedingly rare case in previous literatures. There are no consensus or guideline to safe resection for intracranial lipoma. Uysal et al. [18] reported one surgical rare lipoma involved in the internal auditory canal, intraoperative neuromonitoring was used with brainstem auditory evoked response (BAERs), facial nerve monitoring, motor evoked and somatosensory evoked potentials were also adopted in this patient. However, BAERs were lost because of the highly adhesive nature of the lesion postoperatively, the patient suffered from hearing-lost on the left side, moreover, the right and left facial nerves were noted to have a House-Brackmann Grade 1 and Grade 2 facial palsy, respectively.

21.7 Postoperative Complications

The most common complications following intracranial lipoma resection are related to occurrence of neurological injury. Among 21 patients who underwent surgery reviewed by Tahmouresie et al. [19] only five (23.8%) showed postoperative improvement. There were 10 (47.6%) deaths and one (4.8%) patient developed a severe neurological deficit after operation. Zimmermann et al. [20] reported that microsurgical resection was performed in one rare intracranial lipomas located in the cerebellopontine angle. Postoperatively this patient developed a left glossopharyngeal and hypoglossal nerve paresis. Furthermore she had a mild left-sided hemiparesis from which she recovered within 3 weeks after surgery. Hearing did not improve following operation. Similar complication was occurred in previous literature [18].

One convincing evidence demonstrates that there is an obvious decreasing tendency for lipoma surgery, because only 19% reported improved neurological symptomatology was achieved following operation, while 68% endorsed new or worsened neurological symptoms based on the report of Bigelow et al. [21]. In one large series of 80 lipoma patients involved in cerebellopontine angle and internal auditory canal treated with surgery, new onset of neurological symptoms (including sensorineural hearing loss, headache, facial nerve weakness, facial numbness, or other neurologic sequelae attributable to surgery and/or lipoma) occurred in 28% of surgical patients and in 2% of patients who were observed group. Specifically, hearing loss and facial nerve weakness occurred in 15 (19%) and 13 (16%) of surgical patients. Consequently, surgery for lipoma may be performed less often from the year 2000 (25%) as compared to before 2000 (54%) [22].

21.8 Conclusion

Intracranial lipomas are extremely rare fat-containing lesion which constitute 0.1–0.5% of all intracranial tumors. CT and MRI play a vital role for a differential diagnosis. Moreover, diagnosis accidentally occurs during diagnostic procedures in case of an encephalic disorder. Intracranial lipoma is often accompanied by other cerebral malformations, most commonly corpus callosum anomalies. Headache is the most common symptom of intracranial lipomas and up for 67.48% of all cases. Surgical management is not recommended in the majority of patients, however, surgical therapy for intracranial lipoma is indicated in two following situations: If the lesion progressively increased in size with resulting compression of surrounding structures and develop new neurological deficits; on the other hand, obstructive hydrocephalus caused by the midline lipoma should be treated by surgery immediately. Severe postoperative complications are also kept in mind so as to avoid any aggressive surgical resection.

References

1. Taydas O, Ogul H, Kantarci M. The clinical and radiological features of cisternal and pericallosal lipomas. Acta Neurol Belg. 2020;120(1):65–70.
2. Eghwrudjakpor PO, Kurisaka M, Fukuoka M, Mori K. Intracranial lipomas. Acta Neurochir. 1991;110(3–4):124–8.
3. Yilmaz N, Unal O, Kiymaz N, Yilmaz C, Etlik O. Intracranial lipomas-a clinical study. Clin Neurol Neurosurg. 2006;108(4):363–8.
4. Truwit CL, Barkovich AJ. Pathogenesis of intracranial lipoma: an MR study in 42 patients. AJR Am J Roentgenol. 1990;155(4):855–64.
5. Türk O, Yaldiz C. Incidental intracranial lipomas: assessment of 163 patients. Ideggyogy Sz. 2019;72(3–4):89–92.
6. Chaubey V, Kulkarni G, Chhabra L. Ruptured intracranial lipoma-a fatty outburst in the brain. Perm J. 2015;19(2):e103–4.
7. Kieslich M, Ehlers S, Bollinger M, Jacobi G. Midline developmental anomalies with lipomas in the corpus callosum region. J Child Neurol. 2000;15(2):85–9.
8. Sasaki H, Yoshida K, Wakamoto H, Otani M, Toya S. Lipomas of the frontal lobe. Clin Neurol Neurosurg. 1996;98:27–31.
9. Feldman RP, Marcovici A, Lasala PA. Intracranial lipoma of the sylvian fissure. Case report and review of the literature. J Neurosurg. 2001;94(3):515–9.
10. Romano N, Castaldi A. Imaging of intracranial fat: from normal findings to pathology. Radiol Med. 2021;126(7):971–8.

11. Jabot G, Stoquart-Elsankari S, Saliou G, Toussaint P, Deramond H, Lehmann P. Intracranial lipomas: clinical appearances on neuroimaging and clinical significance. J Neurol. 2009;256(6):851–5.

12. Hughes DS, Osborn RE. Corpus callosal lipoma: report of 2 cases and review of the literature. J Am Osteopath Assoc. 1986 Sep;86(9):564–7.

13. Uchino A, Hasuo K, Matsumoto S, Masuda K. MRI of dorsal mesencephalic lipomas. Clin Imaging. 1993;17(1):12–6.

14. Zee CS, McComb JG, Segall HD, Tsai FY, Stanley P. Lipomas of the corpus callosum associated with frontal dysraphism. J Comput Assist Tomogr. 1981;5(2):201–5.

15. Eghwrudjakpor PO, Kurisaka M, Fukuoka M, Mori K. Intracranial lipomas: current perspectives in their diagnosis and treatment. Br J Neurosurg. 1992;6(2):139–44.

16. Yilmaz MB, Egemen E, Tekiner A. Lipoma of the quadrigeminal cistern: report of 12 cases with clinical and radiological features. Turk Neurosurg. 2015;25(1):16–20.

17. Yilmaz MB, Genc A, Egemen E, Yilmaz S, Tekiner A. Pericallosal lipomas: a series of 10 cases with clinical and radiological features. Turk Neurosurg. 2016;26(3):364–8.

18. Uysal E, Reese J, Cohen M, Curtis D, Shelton C, Couldwell WT. Internal Auditory Canal lipoma: an unusual intracranial lesion. World Neurosurg. 2020;135:156–9.

19. Tahmouresie A, Kroll G, Shucart W. Lipoma of the corpus callosum. Surg Neurol. 1979;11:31–5.

20. Zimmermann M, Kellermann S, Gerlach R, Seifert V. Cerebellopontine angle lipoma: case report and review of the literature. Acta Neurochir. 1999;141(12):1347–51.

21. Bigelow DC, Eisen MD, Smith PG, et al. Lipomas of the internal auditory canal and cerebellopontine angle. Laryngoscope. 1998;108:1459–69.

22. Totten DJ, Manzoor NF, Perkins EL, Labadie RF, Bennett ML, Haynes DS. Cerebellopontine angle and internal auditory canal lipomas: case series and systematic review. Laryngoscope. 2021;131(9):2081–7.

Part II

Incidental Findings of the Spine, Spinal Cord and Spinal Nerves

Spinal Arachnoid Cysts

Rajesh Nair and Girish Menon

22.1　Introduction

Spinal arachnoid cysts (SACs) are benign cerebrospinal fluid (CSF) filled cavities cysts which can occur anywhere along the nervous system and the spine is no exception [1, 2]. First described by Magendie in 1842, SACs account for 1–3% of all benign spinal space-occupying lesions [1]. Seen commonly in the adult population and in thoracic region, their pathogenesis is uncertain and most often idiopathic. SAC cysts can occur in all the three planes—extradural, intradural-extramedullary, and intramedullary and along the nerve roots as well. SAC is often incidental but, may be, produce symptoms by compression of the spinal cord or by traction over the nerve roots. Surgery is indicated in symptomatic patients, but in the absence of large clinical series, the optimal surgical strategy remains unclear. The main goal of surgery is to drain the cyst, relieve the pressure, and prevent reaccumulation—a task easier said than done. Multiple surgical strategies have been proposed, and an individualized customized approach is recommended. Long-term outcome is good despite the risk of recurrence. The fund of knowledge on SAC is currently limited and in need of extensive inputs through large clinical series.

22.2　Classification

SACs have been variably classified based on etiology, histopathology, and location. Yet, the optimal nomenclature and classification of SAC are still unclear and evolving. Based on etiology, SACs are grouped as primary (idiopathic) or secondary (to inflammation, trauma, infection bleeding) [3]. One of the most widely accepted classification is the one by Nabors et al. who classified spinal cysts into three on the basis of their anatomical location and tissue of origin. (Table 22.1) [4]. Type 1 lesions represent extradural cysts and include anterior or lateral meningoceles, synovial cysts, ganglia, ligamentum flavum cysts, and discal cysts [4]. Type 2 cysts

Table 22.1 Classification of spinal cysts (adapted from Nabors et al. [4])

Type	Description
I	Extradural meningeal cysts without spinal nerve root fibers
IA	Extradural meningeal/arachnoid cysts (ACs)
IB	Sacral meningocele
II	Extradural meningeal cysts with spinal nerve root fibers (Tarlov perineural cysts)
III	Spinal intradural ACs

R. Nair · G. Menon (✉)
Department of Neurosurgery, Kasturba Medical College, Manipal Academy of Higher Education, Manipal, Karnataka, India
e-mail: girish.menon@manipal.edu

are extradural meningeal cysts containing nerve root fibers commonly seen in the lumbar and sacral regions [5]. Type 3 cysts represent the true intradural arachnoid cysts (ACs) seen commonly in the posterior spinal subarachnoid space in the thoracic region [4, 6]. Spinal intradural extramedullary cystic lesions also include ependymal cysts, teratogenous cysts, epithelial cysts, neurenteric cysts (NECs), and ACs [7, 8]. Qi et al. advocated another classification strategy and subdivided SAC into five types: intramedullary, subdural extramedullary, subdural/epidural, epidural, and extra spinal [2]. Although epidural SACs are more common than other cyst types, their inclusion as a distinct type of SAC remains controversial as few authors believe that SAC characteristically denotes only the intradural extramedullary cysts.

22.3 Location

In the spine, ACs can be extradural, intradural extramedullary, perineural, or more rarely within the spinal cord. SACs are most commonly seen in the thoracic region followed by lumbar and then cervical segments [8–14]. It is postulated that this may be because the thoracic spine is the longest segment, has a narrow diameter, and patients become symptomatic early due to mass effect on the spinal cord [9]. Extradural SACs are more common than intradural cysts [15, 16]. Similarly, dorsal SACs are more common than ventral SACs except in the cervical region where ventral cysts are more frequent. Sadek et al. in their extensive review of all the 85 primary adult SAC observed that 82% were primarily within the thoracic spine and 93% of those were located within the dorsal aspect [17]. A similar observation was made by Klekamp in their series of 59 cases, the largest series reported so far [3]. The rarity of cervical SAC and absence of sacral SAC (where the septum posticum is absent) further support the theory that these lesions arise from the septum posticum.

22.4 Pathogenesis

The aetiopathogenesis of SAC is not fully known and believed to be multifactorial [18]. In nearly 80% of cases, SAC may be primary (idiopathic) as a distinct cause may not be identified [19]. In the remaining 20%, SAC may occur secondary to trauma, inflammation, hemorrhage, neoplasms, and iatrogenic causes like myelography or spinal surgery.

Several hypotheses have been proposed, both, for the formation and subsequent enlargement of ACs. Perret et al. suggested that primary idiopathic ACs arose from a diverticulum in the septum posticum [9, 20, 21]. The septum posticum is a thin midline arachnoid membrane along the midline dorsal subarachnoid space of the spinal cord which extends from the pial surface to the arachnoid mater and was first described by Magendie. Septum posticum remains indistinct in the cervical region, is better delineated in the cervicothoracic junction, distinct like a clear structure in the thoracic region and ends at the conus medullaris, and remains absent in the sacral region [22–24]. Ventral SACs in the lumbosacral region where septum posticum is deficient may occur due to proliferation of entrapped arachnoid granulations which secrete and give rise to cyst formation [25, 26]. Bassiouni et al. noted that all patients with ventral SACs in their series were younger, had greater craniocaudal extension, and exhibited intracystic tough fibrous septae that were not encountered with primary dorsal lesions [27]. This led to their hypothesis that ventral SACs represent a special subgroup which arise arising after adhesive arachnoiditis due to traumatic subarachnoid hemorrhage [27].

Enlargement of cysts once formed happens due to several possible mechanisms. Formation of an adhesive web which acts as a one-way valve ball valve mechanism between the cyst and sub arachnoid space is one proposed mechanism. Any maneuver which increases intrabdominal and intrathoracic pressure may result an influx into the cyst resulting in its gradual expansion

[12, 28, 29]. Few authors have proposed that an osmotic gradient between the subarachnoid space and the cyst or active secretion by the cells lining the cyst leads to an increase in the size of the SAC [10, 17]. Another interesting concept attributes increase in cyst size to the hydrostatic pressure of cistern terminalis which increases in the erect posture and years of raised hydrostatic pressure may cause the weak wall to gradually expand outwards into the spinal canal space [30]. Recently a novel hypothesis of pathogenesis has been proposed linking CSF flow to cardiac pulsations similar to the Oldfield's theory of syringomyelia formation [17, 31]. CSF's flow, direction, and speed are closely related to systole and diastole [25]. Systolic velocities of CSF in a craniocaudal direction are largest in the thoracic region (25–50 mm/s), almost 4 times greater than in the cervical spine (8–12 mm/s) and double that within the lumbar spine (0–20 mm/s) [25]. In diastole, reversal of flow happens in a caudal to cranial direction. The fast-systolic CSF-velocities within the dorsal CSF space within the thoracic spine can result in a "dissection" within the septum posticum. This gives rise to a focal contained region of turbulent CSF flow that forms the appearance of a cyst with a ball valve inlet [17, 25, 32]. Sadek et al. suggest that this combination of constant and dynamic focal compression on the cord parenchyma due to the alternating intracystic CSF pressures relating to the cardiac cycle gives rise to cord damage [17].

22.5 Clinical Presentation

SACs are reported to be more common among males with a reported predominance of almost 1.8:1 although few studies have observed a female dominance [27, 33–35]. The age of presentation is commonly in the fifth and sixth decade probably related to the fact that the septum posticum thickens with age [22]. Patients with solitary cysts present later in life (mean age, 25.2 years) and those with comorbidities present

earlier (mean age, 16.5 years). It has also been observed that male patients tend to be on average at least 10 years older than their female counterparts [36].

The clinical manifestations correspond with cyst size and the involved spinal levels. Patients commonly present with features of cord compression like gait disturbance (85%), spastic quadriparesis and paraparesis (83.8%), sensory dysfunction (74.2%), and neuropathic pain (55%) [17, 37, 38]. Bowel and bladder dysfunction may be noted in 36–50% of the patients [26, 38, 39]. Since majority of the cysts are located in the thoracic region, dorsal cord compressive symptoms predominate. However, lower cervical segments are more commonly involved in patients with solitary cysts (47.5%) and the lumbosacral region for patients with comorbidities (34%) [40, 41]. These symptoms may present subacutely or chronically or may present acutely following an increase in size during any activity that raises intrathoracic pressure and causes a sudden influx into the cyst [42].

22.6 Radiology/Imaging

MRI is the most definitive investigation of choice for diagnosing a SAC [5, 43]. Plain radiographs, computed tomography scans, and CT myelography can all have complimentary roles. Plain radiographs and computed tomography scans reveal bony anomalies like widening of the spinal canal with erosion and thinning of the pedicles, increased interpedicular distance, scalloping of the posterior vertebral wall, and evidence of instability and deformation [10, 12, 44].

MRI accurately demonstrates the anatomical location and provides a direct visualization of a cystic structure within the spinal canal (Figs. 22.1, 22.2, 22.3, 22.4, 22.5) The characteristic radiographic imaging features of primary SACs include a dorsal location, non-enhancing lesions with signal intensities similar to CSF [39, 43–45]. On contrast, they are non-enhanc-

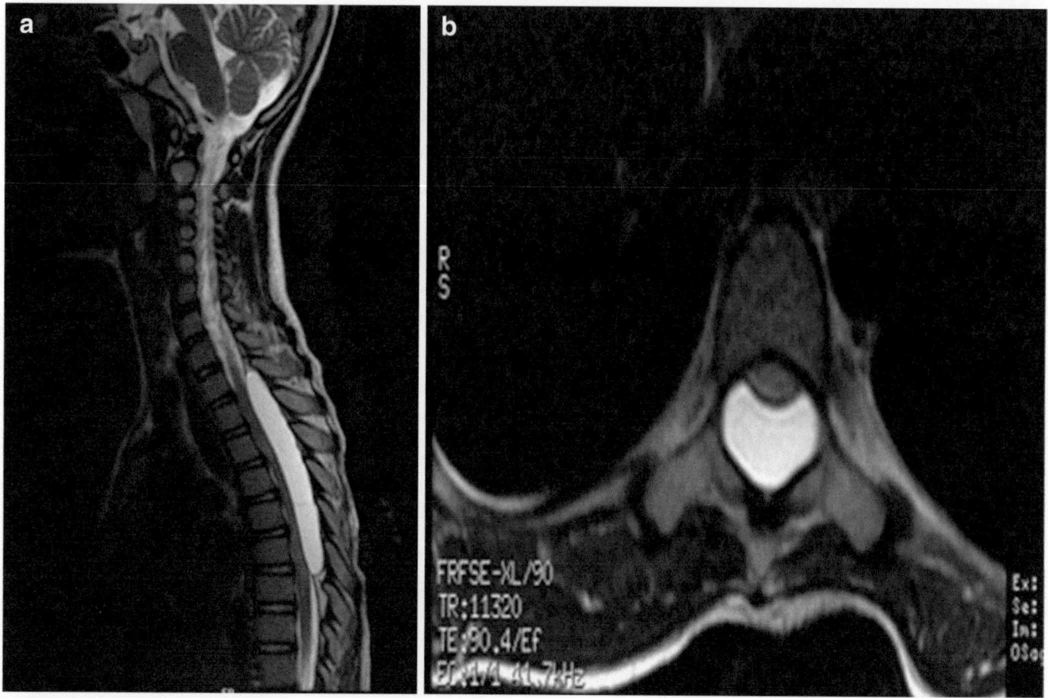

Fig. 22.1 Magnetic resonance imaging (MRI) spine images of a 46-year-old lady (**a**) Sagittal T2-weighted and (**b**) Axial T2-weighted MRIs showing T2 to T8 dorsally located extradural spinal arachnoid cyst (SAC) pushing the spinal cord ventrally

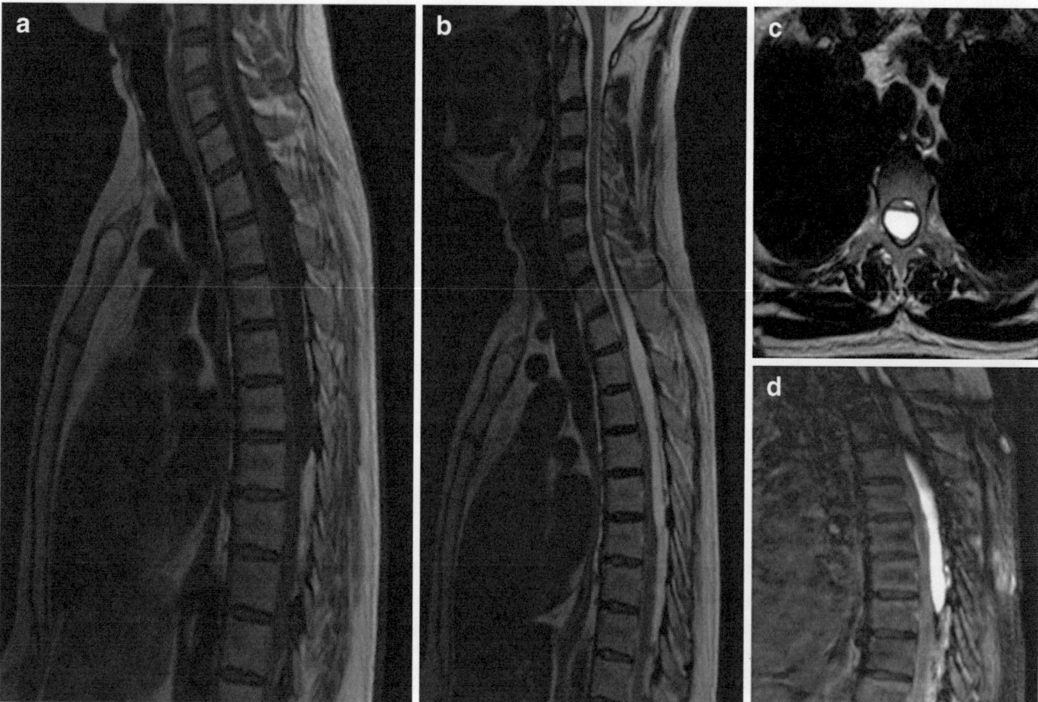

Fig. 22.2 MRI spine images of a 38-year-old lady ((**a**) Sagittal T1-weighted; (**b**) Sagittal T2; (**c**) Axial T2-weighted; and (**d**) Sagittal FLAIR images) showing T2 to T7 dorsally located intradural SAC pushing the spinal cord ventrally

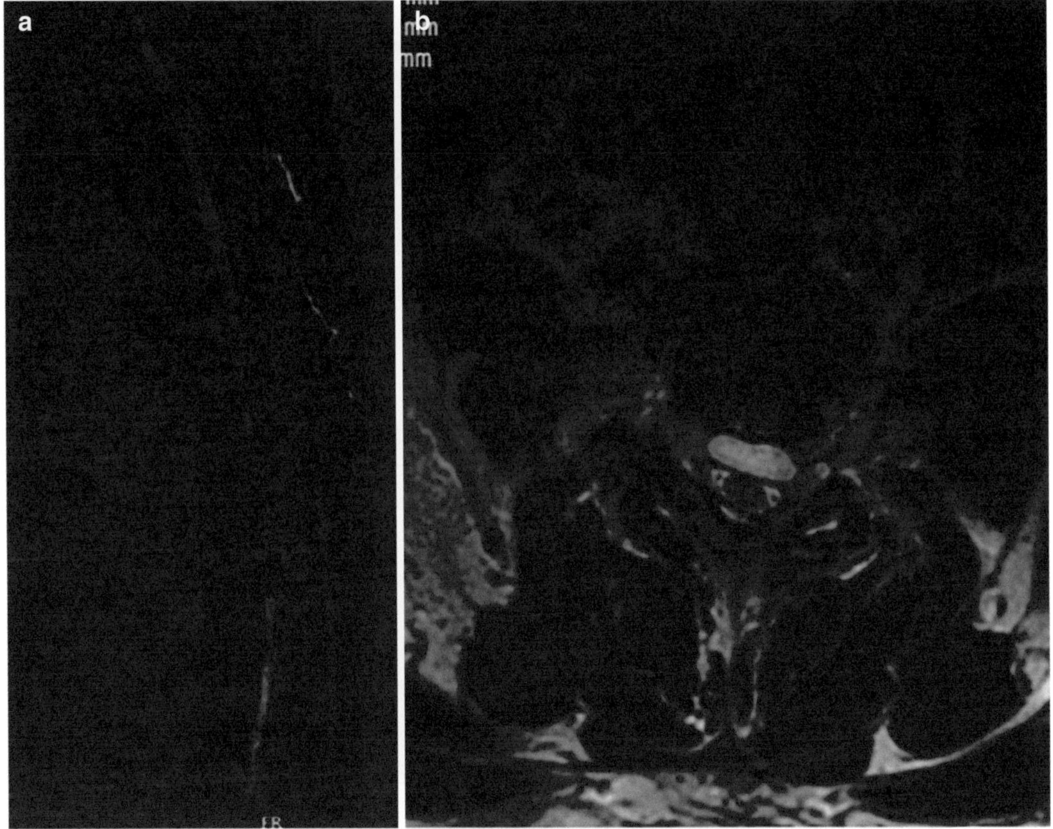

Fig. 22.3 MRI spine images of a 52-year-old male (**a**) Sagittal T2-weighted and (**b**) Axial T2-weighted images showing T2 to T7 ventrally a cervicodorsal intradural SAC pushing the spinal cord ventrally

ing, extramedullary, loculated CSF collections displacing cord or nerve roots. They may span over two to three vertebra and may be associated with a rostral or caudal syrinx in one-third of cases. MRI also helps to clearly delineate focal buckling or compression of the spinal cord, presence of intrinsic cord changes, myelomalacia as well details of surrounding soft tissues which help in differentiating from SAC mimickers [46, 47]. The classic scalpel signs commonly seen with SACs represent the abrupt buckling or change in contour of the spinal cord [10, 12]. Novel high-resolution MRI sequences such as constructive interference in steady states (CISS) and cine-mode steady-state free-precession imaging (SSFP) studies can provide improved visualization of arachnoid webs and can help to localize a defective site by identifying the pulsating turbulent flow void within a defective site [44].

Most intradural SACs communicate freely with the subarachnoid space and opacify on myelography or post myelography CT [48]. CT myelography, however, has the disadvantage of being invasive and is thus a complimentary investigation when the diagnosis is in doubt. CT myelography helps to reliably detect the anatomical location of the cyst, to localize the defect and to gauge the degree of flow of CSF between the cyst and the subarachnoid space [44, 49].

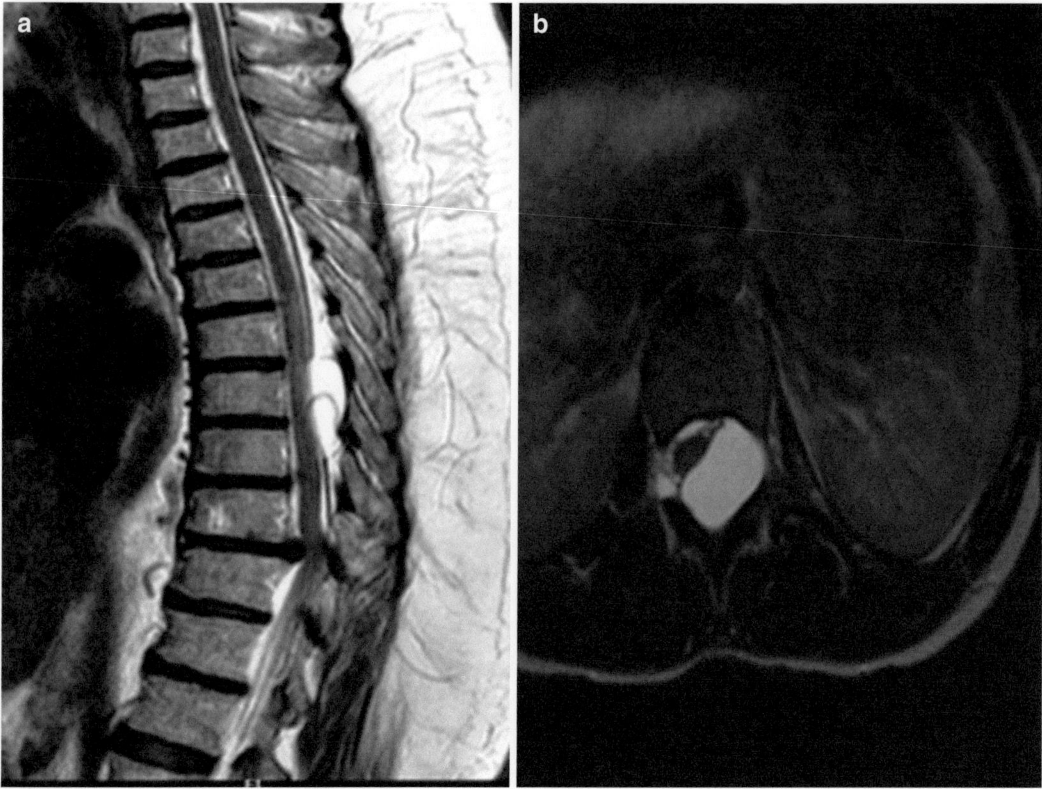

Fig. 22.4 MRI spine images of a 48-year-old male (**a**) Sagittal T2-weighted and (**b**) Axial T2-weighted images showing T7 to T9 septated intradural extramedullary SAC pushing the spinal cord ventrally and to the right. A dorsal disc herniation with cord compression is seen at the level below. This patient gave past history of trauma probably suggesting a post-traumatic inflammatory etiology for the cyst

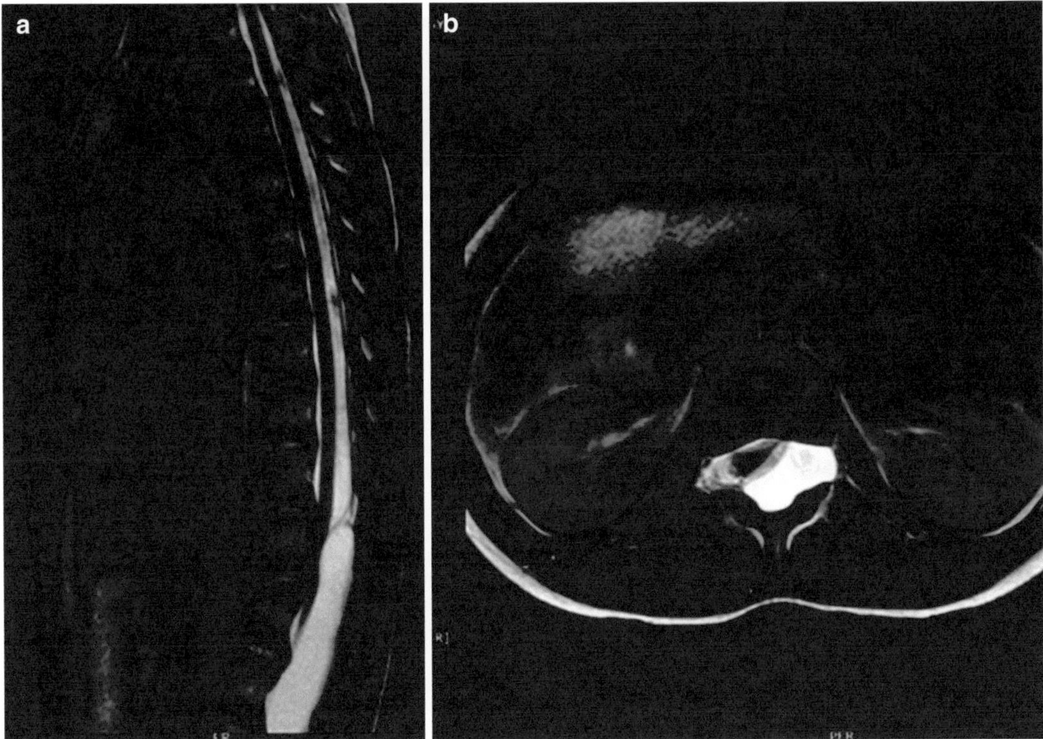

Fig. 22.5 MRI spine images of a 48-year-old male (**a**) Sagittal T2-weighted and (**b**) Axial T2-weighted images showing T9 to L 2 intradural extramedullary SAC pushing the spinal cord ventrally and to the right. The cyst is seen extending laterally into the foramen also

22.7 Differential Diagnoses

Epidural SACs have many differentials which are generally easy to distinguish on radiology. However, two close mimickers of intradural cysts, ventral spinal cord herniation (VSCH) and NEC, pose considerable diagnostic difficulties.

Spontaneous ventral spinal cord herniation refers to herniation of spinal cord through a defect in the ventral dura and is associated with focal atrophy of the spinal cord and anterior displacement of cord. Characteristic distinguishing features include acute angular ventral cord deviation, cord deviation less than two thoracic segments or 3 cm, absence of CSF ventral or ventrolateral to the cord, absence of CSF loculation dorsal to the cord. On post myelography CT, the absence of delayed myelographic CSF opacification dorsal to the cord helps to differentiate this lesion from an intradural SAC [15]. Realizing the challenges in differentiating the two disorders on radiographic imaging, Schultz et al. proposed relying on two indirect signs, namely the contour of dorsal cord indentation on sagittal plane and presence or absence of CSF signal ventral to the cord [19] (Fig. 22.6).

NECs are rare endodermal developmental lesions in the craniospinal axis and account for 0.3–0.5% of all spinal cord tumors. Typically seen in the central cervical region and less commonly in the sacral region, they are present in the second or third decade and are often associated with spina bifida, split-cord malformation, and other visceral anomalies (Arnold). In comparison with SACs, these are thick walled and adherent to adjacent neural structures. MRI signal characteristics vary depending on the intracystic protein content blood products [5, 27]. About 16% of spinal NECs appear isointense compared with CSF, may show hyperintensity on fluid-attenuated

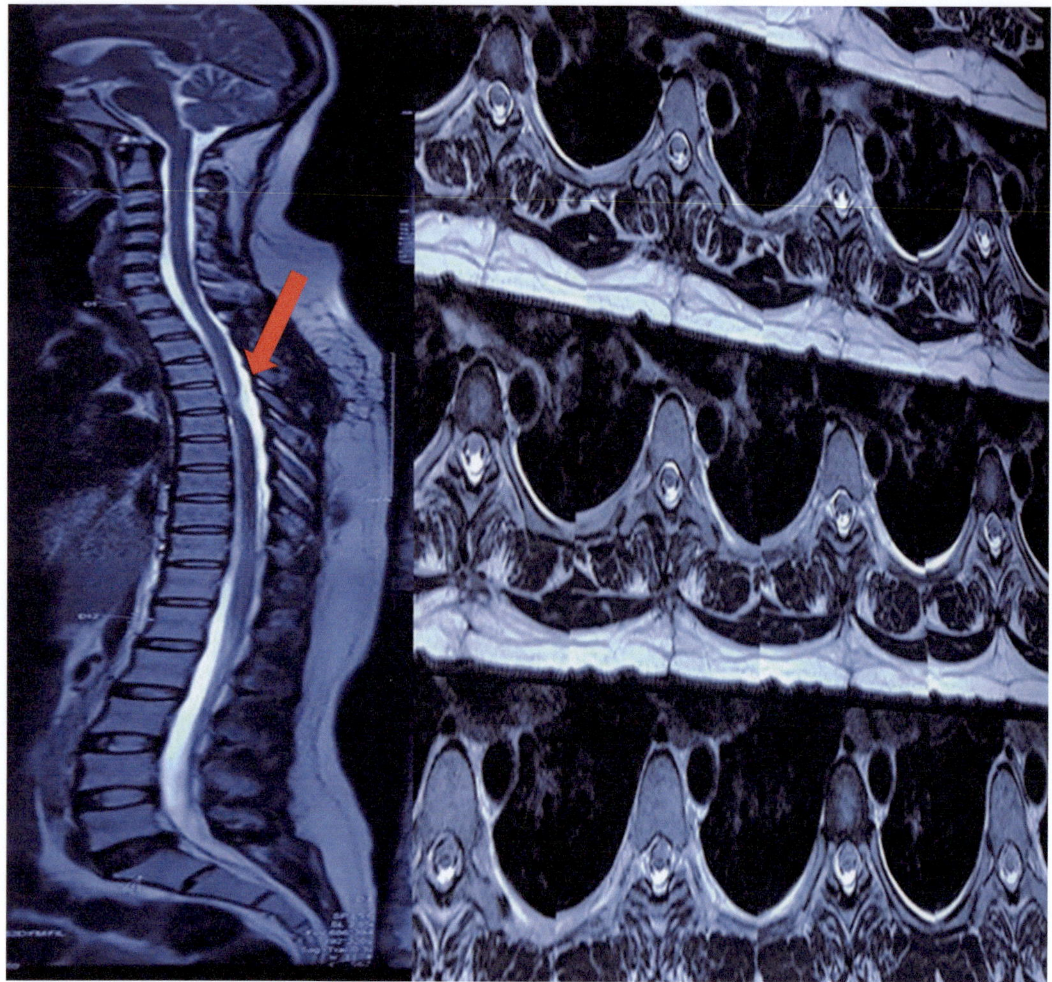

Fig. 22.6 Sagittal T2 and axial T2-weighted MRI images showing a ventral cord herniation at T5–6 level with a posterior SAC mimicker

inversion recovery and mild restriction on diffusion-weighted imaging [50, 51].

Close differentials for extradural cysts include perineural cysts, meningeal cysts, diverticula, dural ectasia, discal cysts, synovial cysts, ganglion cysts, and ligamentum flavum cyst [14]. Perineurial cysts usually occur along the sacral nerve roots, at or distal to the junction of the posterior root and the dorsal ganglion. Generally small and asymptomatic, they may be as large as 3 cm resulting in severe compression of nerve roots. They often occur with clusters and unlike meningeal cysts, at least a part of the lining of perineurial cysts contain nerve fibers. Synovial cyst, most commonly seen at L4-5 levels and L5-S1 have a synovial lining membrane generated from synovium of facet and are associated with underlying spinal instability, facet joint arthropathy, and degenerative spondylolisthesis [20, 52, 53]. Discal cysts result from stressful mechanical loads which result in acute disc herniation, followed by acute degeneration with formation of reactive pseudomembrane. Ganglion cysts are believed to originate from mucinous degeneration within periarticular dense fibrous connective tissue [12]. Ligamentum flavum cyst represents a unique entity being embedded in the inner surface of ligamentum flavum with no epithelial lining and is associated with segmental instability and local stress. Spinal intradural extramedullary cystic lesions like ependymal cysts, teratogenous cysts, epithelial cysts (ACs) have characteristic MRI features which help to differentiate them from SAC [7, 8].

22.8 Management

Asymptomatic arachnoid cysts that cause no pain or mild neurological symptoms/signs and those without mass effect, regardless of their size and spinal location are best treated conservatively with a wait and watch policy [12, 43, 54]. Conservative treatment consists of bed rest, analgesics, physical therapy, bracing, transcutaneous electrical stimulation, epidural or intra-articular steroid injections [55]. Surgery is the treatment of choice for symptomatic patients. Optimal surgical strategy is however a matter of debate, and the common surgical techniques adopted include resection, fenestration, fixation, or placement of a shunt tube. Qi J et al. have proposed an algorithm for SAC as shown in Table 22.2 [2], which provides a broad principle in the surgical management of these lesions.

The initial record of spinal intradural cysts compressing the spinal cord and being successfully treated by surgery was reported by Spiller in 1903 followed by Skoog in 1915 [56, 57]. The main goal of surgery is to relieve nerve root/spinal cord compression, prevent cyst recurrence, and manage instability if any. This is achieved by total resection of the cyst wall, closure of the communication between the cyst and the subarachnoid space and spinal stabilization if required [34, 39]. However, this can be challenging in many instances. The cyst wall might be adherent to neural structures making total excision difficult and hazardous. Cyst wall excision is difficult in case of ventrally located cysts and in situations where the cysts are multiple, extensive, and have multiple septations [10, 26, 58–60]. Identifying the exact site of communication is also a challenge in many patients. Majority of the dorsal SACs and ventral SACs can be approached through a prone position. Anterior ventral SACs may require an anterolateral extension or a conventional anterior cervical approach [61, 62]. Nerve roots within the cyst should be preserved. For lumbar lateralized extradural extraspinal SACs and sacral Tarlov cyst, a transforaminal approach is preferred [63]. Intraoperative ultrasound, electrophysiological monitoring for somatosensory/motor evoked potentials, and anal electromyography are useful operative adjuncts [30, 51, 59, 60, 64]. Preoperative marker X-rays or intraoperative fluoroscopy help to identify the correct vertebral level for surgery [64, 65]. The laminectomy/laminotomy should include one vertebral level above and below the position of the cyst. Safe maximal resection of the cyst wall should be the aim especially in multisegment and post inflammatory SACs. In few cases of extensive cysts or recurrent cysts, other alternative surgical techniques can be used such as stenting, cystic shunting, or simple percutaneous needle aspiration [6, 27, 41, 66]. Water-tight dural closure using a patch and fibrin glue is advisable [67].When the stability of the spine is lessened, surgical stabilization with osteosynthesis/fusion is required.

For extradural arachnoid cysts, the cyst wall should be carefully dissected from the thecal sac, the pedicle isolated ligated, transected, and the cyst removed. Then, the dural defect can usually be sutured closed and reinforced with fibrin glue

Table 22.2 Management algorithm as proposed by Qi et al. [2]

Intramedullary cyst	Cyst wall should be removed, and residual cyst wall should be sutured to the pia mater to obliterate the connection
Subdural extramedullary spinal arachnoid cysts	Cyst wall should be excised carefully assisted with endoscopy to avoid injuries to the spinal cord.
Subdural/epidural cysts	Cyst should be separated from the neck of the cyst, and then tight suturing should be performed after resection of the cyst
Epidural cysts	Ligation of the cervix should be performed, and closure of the dural defect
Intraspinal and extraspinal cysts	Cyst should be removed through enlarged intervertebral foramina

to prevent CSF leakage [35]. Once exposed, cyst fenestration into the subarachnoid space before cystic wall excision followed by meticulous dissection and maximal safe removal of the cyst wall from the adherent dura and neural tissue should be carried out [51]. Few modifications have been suggested by some authors. This includes unilateral managemental approach followed by an excision of the upper pole of the cyst wall in order to create a stoma into the subarachnoid space [68]. Intramedullary cysts are tackled by myelotomy followed by marsupialization/total excision of the cyst. Sun suggested that the residual cyst wall should be sutured to the pia mater to ensure adequate communication between the cyst cavity and the subarachnoid compartment [30].

Recently minimally invasive techniques have been advocated which include use of endoscope for cyst fenestration and communication with the subarachnoid space [33]. CT-scan guided percutaneous aspiration is another minimally invasive method used for perineural/Tarlov cysts in the lumbosacral region [69]. However, percutaneous needle aspiration is an inadequate procedure due to the high rate of cyst recurrence [8, 66, 70].

22.9 Complications

Apart from minor complications like wound infections and dehiscence, postoperative epidural hematoma, the major complications may include cyst recurrence, spinal instability, pseudo meningocele and postoperative kyphosis [64, 65, 71, 72].

Cyst recurrence or insufficient shrinkage of the cyst is seen in less than 12.5% and more commonly seen in intradural forms. Recurrence rates are less for intradural idiopathic cysts (12%) than that of post-hemorrhagic cysts (66%) [8, 17, 64, 73]. Therefore, cysts with multiple septations and those that evolved following bleeding must undergo whenever possible an extended cyst wall resection. Symptomatic recurrence may require redo surgery with cyst-shunting [10, 74, 75]. Long segment cysts may require extensive laminectomy that would be necessary with associated

complications [35, 44, 76]. Laminotomy, minimal skipped laminectomy, selective laminectomy with closure of the dural defect site should be considered in such patients to prevent instability [3, 27, 35, 44] If instability exists and in view of extensive bony erosion/removal appropriate stabilization should be performed. Postoperative CSF leakage and pseudomeningocele should be avoided by careful microscopic surgical techniques, ligation of all fistulas, watertight dural closure, use of dural patch, glue. Even with appropriate operative techniques, residual small cysts cannot be completely avoided and pseudomeningocele formation is often unavoidable.

22.10 Surgical Outcome

Outcome following surgery may be inconsistent and not uniform. Postoperative outcome is good in patients in whom weakness and gait disturbance were the main presenting symptoms [30, 77–79]. Resolution of neuropathic pain, sensory dysfunction, sexual and sphincter disturbances is inconsistent and may happen in less than one-third of the patients following surgery [60]. Radiological improvement with cord expansion is variable and may be seen in 45%–50% [79]. Duration of the symptoms prior to surgery did not correlate with severity or with likelihood of improvement following surgery. Poor outcome prognosticators include multicyclic lesions, presence of pre- and post-operative-syrinxes [80]. Recurrence and reoperation rates vary from 2.5% to 50%. and are more common with post-hemorrhagic cysts (66.7%) than for idiopathic cysts7.8% [2, 3, 81].

22.11 Conclusion

Primary SACs are rare lesions and include a spectrum of lesions. Majority of them are idiopathic and are typically seen within the mid thoracic spine. The exact etiopathogenesis is unclear and is believed to be secondary to dissection within the septum posticum and are propagated secondary to the complex CSF flow dynamics within the thoracic spine. Symptomatology varies from neuropathic pain to myelopathy features and is a result of both static and dynamic compression of the cord parenchyma. Asymptomatic cysts can be observed but symptomatic cyst requires surgical intervention. Optimal surgical technique is debatable but an individualized customized approach is needed. Surgery helps in improvement of few symptoms most notably in motor, gait disturbance but patients need to be followed up to rule out recurrence rates. Large clinical series and studies are needed to provide further insights into this unique pathology.

References

1. Magendie F, Recherchesphysiologiques et cliniques sur le liquide cephalorachidienoucerebro-spinal, Mequignon-Marvisfils; 1842.
2. Qi J, Yang J, Wang GH. A novel five-category multimodal T1-weighted and T2-weighted magnetic resonance imaging-based stratification system for the selection of spinal arachnoid cyst treatment: a 15-year experience of 81 cases. Neuropsychiatr Dis Treat. 2014;10:499–506.
3. Klekamp A. New classification for pathologies of spinal meninges-part 2: primary and secondary intradural arachnoid cysts. Neurosurgery. 2017;81(2):217–29.
4. Nabors, Pait TG, Byrd EB, Karim NO, Davis DO, Kobrine AI, Rizzoli HV. Updated assessment and current classification of spinal meningeal cysts. J Neurosurg. 1988;68(3):366–77.
5. Evans A, Stoodley N, Halpin S. Magnetic resonance imaging of intraspinal cystic lesions: a pictorial review. CurrProblDiagnRadiol. 2002;31:79–94.
6. Noujaim S, Moreng K, Noujaim D. Cystic lesions in spinal imaging: a pictorial review and classification. Neurographics. 2013;3:14–27.
7. Agnoli AL, Laun A, Schönmayr R. Enterogenous intraspinal cysts. J Neurosurg. 1984;61:834–40.
8. Osenbach RK, Godersky JC, Traynelis VC, Schelper RD. Intradural extramedullary cysts of the spinal canal: clinical presentation, radiographic diagnosis, and surgical management. Neurosurgery. 1992;30:35–42.
9. Asamoto S, Fukui Y, Nishiyama M, Ishikawa M, Fujita N, Nakamura S, et al. Diagnosis and surgical strategy for sacral meningeal cysts with check-valve mechanism: technical note. Acta Neurochir. 2013;155(2):309–13.
10. Bond AE, Zada G, Bowen I, McComb JG, Krieger MD. Spinal arachnoid cysts in the pediatric population: report of 31 cases and a review of the literature. J Neurosurg Pediatr. 2012;9:432–41.
11. Cho HY, Lee SH, Kim ES, Eoh W. Symptomatic large spinal extradural arachnoid cyst: a case report. Korean J Spine. 2015;12:217–20.
12. Cho S, Rhee WT, Lee SY, Lee SB. Ganglion cyst of the posterior longitudinal ligament causing lumbar radiculopathy. J Korean Neurosurg Soc. 2010;47(4):298–301.
13. Sun J. Classification, mechanism and surgical treatments for spinal canal cysts. Chinese Neurosurg J. 2016;2 https://doi.org/10.1186/s41016-016-0022-y.
14. Tarlov IM, Bareksei Y, Albanna W, Schirmer M. Spinal perineurial and meningeal cysts. J Neurol Neurosurg Psychiatry. 1970;33(6):833–43.
15. Goyal A, Singh AK, Singh D, Gupta V, Tatke M, Sinha S, et al. Intramedullary arachnoid cyst. Case report. J Neurosurg. 2002;96(suppl):104–6.
16. Lee CH, Hyun SJ, Kim KJ, Jahng TA, Kim HJ. What is a reasonable surgical procedure for spinal extradural arachnoid cysts: is cyst removal mandatory? Eight consecutive cases and a review of the literature. Acta Neurochir. 2012;154(7):1219–27.
17. Sadek AR, Nader-Sepahi A. Spinal arachnoid cysts: presentation, management and pathophysiology. Clin Neurol Neurosurg. 2019;180:87–96. https://doi.org/10.1016/j.clineuro.2019.03.014.
18. Hashizume CT. Cervical spinal arachnoid cyst in a dog. Can Veterinary J La revue vétérinairecanadienne. 2000;41(3):225–7.
19. Schultz A Jr, Steven A, Wessell N, Fischbein CA, Sansur D, Gandhi D, Ibrahimi P. Raghavan, differentiation of idiopathic spinal cord herniation from dorsal arachnoid webs on MRI and CT myelography. J Neurosurg Spine. 2017;26(6):754–9.
20. Khan AM, Girardi F. Spinal lumbar synovial cysts. Diagnosis and management challenge. Eur Spine J. 2006;15(8):1176–82.
21. Perret G, Green D, Keller J. Diagnosis and treatment of intradural arachnoid cysts of the thoracic spine. Radiology. 1962;79:425–9.
22. Di Chiro EL. Timins, supine myelography and the septum posticum. Radiology. 1974;111(2):319–27.
23. Jirout J, Fischer J, Nadvornik F. Anatomical and pneumographic studies on the posterior arachnoid space of the normal thoracic spine. Fortschr Geb Rontgenstr Nuklearmed. 1964;101(4):395–9.
24. Nicholos DS, Weller RO. The fine anatomy of the human spinal meninges. A light and scanning electron microscopy study. J Neurosurg. 1988;69(2):276–82.
25. Fortuna A, La Torre E, Ciappetta P. Arachnoid diverticula: a unitary approach to spinal cysts communicating with the subarachnoid space. Acta Neurochir. 1977;39(3–4):259–68.
26. Garg K, Borkar SA, Kale SS, Sharma BS. Spinal arachnoid cysts - our experience and review of literature. Br J Neurosurg. 2017;31:172–8. https://doi.org/10.1080/02688697.2016.1229747.
27. Bassiouni H, Hunold A, Asgari S, Hubschen U, Konig HJ, Stolke D. Spinal intradural juxtamedullary cysts in the adult: surgical management and out-

come. Neurosurgery. 2004;55(6):1352–9. (discussion 1359–60).

28. Hamamcioglu MK, Kilincer C, Hicdonmez T, Simsek O, Birgili B, Cobanoglu S. Giant cervicothoracic extradural arachnoid cyst: case report. Eur Spine J. 2006;15(S5):595–8.

29. Lesoin F, Rousseau M, Thomas CE III, Jomin M. Post traumatic spinal arachnoid cysts. Acta Neurochir. 1984;70:227–34.

30. Sun JJ, Wang ZY, Teo M, Li ZD, Wu HB, Yen RY, et al. Comparative outcomes of the two types of sacral extradural spinal meningeal cysts using different operation methods: a prospective clinical study. PLoS One. 2013;8(12):e83964.

31. Oldfield EH. Pathogenesis of chiari I – pathophysiology of syringomyelia: implications for therapy: a summary of 3 decades of clinical research. Neurosurgery. 2017;64(CN_suppl_1):66–77.

32. Levy LM, Di Chiro G. MR phase imaging and cerebrospinal fluid flow in the head and spine. Neuroradiology. 1990;32(5):399–406.

33. Endo T, Takahashi T, Jokura H, Tominaga T. Surgical treatment of spinal intradural arachnoid cysts using endoscopy. J Neurosurg Spine. 2010;12(6):641–6.

34. Lee HJ, Cho WH, Han IH, Choi BK. Large thoracolumbar extradural arachnoid cyst excised by minimal skipped hemilaminectomy: a case report. Korean J Spine. 2013;10(1):28–31.

35. Lee SH, Shim HK, Eun SS. Twist technique for removal of spinal extradural arachnoid cyst: technical note. Eur Spine J. 2014;23:1755–60. https://doi.org/10.1007/s00586-014-3393-9.

36. Viswanathan VK, Manoharan SR, Do H, Minnema A, Shaddy SM, Elder JB, Farhadi HF. Clinical and radiologic outcomes after fenestration and partial wall excision of idiopathic intradural spinal arachnoid cysts presenting with myelopathy. World Neurosurg. 2017;105:213–22.

37. Krstacic A, Krstacic G, ButkovicSoldo S. Atypical cause of radiculopathy—intradural spinal arachnoid cyst. Acta Clin Belg. 2016;71:267–8.

38. Wang L, Zhang J, Wu Z, et al. Diagnosis and management of adult intracranial neurenteric cysts. Neurosurgery. 2011;68:44–52.

39. Funao H, Nakamura M, Hosogane N, Watanabe K, Tsuji T, Ishii K, Kamata M, Toyama Y, Chiba K, Matsumoto M. Surgical treatment of spinal extradural arachnoid cysts in the thoracolumbar spine. Neurosurgery. 2012;71(2):278–84; (discussion 284).

40. Paleologos TS, Thom M, Thomas DGT. Spinal neurenteric cysts without associated malformations. Are they the same as those presenting in spinal dysraphism? Br J Neurosurg. 2000;14:185–94.

41. Palma L, Lorenzo ND. Spinal endodermal cysts without associated vertebral or other congenital abnormalities: report of four cases and review of the literature. Acta Neurochir. 1976;33:283–300.

42. Kriss TC, Kriss VM. Symptomatic spinal intradural arachnoid cyst development after lumbar myelography. Case report and review of the literature. Spine. 1997;22:568–72.

43. Netra R, Min L, Shao Hui M, Wang JC, Bin Y, Ming Z. Spinal extradural meningeal cysts: an MRI evaluation of a case series and literature review. J Spinal Disord Tech. 2011;24:132–6.

44. Choi SW, Seong HY, Roh SW. Spinal extradural arachnoid cyst. J Korean Neurosurg Soc. 2013;54:355–8.

45. Oh JK, Lee DY, Kim TY, Yi S, Ha Y, Kim KN, et al. Thoracolumbar extradural arachnoid cysts: a study of 14 consecutive cases. Acta Neurochir. 2012;154:341–8.

46. Krings T, Lukas R, Reul J, Spetzger U, Reinges MH, Gilsbach JM, et al. Diagnostic and therapeutic management of spinal arachnoid cysts. Acta Neurochir. 2001;143:227–35.

47. Silbergleit R, Brunberg JA, Patel SC, Mehta BA, Aravapalli SR. Imaging of spinal intradural arachnoid cysts: MRI, myelography and CT. Neuroradiology. 1998;40:664–8.

48. Buxi TBS, Sud S, Vohra R, Kakkar A, Byotra SP. Giant spinal arachnoid cysts: computed tomography, magnetic resonance imaging and magnetic resonance myelography correlation. AustralasRadiol. 2000;44:216–9.

49. Panigrahi S, Mishra SS, Dhir MK, Parida DK. Giant thoracolumbar extradural arachnoid cyst: an uncommon cause of spine compression. Neurol India. 2012;60:540–2.

50. Preece MT, Osborn AG, Chin SS, Smirniotopoulos JG. Intracranial neurenteric cysts: imaging and pathology spectrum. Am J Neuroradiol. 2006;27:1211–6.

51. Wang MY, Levi AD, Green BA. Intradural spinal arachnoid cysts in adults. Surg Neurol. 2003;60(1):49–55. (discussion 55–6).

52. Aydin S, Abuzayed B, Yildirim H, Bozkus H, Vural M. Discal cysts of the lumbar spine: report of five cases and review of the literature. Eur Spine J. 2010;19(10):1621–6.

53. Trummer M, Flaschka G, Tillich M, Homann CN, Unger F, Eustacchio S. Diagnosis and surgical management of intraspinal synovial cysts: report of 19 cases. J Neurol Neurosurg Psychiatry. 2001;70(1):74–7.

54. Furtado SV, Thakar S, Murthy GK, Dadlani R, Hegde AS. Spinal extradural arachnoid cyst management of complex giant spinal arachnoid cysts presenting with myelopathy. J Neurosurg Spine. 2011;15:107–12.

55. Kato M, Konishi S, Matsumura A, Hayashi K, Tamai K, Shintani K, et al. Clinical characteristics of intraspinal facet cysts following microsurgical bilateral decompression via a unilateral approach for treatment of degenerative lumbar disease. Eur Spine J. 2013;22(8):1750–7.

56. Skoog A. Spinal cord compression from leptomeningeal cysts. With a report of two cases. JAMA. 1915;65:394.

57. Spiller WG. A case of intradural arachnoid cyst with operation and recovery. Trans Coll Physicians Philadelphia. 1913;25:1–18.

58. Baig Mirza A, Bartram J, Sinha S, Gebreyohanes A, Boardman T, Vastani A, et al. Surgical management and outcomes in spinal intradural arachnoid cysts: the experience from two tertiary neurosurgical centres. Acta Neurochir. 2021;164:1217. https://doi.org/10.1007/s00701-021-05027-3.

59. Eroglu U, Bozkurt M, Kahilogullari G, Dogan I, Ozgural O, Shah KJ, et al. Surgical management of spinal arachnoid cysts in adults. World Neurosurg. 2019;122:e1146–52. https://doi.org/10.1016/j.wneu.2018.11.005.

60. Fam MD, Woodroffe RW, Helland L, Noeller J, Dahdaleh NS, Menezes AH, Hitchon PW. Spinal arachnoid cysts in adults: diagnosis and management. A single-center experience. J Neurosurg Spine. 2018;29:711–9. https://doi.org/10.3171/2018.5.SPINE1820.

61. Shrestha P, Shrestha P, Devkota UP. Excision of an anterior intradural arachnoid cyst of the cervical spine through central corpectomy approach. Eur Spine J. 2017;26(Suppl 1):154–7. https://doi.org/10.1007/s00586-017-4973-2.

62. Srinivasan US, Bangaari A, Senthilkumar G. Partial median corpectomy for C2-C3 intradural arachnoid cyst: case report and review of the literature. Neurol India. 2009;57:803–5. https://doi.org/10.4103/0028-3886.59484.

63. Ido K, Matsuoka H, Urushidani H. Effectiveness of a transforaminal surgical procedure for spinal extradural arachnoid cyst in the upper lumbar spine. J Clin Neurosci. 2002;9:694–6. https://doi.org/10.1054/jocn.2002.1138.

64. Moses ZB, Friedman GN, Penn DL, Solomon IH, Chi JH. Intradural spinal arachnoid cyst resection: implications of duraplasty in a large case series. J Neurosurg Spine. 2018;28:548–54. https://doi.org/10.3171/2017.8.SPINE17605.

65. French H, Somasundaram A, Biggs M, Parkinson J, Allan R, Ball J, et al. Idiopathic intradural dorsal thoracic arachnoid cysts: a case series and review of the literature. J Clin Neurosci. 2017;40:147–52. https://doi.org/10.1016/j.jocn.2017.02.051.

66. Petridis AK, Doukas A, Barth H, Mehdorn HM. Spinal cord compression caused by idiopathic intradural arachnoid cysts of the spine: review of the literature and illustrated case. Eur Spine J. 2010;19(S2):124–9.

67. Christophis P, Asamoto S, Kuchelmeister K, Schachenmayr W. "Juxtafacet cysts", a misleading name for cystic formations of mobile spine (CYFMOS). Eur Spine J. 2007;16(9):1499–505.

68. Schmutzer M, Tonn JC, Zausinger S. Spinal intradural extramedullary arachnoid cysts in adults-operative therapy and clinical outcome. Acta Neurochir. 2020;162(3):691–702. https://doi.org/10.1007/s00701-019-04156-0. Epub 2019 Dec 7..

69. Fletcher-Sandersjöö A, Mirza S, Burström G, Pedersen K, KuntzeSöderqvist Å, Grane P, et al. Management of perineural (Tarlov) cysts: a population-based cohort study and algorithm for the selection of surgical candidates. Acta Neurochir. 2019;161:1909–15. https://doi.org/10.1007/s00701-019-04000-5.

70. Spiegelmann R, Rappaport ZH, Sahar A. Spinal arachnoid cyst with unusual presentation. Case report. J Neurosurg. 1984;60:613–6. https://doi.org/10.3171/jns.1984.60.3.0613.

71. Papagelopoulos PJ, Peterson HA, Ebersold MJ, Emmanuel PR, Choudhury SN, Quast LM. Spinal column deformity and instability after lumbar or thoracolumbar laminectomy for intraspinal tumors in children and young adults. Spine (Phila Pa 1976). 1997;22:442–51. https://doi.org/10.1097/00007632-199702150-00019.

72. Yasuoka S, Peterson HA, MacCarty CS. Incidence of spinal column deformity after multilevel laminectomy in children and adults. J Neurosurg. 1982;57:441–5. https://doi.org/10.3171/jns.1982.57.4.0441.

73. Evangelou P, Meixensberger J, Bernhard M, Hirsch W, Kiess W, Merkenschlager A, Nestler U, Preuss M. Operative management of idiopathic spinal intradural arachnoid cysts in children: a systematic review. Childs Nerv Syst. 2012;29:657–64.

74. Carrillo R. Lumbar cerebrospinal fluid drainage for symptomatic sacral nerve root cysts: an adjuvant diagnostic procedure and/or alternative treatment? Technical case report. Neurosurgery. 1998;42:952–3. https://doi.org/10.1097/00006123-199804000-00162.

75. James HE, Postlethwait R. Spinal peritoneal shunts for conditions other than hydrocephalus and pseudotumor cerebri: a clinical report. Pediatr Neurosurg. 2007;43:456–60. https://doi.org/10.1159/000108787.

76. Chynn KY. Congenital spinal extradural cyst in two siblings. Am J Roentgenol. 1967;101(1):204–15.

77. Neulen A, Kantelhardt SR, Pilgram-Pastor SM, Metz I, Rohde V, Giese A. Microsurgical fenestration of perineural cysts to the thecal sac at the level of the distal dural sleeve. Acta Neurochir. 2011;153(7):1427–34.

78. Shi W, Cui DM, Shi JL, Gu ZK, Ju SQ, Chen J. Microsurgical excision of the craniocervical neurenteric cysts by the far-lateral transcondylar approach: case report and review of the literature. Skull Base. 2010;20(6):435–42.

79. Taha H, Bareksei Y, Albanna W, Schirmer M. Ligamentum flavum cyst in the lumbar spine: a case report and review of the literature. J Orthop Traumatol. 2010;11(2):117–22.

80. Griessenauer CJ, Bauer DF, Moore TA 2nd, Pritchard PR, Hadley MN. Surgical manifestations of thoracic arachnoid pathology: series of 28 cases. J Neurosurg Spine. 2014;20:30–40. https://doi.org/10.3171/2013.9.SPINE1323.

81. Mohindra S, Gupta R, Bal A. Intra-dural spinal arachnoid cysts: a short series of 10 patients. Br J Neurosurg. 2010;24:679–83. https://doi.org/10.3109/02688697.2010.504052.

Lipoma of the Filum Terminale

Yuchao Zuo

23.1   Introduction

Lipomas of the filum terminale (LFT) have been defined as an abnormality with fatty deposits in the filum terminale (diameter >2 mm), which is the simplest type of occult spinal dysraphism. The incidental rate of detection of the LFT on magnetic resonance imaging (MRI) ranges 0.24–4% [1–5]. The difference between LFT and caudal type lumbosacral lipoma is whether the caudal end of the conus medullaris is clearly visible on MRI [6]. LFT is a common incidental finding on spinal MRI, and most patients present without associated symptoms [3], the natural history is generally benign for asymptomatic patients.

With the extensive usage of spinal MRI techniques, many incidental asymptomatic LFT are being discovered (Fig. 23.1). FTL with low-lying conus is considered a surgical entity irrespective of symptoms because of its tendency to progress [7]. Surgery for LFT has been considered as a straightforward microsurgical exercise [8]. There is little debate regarding surgery for symptomatic LFT; however, prophylactic surgery for asymptomatic patients still exists controversial [6]. Long-term prospective study of natural history is necessary.

The indications and performance of surgery for the LFT are presented in this chapter that deals mainly with the current techniques applied in the surgical management of LFT. Postoperative complications are also discussed at the end of this chapter.

Y. Zuo (✉)
Department of Neurosurgery, The First Affiliated
Hospital of Zhengzhou University,
Zhengzhou, Henan, China

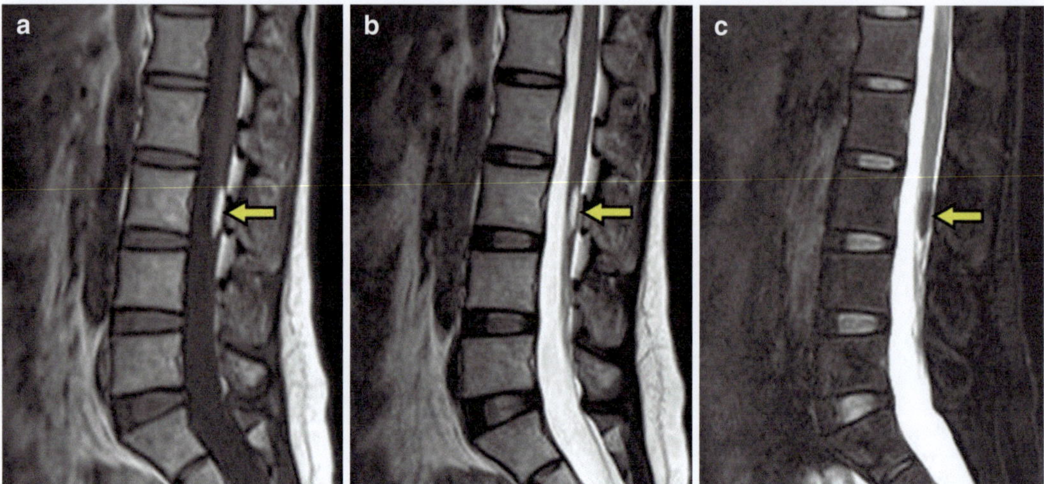

Fig. 23.1 Lipomas of the filum terminale (LFT) was incidentally found in a 30-year-old woman. Typical images on sagittal view of lumbosacral magnetic resonance imaging (MRI). LFT (yellow arrow) showing hypointense signal on T1-weighted MRI image (**a**), hyperintense signal on T2-weighted image (**b**), and low signal on lipid compression image (**c**)

23.2   Preoperative Evaluation

Preoperative evaluation including spinal MRI, clinical presentation, associated syndromes or malformations, skin stigmas, general status, and conus level. The clinical symptoms and neuroimaging evaluation are essential factors that determine the best treatment planning for each patient. If the surgical indication is determined, surgical exploration and decompression by lipoma excision, release of tethered cord, or a combination of these techniques should be considered.

Tamura et al. [9]. reported that cases with the caudal end of conus medullaris below the L2/3 level and symptomatic cases should consider performing surgery. Usami et al. [5] found that the improvement rate of symptoms in symptomatic patients was only about 50%, most symptomatic patients were approximately 8 years old. Meanwhile, 1 in 68 asymptomatic patients developed new symptoms during the postoperative follow-up period, indicating the significance of surgery.

Patients with a deformity or sensorimotor abnormalities of the lower limbs, urinary or defecation disorders, repeated urinary tract infections, and abnormalities noted in the urodynamic study were classified as symptomatic [10]. Surgery is the treatment of choice for symptomatic patients. The surgical indication for asymptomatic patients showing a normal conus level on MRI is controversial.

Surgical therapy for LFT is indicated if the patient demonstrates as following: (1) Obvious neurological deficits caused by tethered cord or syrinx; (2) associated syndromes or symptoms: dysraphism, locoregional syndrome, sphincter dysfunction (dysuria, constipation), neuro-orthopedic disorders (motor weakness, gait disturbance), sensory disturbances, and so on; (3) skin stigmas: fossette in lumbosacral area, intergluteal fold deviation, dermal sinus, cutaneous angioma, and so on; (4) other malformations: diastematomyelia, sacral agenesis, and perineal anomaly, etc.

23.3   Surgical Principles

The main goal of the surgery for LFT is releasing of tethered cord and prevention of tethering recurrence [11, 12]. These goals will be achieved by liberating and resection of filum terminale from surrounding nerves, protecting conus and spinal nerves, partially resecting lipoma, releasing of tethered cord. Patients with comorbidities or an associated syrinx showed a higher risk of untethering procedures for LFT [12].

In surgical practice, however, this is always of some difficult primarily because filum adheres to varying degrees to surrounding neurologic structures; and secondly these patients always combined with some other malformations and the conus levels varied. Usually, intraoperative neuromonitoring is recommended.

In principle, a single-level laminectomy at L5 or S1 was performed. The filum was identified by visual inspection or by intraoperative monitoring, liberated from surrounding nerves.

23.4 Surgical Therapy for LFT

Patients are positioned prone under general anesthesia with supporting rolls on each side [13]. The routine procedure is the L5 laminectomy, and additional partial or complete S1 laminectomy is added in order to expose the dura and then to identify filum terminale. Laminotomy may also be selected for the exposure of the filum, especially in young children.

In cases of spinal bifida occulta, there is no need for laminectomy or laminotomy. Normally, the dural sac ends at the second sacral vertebra. In some circumstances, the spinal cord may continue until the S1 or S2 levels by giving some sacral rootlets, the laminectomy should be performed up to this level. The dura should be opened in the midline and tacked by four sutures bilaterally [13].

Following the dural opening, filum terminale, arachnoid bands, and rootlets should be first observed. Microsurgery with micro-instruments should be used after the dural opening. Filum terminale is a fibrovascular tag containing a large vessel, which becomes smaller across its course in the lumbar subdural space. However, this vessel is not a reliable landmark, because similar vessels can be found on the rootlets or no vessel may be seen on the filum terminale [13].

The most important issue at this time is the differentiation of the neural elements from extra-neural structures. Rootlets and arachnoid bands are mostly confused by the surgeons. The rootlets at the sacral levels are directed to both sides and may be identified by their size and situation. The intraoperative electrophysiological monitoring may be useful for safe surgery, but in the absence of this assortment, good neuroanatomical knowledge is required to preserve the neural structures. The rootlets are retracted laterally by microdissector in order to cut the arachnoid adhesions by microscissors and to expose the filum terminale [13].

In most cases, LFT is thicker than normal, violet in color and is attached to the dura posteriorly in the midline leaving barely no free subarachnoid space for cerebrospinal fluid (CSF) passage. LFT is coagulated and cut after the identification. The practical way to assess the degree of tethering is the immediate cranial movement of LFT right after releasing. This sudden cranial movement of the superior-edge of LFT resembles the movement of the string of a violin. In addition to sectioning the LFT, all connective tissues attached to the caudal part of the spinal cord should be released.

Filum terminale and nerve roots must be free from the surrounding tissues. In cases of dermal sinus, the tracts may be attached to the filum terminale or other fibrous bands, therefore, these structures should also be cut in order to release the spinal cord. Another useful measure of preventing retethering would be performing duraplasty in order to create a potent space allowing passage of CSF between lumbosacral rootlets and dura matter. The only way to prevent a recurrence in a detethered cord is to be certain that the neural elements remain free circumferentially with a patent CSF circulation [13].

23.5 Minimally Invasive Techniques

Besides classical open surgery, minimally invasive techniques involved endoscopic and mini-open approach were also reported [14, 15]. Intraoperative monitoring was introduced using needle electrodes to monitor lumbosacral nerve

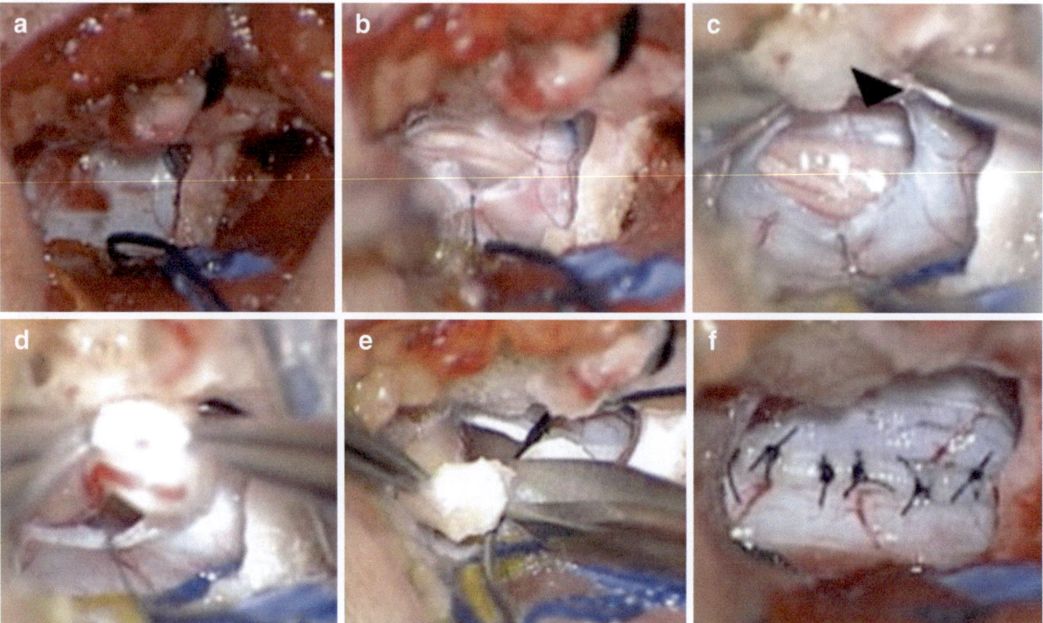

Fig. 23.2 Intraoperative findings of interlaminar approach. (**a**) Ligamentum flavum is incised and the epidural fat tissue is wiped off from the dural surface. (**b**) After dural incision, the arachnoid membrane is tacked to the dural edge. (**c**) Small dissector is inserted into the dural sac toward the posteromedial direction and scoop LFT (*arrow head*). (**d**) The LFT is pulled out from the dural sac. (**e**) The LFT is coagulated and then is sectioned. (**f**) Watertight closure of the dural incision. (Hayashi et al. Minimally Invasive Surgical Approach to Filum Lipoma. Neurol Med Chir (Tokyo). 2018;58(3):132–7)

roots. A 2-cm midline vertical incision was cut over the L4–5. The endoscopic tubular retractor was advanced over sequential dilators down to the ligamentum flavum. An endoscopic system was used for the procedure, and the lamina, ligamentum flavum, and dura were visualized endoscopically. Under endoscopic visualization, a small lumbar 5 laminotomy was performed with the endoscopic drill and the ligamentum flavum was opened with a kerrison rongeur. Then the endoscopic tubular retractor was removed, and an expandable minimally invasive retractor was advanced. The laminotomy was completed, and dural tacking sutures were placed on either side of the midline. The dura was incised vertically, followed by placing endoscope intradurally for visualizing the intrathecal contents. The key portions of the endoscopic procedure were to identify and section the filum terminale. The filum terminale was gentle pulled out of the small dural opening. Confirming that there were no motor responses to stimulating the filum, the filum was coagulated with a bipolar electrocoagulator, then sectioned with a micro-scissor. The dura was closed under microscopic visualization with a single purse string suture in a water-tight fashion.

Recently, Hayashi et al. [11] reported their useful experience of interlaminar approach (Fig. 23.2): A midline 1.5 cm skin incision was performed at the level of the L5 vertebra. After making the skin incision, a periosteal elevator was inserted against the left side of the spinous process to strip the periosteum. Then, the adjacent interspinous ligament was incised to expose the ligamentum flavum. The ligamentum flavum was incised at its midpoint. After minimal electrocoagulation of the epidural fat tissue, the fat tissue was incised and dissected. The exposed dura was incised longitudinally and the arachnoid membrane was tacked to the dural edge, the fatty filum was distinguished by its thickness and pale color, and the yellow color of the fatty tissue. A small dissector was inserted into the dural sac toward the posteromedial direction, and the filum was pulled out. The fatty filum was stimulated, and no evoked electromyographic activity was observed. The filum was coagulated and sectioned. The sectioned filum was usually retracted upward, out of the microscopic field.

23.6 Postoperative Complications

Despite the low rate of postoperative complications following surgery for FTL [5, 7, 11], surgeons should describe these possible problems clearly to the patients and/or their family before surgery. Usami et al. [5] reported these complications in a series of 174 patients, such as infection, cerebrospinal fluid leaks, and pseudomeningocele. Study indicated that the complication of surgery was much lower by the means of intraoperative monitoring [7].

Recurrence of tethering was also observed in some researches. Some postoperative recurrent spinal cord tethering has been reported in FTL patients who have undergone transection of the fatty filum [16]. Ogiwara [16] reported 6 patients in 225 children (2.7%) in whom the filum retethered. Retethering of the spinal cord is a rare condition occurring after the sectioning of a fatty filum terminale [16]. Yong et al. [17] reported 13 patients (8.6%) in 152 patients went on to retether symptomatically at a median time of 23.4 months after the initial procedure.

23.7 Conclusion

LFT in adults likely represents an incidental finding on routine lumbosacral MRI. Special attention for LFT in children is mandatory as it may indicate clinical tethering in otherwise normal appearing lumbosacral spine [1]. Operation for LFT was simple and safe, surgical results were prominent, and the surgery improved the presentation of symptomatic patients and stopped the deterioration of the asymptomatic cases.

Intraoperative monitoring can be used judiciously based on the surgeon's experience. There is no standard protocol for the management of LFT. However, when surgery is discussed, the surgeon should always consider his experience and institutional practice, clinical signs and symptoms, the patient's age and combined conditions, the LFT appearance and its exact location, the relationship between the LFT and contiguous anatomic structures.

References

1. Al-Omari MH, Eloqayli HM, Qudseih HM, Al-Shinag MK. Isolated lipoma of filum terminale in adults: MRI findings and clinical correlation. J Med Imaging Radiat Oncol. 2011;55(3):286–90.
2. Brown E, Matthes JC, Bazan C 3rd, Jinkins JR. Prevalence of incidental intraspinal lipoma of the lumbosacral spine as determined by MRI. Spine (Phila Pa 1976). 1994;19(7):833–6.
3. Cools MJ, Al-Holou WN, Stetler WR Jr, Wilson TJ, Muraszko KM, Ibrahim M, La Marca F, Garton HJ, Maher CO. Filum terminale lipomas: imaging prevalence, natural history, and conus position. J Neurosurg Pediatr. 2014;13(5):559–67.
4. Uchino A, Mori T, Ohno M. Thickened fatty filum terminale: MR imaging. Neuroradiology. 1991;33(4):331–3.
5. Usami K, Lallemant P, Roujeau T, James S, Beccaria K, Levy R, Di Rocco F, Sainte-Rose C, Zerah M. Spinal lipoma of the filum terminale: review of 174 consecutive patients. Childs Nerv Syst. 2016;32(7):1265–72.
6. Arai H, Sato K, Okuda O, Miyajima M, Hishii M, Nakanishi H, Ishii H. Surgical experience of 120 patients with lumbosacral lipomas. Acta Neurochir. 2001;143(9):857–64.
7. Lalgudi Srinivasan H, Valdes-Barrera P, Agur A, Soleman J, Ekstein M, Korn A, Vendrov I, Roth J, Constantini S. Filum terminale lipomas-the role of intraoperative neuromonitoring. Childs Nerv Syst. 2021;37(3):931–9.
8. Morota N, Ihara S, Ogiwara H. New classification of spinal lipomas based on embryonic stage. J Neurosurg Pediatr. 2017;19(4):428–39.
9. Tamura G, Morota N, Ihara S. Impact of magnetic resonance imaging and urodynamic studies on the management of sacrococcygeal dimples. J Neurosurg Pediatr. 2017;20(3):289–97.
10. Nonaka M, Ueno K, Isozaki H, Kamei T, Takeda J, Asai A. Familial tendency in patients with lipoma of the filum terminale. Childs Nerv Syst. 2021;37(5):1641–7.
11. Hayashi T, Kimiwada T, Kohama M, Shirane R, Tominaga T. Minimally invasive surgical approach to filum lipoma. Neurol Med Chir (Tokyo). 2018;58(3):132–7.
12. Kashlan ON, Wilkinson DA, Morgenstern H, Khalsa SS, Maher CO. Predictors of surgical treatment in

children with tethered fibrofatty filum terminale. J Neurosurg Pediatr. 2019:1–8.

13. Solmaz I, Izci Y, Albayrak B, Cetinalp E, Kural C, Sengul G, Gocmez C, Pusat S, Tuzun Y. Tethered cord syndrome in childhood: special emphasis on the surgical technique and review of the literature with our experience. Turk Neurosurg. 2011;21(4):516–21.

14. Potts MB, Wu JC, Gupta N, Mummaneni PV. Minimally invasive tethered cord release in adults: a comparison of open and mini-open approaches. Neurosurg Focus. 2010;29(1):E7.

15. Telfeian AE, Punsoni M, Hofstetter CP. Minimally invasive endoscopic spinal cord untethering: case report. J Spine Surg. 2017;3(2):278–82.

16. Ogiwara H, Lyszczarz A, Alden TD, Bowman RM, McLone DG, Tomita T. Retethering of transected fatty filum terminales. J Neurosurg Pediatr. 2011;7(1):42–6.

17. Yong RL, Habrock-Bach T, Vaughan M, Kestle JR, Steinbok P. Symptomatic retethering of the spinal cord after section of a tight filum terminale. Neurosurgery. 2011;68(6):1594–601; discussion 1601–1592.

Incidental Spinal Cysts of Lumbosacral Region

Anita Jagetia, Shaam Bodeliwala,
and Prashant Bipinchandra Lakhe

24.1 Introduction

The incidentally found cystic lesions in lumbar or sacral region are Tarlov (perineural) cyst, anterior sacral meningocele, and facet cyst.

24.2 Tarlov Cyst

24.2.1 Introduction

Tarlov cyst (TC) was described by Isadore Tarlov in a post-mortem study in the year 1938 in Montreal. It is a type of extradural meningeal cyst arising from perineural space of the posterior sacral roots and ganglia filled with cerebrospinal fluid (CSF) in the sacral spinal canal [1]. Nabors et al. classified meningeal cysts into three types: Type I is extradural meningeal cysts without spinal nerve root fibres; Type II is extradural meningeal cysts with spinal nerve root fibres; and Type III is spinal intradural meningeal cysts [2]. Accordingly, TC is a type II meningeal cyst; however, its main diagnosis is histopathological. Histopathologically, cyst wall consists of membranous tissue with peripheral nerve fibres and ganglionic cells embedded into connective tissue. Presence of spinal nerve root fibres in the cyst wall or in its cavity is characteristic of TC. Voyadzis et al. found nerve fibres in cyst wall in 75% of cases [3].

24.2.2 Pathogenesis

The aetiology of TC formation is unclear. Dilated perineural sheaths are connected with subarachnoid space through micro-connections. "Ball valve theory" states that pulsatile and hydrodynamic unidirectional CSF flow aided by gravitational force fill these cysts. These cysts keep increasing in size and may become symptomatic. Un-valved cysts result due to bidirectional flow of CSF in which CSF circulates in and out of cyst, would cause small and asymptomatic cysts [4]. These cysts are usually multiple. Trauma can lead to interruption of venous drainage in the perineurium and epineurium secondary to hemosiderin deposition. This is associated with inflammation of nerve root, arachnoid proliferation along and around the sacral nerve root and inoculation of fluid. Trauma has been found in about 40% of cases. The presence of nerve fibres, ganglionic cells, or signs of micro-haemorrhage in the form of hemosiderin favours trauma as the cause [5]. Park et al. suggested genetic origin based on their observations of two surgically treated cases of symptomatic sacral TCs in one family [6].

A. Jagetia (✉) · S. Bodeliwala · P. B. Lakhe
Department of Neurosurgery, G.B. Pant Institute of Postgraduate Medical Education and Research,
New Delhi, India

24.2.3 Clinical Presentation

Individuals are often asymptomatic, and these cases are increasingly detected due to rise in magnetic resonance imaging (MRI) screening for backache which may be unrelated to these lesions. Incidence of asymptomatic TC is 1–5% and of symptomatic is approximately 1% or even less [6, 7]. Their presentation is related to S2, S3, and S4 nerve roots. The onset of symptoms may be acute or chronic. It can manifest with symptoms similar to disc prolapse, pelvic pathologies, or other compressive lumbar spine diseases such as low-back pain, sacrococcygeal pain, perineal pain, sciatica, leg weakness, neurogenic claudication, bowel and bladder dysfunction, and sexual dysfunction. Symptoms are exacerbated by coughing, standing, and change of position which may be due to increase in CSF pressure leading to an activation of ball valve mechanism, and symptomatic relief can be achieved in recumbent position. Big cysts can present as backache due to erosion of surrounding sacral bone causing fracture and irritation of the periosteal pain fibres. Confounding conditions like fibromyalgia, degenerative disc disease, reflex sympathetic dystrophy, Chiari malformation surgery, Marfan's syndrome, prior laminectomy and discectomy, prior partial spinal fusion, and prior repair of spinal cord tethering may be associated with TC [8–10].

24.2.4 Preoperative Evaluation

Plain X-ray of lumbosacral spine may be normal or may show localized bone erosion or foraminal enlargement in large cysts. MRI is diagnostic and would show cystic lesion in sacral region with low signal on T1- weighted images and high signal on T2-weighted images similar to CSF. (Fig. 24.1). Size of communication with subarachnoid space should also be defined as this is one of the deciding factors for treatment selection. Scalloping of the sacral vertebral body or posterior elements can be seen on MRI and computed tomography (CT) which is caused by chronic pressure. Conventional MRI cannot differentiate valved and non-valved TCs, it requires intrathecal administration of contrast MRI or CT myelography. Late filling of TCs which can happen even hours after injection of contrast suggests valve mechanism. Myelography is an invasive method, not routinely advocated. These

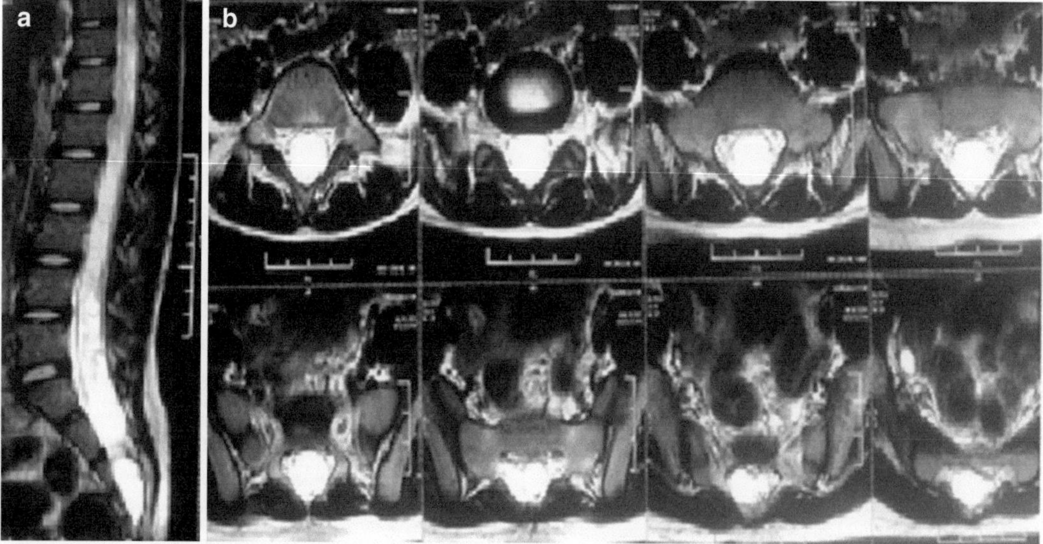

Fig. 24.1 Magnetic resonance imaging (MRI) lumbosacral spine, sagittal (**a**) and axial (**b**) cuts: showing hyperintense Tarlov cyst (TC) at S4–5 level, occupying the spinal canal more on right side

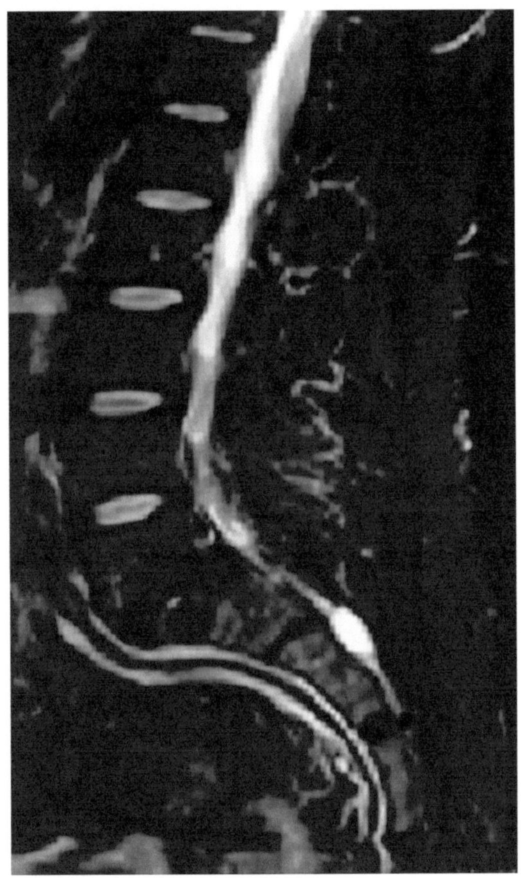

Fig. 24.2 Sagittal MRI lumbosacral spine showing L5-S1 listhesis with TC at S2 level

cysts may be found in association with other spinal diseases such as spondylolisthesis, spinal tumours, lumbar canal stenosis, etc. (Fig. 24.2). CT scan is very useful diagnostic modality as bony details and treatment planning are based on it for aspiration and glue injection [7, 11, 12].

24.2.5 Patient Selection and Treatment

There are no universal guidelines for surgical or conservative management of symptomatic TCs. Patients with severe pain, neurological symptoms, symptomatic patients with cyst >1.5 cm in size, multiple cysts having one with more than 1.5 cm in size are indications for treatment [3, 9, 13].

Conservative treatment with analgesics and physiotherapy is advocated to patients presenting with mild backache. Mitra et al. [4] treated even symptomatic perineural cyst patients with conservative management successfully. Primary pathologies in the form of tumours, disc prolapse, or canal stenosis when associated with TC, main aim is the treatment of primary pathology as TC is often incidental or TC may be the secondary cause of symptoms. Isolated symptomatic TC requires attention. This requires to be carefully evaluated to confirm corelation between clinical and radiological findings.

24.2.6 Surgical Procedures

Primary aim of surgery is to close the communication between the subarachnoid space and cyst wall with or without excision of cyst wall. Alternative way of management is decompression of the cyst by placing the catheter in the sac or subarachnoid space and making CSF diversion to abdominal cavity. However, this is not a preferred method as it is associated with complications related to shunt placement such as malfunction, infection.

There is no consensus for ideal treatment for TC; however, following methods are advocated for symptomatic cases:

1. Minimally invasive treatment:
   (a) CT-guided aspiration with or without instillation of glue: Percutaneous CT-guided aspiration of cyst can alleviate the symptoms but there is tendency for re-accumulation of fluid causing recurrence of symptoms. Recurrence can be prevented by local injection of fibrin glue (Baxter) after aspiration. The contraindication for fibrin glue injection is a wide communication with the thecal sac as injection of fibrin will result in dissemination through CSF resulting in arachnoiditis. Murphy [12] described the CT-guided technique of aspiration as single needle, double needle, or coaxial needle aspiration and glue injection.

Vertebroplasty needly can be used to penetrate the lamina under the CT guidance when doing single needle aspiration, whereas 15 cm long 18 gauze needle can be inserted through the vertebroplasty needle to make it a coaxial system. In two needle technique, one needle is placed in superficial plane and other is in deeper plane. One needle is used to aspirate the fluid, whereas the other is kept open to air so while aspirating the cyst content, through the other needle air will go in the cyst and will keep it visible and expanded. After aspiration, the Tisseel glue (Baxter) in injected into the cavity. The amount of glue injected is similar to the amount of CSF aspirated from the cyst. Before aspiration and injection of glue, the size of communication can be checked by injecting radio-opaque dye in the cyst.

(b) Lumbo-peritoneal shunt: This mode of treatment has been suggested for patients with multiple cysts. Lumbo-peritoneal shunt reduces the CSF pressure rostral to cyst and this in turn would reduce pressure inside the cyst as there is valve mechanism between the subarachnoid space and cyst. This mode of treatment avoids direct manipulation of cyst [14–16].

2. Sacral laminectomy or laminoplasty and microsurgical excision of cyst: Cyst excision should be done precisely avoiding sacrifice of the nerve root. Various other methods are also suggested such as suture the wall of the cyst in a purse string manner, neck ligation, close the communication of the cyst with subarachnoid space, fenestration of cyst in thecal space. Some authors have sacrificed the root without any deficit; however, intraoperative nerve conduction velocity (NCV) and electromyography might help in decision-making. Before closing the dura, cyst cavity may be filled with gelatine sponge with or without fibrin glue, muscle and fat avoiding over packing to avoid future recurrence. Cysto-subarachnoid shunt is an alternative to aiming for excision of sac after performing laminectomy [3, 9, 13, 17–20]. Summary of series reported in literature of cases of TCs is tabulated in Table 24.1.

Table 24.1 Summary of series of Tarlov cyst (TC) patients treated surgically

Study	Number of cases	procedure	Success rate	Complications
Kunz et al. (1999) [21]	8	NA	38%	NA
Mummaneni et al. (2000) [13]	8	SL + CF + Cl	88%	None
Voyadzis et al. (2001) [3]	10	SL + CR + NL + FG + gelfoam	70%	Urinary incontinence
Caspar et al. (2003) [17]	15	SL + CR	87%	None
Lee et al. (2004) [11]	2	CT + NA; SL + CR + NL + Cl	100%	None
Langdown et al. (2005) [22]	3	SL + CR + MP	100%	CSF leak, cauda equina syndrome
Tanaka et al. (2006) [19]	12	SL + CR + Cl|	71%	Prostatitis, posterior fossa bleeding
Zang et al. (2007) [10]	31	CT-NA + FI	80%	Fever, headache
Guo et al. (2007) [9]	11	SL + CR + CI + FG + MP + gelfoam	82%	CSF leak, bladder dysfunction
Park et al. (2008) [6]	2	SL + CR + FG + gelfoam	100%	None
Sajko et al. (2009) [23]	3	CF + FG	100%	None
Neulen et al. (2011) [18]	13	SL + CF + CR	>50%	CSF leak
Murphy et al. (2011) [12]	122	CT + NA &FI; SL + CF + FP	65%;63%	Transient urticaria
Mayur et al. (2015) [24]	3	L/HL + excision/marsupialization with or without glue	100%	CSF leak

Abbreviations: *NA* Not applicable, *SL* Sacral laminectomy, *CF* Cyst fenestration, *Cl* Cyst imbrication, *CR* Cyst resection, *NL* Neck ligation (of cyst), *FG* Fibrin glue, *MP* Muscle patch, *CT-NA & FI* CT-guided needle aspiration and fibrin injection, *L/HL* Laminectomy/hemilaminectomy, *FP* Fat packing

24.2.7 Post-Procedure Outcome

Zhang [10] reported 80% improvement in 31 patients treated with CT-guided aspiration with or without glue injection, whereas a large series of 122 patients treated by Murphy et al. [12] using aspiration followed by glue injection showed 65% improvement and 23% showed symptoms recurrence in 7 months' time. Percutaneous procedures have been found to be associated with development of aseptic meningitis. Open surgery with packing of cavity may cause cauda equina-like symptoms [20]. It may be associated with CSF leak which can be avoided using lumbar drainage for 3–7 days. Symptomatic improvement is seen in 38–100% cases treated by open technique.

Caspar et al. [17] reported improvement in 87% patients with complaints of radicular pain, 90% with sensory, and 10% with motor deficit or bladder and bowel dysfunction. Contrary to this Neurlen et al. [18] suggested no improvement in radicular symptoms as permanent impairment of nerve happens which causes chronic pain because of deafferentation. Patients with multiple cysts or single cyst of >1 cm size and whose symptoms increase by postural changes show improvement following surgery [3].

24.3 Lumbar Facet Cysts

24.3.1 Introduction

Lumbar facet cysts (LFCs) were first described in 1960s as ganglion cyst adjacent to lumbar facet joints [25]. The other nomenclature for this entity is juxta-facet cysts, cystic formation of mobile spine, lumbar intraspinal facet cysts, synovial cysts, and pseudocysts. Christophis et al. [26] described it as cystic malformation of the mobile spine and described heterogenous composition of LFC, in relation to facet joint and in ligamentum flavum. Komp et al. [27] evaluated 94 cysts during endoscopic removal and reported 67% had mucoid, 19% serous, and 14% had haemorrhagic

content. Wilby et al. [28] analysed en block resection specimen in 27 patients, and Kusakabe et al. [29] reviewed 46 specimens. Articular cartilage, bone fragment, fibrinoid, myxoid, and haemorrhagic contents are found in the cyst. Cyst wall contains fibrinoid material, granulation, vessel proliferation, and calcification. LFCs are commonly associated with degenerative spondylolisthesis as adjacent disc, and facet degeneration is found in 54–92% of cases [30–32].

24.3.2 Selection and Preoperative Evaluation

Complete neurological examination including sensory, motor, and reflexes is required to document any neurological deficit. Commonest presentation is radiculopathy (69.6%), followed by low-back pain (48.3%), sensory symptoms (34.6%), and neurogenic claudication (28.2%). There can be sudden deterioration in symptoms which is attributed to facet cyst hematoma. Standing X-ray lumbosacral spine along with full length standing radiograph should be taken to evaluate global alignment and spinopelvic parameters. Dynamic flexion and extension X-rays to see subtle segmental instability. MRI and CT myelography are required to evaluate the neural elements, soft tissue, and bony elements. Commonest location of FC is L4–5 (68%), followed by L3–4 and L5–S1 [33]. Classically, they appear isointense or hypointense inner core on T1-weighted images and hyperintense centre with hypointense rim on T2-weighted sequence of MRI with peripheral ring enhancement on gadolinium contrast administration, however may appear hypointense on T1 and hyperintense on T2-weighted images (Fig. 24.3). Haemorrhage inside the cyst may show various stage blood products. Subacute blood can appear hyperintense because of meth-haemoglobin [34]. Positional MRI protocols increase the detection rate of these cysts as detection rate is 97% in standing position compared to 89% in supine position [35] and is due to increase in cyst size in standing position.

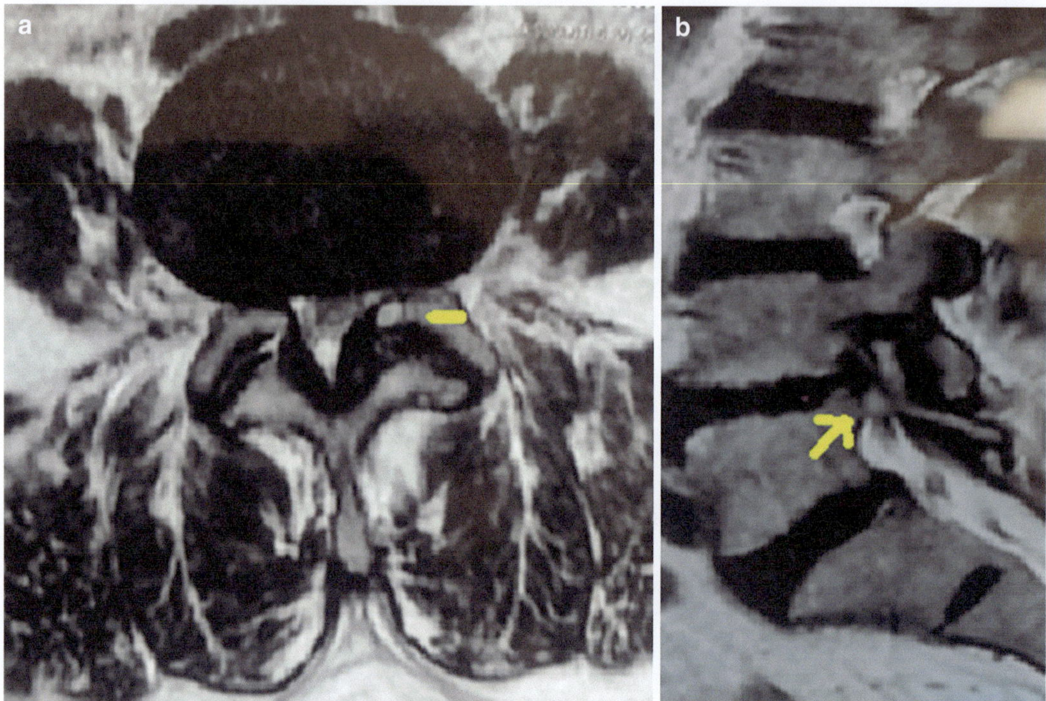

Fig. 24.3 MRI lumbosacral spine axial (**a**) and sagittal (**b**) cuts showing a small facet cyst on left side (arrow yellow coloured) at L4–5 level with no canal compromise

Management: Cysts with mild to moderate symptoms can be managed conservatively using anti-inflammatory drugs, physiotherapy, and lumbar brace.

24.3.3 Minimally Invasive Treatment

Symptomatic patients not relieved by medical management can be managed by C-arm fluoroscopy or CT-guided aspiration or percutaneous rupture of the cyst, and percutaneous steroid injection. Martha et al. [32] studied 101 patients subjected to percutaneous steroid injection and attempted cyst rupture and noted 81% success in rupture of the cyst. They achieved 79% response to treatment and 54% required surgery for persistent symptoms. High or intermediate signal on MRI suggests that high fluid composition of cyst and percutaneous rupture rates of these cysts are higher than hypointense cyst which suggests gelatinous or calcified composition of cyst. Aspiration method does not require extensive ligament and muscle dissection therefore less likely to cause instability.

24.3.4 Surgical Intervention

Surgical intervention is reserved for patient's refractory to conservative treatment or presenting with radiculopathy or neurogenic claudication, cauda equina syndrome. It includes laminectomy or hemilaminectomy with medial facetectomy and partial or complete cyst excision, root decompression which may or may not be followed by fusion. Laminotomy can also be considered in place of laminectomy. Cyst is caught with allies or tooth forceps, dissected off the dura and one may leave a thin wall of cyst adherent to dura to avoid dural tear. Any sign of instability should prompt for spinal fixation. If it is associated with central canal stenosis, bilateral root decompression is required. Endoscopic interlaminar, transforaminal approaches can be used to excise the cyst.

24.3.5 Postoperative Complications

Complications associated with LFC excision are iatrogenic spondylolisthesis, dural tear, CSF leak, deep vein thrombosis, and re-surgery. These cysts are often adherent to dura, which makes complete excision either difficult or attempt to excise leads to dural tear. Dural tear can happen during revision surgery for subsequent fixation due to mechanical instability following cyst excision. Epstein [36] noted 16.7% incidence of CSF fistula formation in patients subjected to revision surgery for instability versus 3.8% without revision. This is perhaps due to adhesions to dura which occurs in 50–55% of cases [37]. To avoid this complication to happen, partial cyst excision is recommended in cases where cyst is densely adherent to dura. Fusion at the time of cyst excision may decrease the rate LFC recurrence and mechanical back pain, however risk of adjacent segmental disease and pseudo-arthrosis should be considered. Compared with hemilaminectomy, instrumentation with facetectomy is associated with increases hospital stay (2.9 vs 5.8 days), dural tear (3.9 vs 21.4 days), intraoperative blood loss (125 mL vs 600 mL), and wound infection rate (0 vs 7.1%) [33].

24.4 Anterior Sacral Meningocele

24.4.1 Introduction

Anterior sacral meningocele (ASM) is a rare form of spinal cystic pathology which can be congenital or acquired. It was first described by Bryant in the year 1837 [38]. Wall of the sac is double layered consisting of outer dura and inner arachnoid which protrudes through the anterior sacral defect into retroperitoneal presacral space from the sacral spinal canal [39]. It is commoner in females with the female and male ratio is 4:1. The sac can be incidentally detected during a vaginal or rectal digital examination for obstetric and gynaecological problems such as dystocia, dyspareunia and sometimes diagnosed during antenatal examination [40]. It can happen due to spinal dysraphism or dysplasia of sacral foramina [41, 42].

24.4.2 Patient Selection and Preoperative Evaluation

The manifestation of the disease is nonspecific. It can present as constipation, pain abdomen, urinary retention, incontinence or urgency, postural headaches, and radiculopathy. These symptoms are produced by the pressure exerted by the mass on pelvic organs, sacral nerve roots. Headache is due to alternating intracranial hypertension or hypotension which is caused by the CSF flowing through the communication into the subarachnoid space from the ASM or inversely. Neurological examination may reveal perineal hypoesthesia and anal sphincter hypotonia. Clinical syndromes associated with this disease is Currarino syndrome (combination of presacral mass, sacral defect, and an anorectal malformation also known as.

Currarino's triad) [40] which is a X-linked autosomal dominant disorder. Other diseases such as Marfan syndrome, connective tissue dysplasia, and bone abnormalities may also cause dural herniation and sacrum dysplasia. Other systemic association are duplication of urogenital tracts, anorectal malformations, uterus duplication, lipomas, and teratocarcinoma [43, 44].

Rectal and pelvic examination may reveal a smooth cystic mass. Plain X-ray lumbosacral spine would show sacral deformity known as scimitar sacrum also known as sickle-shaped sacrum or hemi-sacral agenesis. This occurs due to chronic pressure on sacrum and coccyx leading to erosion of both. CT and preferably 3D-CT would reveal sacral agenesis, bony abnormality, however it cannot delineate the size of communication between sac and subarachnoid space. It can be detected while doing ultrasound (US) for any pelvic symptoms, US can be a cheaper tool to follow these patients postoperatively to assess complete excision and recurrence. MRI is essen-

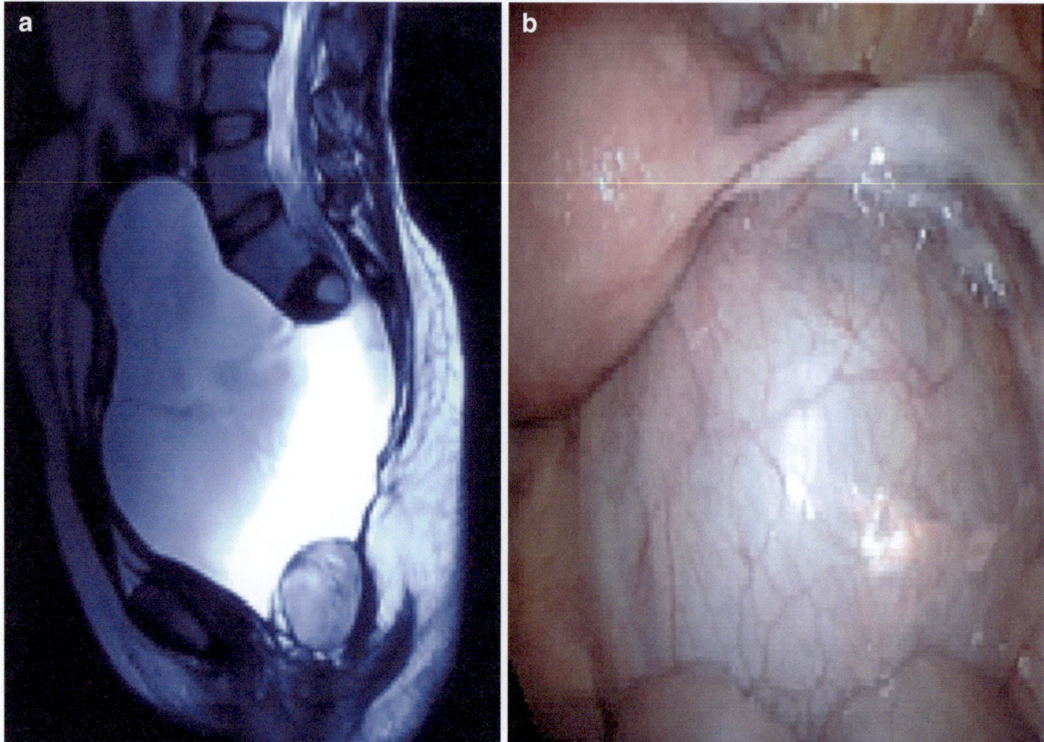

Fig. 24.4 (a) MRI pelvis showing a well-defined cerebrospinal fluid intensity lesion of approximately 12 × 12 × 19 cm in the presacral space with bifid sacrum and hypoplastic lower sacral bodies, displacing rectum, uterus and bladder anteriorly with intraspinal extension suggestive of anterior sacral meningocele. Sac contains solid part at posteroinferior region. (b) Intraoperative picture showing a large retroperitoneal mass bulging anterosuperiorly displacing the uterus

tial investigation and would reveal CSF intensity herniation of dural sac from anterior aspect of sacrum protruding into retroperitoneal space (Fig. 24.4a). Associated anomalies such as teratoma, epidermoid, other pelvic lesions, even bony details can also be identified.

24.4.3 Surgical Principles

Conservative treatment can be offered to those with small and asymptomatic cyst without any associated tumour. However, it should be kept in mind that this can cause death in females if not treated timely as it may cause pelvic obstruction during labour and rupture of it may cause meningitis.

The aim of surgery is to obliterate the communication between the subarachnoid space and the cyst, decompress the pelvis through drainage and excision of the sac, resect the associated tumour if any, and detether the spinal cord if necessary [40, 45]. Management of this entity may involve multiple specialty such as general surgeon, spine surgeon, obstetrics and genecology surgeon, and gastro-surgeon. Different approaches are described for the treatment of ASM such as transrectal or transvaginal aspiration, dorsal trans-sacral approach, and ventral transabdominal-transpelvic approach (for large intraabdominal lesion and a sac with large pedicles.) Other approaches are inferior presacral approach, oblique para-sacral approach of Demel and Coqui [46]. Posterior transsacral approach was advocated by Adson in 1938 and is most familiar approach to neurosurgeon with low complication rate [40]. Lumbar-peritoneal shunt is the minimally invasive procedure which can be offered; however, it is associated with all the complications related to shunt. Endoscopic/laparoscopic approach (Fig. 24.4b) is less invasive, does not require laminectomy, communication is obliterated and defect filled with fat grafts. Anterior transabdominal laparoscopic excision and repair can be done with the help of gastro-surgeons [47].

24.4.4 Postoperative Complications

Transrectal or transvaginal aspiration is associated with high mortality due to increased risk of severe complications such as meningitis, CSF fistula, and even death [48]. The transabdominal approaches are associated with risk of bowel injury or CSF leak [47]. There can be recurrence of cyst, so patient should be followed up in post-operative period.

24.5 Conclusion

First line of treatment of symptomatic TC and LFC is minimally invasive procedures. Symptomatic TC patients are assessed for size of communication between cyst and the subarachnoid space. Small communication cyst can be treated with CT-guided aspiration and glue injection. Patients who are not the candidates for aspiration such as with intraoperative detection of a high rate of refilling of cyst with CSF can be treated with laminectomy or laminoplasty, cyst fenestration, and fat packing. Other patients who do not improve, or have recurrent pain following aspiration/fibrin injection or surgery, can be re-evaluated for possible repeat aspiration/fibrin injection, surgery. Complete excision of LFC may not be possible many a times, which can be treated with partial excision. Excision to be followed by fixation or not is controversial, however studies report that fixation reduces the chances of recurrence and take care of backache. Small ASM also requires attention as it can be dangerous to have these in women of child bearing age. Both open and endoscopic or laproscopic excision and repair of ASM can be offered depending on the expertise available.

References

1. Tarlov IM. Cysts of the sacral nerve roots; clinical significance and pathogenesis. AMA Arch Neurol Psychiatry. 1952;68(1):94–108.
2. Nabors MW, Pait TG, Byrd EB, Karim NO, Davis DO, Kobrine AI, et al. Updated assessment and current classification of spinal meningeal cysts. J Neurosurg. 1988;68:366–77.
3. Voyadzis JM, Bhargava P, Henderson FC. Tarlov cysts: a study of 10 cases with review of the literature. J Neurosurg. 2001;95(1 Suppl):25–32.
4. Mitra R, Kirpalani D, Wedemeyer M. Conservative management of perineural cysts. Spine (Phila Pa 1976). 2008;33(16):E565–8.
5. Nishiura I, Koyama T, Handa J. Intrasacral perineurial cyst. Surg Neurol. 1985;23:265–9.
6. Park HJ, Jeon YH, Rho MH, Lee EJ, Park NH, Park SI, et al. Incidental findings of the lumbar spine at MRI during herniated intervertebral disk disease evaluation. AJR Am J Roentgenol. 2011;196:1151–5.
7. Paulsen RD, Call GA, Murtagh FR. Prevalence and percutaneous drainage of cysts of the sacral nerve root sheath (Tarlov cysts). AJNR Am J Neuroradiol. 1994;15:293–9.
8. Acosta FL Jr, Quinones-Hinojosa A, Schmidt MH, Weinstein PR. Diagnosis and management of sacral Tarlov cysts. Case report and review of the literature. Neurosurg Focus. 2003;15(2):E15.
9. Guo D, Shu K, Chen R, Ke C, Zhu Y, Lei T. Microsurgical treatment of symptomatic sacral perineurial cysts. Neurosurgery. 2007;60:1059–66.
10. Zhang T, Li Z, Gong W, Sun B, Liu S, Zhang K, et al. Percutaneous fibrin glue therapy for meningeal cysts of the sacral spine with or without aspiration of the cerebrospinal fluid. J Neurosurg Spine. 2007;7:145–50.
11. Lee JY, Impekoven P, Stenzel W, Löhr M, Ernestus RI, Klug N. CT-guided percutaneous aspiration of Tarlov cyst as a useful diagnostic procedure prior to operative intervention. Acta Neurochir. 2004;146:667–70.
12. Murphy KJ, Nussbaum DA, Schnupp S, Long D. Tarlov cysts: an overlooked clinical problem. Semin Musculoskelet Radiol. 2011;15:163–7.
13. Mummaneni PV, Pitts LH, McCormack BM, Corroo JM, Weinstein PR. Microsurgical treatment of symptomatic sacral Tarlov cysts. Neurosurgery. 2000;47:74–9.
14. Bartels RH, van Overbeeke JJ. Lumbar cerebrospinal fluid drainage for symptomatic sacral nerve root cysts: an adjuvant diagnostic procedure and/or alternative treatment? Technical case report. Neurosurgery. 1997;40:861–5.
15. Ju CI, Shin H, Kim SW, Kim HS. Sacral perineural cyst accompanying disc herniation. J Korean Neurosurg Soc. 2009;45:185–7.
16. Morio Y, Nanjo Y, Nagashima H, Minamizaki T, Teshima R. Sacral cyst managed with cyst-

subarachnoid shunt: a technical case report. Spine (Phila Pa 1976). 2001;26:451–4.

17. Caspar W, Papavero L, Nabhan A, Loew C, Ahlhelm F. Microsurgical excision of symptomatic sacral perineurial cysts: a study of 15 cases. Surg Neurol. 2003;59:101–6.

18. Neulen A, Kantelhardt SR, Pilgram-Pastor SM, Metz I, Rohde V, Giese A. Microsurgical fenestration of perineural cysts to the thecal sac at the level of the distal dural sleeve. Acta Neurochir (Wien). 2011;153:1427–34.

19. Tanaka M, Nakahara S, Ito Y, Nakanishi K, Sugimoto Y, Ikuma H, et al. Surgical results of sacral perineural (Tarlov) cysts. Acta Med Okayama. 2006;60:65–70.

20. Ishii K, Yuzurihara M, Asamoto S, Doi H, Kubota M. A huge presacral Tarlov cyst. Case report. J Neurosurg Spine. 2007;7:259–63.

21. Kunz U, Mauer UM, Waldbaur H. Lumbosacral extradural arachnoid cysts: diagnostic and indication for surgery. Eur Spine J. 1999;8:218–22.

22. Langdown AJ, Grundy JR, Birch NC. The clinical relevance of Tarlov cysts. J Spinal Disord Tech. 2005;18:29–33.

23. Sajko T, Kovać D, Kudelić N, Kovac L. Symptomatic sacral perineurial (Tarlov) cysts. Coll Antropol. 2009;33:1401–3.

24. Sharma M, Velho V, Mally R, Khan SW. Symptomatic lumbosacral perineural cysts: a report of three cases and review of literature. Asian J Neurosurg. 2015;10(3):222–5.

25. Kao CC, Uihlein A, Bickel WH, Soule EH. Lumbar intraspinal extradural ganglion cyst. J Neurosurg. 1968;29(2):168–72.

26. Christophis P, Asamoto S, Kuchelmeister K, Schachenmayr W: "Juxtafacet cysts," a misleading name for cystic formations of mobile spine (CYFMOS). Eur Spine J 2007; 16(9):1499–1505.

27. Komp M, Hahn P, Ozdemir S, et al. Operation of lumbar zygapophyseal joint cysts using a full-endoscopic interlaminar and transforaminal approach: prospective 2-year results of 74 patients. Surg Innov. 2014;21(6):605–14.

28. Wilby MJ, Fraser RD, Vernon-Roberts B, Moore RJ. The prevalence and pathogenesis of synovial cysts within the ligamentum flavum in patients with lumbar spinal stenosis and radiculopathy. Spine (Phila Pa 1976). 2009;34(23):2518–24.

29. Kusakabe T, Kasama F, Aizawa T, Sato T, Kokubun S. Facet cyst in the lumbar spine: radiological and histopathological findings and possible pathogenesis. J Neurosurg Spine. 2006;5(5):398–403.

30. Lyons MK, Atkinson JL, Wharen RE, Deen HG, Zimmerman RS, Lemens SM. Surgical evaluation and management of lumbar synovial cysts: the Mayo Clinic experience. J Neurosurg. 2000;93(1 suppl):53–7.

31. Parlier-Cuau C, Wybier M, Nizard R, Champsaur P, Le Hir P, Laredo JD. Symptomatic lumbar facet joint synovial cysts: clinical assessment of facet joint steroid injection after 1 and 6 months and long-term follow-up in 30 patients. Radiology. 1999;210(2):509–13.

32. Martha JF, Swaim B, Wang DA, et al. Outcome of percutaneous rupture of lumbar synovial cysts: a case series of 101 patients. Spine J. 2009;9(11):899–904.

33. Boody BS, Savage JW. Evaluation and treatment of lumbar facet cysts. J Am Acad Orthop Surg. 2016;24(12):829–42.

34. Miyatake N, Aizawa T, Hyodo H, Sasaki H, Kusakabe T, Sato T. Facet cyst haematoma in the lumbar spine: a report of four cases. J Orthop Surg (Hong Kong). 2009;17(1):80–4.

35. Niggemann P, Kuchta J, Hoeffer J, Grosskurth D, Beyer HK, Delank KS. Juxtafacet cysts of the lumbar spine: a positional MRI study. Skelet Radiol. 2012;41(3):313–20.

36. Epstein NE. Lumbar laminectomy for the resection of synovial cysts and coexisting lumbar spinal stenosis or degenerative spondylolisthesis: an outcome study. Spine (Phila Pa 1976). 2004;29(9):1049–55.

37. Scholz C, Hubbe U, Kogias E, Klingler JH. Incomplete resection of lumbar synovial cysts: evaluating the risk of recurrence. Clin Neurol Neurosurg. 2015;136:29–32.

38. Villarejo F, Scavone C, Blazquez MG. Anterior sacral meningocele: review of literature. Surg Neurol. 1983;19:57–71.

39. Somuncu S, Aritürk E, İyigün Ö, et al. A case of anterior sacral meningocele totally excised using the posterior sagittal approach. J Pediatr Surg. 1997;32:730–2.

40. Shedid D, Roger EP, Benzel EC. Presacral meningocele: diagnosis and treatment. Semin Spine Surg. 2006;18:161–7.

41. Gilete-Tejero IJ, Ortega-Martínez M, Mata-Gómez J, et al. Anterior sacral meningocele presenting as intracystic bleeding. Eur Spine J. 2018;27:276–80.

42. Wilkins RH. Lateral and anterior spinal meningoceles. In: Wilkins RH, Rengachary SS, editors. Neurosurgery, vol. III. 2nd ed. New York: McGraw-Hill; 1996. p. 3521–6.

43. Krivokapić Z, Grubor N, Micev M, et al. Anterior sacral meningocele with Presacral cysts: report of a case. Dis Colon Rectum. 2004;47:1965–9.

44. Kole MJ, Fridley JS, Jea A, et al. Currarino syndrome and spinal dysraphism. J Neurosurg Pediatr. 2014;13:685.

45. Schijman E, Rugilo C, Sevlever G, et al. Anterior sacral meningocele. Childs Nerv Syst. 2005;21:91–3.

46. Manson F, Comalli-Dillon K, Moriaux A. Anterior sacral meningocele: management in gynecological practice. Ultrasound Obstet Gynecol. 2007;30:893–6.

47. Jeon BC, Kim DH, Kwon KY. Anterior endoscopic treatment of a huge anterior sacral meningocele: technical case report. Neurosurgery. 2003;52(1231–3):1233–4.

48. Tani S, Okuda Y, Abe T. Surgical strategy for anterior sacral meningocele. Neurol Med Chir (Tokyo). 2003;43(4):204–20.

Batuk Diyora and Kavin Devani

25.1 Introduction

The incidental radiological finding is defined as an abnormal lesion that is unrelated to the primary pathology for which the imaging was requested [1]. Since the advent of advanced imaging techniques, increasing anxiety among the citizens, and increased accessibility of imaging methods, an increasing number of patients are over investigated [2]. As a result, we encounter more clinically insignificant lesions unrelated to why the scan was primarily done, making the patient anxious and unnecessary intervention. It can also lead to failure to identify the severe condition, masqueraded by the incidental finding causing the diagnostic delay. Thus, it becomes inevitable for all to have adequate knowledge about such lesions as many such lesions are asymptomatic and clinically insignificant. Lower back pain is the commonest complaint when a patient consults a physician [3]. Following clinical examination of such patients, radiological imaging is asked for. Also, patients with trauma undergo thorough spinal imaging replacing basic imaging using radiography. As a result of such imaging, many incidental lesions are detected.

Incidental spinal lesions are divided into intraosseous vertebral lesions and intraspinal lesions. The vertebrae comprise of the most common site. Almost 70–80% of incidentally detected lesions are located in vertebrae [4]. Vertebral hemangiomas, intraosseous tumors, and metastasis comprise of intraosseous vertebral lesions. Intraspinal lesions are comparatively less common. They can further be divided into either extradural or intradural locations. Intraspinal, extradural lesions consist of Tarlov cysts, fibrolipoma, tethered cord, and thickened filum terminale [5]. Intraspinal, intradural lesions composed of meningioma, schwannoma, neurofibroma, and intramedullary lesions like myxopapillary ependymoma [6]. Computed tomography (CT) and magnetic resonance imaging (MRI) play a crucial role in their diagnosis. CT scan helps differentiate the lesions affecting the vertebral column and demonstrates the amount of destruction caused by the lesion and instability. MRI helps to delineate the location of the lesion along with its detailed characteristics. Often times, there are instances when the patient is screened for disc prolapse, and a tumor is found adjacent to the herniated disc [7]. Also, these tumors can be incidentally discovered during the latent period when they are in their growing state [8]. Thus, one must keep a timely follow-up of such lesions and intervene at the right time before any permanent neuro deficit sets in.

Park et al. published one of the largest series of MRIs of 1268 patients; only 8.4% of patients had incidental findings, out of which none of the

B. Diyora (✉) · K. Devani
Department of Neurosurgery, LTMMC <MG Hospital, Sion Hospital, Mumbai, Maharashtra, India

M. Turgut et al. (eds.), *Incidental Findings of the Nervous System*,
https://doi.org/10.1007/978-3-031-42595-0_25

patients had any tumors. Less than 0.05% of patients are found to have incidental tumors [9–11]. MRI characteristics of these lesions give a fair idea of how aggressive a tumor is going to be. Iso to hypodense tumors with hyperintensity and rim enhancement on post gadolinium contrast administration are slow-growing tumors, whereas hyperdense and hyperintense tumors grow rapidly [10]. The management of these tumors depends on their size and neurological symptoms. Smaller tumors can initially be followed with regular imaging until significant growth is observed. Stereotactic radiosurgery is gaining popularity as a non-operative treatment option. Patients readily accept it, who do not wish to undergo surgical intervention. They lead to tumor shrinkage over 34 to 36 months and resolution of the symptoms [12].

25.2 Spinal Meningioma

Meningiomas are the most common tumors which a neurosurgeon encounters. They are dural-based, benign, slow-growing, extra-axial neoplasm which arises from the arachnoid cap cells or the meningothelial cells. They can be present anywhere along the craniospinal axis. They usually manifest during the fourth to seventh decade and show female predominance [13]. Of all the meningioma encountered along the craniospinal axis, spinal meningioma accounts for 12% of these lesions [14]. They are commonly found along the spinal axis in the thoracic (67–84%) region, followed by the cervical (14–27%) and the lumbar region(2–14%) [15, 16] Symptomatic lesions usually present with local and radicular pain (27.6%). They also present with the motor deficit (84%), sensory deficits (63%), and gait disturbances. Uncommonly they can present with bowel and bladder disturbances (23.3%) [17]. However, patients in whom these lesions are incidentally detected are usually asymptomatic or have mild backache. MRI is the gold standard investigation for their management. These tumors are extra-axial, T1 isointense to hypointense, and T2 hyperintense lesions, with intense post-contrast enhancement. A dural tail is associated with these lesions. However, certain meningioma, smaller in size, are detected incidentally while investigating for some other pathology (Fig. 25.1), viz. trauma, or while screening neurofibromatosis patients. Ideally, the management goals of meningioma are spi-

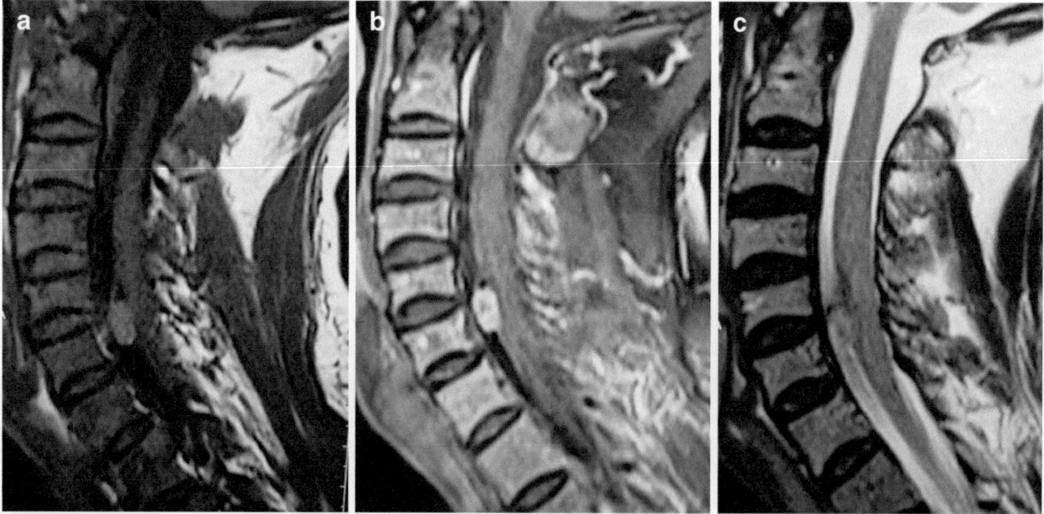

Fig. 25.1 Magnetic resonance imaging (MRI) of cervical spine sagittal view showing contrast enhancing lesion at the level of C5–6 (**b**) which appears iso to hyperintense on T1-weighted images (**a**) and iso to hyperintense on T2-weighted images (**c**) suggestive of meningioma

nal cord decompression and complete tumor removal. Recent advancements have led to minimally invasive spine procedures via endoscopic or microsurgical tubular system. The tumor via these techniques is approached via para-spinal approach, and a hemilaminectomy centered over the lesion is done, preserving the para-spinal scaffold of the muscles, facet, and tension bands [18]. Also, intraoperative neuromonitoring should be performed whenever feasible [19]. Some of the most significant post-operative complications include cerebrospinal fluid (CSF) leak and secondary meningitis. About 80% of the patients achieve complete recovery post-surgery, whereas the rest of the patients have some of the other deficits or deterioration [20].There have been reports that the meningioma has spontaneously regressed for unknown reasons [21]. Small incidentalomas can be managed conservatively. The treating physician should examine the patients in detail and carefully look for signs of early myelopathy where the patient may not have any clinical symptoms. So patients without clinical symptoms but the presence of subtle signs of myelopathy with the sizable lesion, it is wise to consider for surgical intervention. For patients without clinical symptoms and signs, it is absolutely necessary for the treating physician to explain the patient and family as well as referring physician in detail. Patients and referring physician should be counseled about the incidental nature of the tumor, absence of clinical symptoms and signs related to it, their natural course and rate of progress, observation for red flag signs and frequent follow-up. However, surgical intervention is also warranted if the lesion is large enough to cause significant compression or neurological deficit.

However, surgical intervention is warranted if the lesion is large enough to cause significant compression or neurological deficit. It is proposed by Raimund et al. that the annual growth rate of meningioma is 0.5–21%, with a median rate of 3.6% [22]. According to a study by Makoto et al., the annual growth rates were less than 1 cm^3/year [15]. Considering the slower growth rates, one can expectantly manage smaller, incidentally found, asymptomatic meningiomas.

25.3 Schwannoma

Schwannoma, neurinomas, or neurilemmomas are benign, encapsulated, slow-growing, extra-axial nerve sheath tumors originating from Schwann cells. They can occur anywhere in the central or peripheral nervous system [23]. According to the report by Michael et al., these lesions are common in the cervical region (44%) followed by the lumbosacral area (40%), with only 16% cases encountered at the thoracic level [24]. Most spinal schwannomas are intradural; however, 30% of these tumors extend along the nerve root and are located extradural [25]. They can be classified according to Modified Shridhar Classification [26]. Approximately 90% of lesions are single and sporadic, and only 4% are associated with neurofibromatosis (NF) type 2. About 5% of tumors are multiple and do not show any association with NF type 2 [27]. Their presentation is varied and depends on their location. They can present with radiculopathy, followed by paraesthesia and motor deficits. The sacral region schwannomas can present with sacral paraesthesia and dysesthesia, constipation, urinary retention, or incontinence [28]. They affect the sensory nerves, and 75% appear in the sensory dorsal roots. They have a strong association with NF type 2 [29]. Benign lesions are isointense on T1-weighted images and hyperintense on T2-weighted images with intense post-contrast enhancement [29]. Sacral schwannomas spread anteriorly and posteriorly, due to which they present late. Often patients are investigated for bowel or bladder complaints that initially have resulted because of anterior extension of the tumor, leading to accidental detection of these tumors [27].They warrant surgical excision almost all the time. Post-operatively, the neurological deficits persist to a lesser or greater degree. Togral et al. have documented a case of a 42-year-old female who had presented with left upper quadrant abdominal pain. A mass was identified on abdominal ultrasound. CT scan and MRI of the lumbosacral spine were requested, and she was found to have a giant invasive sacral schwannoma [30].

Spinal schwannoma has a different growth rate. Ogawa et al. reported an absolute growth of

139 mm³ per year and a relative growth rate of 2.3% ± 5.5% [24]. An idea of its aggressivity can be obtained from its MRI appearance. Those lesions which are homogenously hyperintense on T2-weighted images are hypocellular lesions, and they gradually transform and develop cystic changes. Such lesions can be followed up as they don't grow rapidly. Other lesions, which are isointense or heterogeneously hyperintense on T2-weighted images and showed homogenous enhancement on post-contrast T1-weighted images, are hypercellular and have associated cystic changes. Such lesions may undergo rapid expansion and warrant surgical excision [24]. There were instances when patients who underwent imaging for herniated discs were found to have a co-existing intradural schwannoma. For patients presenting with signs of upper and lower motor neuron lesions, one should suspect the tumors. In such cases, preoperative detection of such lesions positively impacts the outcome of the surgical intervention, as significant improvement is noted after the excision of both the lesions [31]. Surgical intervention always remains the primary option for symptomatic spinal schwannomas. However, the course of management of asymptomatic spinal schwannoma is unclear.

25.4 Spinal Metastasis

Spinal metastasis is is the most common spinal tumor. They usually present with bony involvement and occasionally also involve the spinal cord. They are most commonly encountered in the thoracic, followed by the lumbar and cervical region [30]. Primaries from breast, lung, prostate, kidney, gastrointestinal tract, and thyroid are known to metastasize to the spine in decreasing order. Often time patients only present with excruciating localized back pain. While evaluating such patients by doing MRI and CT imaging, one finds lytic or sclerotic lesions in the vertebrae with varying degrees of spinal cord compromise. Osteoblastic metastasis exhibits a hypointense appearance on T1- and T2-weighted images. Mixed sclerotic and lytic lesions are isointense on T1-weighted images and hypo to hyperintense

on T2-weighted images. Purely lytic metastasis is hypointense on T1-weighted images and hyper to isointense on T2-weighted images. They also show enhancement post-contrast administration [32]. Such incidental findings often lead to the discovery of the primary lesions.

Dual Energy X-Ray Absorptiometry (DEXA) is a gold standard method to study the bone mineral density (BMD). It is a screening tool used in elderly patients and post-menopausal females. It calculates the BMD at the lumbar spine from L1-L4 levels, femoral neck, and hip joint. Patients with raised BMD at these levels are suspected of having osteoblastic metastasis during such screening. On encountering such suspicious lesions, the patients should be advised to undergo CT and MRI scans. If lesions are confirmed on imaging, a religious search for the primary lesion, breast in females, and prostate in males should be carried out [33].

Further management is tailored according to the patient's needs and condition. The primary aim of any intervention is to maintain biomechanical stability and preserve neurological function [3]. If the patient is in good condition, with osteolytic metastasis, slowly progressive systemic disease, one must aim for anterior epidural decompression via anterior approach with vertebral body replacement and adjunctive therapy in the form of radiotherapy and chemotherapy. If the patient has pathological pain and a debilitating condition, kyphoplasty with biopsy and adjunctive radiotherapy and chemotherapy should be advised. In patients with osteoblastic metastasis, epidural compression and radiculopathy without instability should be subjected to only decompression and adjunctive radio-chemotherapy.

25.5 Ependymoma

Ependymomas are malignant tumors that arise from the lining of the ventricles or central canal of the spinal cord and are encountered in the intramedullary space. Histopathologically, they are divided into two main types—myxopapillary and cellular variety. The cellular variety of ependymoma is usually located in the cervical cord. In contrast, the myxopapillary variety is exclusively encountered in the conus medullaris and filum terminale and can be found incidentally [34]. In the lumbosacral region, they occur in the sacrum, presacral space, or dorsal sacral subcutaneous tissue. They have male predominance and are usually present in the fourth decade [35].They present with backache, radiculopathy, bladder, and bowel involvement. When the lesion is small, it might not cause enough symptoms. Such lesions might catch the attention when the patients are being investigated for other benign pathology. Occasionally patient can have multiple lesions in the entire spinal axis, and all may not be symptomatic (Fig. 25.2). They should be adequately imaged. MRI is the gold standard investigation for their evaluation. They are T1 isointense, and some substances like bleeding calcification can lead to a hyperintense appearance on T1-weighted imaging. The lesion is T2 hyperintense and shows enhancement post-contrast administration [36]. This lesion almost always warrants surgical intervention, even if

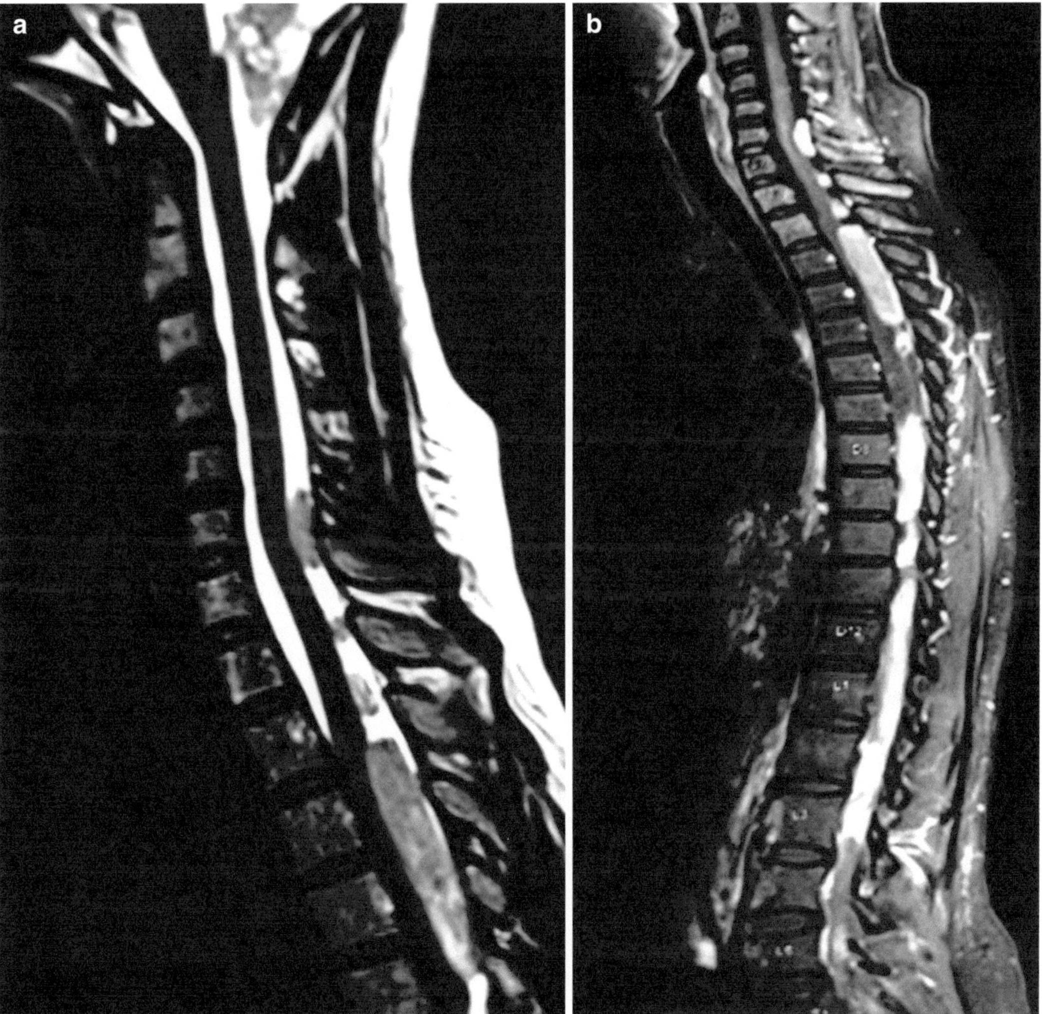

Fig. 25.2 MRI of cervicothoracic spine T2-weighted image sagittal view (**a**) showing multiple hypointense lesions at the C6-C7 level and D1-D5 level. MRI of the whole spine T1-weighted post-contrast image (**b**) showing multiple contrast enhancing lesions at lower cervical, thoracic, and lumbar levels

they are incidentally detected, followed by adjuvant therapy. These lesions should be aggressively treated as they tend to metastasize to other organs like lungs predominantly [36].

25.6 Neurofibromatosis and Associated Tumors

Neurofibromatosis is the most common neurocutaneous syndrome resulting from a mutation in the tumor suppressor genes, neurofibromin, and merlin, located on chromosomes 17q11.2 and 22q12 in neurofibromatosis type 1 and neurofibromatosis type 2, respectively. They are associated with multiple space-occupying lesions in the brain and spinal cord. NF-1 is associated with gliomas, predominantly low-grade pilocytic.

NF-1 can present with pheochromocytoma, myelodysplastic syndrome, osteosarcoma, and rhabdomyosarcoma outside the nervous system. NF-2 patients can develop multiple schwannomas, meningiomas, and ependymomas anywhere along the craniospinal axis. Among all vestibular schwannomas are most common.

These patients usually present with symptoms associated with cranial tumors. But before we intervene for cranial lesions, the patient must undergo whole spine screening. In patients with NF-1, symptomatic spinal cord tumors are encountered in 2% population. They usually present with impairment of sensation, pain, and paralysis. Patients with NF-2 have higher symptomatic affliction with spinal tumors up to 30–40%. These tumors seldom cause any neurological deficit in young patients when detected while screening (Fig. 25.3). They are known to cause neurological deficits in the geriatric age-group. In neurofibromatosis, 20% of tumors are astrocytic tumors, 3–4% are ependymomas, and 25–30% are meningiomas [15]. In such asymptomatic cases, counseling of the patients and family members is of utmost importance. They should be warned about possible symptoms and signs of such lesions and asked for an early follow-up.

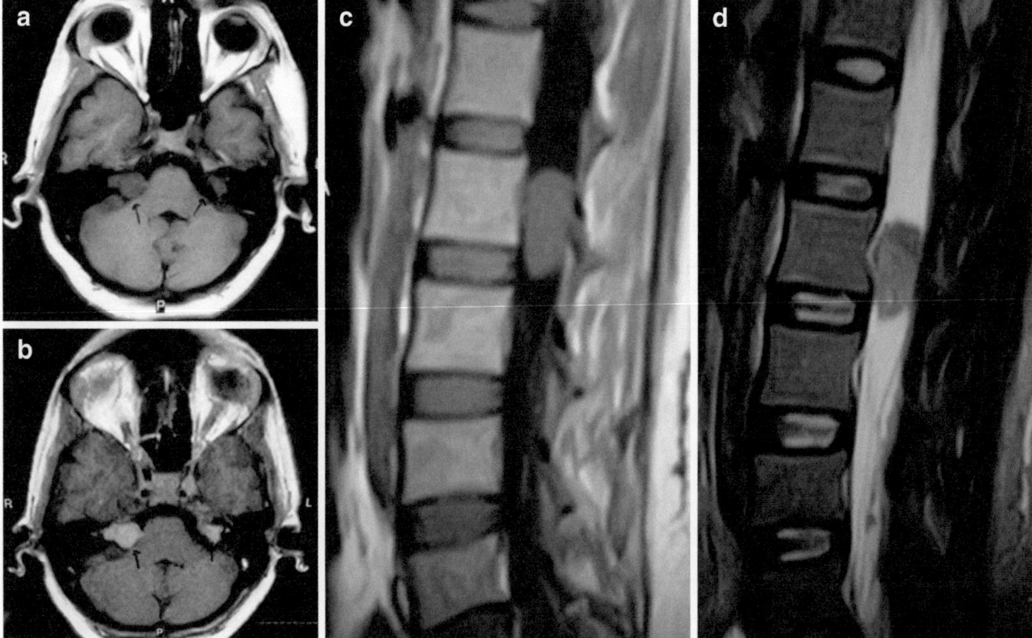

Fig. 25.3 MRI of brain axial view; T1-weighted image showing hypointense lesion at both cerebellopontine angles, extending into internal acoustic meatus causing its widening (**a**) and post-contrast image showing intensely enhancing lesion at both cerebellopontine angles (**b**), extending into internal acoustic meatus. MRI lumbar spine sagittal section showing a single, oblong, intradural, mass lesion at L2–L3 level which appears isointense on T1-weighted images (**c**) and hypointense on T2-weighted images (**d**)

25.7 Vertebral Hemangioma

Hemangioma (L. "angio" plus "oma") is a condition that is characterized by enlargement or proliferation of new blood vessels. Vertebral hemangioma is characterized by abnormal proliferation of capillary and venous structures [37]. They are the most common primary tumor of the spine [38]. They have been detected in 11% of patients at general autopsy [30]. They are commonly encountered in the older population and have slight female preponderance. They are commonly encountered in patients when investigated for thoracic and lumbar spine pathologies [34].They are usually asymptomatic; however, few patients can present with vague symptoms like varying degrees of back pain. Some lesions extending to the neural foramina or spinal canal can present with the neurogenic spine [39]. Less than 1% of these lesions are also associated with the pathologic fracture of the vertebral body and resulting in myelopathy or radiculopathy due to cord compression by the osseous fragments. The exact etiology which incites this abnormal proliferation of new blood vessels is unknown. The progression of the pathology is similar to the hemangiomas that occur elsewhere in the body. These lesions proliferate and erode the bone and can sometimes erode into the spinal canal. The most common presentation is that of localized and dull back pain. Advanced lesions can present with radiating pain or radiculopathies. There are two varieties of hemangiomas: cavernous and capillary hemangioma. Cavernous hemangioma involves large blood vessels, whereas capillary hemangioma involves thin-walled capillary vessels which are separated by a normal bone. The bone surrounding the lesion exhibits osteolysis [40].

Imaging helps evaluate the lesion size, site, extent, and degree of the lysis of the surrounding bone. The cord compression, foraminal narrowing, or nerve root compression should be evaluated. Cavernous hemangiomas have coarse vertical striations or honeycomb appearance on the plain radiograph, polka dot appearance on the CT imaging, and multiple flow-voids on MRI. Capillary types of hemangiomas have vertical striations on the plain radiograph with varying amounts of bone resorption, as appreciated on the CT imaging. They exhibit isointense and hyperintense signals on T1-weighted and T2-weighted imaging, respectively [1, 41].

Most of these lesions are without any symptoms so that they can be managed conservatively. Often these lesions are innocent bystanders. Thus, an aggressive search of other pathologies like metastasis or Paget's disease should be carried out before they are declared culprits. However, in severely symptomatic patients in whom hemangioma is causing severe discomfort, there are various methods to treat these lesions. Endovascular embolization has shown promising results to relieve the cord compression resulting from these lesions [41]. Other options include percutaneous vertebroplasty [42] and transpedicular ethanol injection [38].Given that these lesions are radiosensitive, radiotherapy has also been proposed in their management [38].

25.8 Tarlov Cyst

Tarlov cysts, also known as the perineural cyst, are CSF-filled saccular cysts formed within the sacral spinal canal outside the dura in the nerve roots of the lower spine, especially in the sacral region. They are formed within the nerve root sheath of the dorsal root ganglion. Tarlov first documented them in 1938 in one of the autopsy specimens [43]. Their incidence is thought to be between 1% and 5% [43, 44]. Nabors et al. have classified spinal meningeal cysts into three types [45]: Type 1—Extradural meningeal cysts without spinal nerve root fiber, Type 2—Extradural meningeal cysts with spinal nerve root fibers, which is Tarlov cyst, and Type 3—Spinal intradural meningeal cysts. It is a must for the presence of the spinal nerve root fibers in the cyst wall for the cyst or in its cavity for them to be labeled as the Tarlov cyst [46].

The various hypothesis has been postulated in the pathogenesis of the Tarlov cysts. It is believed that inflammation of the nerve root followed by inoculation of the fluid, arachnoid proliferation around the sacral nerve root, hampering of venous drainage in the perineurium and epineurium [47].Congenital causes and trauma are also thought to cause these cysts [12].

Most of these cysts are asymptomatic cysts. Occasionally, they may present vague complaints like lower backache, peri-anal pain, and motor symptoms, such as lower limb muscle weakness. They may also lead to neurogenic claudication, bowel, and bladder dysfunction. These symptoms exaggerate when the patient does any straining activity and relieves when the patient lies in the recumbent position [45, 48]. MRI is the investigation of choice for these lesions. They help to delineate the detailed anatomy and relation with the nerve roots. They appear as cystic lesions, which are hypointense on T1-weighted and hyperintense on T2-weighted images.

Occasionally several lobules of the cyst are found along with associated scalloping of the vertebrae. Usually, plain radiograph does not contribute to their diagnosis. Occasionally one may find the erosion of the spinal canal or the neural foramen. CT scan helps to better understand the bony changes [49].

Not all Tarlov cysts warrant treatment. When incidentally found, a religious search for other pathology to find the primary lesion should be carried out (Fig. 25.4). Most of these cysts are managed conservatively by expectant management. However, in some of these cysts, if the pain is inevitable, medical management with analgesics and steroids is administered [48, 50]. Often, this leads to complete resolution of the symptoms. CT-guided aspiration is another option for their management. However, they are associated

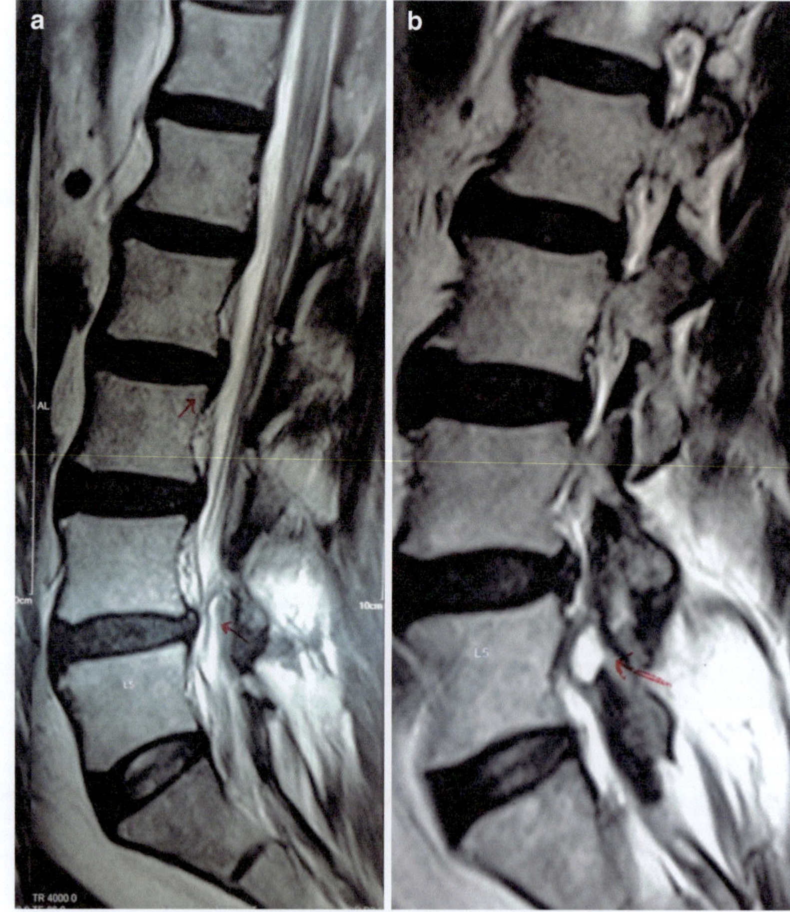

Fig. 25.4 MRI of lumbar spine T2-weighted Images sagittal section showing diffuse herniation of discs at multiple levels along with a hyperintense cystic lesion at L4-L5 level (**a**) and a well-defined sub centimetric sized hyperintense lesion in the thecal sac at the midbody level of L5 vertebrae suggestive of Tarlov cyst (**b**)

with higher re-accumulation rates. Subsequently, post aspiration fibrin glue has been injected to prevent re-accumulation [21, 44]. Surgical interventions often aim at reducing the CSF pressure. Thus, surgeries like lumbo-peritoneal shunt have been performed in patients with symptomatic Tarlov cysts [51]. Some authors have also suggested cystoperitoneal shunt for their management [6, 51].

25.9 Fibro-lipoma of the Filum Terminale

Fibro-lipoma of the filum terminale is, also known as filum terminale lipomas, is the type of lumbosacral lipoma in which the fat is entirely in the filum and is entirely separated from the conus medullaris. These are also incidentally found on imaging, and their clinical significance is questionable. Though extremely uncommon, they can present with symptoms like back pain, radiculopathy, urinary symptoms, and/ or sensory symptoms [52]. MRI is the investigation of choice, and they give a linear fat signal on T1-weighted images. The size of the filum is normal. If the size of the filum is more than 2 mm, then the diagnosis of intraspinal lipoma is made. They are usually managed conservatively. However, untethering is performed in indicated cases in which no other cause has been attributed to the patients' symptoms [16].

25.10 Synovial Cysts

Synovial cysts are abnormal fluid-filled sacs in the joints in the spine. They were first described by Baker in 1885 [53]. They can occur at any joint in the body. In the spine, they can present at any level, with the maximum incidence in the lumbar spine at L4-L5 level, which is the area of maximum mobility [51]. They are predominantly seen in females, and the mean age of their presentation is 60 years [51, 54]. Their incidence is less than 0.5% of the general population. They are usually asymptomatic unless they extend into the epidural space and cause nerve root or cord compression, leading to symptoms like radiculopathy, neurogenic claudication, and occasional sensory deficits [55]. MRI is the investigation of choice. They appear as well-circumscribed, extradural hypo to isointense on T1- and T2-weighted images, and their signal intensity is similar to that of CSF with hypointense cyst wall. The cyst wall enhances post gadolinium contrast administration [56]. Since most of these lesions are asymptomatic, expectant management is preferred in patients with mild symptoms; analgesics, steroids, and puncture and aspiration of the cyst have also been advocated [57]. In patients with intractable pain and neurological deficits because of these lesions, excision of the cyst should be performed with or without fusion procedures [58].

25.11 Sacral Meningocele

A sacral meningocele is a form of spinal dysraphism, which is defined as a protrusion of the spinal meninges through the foramina or vertebral column. There is no predilection toward any specific gender [59].Often they are encountered in female patients when they undergo pelvic examination. They present between the third to fifth decade of life. They are associated with malformations like imperforate anus, bicornuate uterus, spina bifida, and sacral bony defects. The meningocele cavity communicates with the spinal canal with a narrow communication. The sacral nerve usually lies within the cystic cavity adjacent to the cyst, getting compressed against the bony wall. They are asymptomatic. However, they can present with constipation, defecation problems, and neurological symptoms like back pain and radiculopathy [60]. These lesions can be diagnosed on a plain radiograph. The scimitar sign is the most characteristic sign, which denotes a smooth, uniform, unilateral sacral defect simulating the shape of an Arabic saber [61]. MRI is the best investigation for such lesions. They appear as intradural, extra-medullary T1 and T2 hyperintense lesions [62].In asymptomatic patients, they can be managed expectantly. However, in symptomatic patients, posterior laminectomy is followed by obliterating the communication between the meningocele and spinal subarachnoid space and untether if necessary [63]. The laparoscopic approach is more in favor these days [64].

25.12 Conclusion

In this era, with several diagnostic modalities, easy accessibility to the common strata and over the investigation of simple symptoms have skyrocketed the detection of several incidental findings which often times are irrelevant to patient's complaints. These unexpected findings are like a double-edged sword. They cause a burden on the resources, increase patient's anxiety, and can even lead to overtreatment of seemingly benign lesions. However, these incidentally detected findings are beneficial at times as they can lead to timely treatment of certain conditions. Now the onus lies upon the radiologist to detect, characterize, and report any relevant incidental finding.

References

1. Gaston A, Loredo JD, Assouline E, Combes C, Meder JF. Compressive vertebral hemangiomas. Value of imaging for diagnosis and definition of treatment. Neurochirurgie (Fre). 1898;35:275–83.
2. Wagner SC, Morrison WB, Carrino JA, Schweitzer ME, Nothnagel H. Picture archiving and communication system: effect on reporting of incidental findings. Radiology. 2002;225:500–5. https://doi.org/10.1148/radiol.2252011731.
3. Friedman BW, et al. Diagnostic testing and treatment of low back pain in US emergency departments. A national perspective. Spine. 2010;35(24):E1406–E141. https://doi.org/10.1097/brs.0b013e3181d952a5.
4. Arnautovic A, Arnautovic KI. Extramedullary intradural spinal tumors. Contem Neurosurg. 2014;36:1–8. https://doi.org/10.1097/01.CNE.0000448459.65797.ce.
5. Kousttais S, O'Halloran PJ, Hassan A, Brett F, Young S. Incidental primary intradural carcinoid tumor in a patient with lumbar radiculopathy. World Neurosurg. 2017;105:1042.e11–4. https://doi.org/10.1016/j.wneu.2017.06.179.
6. Ju CI, Shin H, Kim SW, Kim HS. Sacral perineural cyst accompanying disc herniation. J Korean Neurosurg Soc. 2009;45:185–7.
7. Ciftdemir M, Kaya M, Selcuk E, Yalniz E. Tumors of the spine. World J Orthop. 2016;7(2):109–16. https://doi.org/10.5312/wjo.v7.i2.109.
8. Ahad A, Elsayed M, Tohid H. The accuracy of clinical symptoms in detecting cauda equina syndrome in patients undergoing acute MRI of the spine. Neuroradiol J. 2015;28:438–42. https://doi.org/10.1177/1971400915598074.
9. Aich RK, Deb AR, Banerjee A, Karim R, Gupta P. Symptomatic vertebral hemangioma: treatment with radiotherapy. J Cancer Res Ther. 2010;6(2):199–203. https://doi.org/10.4103/0973-1482.65248.
10. Baker WM. Formation of synovial cysts in connection with joints. St Bartholomews Hospital Reports. 1885;21:177–90. PMID: 8119018
11. Birch BD, McCormick PC, Resnick DK. Intradural extramedullary spinal lesions. In: Benzel EC, editor. Spine surgery techniques, complications avoidance, and management, vol. 2. Philadelphia: Elsevier; 2005. p. 948–60. https://doi.org/10.1148/rg.2019180200.
12. Voyadzis JM, Bhargava P, Henderson FC. Tarlov cysts: a study of 10 cases with review of the literature. J Neurosurg. 2001;95(1 Suppl):25–32. https://doi.org/10.3171/spi.2001.95.1.0025.
13. Trapp C, Farage L, Clatterbuck RE, Romero FR, Rais-Bahrami S, Long DM, et. Al. Laparoscopic treatment of anterior sacral meningocele. Surg Neurol. 2007;68(4):443–8.; discussion 448. https://doi.org/10.1016/j.surneu.2006.11.067.
14. Hallinan JT, Hegde AN, Lim WE. Dilemmas and diagnostic difficulties in meningioma. Clin Radiol. 2013;68(8):837–44. https://doi.org/10.1016/j.crad.2013.03.007.
15. Mautner VF, Tatagiba M, Lindenau M, Fünsterer C, Pulst SM, Baser ME, Kluwe L, Zanella FE. Spinal tumors in patients with neurofibromatosis type 2: MR imaging study of frequency, multiplicity, and variety. AJR Am J Roentgenol. 1995;165(4):951–5. https://doi.org/10.2214/ajr.165.4.7676998.
16. Makoto Nakamura MD, Florian Roser MD, Michel J, Jacobs C, Samii M. The natural history of incidental meningiomas. Neurosurgery. 2003;53(1):62–71. https://doi.org/10.1227/01.NEU.0000068730.76856.58.
17. Solero CL, Fornari M, Giombini S, Lasio G, Oliveri G, Cimino C, Pluchino F. Spinal meningiomas: review of 174 operated cases. Neurosurgery. 1989;25(2):153–60.
18. Tumialán LM, Theodore N, Narayanan M, Marciano FF, Nakaji P. Anatomic basis for minimally invasive resection of Intradural extramedullary lesions in thoracic spine. World Neurosurg. 2018;109:e770–7. https://doi.org/10.1016/j.wneu.2017.10.078.
19. Ghadirpour R, Nasi D, Iaccarino C, Giraldi D, Sabadini R, Motti L, Sala F, Servadei F. Intraoperative neurophysiological monitoring for intradural extramedullary tumors: why not? Clin Neurol Neurosurg. 2015;130:140–9. https://doi.org/10.1016/j.clineuro.2015.01.007.

20. Sandalcioglu IE, Hunold A, Müller O, Bassiouni H, Stolke D, Asgari S. Spinal meningiomas: critical review of 131 surgically treated patients. Eur Spine J. 2008;17(8):1035–41. https://doi.org/10.1007/s00586-008-0685-y.

21. Mitra R, Kirpalani D, Wedemeyer M. Conservative management of perineural cysts. Spine (Phila Pa 1976). 2008;33:E565–8. https://doi.org/10.1097/BRS.0b013e31817e2cc9.

22. Firsching RP, Fischer A, Peters R, Thun F, Klug N. Growth rate of incidental meningiomas. J Neurosurg. 1990;73(4):545–7. https://doi.org/10.3171/jns.1990.73.4.0545.

23. Gottfried ON, Gluf W, Quinones-Hinojosa A, Kan P, Schmidt MH. Spinal meningiomas: surgical management and outcome. Neurosurg Focus. 2003;14(6):e2. https://doi.org/10.3171/foc.2003.14.6.2.

24. Ando K, Imagama S, Ito Z, et al. How do spinal schwannomas progress? The natural progression of spinal schwannomas on MRI. J Neurosurg Spine. 2016;24:155–9. https://doi.org/10.3171/2015.3.SPINE141218.

25. Klimo P Jr, Rao G, Schmidt RH, Schmidt MH. Nerve sheath tumors involving the sacrum, case report, and classification scheme. Neurosurg Focus. 2003;15:E12. https://doi.org/10.3171/foc.2003.15.2.12.

26. Park SC, Chung SK, Choe G, Kim HJ. Spinal intraosseous schwannoma: a case report and review. J Korean Neurosurg Soc. 2009;46:403–8.

27. Li P, Zhao F, Zhang J, Wang Z, Wang X, Wang B, Yang Z, Yang J, Gao Z, Liu P. Clinical features of spinal schwannomas in 65 patients with schwannomatosis compared with 831 with solitary schwannomas and 102 with neurofibromatosis type 2: a retrospective study at a single institution. J Neurosurg Spine. 2016;24(1):145–54. https://doi.org/10.3171/2015.3.SPINE141145.

28. Alfieri A, Campello M, Broger M, Vitale M, Schwarz A. Low-back pain as the presenting sign in a patient with a giant, sacral cellular schwannoma: 10-year follow up. J Neurosurg Spine. 2011;14:167–71. https://doi.org/10.3171/2010.10.SPINE1015.

29. Louis DN, Perry A, Reifenberger G, von Deimling A, Figarella-Branger D, Cavenee WK, Ohgaki H, Wiestler OD, Kleihues P, Ellison DW. The 2016 World Health Organization classification of tumors of the central nervous system: a summary. Acta Neuropathol. 2016;131(6):803–20. https://doi.org/10.1007/s00401-016-1545-1.

30. Togral G, Arikan M, Hasturk AE, Gungor S. Incidentally diagnosed giant invasive sacral schwannoma. Its clinical features and surgical management without stability. Neurosciences (Riyadh). 2014;19(3):224–8.

31. Baek S, Kim C, Chang H. Intradural schwannoma complicated by lumbar disc herniation at the same level: a case report and review of the literature. Oncol Lett. 2014;8:936–8. https://doi.org/10.3892/ol.2014.2181.

32. Mundy GR. Metastasis to bone: causes, consequences, and therapeutic opportunities. Nat Rev Cancer. 2002;2(8):584–93. https://doi.org/10.1038/nrc867.

33. Mehta SD, Sebro R. Random forest classifiers aid in the detection of incidental osteoblastic osseous metastases in DEXA studies. Int J Comput Assist Radiol Surg. 2019;14(5):903–9. https://doi.org/10.1007/s11548-019-01933-1.

34. Guillevin R, Vallee JN, Lafitte F, et-al. Spine metastasis imaging: a review of the literature. J Neuroradiol. 2007;34(5):311–21. https://doi.org/10.1016/j.neurad.2007.05.003.

35. Abul-kasim K, Thurnher MM, Mckeever P, et-al. Intradural spinal tumors: current classification and MRI features. Neuroradiology. 2008;50(4):301–14. https://doi.org/10.1007/s00234-007-0345-7.

36. Fassett DR, Schmidt MH. Lumbosacral ependymomas: a review of the management of intradural and extradural tumors. Neurosurg Focus. 2003;15(5):E13. https://doi.org/10.3171/foc.2003.15.5.13.

37. Pastushyn AI, Slin'ko EI, Mirzoyeva GM. Vertebral hemangiomas: diagnosis, management, natural history and clinicopathological correlates in 86 patients. Surg Neurol. 1998;50(6):535–47. https://doi.org/10.1016/s0090-3019(98)00007.

38. Doppman JL, Oldfield EH, Heiss JD. Symptomatic vertebral hemangiomas: treatment by means of direct intralesional injection of ethanol. Radiology. 2000;214:341–8. https://doi.org/10.1148/radiology.214.r00fe46341.

39. Vinay S, Khan SK, Braybrooke JR. Lumbar vertebral haemangioma causing pathological fracture, epidural haemorrhage, and cord compression: a case report and review of the literature. J Spinal Cord Med. 2011;34(3):335–9. https://doi.org/10.1179/2045772311y.00000004.

40. Gray F, Gherardi R, Benhaiem-Sigaux N. Vertebral hemangioma. Definition, limitations, anatomopathologic aspects. Neurochirurgie. 1989;35(5):267–9.

41. Laredo JD, Assouline E, Gaston A, Gelbert F, Mezland JJ. Radiological features differentiating compressive and asymptomatic vertebral hemangiomas. Neuro-Chirurgie (Fre). 1989;35:284–8.

42. Hao J, Hu Z. Percutaneous cement vertebroplasty in the treatment of symptomatic vertebral hemangiomas. Pain Physician. 2012;15(1):43–9.

43. Tarlov IM. Perineural cysts of the spinal nerve roots. Arch Neurol Psychiatr. 1938;40:1067–74. https://doi.org/10.1001/arch-neuropsyc.1938.02270120017001.

44. Park HJ, Jeon YH, Rho MH, Lee EJ, Park NH, Park SI, et al. Incidental findings of the lumbar spine at MRI during herniated intervertebral disk disease evaluation. AJR Am J Roentgenol. 2011;196:1151–5. https://doi.org/10.2214/ajr.10.5457.

45. Paulsen RD, Call GA, Murtagh FR. Prevalence and percutaneous drainage of cysts of the sacral nerve root sheath (Tarlov cysts). AJNR Am J Neuroradiol. 1994;15:293–9.

46. Nabors MW, Pait TG, Byrd EB, Karim NO, Davis DO, Kobrine AI, et al. Updated assessment and current classification of spinal meningeal cysts. J Neurosurg. 1988;68:366–77. https://doi.org/10.3171/jns.1988.68.3.0366.
47. Neulen A, Kantelhardt SR, Pilgram-Pastor SM, Metz I, Rohde V, Giese A. Microsurgical fenestration of perineural cysts to the thecal sac at the level of the distal dural sleeve. Acta Neurochir. 2011;153:1427–34. https://doi.org/10.1007/s00701-011-1043-0.
48. Nishiura I, Koyama T, Handa J. Intrasacral perineurial cyst. Surg Neurol. 1985;23:265–9. https://doi.org/10.1016/0090-3019(85)90093-x.
49. Langdown AJ, Grundy JR, Birch NC. The clinical relevance of Tarlov cysts. J Spinal Disord Tech. 2005;18:29–33. https://doi.org/10.1097/01.bsd.0000133495.78245.71.
50. Murphy KJ, Nussbaum DA, Schnupp S, Long D. Tarlov cysts: an overlooked clinical problem. Semin Musculoskelet Radiol. 2011;15:163–7. https://doi.org/10.1055/s-0031-1275599.
51. Bartels RH, van Overbeeke JJ. Lumbar cerebrospinal fluid drainage for symptomatic sacral nerve root cysts: an adjuvant diagnostic procedure and/or alternative treatment? Technical case report. Neurosurgery. 1997;40:861–5. https://doi.org/10.1097/00006123-199804000-00162.
52. Morio Y, Nanjo Y, Nagashima H, Minamizaki T, Teshima R. Sacral cyst managed with cyst-subarachnoid shunt: a technical case report. Spine (Phila Pa 1976). 2001;26:451–3. https://doi.org/10.1097/00007632-200102150-00025.
53. Brown E, Matthes JC, Bazan C 3rd, Jinkins JR. Prevalence of incidental intraspinal lipoma of the lumbosacral spine as determined by MRI. Spine. 1994;Phila Pa 1976(19):833–6. https://doi.org/10.1097/00007632-199404000-00018.
54. Khan AM, Girardi F. Spinal lumbar synovial cysts. Diagnosis and management challenge. Eur Spine J. 2006;15(8):1176–82.
55. Liu SS, Williams KD, Drayer BP, Spetzler RF, Sonntag VK. Synovial cysts of the lumbosacral spine: diagnosis by MR imaging. AJR. 1990;154:163–6. https://doi.org/10.2214/ajr.154.1.2104702.
56. Pirotte B, Gabrovsky N, Massager N, Levivier M, David P, Brotchi J. Synovial cysts of the lumbar spine: surgery-related results and outcome. J Neurosurg. 2003;99(1 Suppl):14–9. https://doi.org/10.3171/spi.2003.99.1.0014.
57. Knox AM. Fon GT the appearances of lumbar intraspinal synovial cysts. Clin Radiol. 1991;44(6):397–401. https://doi.org/10.1016/s0009-9260(05)80658-0.
58. Lyons MK, Atkinson JL, Wharen RE, Deen HG, Zimmerman RS, Lemens. Surgical evaluation and management of lumbar synovial cysts: the Mayo Clinic experience. SM. J Neurosurg. 2000;93(1 Suppl):53–7. https://doi.org/10.3171/spi.2000.93.1.0053.
59. Métellus P, Flores-Parra I, Fuentes S, Dufour H, Adetchessi T, Do L, et. Al. A retrospective study of 32 lumbar synovial cysts. Clinical aspect and surgical management. Neurochirurgie. 2003;49(2–3 Pt 1):73–82. https://doi.org/10.1097/BRS.0b013e31817e2cc9.
60. Dahlgren RM, Baron EM, Vaccaro AR. Pathophysiology, diagnosis, and treatment of spinal meningoceles and arachnoid cysts. (dissertation) Philadelphia, PA: Department of Orthopaedic Surgery, Thomas Jefferson University; 2007. doi: https://doi.org/10.1053/j.semss.2006.06.003.
61. North RB, Kidd DH, Wang H. Occult, bilateral anterior sacral and intrasacral meningeal and perineurial cysts: case report and review of the literature. Neurosurgery. 1990;27(6):981–6. https://doi.org/10.1097/00006123-199012000-00020.
62. Kovalcik PJ, Burke JB. Anterior sacral meningocele and the scimitar sign. Report of a case. Dis Colon Rectum. 1988;31(10):806–7. https://doi.org/10.1007/bf02560112.
63. Sachdev S, Dodd RL, Chang SD, et al. Stereotactic radiosurgery yields long-term control for benign intradural, extramedullary spinal tumors. Neurosurgery. 2011;69:533–9. https://doi.org/10.1227/NEU.0b013e318218db23.
64. Shimizu H, Tominaga T, Takahashi A. Cine magnetic resonance imaging of spinal intradural arachnoid cysts. Neurosurgery. 1997;41:95–100. https://doi.org/10.1097/00006123-199707000-00020.

Incidental Spinal Vascular Malformations

Parth A. Jani, Manjul Tripathi, Chirag K. Ahuja, and Sunil K. Gupta

26.1 Introduction

Spinal vascular malformations are rare lesions described in literature and have gathered great interest and attention in the post-imaging era of the twentieth and twenty-first centuries. They comprise of true congenital/inborn malformations such as cavernomas or arteriovenous malformations (AVM) and acquired pathologies such as dural arteriovenous fistulas (DAVF). The first description of a spinal AVM was by Gaupp in 1888 [1]. In 1911, Krause reported the first excision of spinal DAVF [2]. Three years later in 1934, Ellsberg described the resection of epidural vein as treatment for the same. In 1943, Wyburn–Mason described their large series of 110 patients with two main types of spinal vascular lesions—venous angiomas and AVMs [3]. With the advent of angiography in 1960s, Oldfield et al. described 3 main types of spinal AVMs—single coiled vessel fistula, glomus AVMs with clear nidus, and juvenile AVMs with diffuse and extensive nidus [4]. The classification systems and description of these rare entities have evolved over the last

5 decades. In the pre-imaging era, all spinal vascular malformations were considered to be the same or at least of a single general type of disease. The widespread use of magnetic resonance imaging (MRI) and selective spinal angiography has challenged this notion, and significant progress has been made in understanding the anatomy and the pathophysiology of these vascular malformations.

26.2 Epidemiology and Classification

It is the rarity of spinal vascular lesions that keep their true incidence and prevalence under the dark. Overall, spinal AVMs share 3–4% of the entire intradural spinal cord space occupying lesions (Fig. 26.1) [5]. Spinal DAVFs comprise of 70% of these rare lesions and are the commonest spinal vascular malformations (Fig. 26.1) [1]. They have an incidence of 5–10 per million population [6]. These DAVFs are acquired vascular lesions with five times higher incidence in males as compared to females. Spinal DAVF usually present in the age-group of 55–60 years and are mostly thoracolumbar in location [7]. In contrast to the cranial DAVFs, only 4% spinal DAVF have an associated history of trauma and DAVFs are rarely asymptomatic [7]. Capillary telangiectasias are congenital lesions but in contrast to the brain they have not been described in

P. A. Jani · M. Tripathi · S. K. Gupta (✉)
Department of Neurosurgery, Postgraduate Institute of Medical Education and Research, Chandigarh, India

C. K. Ahuja
Department of Neuroradiology, Postgraduate Institute of Medical Education and Research, Chandigarh, India

© The Author(s), under exclusive license to Springer Nature Switzerland AG 2023
M. Turgut et al. (eds.), *Incidental Findings of the Nervous System*,
https://doi.org/10.1007/978-3-031-42595-0_26

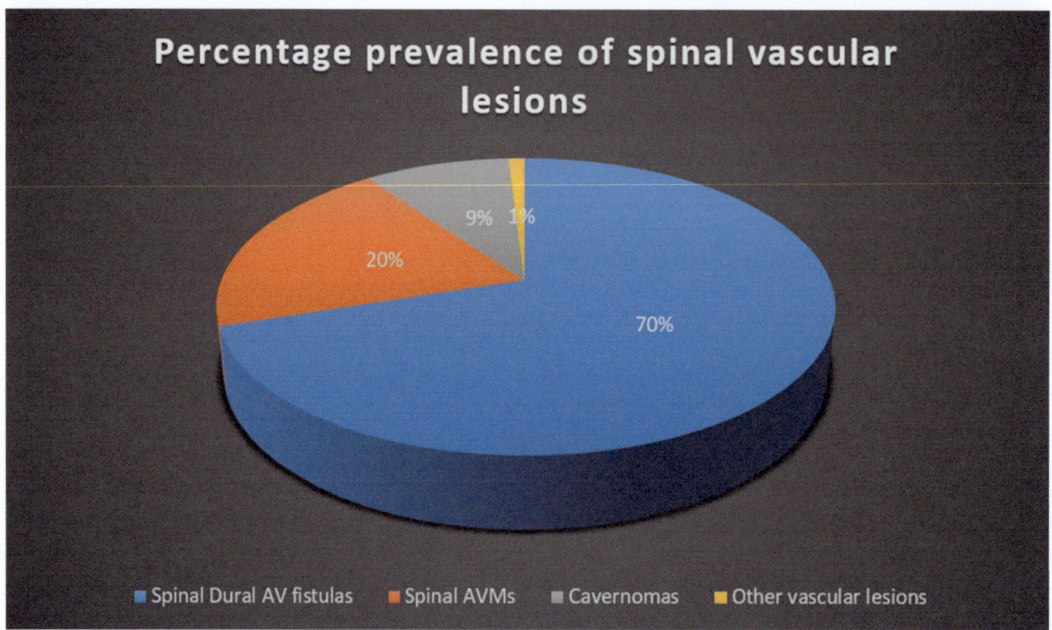

Fig. 26.1 Percentage prevalence of spinal vascular lesions (*AVM* Arteriovenous malformation, *DAVF* Dural arteriovenous fistula)

the spine hence will not be discussed further in this chapter [8].

Spinal AVMs represent 20–30% of the vascular lesions and have been further classified into glomus and juvenile AVMs, with the former being the most common subtype. They can be located superficially on the surface of the spinal cord or deep within the cord parenchyma. In rare cases, they may extend to both compartments. Owing to their congenital origin, these lesions are more prevalent in younger age-groups (<30 years) [5]. Occasionally, they may be associated with inherited disorders like hereditary hemorrhagic telangiectasias [9], familial cutaneous hemangiomas, Klippel-Trenaunay-Weber syndrome [10], familial cerebral cavernous hemangioma [11], etc. Spinal AVMs show no sex predilection. Spinal AVMs are either supplied by sulcal arteries originating from anterior spinal artery (ASA) or by perforating pial arteries derived from vasa-corona supplemented by dorsal lateral arteries and small branches from the ASA [12].

Cavernous malformations of the spinal cord comprise about 9–12% of all spinal pathologies. 27% of the patients with spinal cord cavernomas have an associated intracranial cavernoma, and 45% of these subset of patients has a positive family history [13].

26.3 Classification of Spinal Vascular Malformations

Multiple classification systems have evolved overtime. From the neurosurgeon's perspective, the following classification systems have been described and modified subsequently (Table 26.1).

(i) Classification by Anson and Spetzler-1992 [14]
(ii) Modified classification of spinal vascular lesions by Spetzler et al 2002 [15]

Table 26.1 Classification schemes of spinal vascular malformations

Classification spinal vascular malformations (Anson and Spletzer-1992)		
Type 1	Dural Arterio-venous Fistula	
Type 2	Intramedullary Glomus Arteriovenous Malformations	
Type 3	Extensive AVM extending into vertebral body and para-spinal muscles	
Type 4	Pial Arteriovenous fistula	Type A: single feeder with moderate venous hypertension Type B: more feeders with increased flow and dilated veins. Type C: Giant, High Flow lesions with a markedly distended venous network
Modified classification of Spinal Vascular Lesions by Spletzer et al. (2002).		
I. Neoplasms-	Hemangioblastomas, Cavernous Malformations.	
II. Spinal Aneurysms.		
III. ArteriovenousLesions-		
A. Arteriovenous Fistulas	1. Extra Dural	
	2. Intradural- Ventral	A. Single feeding artery from ASA, B. Primary large feeder from ASA, + Multiple feeders from adjacent arteries, C. Giant fistulas with multiple small feeders from adjacent arteries
	3. Intradural- Dorsal	
B. Arteriovenous malformations:	1. Extradural-intradural.	
	2. Intradural—compact nidus	
	3. Intradural diffuse nidus	
	4. Intramedullary-extramedullary	

AVM Arteriovenous malformation, *ASA* Anterior spinal artery

26.4 Pathophysiology of Spinal Vascular Malformations

Three main pathophysiological processes are involved in causing clinical deterioration among patients suffering from spinal dural AVFs and AVMs [4, 16, 17], namely

(i) Venous hypertension.
(ii) Arterial steal phenomena.
(iii) Hemorrhage—subarachnoid hemorrhage (SAH).

26.5 Clinical Presentation and Natural History

Most common clinical presentation of spinal AVFs and AVMs consists of progressive motor weakness, sensory impairment, sphincter distur-

bances, and localized pain [18, 19]. Depending on the type of vascular malformation, initial symptoms may also be attributable to intramedullary or SAHs. Spinal SAH is more frequently observed in AVMs as compared to AVFs. An acute bleed such as SAH leads to early diagnosis owing to the acute onset of the symptoms. On the contrary, venous congestion causing chronic myelopathy frequently leads to unspecific initial neurological symptoms on a prolonged duration of time that render an early diagnosis confusing and difficult [8].

Spinal AVFs may present with non-specific back pain to severe motor weakness, sensory disturbances, and micturition problems [18, 19]. The arteriovenous shunt is located in the dura matter of a proximal root sleeve typically directly underneath the pedicle where the arterial blood from a radiculomeningeal artery enters into a radicular vein. The increase in spinal venous pressure diminishes the arteriovenous pressure gradient which leads to a decreased drainage of normal spinal veins causing venous congestion with intramedullary edema. This is usually localized at the lower cord and conus leading to chronic hypoxia and progressive myelopathy [18]. Motor deficits are the commonest mode of presentation and the most responsive to the treatment [20]. Incidental detection or presentation with minor symptoms like isolated back pain is an extremely rare phenomena for spinal dural AVF and not commonly seen. Spinal AVFs most commonly involve lower thoracic and lumbar spine, with clear male predominance (80%) in an age-group of 55–60 years. Spinal AVFs are "slow flow fistulas" unlike their cranial counterparts and therefore paradoxically less likely to present with hemorrhage (SAH/epidural hemorrhages). From a clinical point of view, spinal arteriovenous fistulas are the most misdiagnosed entities. They mimic spinal degenerative disease, polyneuropathy, neoplasm, or infections and only a careful clinical analysis with selective imaging will result in the correct diagnosis of the disease [20].

Patients report progressive worsening of symptoms with Valsalva maneuver, physical exercise, and postural modifications, as increased intraabdominal and intrathoracic pressure also increases intraspinal venous pressure which aggravates venous hypertension [21]. Pregnancy also precipitates these physiological changes and paves way to the diagnosis of these asymptomatic lesions.

26.6 Spinal Arteriovenous Malformations

Since these vascular lesions are "high flow high pressure lesions," they are more likely to present with hemorrhages (SAH or hematomyelia). Sudden onset of severe back pain radiating along the nerve root at the level of the lesion is the commonest presentation. Patients without hemorrhage present with a slowly progressive neurological decline in terms of motor, sensory, and bladder disturbances [5]. Upper dorsal spine and cervical spine are the most common regions involved, with an age-group of 15–40 years. There is no exacerbation of the clinical symptoms with physical activity or Valsalva maneuver. The presentation is location specific, and patients harboring conus medullaris AVMs frequently present with cauda equina syndrome [22]. Contrary to spinal DAVFs, spinal AVMs tend to get symptomatic in younger age. The high flow shunts present in some perimedullary fistula can even lead to cardiac insufficiency hence immediate postnatal presentation. Conus medullaris AVMs may present with both upper and lower motor neuron symptoms. Elimination of the mass effect on descending roots of the cauda equina can be associated with striking clinical improvement.

Spinal Cavernous Malformation: The clinical presentation of these lesions may follow any of the following patterns [13]:
1. Discrete neurological deficits—acute episodic progression over months to years
2. Slowly progressive decline in function over months to years
3. Acute onset and rapid progression
4. Acute mild symptoms with slow progression of symptoms
5. Incidentally detected while screening for other complaints or in patients with familial cavernomatosis

Due to compact volume of spinal cord, cavernomas of spinal cord are more likely to be symptomatic than their cerebral counterparts. Zevgaridis et al. in their review article reviewing 117 spinal cavernomas published via 48 studies, noted that, all patients showed a progressive decline in neurological deficits, no patient had asymptomatic cavernoma [13].

Natural History: 50% of the spinal DAVFs and spinal AVMs become severely disabled within 3 years of onset of motor symptoms, and thus have an unfavorable course in the natural history. Sudden neurological deteriorations occur secondary to hemorrhages (SAH $\gg$ Hematomyelia) while progressive myelopathy symptoms occur secondary to chronic venous hypertension [23].

Despite the latest imaging advances, the diagnosis lags the clinical deterioration in most of the cases thereby paradoxically reducing the chances of these lesions getting detected incidentally.

26.7 How Common Are Incidental Spinal Cavernomas?

The overall prevalence of spinal cord cavernomas has risen following MRI era of diagnostic imaging, so much that in general population the prevalence is estimated to be close to 5% in adults and 1% in children [24]. However, these lesions are rarely asymptomatic due to the high density of the eloquent neural tissue in spinal cord parenchyma. Lesions are detected asymptomatically in only 0.9% adult population.

26.8 Which Spinal Vascular Malformations Are More Commonly Seen Incidentally?

Due to the paucity of literature in this direction, and the rarity of these vascular lesions, the exact prevalence and incidence of these vascular malformations have not been described in the literature. Most of the large case series and review articles of spinal cord cavernoma or tumors (hemangioblastomas) comprise of all the symptomatic lesions. Spinal dural AVFs and spinal AVMs have already been described to present with clinical deterioration even before the diagnosis of these lesions.

Apparently, only the incidentally detected spinal cord cavernomas and hemangioblastomas as detected by screening in familial syndromes seem to be the commonest spinal vascular malformations.

26.9 Radiologic Evaluation of Spinal Vascular Lesions (Table 26.2)

While MRI is the first-choice diagnostic modality for the suspected spinal vascular malformations, the definite diagnosis and the therapeutic approach are usually decided only after definite digital subtraction angiography (DSA).

Spinal DAVFs: MRI spine classically shows spinal cord edema with perimedullary vessels [3]. Ill-defined, predominantly central medullary, increased T2 signal secondary to venous congestion, may span multiple segments of spinal cord. In cases with chronic venous congestion, mild contrast enhancement can be seen. Arterialized veins are seen as large flow voids on T2-weighted images. The edema is often accompanied by a hypointense rim most likely representing deoxygenated blood within the dilated capillary vessels surrounding the congestive edema [3].In rare cases, the cord is swollen and can demonstrate contrast enhancement as a sign of chronic venous congestion. In cases of persistent edema, myelomalacia may ensue. The perimedullary vessels are often dilated, coiled, and typically seen on T2-weighted images as flow voids [25].

Spinal DSA remains the gold standard for diagnosing DAVF (Fig. 26.2); however, evaluation with an magnetic resonance angiography may guide selective angiography of the involved region, aiding the diagnosis and saving patient from a complete spinal angiography. The common angiographic features are early venous filling, dilated peri medullary veins, contrast stasis in anterior spinal arteries, and radiculomedullary arteries [26].

Spinal AVMs: MRI spine is a highly sensitive investigation for AVMs. Nidus with serpentine flow voids, with/without an increased signal on T2 MRI representing edema [27]. Spinal DSA (Figs. 26.3 and 26.4) is vital in planning management and detailed evaluation as it adds finer details like feeding artery, draining veins, intra-nidal aneurysms, and exact span of the lesion location—dorsal/ventral, diffuse/compact nidus [12].

Table 26.2 Diagnostic algorithms for spinal vascular malformations

Screening cohorts for spinal Vascular Malformations-	Clinical presentation of – (acute onset/gradually progressive)
• Multiple intracranial cavernomas. • Familial cavernomatosis with CCM-1, CCM-2, CCM3 mutations. • Von-Hippel Lindau disease with intracranial HGBS and retinal angiomas.	• Walking Disturbances-Para paresis, etc. • Sensory disturbances- paresthesia, persistent pain in back. • Micturition disturbances. • Anal sphincter disturbances. • Erectile dysfunction Clinical examination and spinal cord segment level localization.

MRI Spine (plain +contrast) with T2 sagittal whole spine screening.

T1- Hypo-Iso-Intense solid cystic **T2**- Iso-Hyper-intense, focal flow voids, hemosiderin capping, **T1C+-** Tumour nodule enhances vividly.	**T1, T2**- Rounded regions with heterogeneous signal intensity with blood products of varying ages.	**T2-** Serpentine /tangle of blood vessels (seen as flow voids) in epidural/Intradural /intramedullary spaces
• Intramedullary component with 2/3 rd having a dorsally exophytic component. • Associated tumour cyst/syrinx in 50-100% • *THORACIC CORD(50%) > CERVICAL CORD(40%)*	*"Popcorn Appearance"* **GRADIENT ECHO**- blooming + **T1C+-** no/minimal enhancement.	+/- T2 Signal hyper-intensities
HEMANGIOBLASTOMA	**Spinal Cavernomatous Malformation**	**? Spinal Dural AVFs ? Spinal AVMs.**

DIAGNOSTIC DIGITAL SUBSTRACTION ANGIOGRAPHY

Arterial phase	**NIDUS/FISTULA characteristics**	**Venous phase**
• Lesion delineation. • Single/multiple arterial feeders from ASA/PSA in A-P views. • Intrinsic/extrinsic cord feeders. • Calibre of feeding vessels- larger branches going in to fistula- direct fistulas, smaller branches- indirect fistulas. • Aneurysms with AVMs - flow related or dysplastic. • AN with radicular arteries- show multiple haemorrhages.	•Nidus delineation poor- vascular anastomoses and channels seen. Commonly- •Fistulas from ASA are high flow- "macro AFs" •Dorsal AVFs are "Micro AVFs" •Filum terminale AVFs- "micro AFs"	**AVMs-** venous pouches, ectasias, kinking of vein, Mechanical compression of the spinal cord inside canal. Radicular veins are patent **AVFs-** thrombosis of the radicular veins, congestion of the radicular veins

ASA Anterior spinal artery, *AVF* Arteriovenous fistula, *AVM* Arteriovenous malformation, *CCM* Cerebral cavernous malformations, *DSA* Digital subtraction angiography, *HGBS* Hemangioblastomas, *PSA* Posterior spinal artery

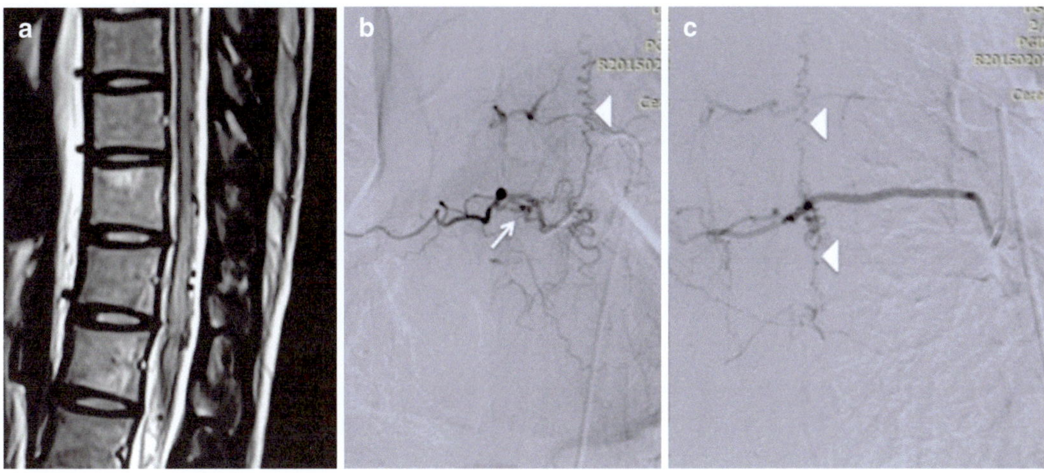

Fig. 26.2 Spinal DAVF: Sagittal T2-weighted magnetic resonance imaging (MRI) (**a**) shows flow voids along the dorsal surface of the spinal cord with T2 hyperintense signal changes in the cord parenchyma signifying congestive venous changes. Frontal (**b**) and lateral (**c**) digital subtraction angiography (DSA) images demonstrating the DAVF (arrow) with draining venous channels (arrowheads)

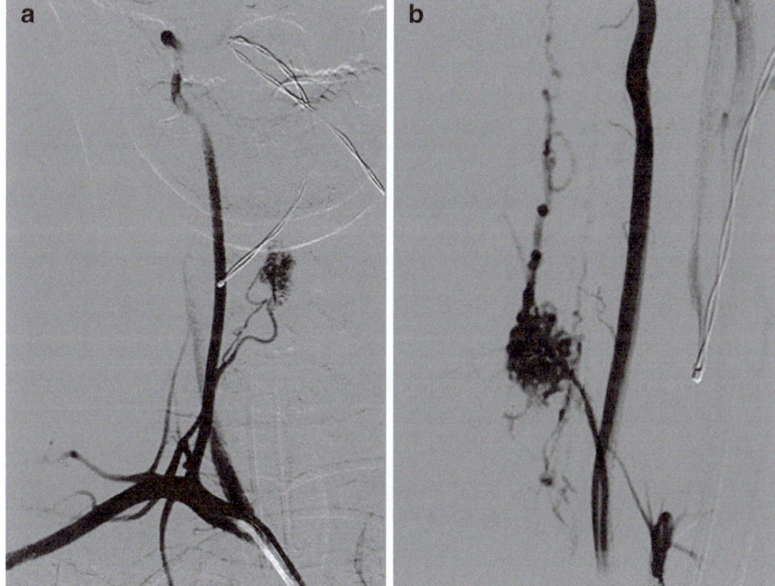

Fig. 26.3 Spinal cord AVM: Frontal (**a**) and lateral (**b**) DSA images depicting a compact nidus within the cervical spinal cord receiving arterial feeders form the ascending cervical branch of the thyrocervical trunk

Spinal Cavernomas: MRI spine is the diagnostic imaging of choice due to their angiographically occult nature. Heterogeneous appearance is seen on T1- and T2-weighted images with a surrounding halo on T2 due to hemosiderin ring. Heterogeneous hypo-hyper intensities often impart a "popcorn like appearance" on MRI. 25% of these lesions may show developmental venous anomaly on DSA (Fig. 26.5) [28].

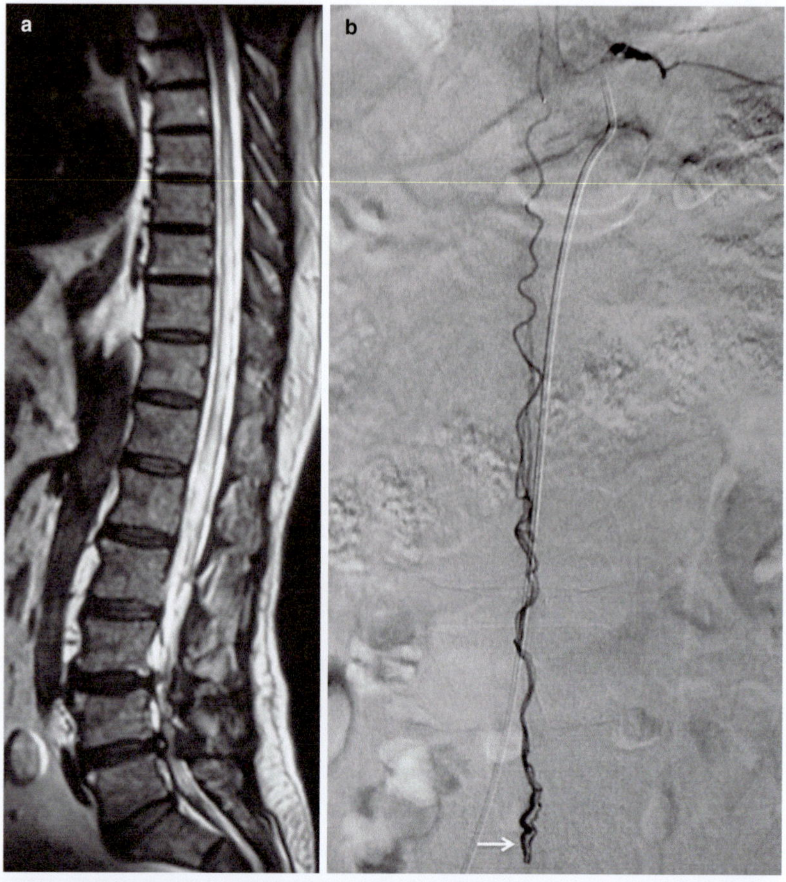

Fig. 26.4 Spinal perimedullary AVF (Type IV): (**a**) Sagittal MRI depicting myelopathic changes in the dorsal cord seen as T2 hyperintense signal. Frontal DSA (**b**) image shows the site of perimedullary AV fistula (arrow)

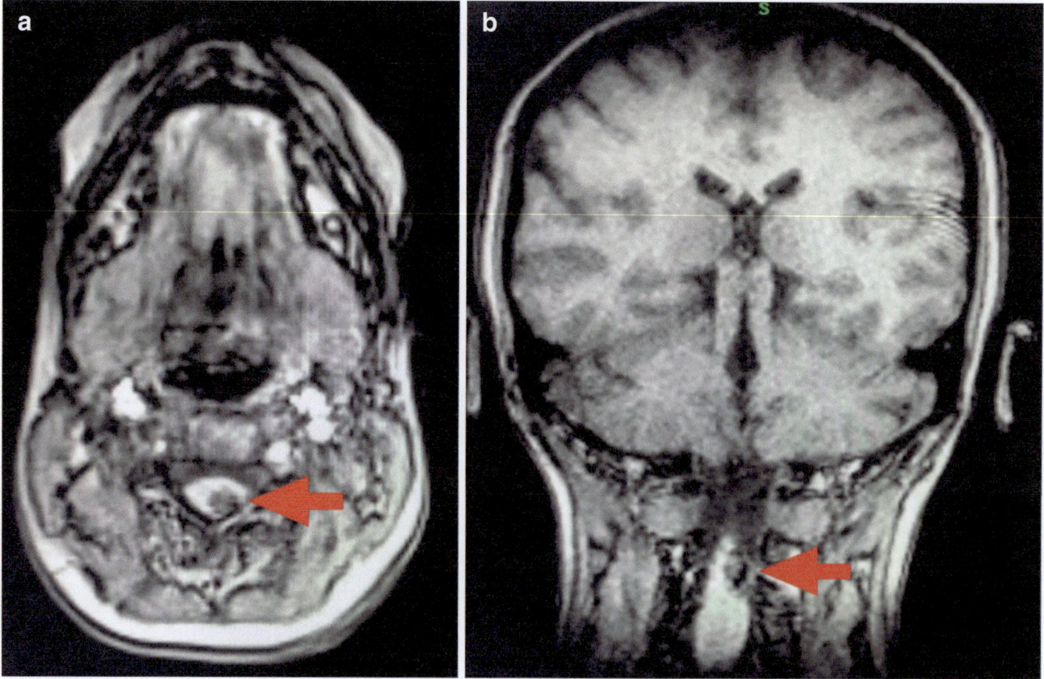

Fig. 26.5 Incidentally detected cavernous malformation (red arrow) in cervical spine in a 24 years old female. (**a**): Axial and (**b**) Coronal T2 weighted images

26.10 Management (Tables 26.3 and 26.4)

26.10.1 Rationale for Management of Incidental Spinal Vascular Malformations

In view of rare discovery of an asymptomatic spinal vascular malformation, the management becomes a controversial issue. The diagnosis can be ascertained in its entirety with emphasis on the extent of the lesion, radiological evidence of prior asymptomatic bleed, or neural injury on currently available sophisticated radiological parameters. The management is decided by the perceived natural history of the particular lesion in relation to the age of the patient, and geographical location in the spine. There are no standard guidelines to help management of asymptomatic incidentalomas. Hence the treatment needs to be tailored individually with a balanced approach and detailed discussion with the patient with the emphasis on paucity in the literature on established management protocols. Till then management of incidental spinal vascular malformations would remain a Sophie's choice.

Spinal Dural AVFs:-Treatment options comprise of—*endovascular, open surgery,* or *combination of both* the modalities. Broadly speaking, endovascular techniques have replaced open surgery and emerged as the main stay treatment for SDAVFs [26]. Endovascular treatment is specifically targeted at identifying the exact fistula anatomy, the arterial feeder, the fistula, and the draining vein. A superselective catheterization of the feeding arteries is vital to achieve this anatomical clarity. After this, the goal is to occlude the fistula and the proximal part of the draining vein with a liquid embolic agent. Failure to include the proximal portion of the draining vein may result in recurrence.

In cases of doubtful embolization or failed occlusion, a radio-opaque coil may be placed to locate the fistula under fluoroscopic guidance in an open rescue surgery [29]. Neurophysiological monitoring is often used as an adjuvant tool during the endovascular and open approaches.

Open surgical obliteration of spinal DAVFs is a straightforward approach with a reported obliteration of 98%. Exact preoperative localization is of utmost importance. General surgical considerations include patient in prone position on Wilson's frame, maintaining a mean arterial pressure of 60–80 mmHg. A radio-opaque fiducial marker may aid in further localization, and lamino-spinal complex is removed with a high-speed drill in a single piece and preserved so as to repair with laminoplasty later on. An intraoperative indocyanine green (ICG)-angiography is very useful in identifying the feeder arteries and draining vein. Bipolar cautery is used to coagulate the arterialized vein. Normalization of the venous pressures is seen as these veins turn from red to blue [30]. ICG angiogram is a useful intraoperative adjunt to judge the obliteration and flow. Pathology-specific operative considerations are given in the following Table 26.4.

Table 26.3 Microsurgical management of spinal dural arterio-venous fistulas

Subtype	Technical pearls in surgery
1. Intradural Dorsal Arteriovenous Fistula	• Most common site- laterally near the root entry zone dorsally. • Dura-arachnoid opened- anchored, arterialized vein identified. • *Check ICG-* to confirm arterialized vein. • *Sharp dissection* of the arterialized vein proximally near the fistula. Vein coagulated and cut as proximal as possible to avoid venous congestion. • Inner Dural surface at the fistulous point is inspected for other feeders, and coagulated if any.

(continued)

Table 26.3 (continued)

Subtype	Technical pearls in surgery
2. Intradural Ventral Arteriovenous fistula	• Anterior, Posterior, Postero-lateral approaches. • Surgery is only indicated in type A and some type B. very risky for type C. • Difficult to approach—*ventral location, close proximity to anterior spinal artery.* • ICG confirmation of the fistulous connection. • Junction between Anterior spinal artery and the feeding vessel is identified and clip ligated. • Avoid use of bipolar to prevent damage to ASA. • Anterior approach- vertebral column reconstruction Required-Endovascular intervention preferred.
3. Extra-Dural Arteriovenous fistula	• Epidural fistula. • Fistula between—extradural branch of radicular artery and epidural venous plexus. • Check ICG—identifying the fistulous connection. • Fistulous connection clipped or coagulated.

ICG Indocyanine angiography

Table 26.4 Proposed management algorithm for incidental spinal vascular malformations

Incidentally Detected Spinal Vascular Malformation-Subtype specific Management

Spinal Cavernomatous Malformations	Hemangioblastoma	Spinal Dural Arterio-venous fistula	Spinal Arterio-Venous Malformation
Asymptomatic- observation with sequential MRI.	*Asymptomatic-* observation with sequential MRI.	**Asymptomatic-** ? endovascular glue embolization (in view of safety of endovascular approach over surgery)	*Glomus type-* **Asymptomatic**—observation with sequential DSA and imaging. **Symptomatic/progression**—Surgery/embolization.
Surgical intervention for symptomatic cases or Progression	*Surgical intervention* for symptomatic cases or Progression	*Symptomatic or Progression-* Surgical ligation of the fistula/ endovascular obliteration/ hybrid	*Juvenile type-* **Asymptomatic**—observation **Symptomatic/progression**—Hybrid approach-embolization + surgery.

26.11 Spinal Arteriovenous Malformations

26.11.1 Intramedullary Spinal Arteriovenous Malformations

Surgical excision of intramedullary spinal AVM is the gold standard treatment, but because of the surgical challenges involved, in excising these thin-walled high flow lesions which may bleed profusely intraoperatively, embolization as stand-alone therapy and in combination to surgery has emerged as safer and preferred treatment modality [5, 30, 31].

• Preoperative DSA is must in all the cases. Relation of spinal AVM to ASA is noted. If not seen distinctly, embolization of the vessels is avoided. In a classical posterior approach, patient is made prone, a midline incision is taken, a liberal laminectomy is done keeping the spino-laminar complex intact (which can be later replaced and fixed for laminoplasty) and dura is exposed. Apart from the spinal angiography, preoperative fiducial marker/glue embolization for localization. Intraoperative localization is done with following clues—increased vascularity over the dura, intraoperative ICG to see the arterial feeders, AVM nidus, and the draining vein.

- Arterial feeders and fistulous communication are the ones coagulated initially in dural AVFs, whereas in spinal AVMs, it is very important to preserve these arterial feeders, especially at the dural entry zone, as they may be feeding the anterior spinal arteries. For instance, in lower thoracic cord AVMs, the artery of Adamkiewicz is identified and preserved. Sectioning the dentate ligament augments the manipulation of the spinal cord in the canal, increasing the antero-lateral exposure.
- AVM nidus is devascularized and resected circumferentially at the pial surface. In patients with surfacing AVMs, the approach is direct.
- In deeper locations, usually a midline myelotomy is done to identify the nidus and then excised. Another myelotomy approaches include anterior midline, dorsal root entry zone, and lateral. Dorsal nerve roots may be sacrificed in demanding situations.
- Large venous varices can be coagulated to gain space for circumferential dissection, inflow arterial feeders are skeletonized and coagulated/clip ligated before attacking draining veins.
- Check ICG should be routinely performed at multiple stages during the resection to ensure safe identification of arterial feeders and avoid clipping the draining veins early in the course of surgery.
- Perinidal dissection is safer than intra-nidal or deeper dissections in the cord parenchyma to preserve spinal nuclei and tracts. Concept is to work in the gliotic perinidal tissue which immediately surrounds AVM nidus, to prevent breaching the normal cord parenchyma [30].
- In contrast to the cranial AVMs, in which complete resection is important, and partial resection does not alter the natural history of bleeding and deficits, in complex spinal AVMs, partial resection and leaving the embolized portions of AVM do not lead to significant bleeding, infarctions, or neurological deterioration.
- Post resection, hemostasis is done, myelotomy is closed, and dural closure is performed. Lamino-spinal complex is fixed with screws and miniplates.

Extradural–Intradural AVMs: Previously known as juvenile AVMs, these AVMs are metameric in distribution and involve neural structures, bone, soft tissue, at the spinal level and are the most complex category to manage both surgically and endovascularly.

- Surgical policy—devascularization of these lesions by coagulating the large feeding vascular pedicles thereby reducing the venous hypertension, and venous congestion.
- Decompressing the spinal nerves and cord by compressing elements.
- Endovascular treatment remains a safer option, with staged embolization of various arterial feeders.
- Treatment is palliative due to the complex nature of these lesions. There is no consensus guidelines for the management of an asymptomatic AVM since data concerning spontaneous prognosis are not available. However, in consensus, symptomatic AVMs should be treated since therapy ameliorates the prognosis of the patient.

26.11.2 Conus Medullaris-Arteriovenous Malformations

These rare lesions have the following peculiarities [22]:-

- Multiple arterial feeders from both anterior and posterior spinal arteries.
- Highly likely to be symptomatic, presenting commonly as cauda equine syndrome or conus medullaris syndrome.

- AVM nidus, arteriovenous shunts, and large dilated venous varices all three can be present pathologically in these lesions.
- Due to these complexities, both endovascular treatment and open surgical approach are required in these notorious lesions. Aggressive combined approach is the only salvage treatment modality for these lesions.
- Preoperative angiography, with aggressive embolization of anterior and posterior feeder vessels followed by surgical resection of the nidus, or engorged veins.
- Surgical approach in prone position is a classical posterior approach to conus medullaris, as described before.
- In patients with a compact nidus, surgical principles are same as described for intramedullary AVMs.

26.11.2.1 Spinal Cavernomas

Treatment of symptomatic spinal cavernomas offers an improvement in prognosis. Microsurgical treatment is recommended for symptomatic spinal cord cavernomas [13, 32, 33].

26.11.3 Follow-up

Routinely a follow-up imaging should be done immediately after resection, and subsequently at 1, 3, 5, and 10 years post-operatively to rule out any possibility of recurrence. In patients which show recurrence of the symptoms, a repeat MRI imaging should be done to rule out tethering of the spinal cord.

26.11.4 Outcome

These spinal vascular lesions spinal DAVFs, AVMs, are rare lesions. Both surgery and endovascular treatments have shown comparable outcomes. Early study by Logue et al. including 24 patients treated primarily by surgery (embolization was used as an adjunct in one case) has shown a 62% improvement in gait among all 24 patients; however, only 22% showed improve-

ment in bladder control. A similar conclusion was drawn in a study by Symon et al. in 46 patients which showed improvement in motor symptoms in 69% of the patients [34]. In spinal AVFs, the success rates of endovascular therapy have been reported to vary between 25 and 75% where surgical success rates are close to 95%. During follow-up after complete occlusion of the fistula, 2/3rd of all patients experience improvement in their motor symptoms while only 1/3 report an improvement of their sensory complaints. Sexual dysfunctions and sphincter disturbances are mostly irreversible [35].

The obliteration rate with surgery is as high as 100%, with improvement in 91% of the patients. In comparison, the endovascular treatment obliteration rates are widely variable and range from 30 to 90%. Recanalization rates are also reportedly high in the later. Considering the functional outcome, Velat et al. showed that 70 percent were functionally independent, at long-term follow-up after surgical resection of intramedullary AVMs, with a 75% obliteration rate [36].

26.11.5 Spinal Cavernomas— Treatment Strategies

Watchful observation is usually the strategy for incidental cavernomas due to narrow margin of safety in spinal cord as compared to brain. The re-bleeding rates of spinal cavernomas are supposed to be higher than 10% demanding treatment of the lesion [32, 33].

- Surgical resection remains the mainstay of the treatment for patients presenting with severe deterioration, or patients showing a progressive neurological decline and myelopathy.
- Posterior approaches like laminoplasty and hemilaminectomy are the mainstay for these benign lesions.
- Goal of the surgery is complete resection, as the residual lesion may result in multiple hemorrhages. In cavernomas with developmental venous anomaly, the venous drainage must be preserved in all circumstances to avoid any bleed due to the lack of the draining channel.

- After opening dura, cavernomas can be visualized with hemosiderin staining or bluish tinge of pia.
- In contrast to the surgical principles of cerebral cavernoma, in spinal cavernomas the hemosiderin ring should be left in situ to avoid cord parenchymal injury and neurological deficit.

26.12 Conclusion

Spinal vascular malformations are extremely rare. The prevalence of incidental spinal vascular malformations is now on increasing trend in the post imaging era reaching close to 5% in adults and 1% in children. Therefore their understanding is vital for neurosurgeons. Spinal cord cavernomas and tumours (e.g. hemangioblastomas) are the most common incidental spinal vascular malformations, followed by spinal DAVFs and AVMs. Later are more likely to present symptomatically. Treatment needs to be tailored individually with a balanced approach considering various factors like patient characteristics, clinical status, radiological type and architecture and location of the lesion. *Watchful observation is usually the strategy for incidental cavernomas, tumours, spinal AVMs. Endovascular treatment is a safer alternative to observation for spinal DAVFs. Micro-neurosurgery remains the gold standard treatment for all patients with disease progression on conservative regimen.* Endovascular intervention has emerged as a safer alternative to microsurgery for spinal AVMs and AVFs, however micro neurosurgery still has a much higher obliteration rate and least recurrence rate.

References

1. Gaupp J. Hamorrhoiden der Pia Mater Spinalis im Gebiet des Lendenmarks. Beitr Pathol. 1888:516–8.
2. Krause F. Chirurgie des Gehirns und Rückenmarks. Berlin: Urban & Schwarzenberg; 1911.
3. Wyburn-Mason R. The vascular abnormalities and tumours of the spinal cord and its membranes. St. Louis: CV Mosby; 1943.
4. Oldfield EH, Di Chiro G, Quindlen EA, Rieth KG, Doppman JL. Successful treatment of a group of spinal cord arteriovenous malformations by interruption of dural fistula. J Neurosurg. 1983;59(6):1019–30.
5. Rosenblum B, Oldfield EH, Doppman JL, Di Chiro G. Spinal arteriovenous malformations: a comparison of dural arteriovenous fistulas and intradural AVM's in 81 patients. J Neurosurg. 1987;67(6):795–802.
6. Da Costa L, Dehdashti AR, terBrugge KG. Spinal cord vascular shunts: spinal cord vascular malformations and dural arteriovenous fistulas. Neurosurg Focus. 2009;26(1):E6. https://doi.org/10.3171/FOC.2009.26.1.E6. PMID: 19119892.
7. Jellema K, Canta LR, Tijssen CC, van Rooij WJ, Koudstaal PJ, van Gijn J. Spinal dural arteriovenous fistulas: clinical features in 80 patients. J Neurol Neurosurg Psychiatry. 2003;74(10):1438–40.
8. Bostroem A, Thron A, Hans FJ, Krings T. Spinal vascular malformations—typical and atypical findings. Zentralbl Neurochir. 2007;68(4):205–13.
9. Poisson A, Vasdev A, Brunelle F, Plauchu H, Dupuis-Girod S, French Italian HHT, network. Acute paraplegia due to spinal arteriovenous fistula in two patients with hereditary hemorrhagic telangiectasia. Eur J Pediatr. 2009;168(2):135–9.
10. Alexander MJ, Grossi PM, Spetzler RF, McDougall CG. Extradural thoracic arteriovenous malformation in a patient with Klippel-Trenaunay-weber syndrome: case report. Neurosurgery. 2002;51(5):1275–8; discussion 1278–1279.
11. Hu M-H, Wu C-T, Lin K-L, Wong AM-C, Jung S-M, Wu C-T, et al. Intramedullary spinal arteriovenous malformation in a boy of familial cerebral cavernous hemangioma. Childs Nerv Syst. 2008;24(3):393–6.
12. Biondi A, Merland JJ, Hodes JE, Pruvo JP, Reizine D. Aneurysms of spinal arteries associated with intramedullary arteriovenous malformations. I. Angiographic and clinical aspects. AJNR Am J Neuroradiol. 1992;13(3):913–22.
13. Zevgaridis D, Medele RJ, Hamburger C, Steiger HJ, Reulen HJ. Cavernous haemangiomas of the spinal cord. A review of 117 cases. Acta Neurochir. 1999;141(3):237–45.
14. Anson JA, Spetzler RF, Anson J, Spetzler R. Classification of spinal arteriovenous malformations and implications for treatment. BNI Quarterly. 1992;(8):2–8.
15. Spetzler RF, Detwiler PW, Riina HA, Porter RW. Modified classification of spinal cord vascular lesions. J Neurosurg. 2002;96(2 Suppl):145–56.
16. Berenstein A, Lasjaunias P, terBrugge K, Lasjaunias PL. Surgical neuroangiography: clinical and endovascular treatment aspects in adults, vol. 2. New York: Springer; 2004. p. 847–72.
17. Eskandar EN, Borges LF, Budzik RF, Putman CM, Ogilvy CS. Spinal dural arteriovenous fistulas: experience with endovascular and surgical therapy. J Neurosurg. 2002;96(2 Suppl):162–7.
18. Criscuolo GR, Oldfield EH, Doppman JL. Reversible acute and subacute myelopathy in patients with dural

arteriovenous fistulas. Foix-Alajouanine syndrome reconsidered. J Neurosurg. 1989;70(3):354–9.

19. Fugate JE, Lanzino G, Rabinstein AA. Clinical presentation and prognostic factors of spinal dural arteriovenous fistulas: an overview. Neurosurg Focus. 2012;32(5):E17.

20. Jellema K, Tijssen CC, van Gijn J. Spinal dural arteriovenous fistulas: a congestive myelopathy that initially mimics a peripheral nerve disorder. Brain. 2006;129(Pt 12):3150–64.

21. Berenstein A, Lasjaunias P, terBrugge K. Spinal dural arteriovenous fistulae. In: Surgical neuroangiography: Vol 2 Clinical and endovascular treatment aspects in adults. New York: Springer; 2004. pp. 847–72.

22. Wilson DA, Abla AA, Uschold TD, McDougall CG, Albuquerque FC, Spetzler RF. Multimodality treatment of conus medullaris arteriovenous malformations: 2 decades of experience with combined endovascular and microsurgical treatments. Neurosurgery. 2012;71(1):100–8.

23. Cenzato M, Debernardi A, Stefini R, D'Aliberti G, Piparo M, Talamonti G, et al. Spinal dural arteriovenous fistulas: outcome and prognostic factors. Neurosurg Focus. 2012;32(5):E11.

24. Cosgrove GR, Bertrand G, Fontaine S, Robitaille Y, Melanson D. Cavernous angiomas of the spinal cord. J Neurosurg. 1988;68(1):31–6.

25. De Marco JK, Dillon WP, Halback VV, Tsuruda JS. Dural arteriovenous fistulas: evaluation with MR imaging. Radiology. 1990;175(1):193–9.

26. Jellema K, Sluzewski M, van Rooij WJ, Tijssen CC, Beute GN. Embolization of spinal dural arteriovenous fistulas: importance of occlusion of the draining vein. J Neurosurg Spine. 2005;2(5):580–3.

27. Doppman JL, Di Chiro G, Dwyer AJ, Frank JL, Oldfield EH. Magnetic resonance imaging of spinal arteriovenous malformations. J Neurosurg. 1987;66(6):830–4.

28. Barnwell SL, Dowd CF, Davis RL, Edwards MS, Gutin PH, Wilson CB. Cryptic vascular malforma-tions of the spinal cord: diagnosis by magnetic resonance imaging and outcome of surgery. J Neurosurg. 1990;72(3):403–7.

29. Britz GW, Lazar D, Eskridge J, Winn HR. Accurate intraoperative localization of spinal dural arteriovenous fistulae with embolization coil: technical note. Neurosurgery. 2004;55(1):252–4; discussion 254–255.

30. Kim LJ, Spetzler RF. Classification and surgical management of spinal arteriovenous lesions: arteriovenous fistulae and arteriovenous malformations. Neurosurgery. 2006;59(5 Suppl 3):S195–201; discussion S3–13.

31. Ausman JI, Gold LH, Tadavarthy SM, Amplatz K, Chou SN. Intraparenchymal embolization for obliteration of an intramedullary AVM of the spinal cord. Technical note. J Neurosurg. 1977;47(1):119–25.

32. Endo T, Aizawa-Kohama M, Nagamatsu K, Murakami K, Takahashi A, Tominaga T. Use of microscope-integrated near-infrared indocyanine green videoangiography in the surgical treatment of intramedullary cavernous malformations: report of 8 cases: clinical article. SPI. 2013;18(5):443–9.

33. Kharkar S, Shuck J, Conway J, Rigamonti D. The natural history of conservatively managed symptomatic intramedullary spinal cord Cavernomas. Neurosurgery. 2007;60(5):865–72.

34. Logue V. Angiomas of the spinal cord: review of the pathogenesis, clinical features, and results of surgery. J Neurol Neurosurg Psychiatry. 1979;42(1):1–11.

35. Behrens S, Thron A. Long-term follow-up and outcome in patients treated for spinal dural arteriovenous fistula. J Neurol. 1999;246(3):181–5.

36. Velat GJ, Chang SW, Abla AA, Albuquerque FC, McDougall CG, Spetzler RF. Microsurgical management of glomus spinal arteriovenous malformations: pial resection technique: clinical article. J Neurosurg Spine. 2012;16(6):523–31.

Asymptomatic Hydromyelia and Syringomyelia

27

Suyash Singh, Amit Shukla,
Ashutosh Kumar Mishra, and Sanjay Behari

Abbreviations

CSF   Cerebrospinal fluid
MRI   Magnetic resonance imaging

27.1   Historical Vignettes

Ollivier d' Angers termed "Syringomyelia" in context with a developmental anomaly in 1824 as "dilated central canal." The understanding and description of syringomyelia subsequently modified several times thereafter. "Syrinx" is a Greek word meaning "tube" and "myelos" means "marrow." Stilling et al. used the term "hydromyelia" for the same "dilated central canal" and "syringomyelia" for a separate cavity inside the gray matter of spinal cord. In 1888, Chiari hypothesized that all the cavities are interconnected and there is no pathophysiological difference between the two terms. Virchow et al. and Pick et al. also backed Chiari for his hypothesis. Thereafter, Ballantine et al. coined the term "syringohydromyelia" in order to get rid of the confusion [1].

S. Singh · A. Shukla · A. K. Mishra
Department of Neurosurgery, All India Institute of
Medical Sciences, Raebareli, Raebareli, U.P., India

S. Behari (✉)
Department of Neurosurgery, Sanjay Gandhi Post
Graduate Institute of Medical Sciences,
Lucknow, U.P., India

27.2   Definition

Syringomyelia is a heterogeneous disorder characterized by abnormal fluid-filled cavities within the spinal cord. Syringomyelia is primary or idiopathic when it is not associated with abnormalities at the level of foramen magnum or with other infective, congenital, traumatic, or neoplastic etiologies. We believe that there is a minor etiological and pathological difference between the two entities; dilation of the central canal due to alterations in the cerebrospinal fluid (CSF) dynamics is termed as syringomyelia, whereas formation of cavities inside the gray matter of the spinal cord after the development of an infective, traumatic, or neoplastic pathology should be termed as "hydromyelia" (the cavities may be interconnected but not connected to the central canal) or "syringohydromyelia" (when cavities are connected to the central canal). In context to this chapter, we will use terms "syringomyelia" broadly for all types of dilated cavities. Syringomyelia may be detected at radiological imaging incidentally or during screening, i.e., asymptomatic syringomyelia (AS), or it may associated with neurological symptoms and deficits. The exact incidence of AS is variably reported in literature because once it was considered as a "rare" clinical entity. It is, however, more often found with advancement in the modern radiology. The axial diameter of the central canal is 2–4 mm, which usually decreases with age; and anything diameter more than that is considered to be representative of syringomyelia or hydromyelia [2–6].

27.3 Etiology

In a radiological study by Sukushima et al. (Japan), the prevalence of syringomyelia was found to be 1.94 per 100000; and the prevalence of AS was 22.6% [7]. Therefore, management of the syrinx before symptoms are obvious becomes an important matter of concern and debate. Various studies have shown that the symptomatology of syringomyelia is reversible only when intervention is done at an early stage; but no level I evidence exists for the timing as well as the need for intervention for AS. Syringomyelia is associated with traumatic, infective, neoplastic, and congenital pathologies. These include:

Congenital Malformations
(a) Chiari malformation
(b) Dandy Walker malformation
(c) Tonsillar herniation with Apert's syndrome, achondroplasia, and Crouzon's syndrome
(d) Noonan syndrome
(e) Cranio-vertebral junction anomalies like pannus or basilar invagination

Iatrogenic
(a) Secondary to lumbo-peritoneal shunt
(b) Secondary to spinal tumor excision
(c) Secondary to extradural surgeries like lumbar or cervical disc surgery
(d) Post radiation manifestation

Spinal dysraphism
(a) Tethered cord syndrome
(b) Myelo-meningocele
(c) Split cord malformation
(d) Spinal dermoid
(e) Neurenteric cyst

Traumatic Spinal Injury
(a) Cord bleed
(b) Bony spinal injury

Infective
(a) Tuberculous arachnoiditis or myelitis
(b) Post viral or bacterial arachnoiditis

Neoplastic
(a) Primary spinal cord tumors (intramedullary or extramedullary)
(b) Metastatic spinal tumors
(c) Lymphoma

Before the advent of magnetic resonance imaging (MRI) studies, the incidence of syringomyelia associated with Chiari malformation has been reported between 20 and 70% in textbooks. Studies using MRI for screening have shown a much higher incidence (up to 85–88%). Similarly, AS is often associated with arachnoiditis. The arachnoiditis may be related to bacterial meningitis, subarachnoid hemorrhage, tuberculosis, syphilitic pachymeningitis, trauma, injected radio-opaque dyes or spinal anesthetic injections, or viral acute myelitis [8–12].

27.4 Asymptomatic vs Non-bothering Symptomatic Syringomyelia

Sometimes the presence of the syrinx may be mildly symptomatic but not interfering with the daily activities of the patient. This is alarming for a clinician as serial radiological follow-up is required for years. Mild back pain, sometimes diffuse non-localizing or dysesthetic burning pain is present and these patients are often treated for the coexisting degenerative spondylosis. It is important to note here that the size of the syrinx cavity has not been found to be clinically correlating with the symptomatology [12, 13]. These patients may further progress to:

(a) Spastic paraparesis or quadriparesis according to the location of syrinx
(b) Scoliosis
(c) Bulbar involvement with cranial progression of syrinx (syringobulbia)
(d) Bladder manifestations

27.5 Investigations Needed for Incidentally Detected Asymptomatic Syringomyelia

Apart from a meticulous radiological follow-up, patients with AS associated with etiologies discussed above should be investigated further to document the subtle neurological deficits. F-wave latencies in the upper limbs are prolonged if syrinx is present at the C8-T1 level. Electromyography studies may show chronic partial denervation. Although the fluid aspiration did not show any promising correlation, however the protein level in the syringomyelia fluid ranges from 0.35 to 3.9 g/L with a yellowish discoloration. Clinical progression of the disease is highly variable:

(a) Some patients show clinical progression for years and then remain static.
(b) Some patients remain asymptomatic for a long time and then show sudden deterioration with a trivial trigger point history.
(c) A few patients show a continuous slow deterioration.

The maximum reported latent period between the initial inflammatory event and that of the development of syringomyelia is 30-years. Contrast-enhanced MRI should be done especially in cases of syringomyelia associated with a neoplastic etiology. These patients needed an early intervention, even in the asymptomatic stage.

27.6 Differential Diagnosis of Syringomyelia

(a) Spinal intramedullary cyst
(b) Myelomalacia
(c) Arachnoid cyst
(d) Glio-ependymal cyst
(e) Persistent or residual central spinal canal

27.7 Histology of Syrinx

The syrinx cavity is lined by ependymal or sometimes fibrillary glial tissue (with Rosenthal fibers). The shape and lining of the syrinx wall may vary individually according to the vertebral level of the pathology and the nature of pathology. Vascular changes like hyalinized and thickened vessels, edema or hemorrhage may be seen around the syrinx wall. Not unusually, aberrant nerve fibers may be seen in the wall of the cavity. As these syrinxes are usually manifestations of a dilated central canal and the motor-sensory fiber tracts cross at a certain distance, paracentral dissections are only occasionally present.

27.8 Pathogenesis

Giner et al. highlighted two physics principles explaining the formation of syrinx in the spinal cord [5]
1. Bernoulli's principle—Increase in CSF flow speed due to the narrow channel, resulting in decreased pressure in that region
2. Venturi effect—A fluid flowing at a high speed creates a suction effect

The combined effects of the above two principles result in the dilation of the parenchyma below the level of obstruction.

Other established theories in literature for the possible explanation of pathogenesis of syringomyelia are as follows [14–18]:

(a) *Post-operative syrinx*
   It is not unusual to find AS in follow-up MRI scans post-intramedullary tumor surgery or traumatic spinal cord injury (SCI) surgery. It is hypothesized that post-surgical scarring of peri-dural tissues or the cord atrophy after damage to the microvasculature lead to compression or decrease of the central canal diameter. This

decrease in canal size leads to alteration in CSF dynamics locally, and consequently, the dilation of canal (as a result of gradual increase in hydrostatic pressure) cranially and caudally.

(b) *Gardner's water hammer effect theory*

Gardner et al. proposed that the pathological transmission of arterial pulsations from the choroid plexus to the central canal of the spinal cord leads to dilation of the canal, and hence, to the formation of syringomyelia. The low protein content found in aspirated fluid from the syringomyelic cavity is an indirect evidence supporting Gardner's theory. Furthermore, it is known that the central canal is lined by "high water containing" gray matter compared to "white matter" lined ventricles; therefore, the central canal dilates to form syringomyelia at the same low pressure when ventricles are not seen dilated.

(c) *William's ball valve mechanism sump effect theory*

William et al. believe that cerebellar tonsils act as a one-way valve allowing CSF to enter the cisterna magna during the Valsalva maneuver (coughing, straining, etc.) and prevent the fluid from reentering the spinal canal. Physiologically, the spinal cord is slightly pushed cranially during the Valsalva maneuver. Any pathological or congenital change at the cranio-vertebral junction or the presence of hindbrain malformation lead to loss of this ball valve mechanism, and a pressure difference is created between the posterior fossa and the spinal canal. Once the CSF physiological dynamics (fourth ventricle—cisterna magna—thecal sac) is lost, the only possible opening left is the central canal. A suck-in or sump effect is created which forces the CSF to enter the central canal, thereby dilating it.

(d) *Non-communicating syringomyelia*

Both the Gardner's and William's theories revolve around the communicating syringomyelia but autopsy studies have found that adhesions are present near the tonsils or the obex and often these hindbrain cavities are non-communicating. It is therefore, proposed that the fluid inside the non-pulsatile syrinx cavity of the spinal cord gray matter comes from the dorsal root entry zone or perivascular spaces around the syrinx wall.

(e) *Congenital origin of syringomyelia*

Muthukumar [19] and Li et al. [20] proposed that a single embryological insult results in both the development of the syrinx and also occult spinal dysraphism formation. Pang hypothesized that complete lack of retrogressive differentiation leads to an extremely low conus medullaris with persistent terminal syrinx or terminal ventricle [21]. Some authors believe that failure of development of a connection between the terminal ventricle and the central canal leads to a pathological dilation of the terminal ventricle. In a contrasting view, Iskandar et al. proposed that the above embryological basis explains only the development of asymptomatic smaller or low pressure syrinx cavities; high pressure syrinx cavities of the cord may be due to the development of ischemia secondary to cord tethering.

(f) *Ball and Dayan's infiltration theory, Oldfield's piston theory, and Heiss theory* revolve around the trans-medullary infiltration of CSF through the perivascular space. Blockage of subarachnoid space leads to increase in cerebrospinal fluid pressure. This pressure further augments during the systole phase of the cardiac cycle; and with each systole, the fluid travels through perivascular spaces into the gray matter of spinal cord and thereby leads to the formation of syringomyelia.

27.8.1 Idiopathic Syringomyelia

Syringomyelia is called primary or idiopathic when it is not associated with abnormalities at the level of foramen magnum or other infective, congenital, traumatic, or neoplastic etiologies. The controversy with this terminology increased after acceptance of a new subtype of Chiari as "Chiari Type-0", wherein only syringomyelia (and not tonsillar herniation) is seen and the pathology subsides after surgical intervention. Invasive myelography or non-invasive cine-MRI may help in differentiating idiopathic syringomyelia with secondary forms. Nakamura et al. further classified idiopathic syringomyelia into two types: first is a "localized" type, which represents congenital enlargement of the central canal, and can be managed conservatively; the second is the "extended" type, which causes progressive neurologic dysfunction, and may need surgical intervention [22]. Localized idiopathic syrinx, which remain asymptomatic, extends from 2 to 3 vertebrae. Long-term radiological follow-up is required for AS.

27.8.2 Asymptomatic Syringomyelia Associated with Spinal Dysraphism

The occult or spinal dysraphic state or the overt spinal dysraphism 'aperta' leads to congenital defect with tethering of the spinal cord, either because of a thick filum terminale or due to adherence of nerve roots or cord elements to the aberrant fatty tissue of lipomeningocele. This tethering of cord is followed by stretching of the lower end of the spinal cord, as the child grows in height. Due to this, two critical events may occur:

(a) Micro-hemorrhagic changes inside the gray matter of spinal cord
(b) Alteration in local CSF dynamics

Another possible explanation by Pang et al. is the unified theory of origin [21]. This proposes that a single genetic change leads to both the phenotype of spina bifida cystica and syringomyelia. In his review of syringomyelia in tethered cord patients, Lee et al. found that nearly 12% of patients with syringomyelia have occult spinal dysraphism of the various types (20–65%

in literature). Myelomeningocele and split cord malformation are reported to be the most commonly associated types dyraphic states associated with the formation of an AS. Syrinx formation or enlarged central canal in the caudal most portion of spinal cord is known as persistent terminal ventricle (Figs. 27.1 and 27.2). One important point to highlight herein is that it is very difficult to ascertain whether symptoms arising are due to the dysraphic state or due to syringomyelia. In usual clinical practice, dysraphism is taken care of while syrinx is left to spontaneous resolution. In a few cases, where the syrinx does not resolve, such patients need syringostomy or the theco-peritoneal shunt [23].

27.8.3 Syringomyelia Associated with Spinal Tumors

The pathogenesis and association of syringomyelia with respect to spinal tumors need a separate mention. It has been found in dynamic magnetic resonance imaging scans that the syrinx cavity associated with a neoplastic etiology is usually non-pulsatile in comparison to the pulsatile syrinx associated with a hindbrain or craniovertebral junction anomaly. Historically, it was believed that both the abnormal syrinx cavity and the tumor arise from abnormal glial and mesodermal tissues. Abnormal glial proliferation leads to degeneration and subsequently to cavity formation. Later on, Gardner et al. highlighted that the syrinx cavity in tumors is a mere tumor cavity, as in cystic tumors of the brain. Other pathogenesis postulated include:

(a) Inference of tumor with vascular supply of the spinal cord leading to micro-infarcts
(b) Intra-tumoral hemorrhages
(c) Tissue fluid drainage or tumor secreting fluid or the formation of a transudate
(d) Peri-tumoral edema blocking local CSF dynamics
(e) Increased spinal venous pressure leading to influx of CSF into the perivascular spaces

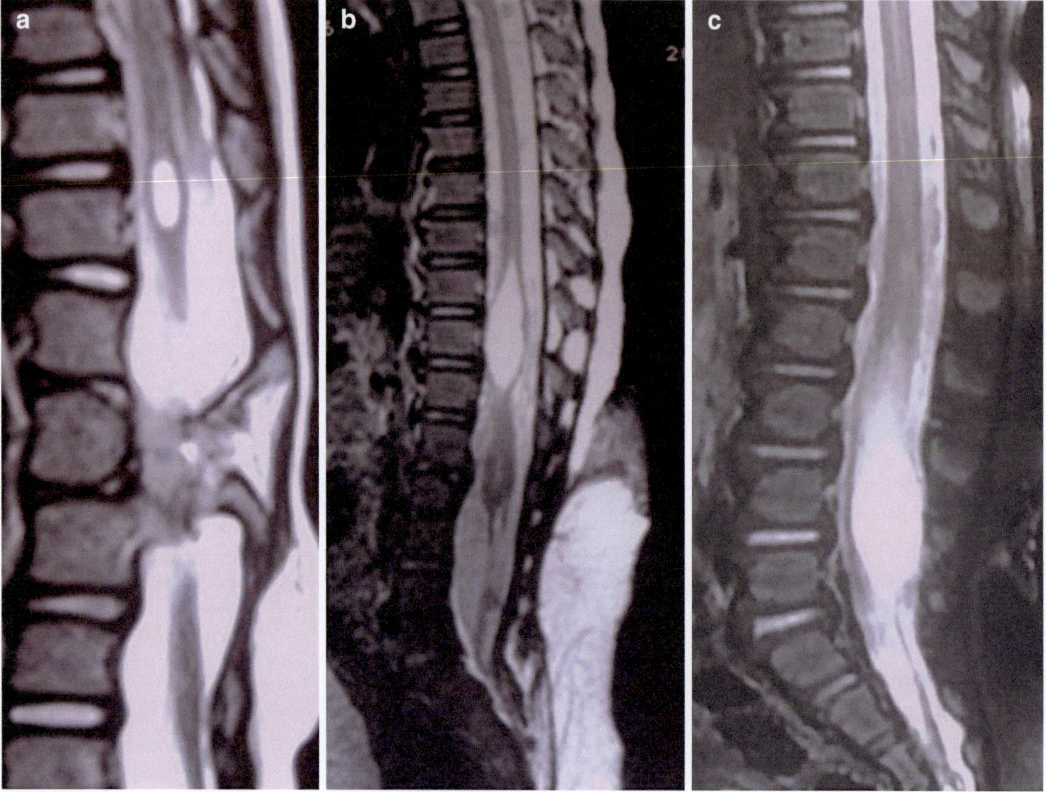

Fig. 27.1 (a–c) A patient with diastematomyelia with syringomyelia at the level of conus (terminal ventricle) that was complete asymptomatic

The exact pathogenesis of the appearance of AS long after tumor excision as well as the resolution of syringomyelia after tumor excision is not present in literature. Some authors believe that the formation of surgical iatrogenic adhesions and the presence of cord tethering is the likely etiology.

Similar explanation has been given for post-traumatic syringomyelia, in which adhesions or cord tethering lead to the traction of tonsils cranially. Subsequently alteration in the CSF dynamics occurs leading to syringomyelia formation. Some authors have found that cord atrophy is a common occurrence after trauma. This may be due to the associated micro-infarcts or hemorrhagic degeneration. Thus, formation of a post-traumatic degenerative cavity may be proposed as the pathophysiology for syringomyelia formation [2, 3].

27.8.4 Iatrogenic Syringomyelia

Kurzbuch et al. reviewed case reports on iatrogenic syringomyelia and found that the following surgeries are associated with post-operative syringomyelia [24]:

- Shunt surgeries like ventriculo-peritoneal shunt, lumbo-peritoneal shunt, cysto-peritoneal shunt, and subdural-peritoneal shunt.
- Suboccipital craniotomy or surgery for Chiari malformation.
- Craniosynostosis surgery.
- Intracranial tumor surgery.

In the same study, it was also found that the mean time of manifestation of the iatrogenic syringomyelia after cranial surgery was 5.7-

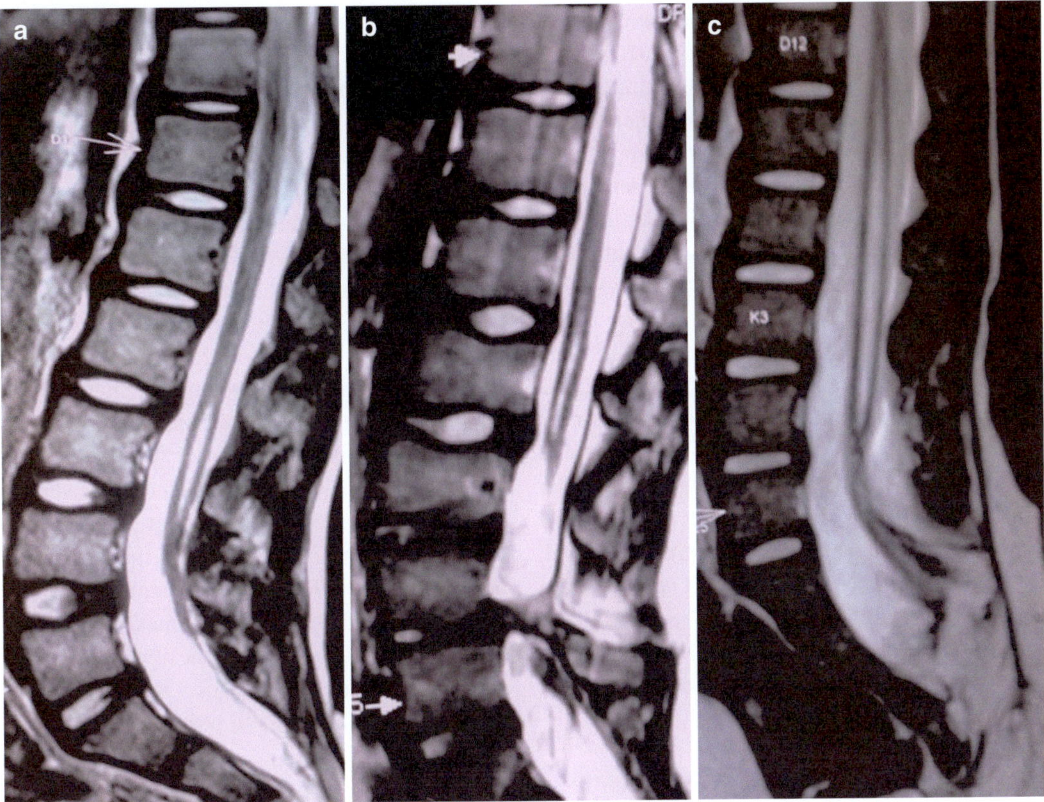

Fig. 27.2 (**a–c**) A patient with symptomatic holocord syringomyelia with tethered cord in the lumbosacral region

years (range of 0.1–51-years). Three structural risk factors for the formation of iatrogenic-induced syringomyelia are post-operative intracranial scarring, shunt malfunction, and mass effect on the foramen magnum. Kersey et al. reported a case of lumbar-peritoneal shunt, wherein, iatrogenic syringomyelia developed after the patient became pregnant. It was hypothesized that the raised intra-abdominal pressure is transmitted to the perivascular spaces leading to the formation of cavitation [25]. Similar iatrogenic syrinx is seen after the excision of intramedullary tumors like astrocytoma or ependymoma. After excision or decompression of these tumors, two possibilities occur: (a) the cavity is filled with fluid with an increased protein content. This fluid is thicker than the surrounding CSF and thereby has increased tendency to form adhesions or arachnoidal bands. Hence, these adhesive bands either lead to cord

tethering or alteration in CSF dynamics; (b) after an intramedullary decompression, microvasculature changes leads to small infarcts and micro-hemorrhages that may progress to the formation of syrinx.

27.8.5 Post-infective Syringomyelia

Asymptomatic syrinx is occasionally found associated with post bacterial, viral, or tuberculous myelitis or arachnoiditis [6]. It is estimated that around 10% of patients with tuberculous meningitis have some form of spinal cord involvement. The parasite cysticercosis has also been reported to be associated with arachnoiditis. Parasitic infestation may lead to myelin/axon damage and necrosis or cavitation formation. Sabrina et al. in their series explained the various mechanisms of infectious/inflammatory myelitis associated with syringomyelia. This includes (a) the development of an inflammatory state leading to narrowing of the subarachnoid space, (b) the initiation of intrinsic mechanisms related to the inflammatory process like blood–spinal cord barrier breakdown, accumulation of extracellular edema, and venous congestion that contribute to the increase in interstitial pressure. Arterial vasculitis has been a characteristic feature of tuberculous meningitis. Similar arterial vasculitis is seen in the spinal cord along with constrictive fibrosis, ischemia, and subsequent syrinx formation. These infections lead to inflammation of the arachnoid matter, which becomes thick and adherent. Several cases have been reported showing similar arachnoid inflammation after the usage of oil-based contrast agents [11, 12]. Quencer et al. described a number of patients in whom arachnoiditis was totally asymptomatic. Some authors have reported a rare form of chronic inflammatory familial arachnoiditis which runs in the Japanese population.

There are three main stages of arachnoiditis
1. Radiculitis stage: The spinal nerve roots are inflamed in response to a pathological event, and the subarachnoid space is encroached upon by the swollen nerve roots. Deposition of collagen fibrils begins.
2. Arachnoiditis: The scar tissue increases, and the nerves begin to adhere to each other and the dura.
3. Adhesive arachnoiditis: In the third stage, there is complete encapsulation of the nerve roots by the scar tissue. This scarring prevents contact with the surrounding spinal fluid, thereby impeding CSF dynamics around the affected area. The isolated nerve roots are, therefore, starved of oxygen and nutrients and the waste products of metabolism accumulate all around.

The problem of iatrogenic drug- or dye-induced arachnoiditis is on the rise. Anesthetic drugs in epidural space, steroid injections for the treatment of spondylosis, the myelogram dye, and the chemotherapeutic agents instilled into the spinal subarachnoid space are the prime examples.

27.8.6 Posttraumatic Syringomyelia

Symptomatic posttraumatic syringomyelia is a rare complication or sequelae after SCI. It occurs in 1 to 4% of patients who have developed spinal cord injury; however, an asymptomatic syrinx is more prevalent and may represent a focal area of liquefaction necrosis of the spinal cord. The reported incidence has been as high as 51% with majority being in the cervical location. The pathogenesis is similar to infective arachnoiditis with the causative event being a traumatic etiology. Spinal cord inflammation, edema, hematoma, liquefaction, intracellular lysosome-content release, ischemia, necrosis, or arterial and venous occlusion may all in different degrees contribute to the formation of a syrinx. In their series of posttraumatic SCI patients, Biyani and Curati et al. suggest that complete spinal cord lesions double the risk of development of clinical syringomyelia. Other risk factors included spinal canal stenosis (>25%) and posttraumatic kyphosis (>15°) [7, 9, 10].

27.8.7 Do We Need Surgical Intervention for Asymptomatic Syringomyelia?

The need of surgical intervention at the asymptomatic stage is still controversial and a topic of debate. The time duration is unpredictable when any asymptomatic patient may become symptomatic. Various authors have concluded that early intervention is warranted for syringomyelia as chances of reversing the symptoms are possible only when timely surgical intervention has been done [7, 14]. The primary objective in the management of syringomyelia is to treat the underlying causative pathology. If the condition do not subside, then syrinx cavity may need to be managed by diverting the spinal CSF to an alternate pathway using a CSF diversion procedure. This may be a justification for the surgical management of AS also. However, treatment is usually unsatisfactory and none of the available options has shown a promising and an acceptable outcome [26].

27.9 Conclusion

AS is an uncommon clinical entity that usually affects young adults and may or may not progress to symptomatic myelopathy. The size of the syrinx cavity usually does not show any correlation with the symptoms and severity. Early intervention may lead to a cessation in the disease progression.

References

1. Roy AK, Slimack NP, Ganju A. Idiopathic syringomyelia: retrospective case series, comprehensive review, and update on management. Neurosurg Focus. 2011;31(6):E15. https://doi.org/10.3171/2011.9.FOCUS11198.
2. Hamlat A, Le Strat A, Boisselier P, Brassier G, Carsin-Nicol B. Asymptomatic syringomyelia in the course of medulloblastoma. Pediatr Neurosurg. 2005;41(5):258–63. https://doi.org/10.1159/000087485.
3. Zhou JJ, Xu JF, Zheng XN, Peng GP. Asymptomatic syringomyelia accompanied with metastatic cerebellar and spinal intramedullary lymphoma: a case report. Medicine (Baltimore). 2017;96(46):e8593. https://doi.org/10.1097/MD.0000000000008593.
4. Pasoglou V, Janin N, Tebache M, Tegos TJ, Born JD, Collignon L. Familial adhesive arachnoiditis associated with syringomyelia. AJNR Am J Neuroradiol. 2014;35(6):1232–6. https://doi.org/10.3174/ajnr.A3858.
5. Giner J, Pérez López C, Hernández B, Gómez de la Riva Á, Isla A, Roda JM. Update on the pathophysiology and management of syringomyelia unrelated to Chiari malformation. Neurologia (Engl Ed). 2019;34(5):318–25. https://doi.org/10.1016/j.nrl.2016.09.010.
6. Wen N, Zhao F, Zhu Y, Jia F, Wan C, Wen Y. Acute development of syringomyelia following TBM in a pediatric case. BMC Pediatr. 2021;21(1):36. https://doi.org/10.1186/s12887-021-02493-7.
7. Sakushima K, Tsuboi S, Yabe I, Hida K, Terae S, Uehara R, Nakano I, Sasaki H. Nationwide survey on the epidemiology of syringomyelia in Japan. J Neurol Sci. 2012;313(1–2):147–52. https://doi.org/10.1016/j.jns.2011.08.045.
8. Koyanagi I, Iwasaki Y, Hida K, Houkin K. Clinical features and pathomechanisms of syringomyelia associated with spinal arachnoiditis. Surg Neurol. 2005;63(4):350–5. https://doi.org/10.1016/j.surneu.2004.05.038.
9. Biyani A, el Masry WS. Post-traumatic syringomyelia: a review of the literature. Paraplegia. 1994;32(11):723–31. https://doi.org/10.1038/sc.1994.117.
10. Kleindienst A, Engelhorn T, Roeckelein V, et al. Development of pre-syrinx state and syringomyelia following a minor injury: a case report. J Med Case Rep. 2020;14:223. https://doi.org/10.1186/s13256-020-02568-6.
11. Brammah TB, Jayson MI. Syringomyelia as a complication of spinal arachnoiditis. Spine (Phila Pa 1976). 1994;19(22):2603–5. https://doi.org/10.1097/00007632-199411001-00019.
12. Abel TJ, Howard MA, Menezes A. Syringomyelia and spinal arachnoiditis resulting from aneurysmal subarachnoid hemorrhage: report of two cases and review of the literature. J Craniovertebr Junction Spine. 2014;5:47–51.
13. Stoodley MA, Gutschmidt B, Jones NR. Cerebrospinal fluid flow in an animal model of noncommunicating syringomyelia. Neurosurgery. 1999;44(5):1065–75. https://doi.org/10.1097/00006123-199905000-00068.
14. Batzdorf U. Primary spinal syringomyelia. J Neurosurg Spine. 2005;3:429–35.
15. Heiss JD, Suffredini G, Smith R, DeVroom HL, Patronas NJ, Butman JA, et al. Pathophysiology of persistent syringomyelia after decompressive craniocervical surgery. J Neurosurg Spine. 2010;13:729–42.
16. Oldfield EH, Muraszko K, Shawker TH, Patronas NJ. Pathophysiology of syringomyelia associated with Chiari I malformation of the cerebellar tonsils. Implications for diagnosis and treatment. J Neurosurg. 1994;80:3–15.
17. Williams B. Simultaneous cerebral and spinal fluid pressure recordings. 2. Cerebrospinal dissociation with lesions at the foramen magnum. Acta Neurochir (Wien). 1981;59:123–42.
18. Chang HS, Nakagawa H. Hypothesis on the pathophysiology of syringomyelia based on simulation of cerebrospinal fluid dynamics. J Neurol Neurosurg Psychiatry. 2003;74(3):344–7. https://doi.org/10.1136/jnnp.74.3.344.
19. Muthukumar N. Terminal syringomyelia communicating with a spinal dermal sinus. J Clin Neurosci. 2007;14(7):688–90. https://doi.org/10.1016/j.jocn.2006.02.013.
20. Li YD, Therasse C, Kesavabhotia K, Lamano JB, Ganju A. Radiographic assessment of surgical treatment of post-traumatic syringomyelia. J Spinal Cord Med. 2021;44(6):861–9.
21. Pang D, Dias MS, Ahab-Barmada M. Split cord malformation: part I: a unified theory of embryogenesis for double spinal cord malformations. Neurosurgery. 1992;31(3):451–80. https://doi.org/10.1227/00006123-199209000-00010.
22. Nakamura M, Ishii K, Watanabe K, Tsuji T, Matsumoto M, Toyama Y, Chiba K. Clinical significance and prognosis of idiopathic syringomyelia. J Spinal Disord Tech. 2009;22(5):372–5. https://doi.org/10.1097/BSD.0b013e3181761543.

23. Rangari K, Das KK, Singh S, Kumar KG, Bhaisora KS, Sardhara J, et al. Type I Chiari malformation without concomitant bony instability: assessment of different surgical procedures and outcomes in 73 patients. Neurospine. 2021;18(1):126–138.

24. Kersey J, Cato-Addison W, Holliman D. Iatrogenic syringomyelia secondary to lumboperitoneal shunt altered by the raised intra-abdominal pressure of pregnancy. Br J Neurosurg. 2017;32(6):684–5. https://doi.org/10.1080/02688697.2017.1297369.

25. Kurzbuch AR, Magdum S. Iatrogenic syringomyelia postcranial surgery in pediatric patients: systematic review and illustrative case. Childs Nerv Syst. 2021;37(9):2879–90. https://doi.org/10.1007/s00381-021-05268-8.

26. Arora P, Behari S, Banerji D, Chhabra DK, Jain VK. Factors influencing the outcome in symptomatic Chiari I malformation. Neurol India. 2004;52(4):470–4.

Intraspinal Lipoma

28

Yan Hu

28.1 Introduction

Spinal lipoma is a rare congenital benign tumor. The source of the lipoma is not clear, intradural various tissues except on the pia mater spinalis found a small amount of mature adipose tissue, there is no other adipose tissue, and abnormal embryonic original meningeal residues and adipose differentiation, often with other congenital malformation, such as fat tissue in vertebral canal, disturbing the normal closure of nerve groove, can be combined with spina bifida, myelomeningocele, spinal cord tethered, subcutaneous lipoma, and fur sinus. Intramedullary lipomas are rare lesion. Most of them originate under the spinal cord membrane and grow outward to form subdural lipomas, usually located near the dorsal midline of the spinal cord and involved in multiple vertebral segments. Dural sac defect and skin abnormality are not found in the cervical and thoracic lipomas. Patients in the lumbosacral spinal canal are often accompanied by dural defects, myelomeningocele, myelome-ningocele, and other developmental malformations, as well as subcutaneous lipoma and fur sinus [1].

28.2 Patient Selection and Preoperative Evaluation

For serendipitous intraspinal lipoma, regular follow-up is usually recommended without excessive clinical intervention if the patient has no obvious clinical symptoms. For pediatric patients, most surgeons advocate the need for early preventive surgery. Aggressive lipoma resection seems to provide better long-term protection against symptomatic recurrence than partial resection [2]. Because of the spinal canal lipoma grew more slowly, more is located in the spinal cord dorsal. Consequently, the majority of patients with progressive numbness and paresthesia for common symptoms. Duration of symptoms is usually longer which results in the majority of patients ignore to the progression of the symptoms. As the tumor increases its compression on the spinal cord tumors becomes largely serious, can appear across the spinal cord lesions [3]. Preoperative plain X-ray examination of such patients shows that erosion of the vertebral body and its accessory structures or accompanied by spina bifida, meningocele, and other malformations are often observed. CT examination shows uniform low-density changes of the

Y. Hu (✉)
Department of Neurosurgery, The First Affiliated Hospital of Zhengzhou University,
Zhengzhou, Henan, People's Republic of China

International Joint Laboratory of Nervous System Malformations, The First Affiliated Hospital of Zhengzhou University,
Zhengzhou, Henan, People's Republic of China
e-mail: fcchuy@zzu.edu.cn

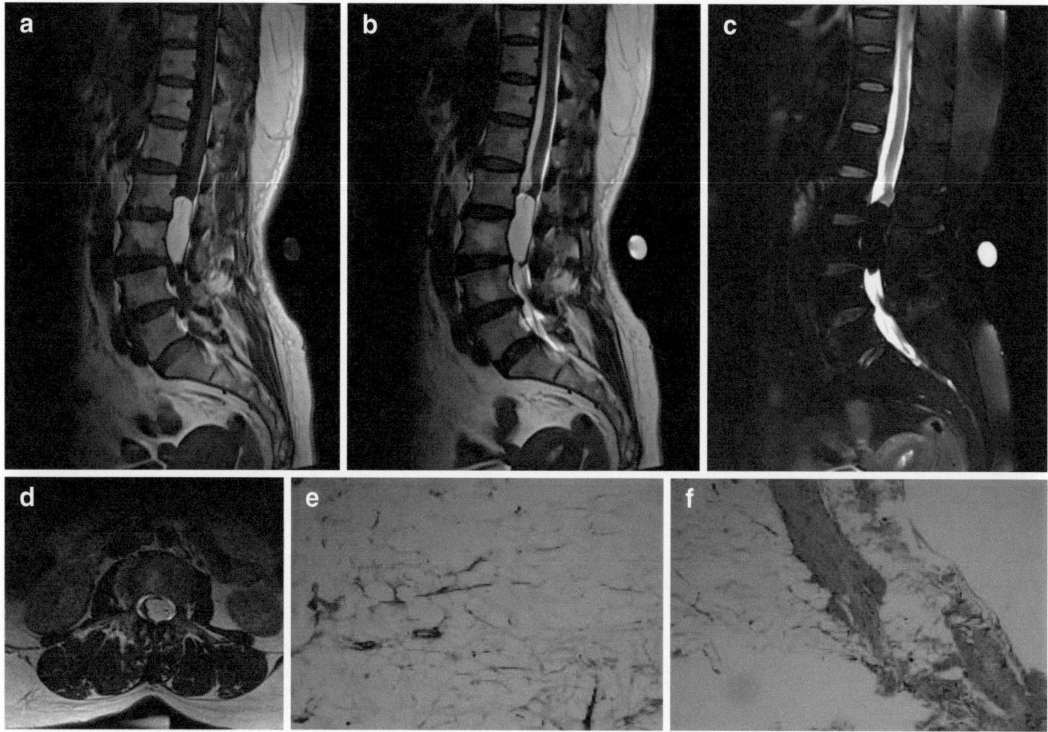

Fig. 28.1 (**a**) Preoperative MRI T1WI showed short T1 signal in the subdural of L2–4 spinal canal; (**b**) preoperative MRI T2WI showed long T2 signal in the subdural of L2–4 spinal canal; (**c**) preoperative MRI fat suppression examination showed L2–4 signal inhibition; (**d**) preoperative MRI T2WI axial position showed tumor space occupying effect; (**e**, **f**) pathological examination showed that the tumor was composed of fat and fibrous tissue (HE 10 × 40)

tumor, with CT value of 70–120 HU, clear edge and no enhancement is found after enhancement [4]. The subdural lesions is parallel to the long axis of the spinal cord, and the adjacent subdural space is widened. The spinal cord is deformed and displaced under compression. MRI showed typical fat signals of short T1 and long T2, and lipoma could be confirmed by fat suppression imaging. There is no enhancement of the lesion on enhanced scan, and when the lesion is large, it could wrap around adjacent blood vessels and nerve components, that is, blood vessels passed through the lesion, presenting linear enhancement [5]. Part of the lesions can infiltrate into the medullary, and fat components with short T1 and long T2 signals can be seen, and the signals can be uniform or mixed. The high signal of the lesion, low signal of the lipid suppressive sequence, and no enhancement signs are important imaging evidence for the diagnosis of the spinal lipoma (Fig. 28.1), which should be distinguished from dermoid cysts and teratoma which also contain fat. T1WI with high signal should be differentiated from subacute hemorrhagic lesions, melanoma, enterogenous cysts, and epidermoid cysts. At present, MRI examination is the best diagnostic method of intraspinal lipoma.

28.3 Principles of Surgery

When we have to perform surgical intervention on patients, it should be noted that for lipomas located in the cervical or thoracic spinal cord, the operation is still full of risks. If the tumor is closely adhered to the soft membrane of the spinal cord or the spinal nerve, it is not advisable to force total resection. During the operation, nerve electrophysiological monitoring is used to avoid accidental injury or excessive damage to the

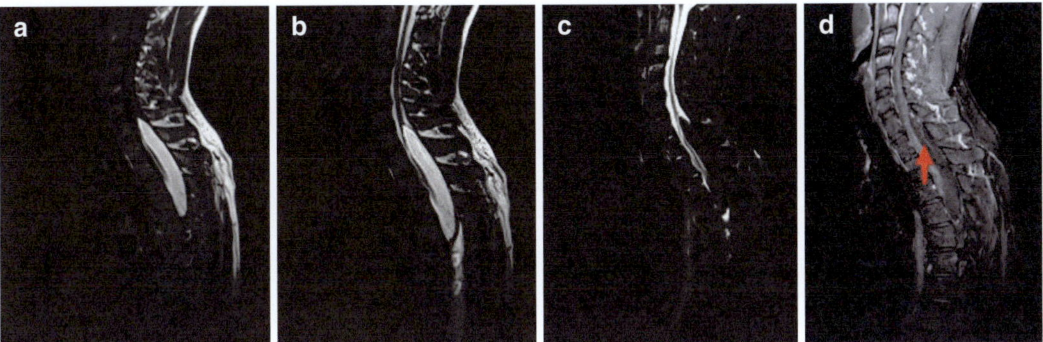

Fig. 28.2 (**a**) Preoperative MRI T1WI showed short T1 signal in C6–T5 spinal canal and subdural; (**b**) preoperative MRI T2WI showed long T2 signal in C6–T5 spinal canal and subdural; (**c**) preoperative MRI fat suppression examination showed C6–T5 signal inhibition; (**d**) preoperative MRI sagittal enhancement showed linear enhanced vascular shadow in lipoma

nerve tissue. The soft membrane of the spinal cord was cut under the microscope, and yellow fatty tissue was visible. Some tumors have hard and tough texture and rich blood supply. It is difficult to remove the tumor by conventional microscopy. It is better to use electromagnetic knife or contact laser knife to remove the tumor and avoid damaging the spinal cord and nerve root (Fig. 28.2). Daisuke Tateiwa reported a case of an intraspinal extradural lipoma with spinal epidural lipomatosis, the made an extensive review of several studies. Although only partial or majority resection is performed, the clinical symptoms are often improved to a certain extent after decompression with the removal of the lamina and the extension of the dural repair [6].

28.4 Diagnosis and Treatment of Epidural Lipoma

Adipose tissue is widely found in the epidural space, covering the dura mater and nerve roots under normal physiological conditions, especially in areas of high mobility in the spine, where it lubricates and protects surrounding tissues. In some pathological states, the local and spatial distribution of epidural fat will change, such as spinal epidural lipomatosis (SEL). Due to the compression of spinal cord and nerve root by increased fat in the spinal canal, it usually presents with a variety of neurological symptoms, including severe lumbago and leg pain, paresthesia, and bladder dysfunction [7]. Of course, the treatment of epidural lipomatosis is mainly targeted at the etiology, such as reducing steroid hormones, reducing body fat rate, regulating fat metabolism, and other conservative treatment methods. Surgical treatment is not the first choice. The purpose is to relieve the pressure of excess fat on nerve roots and relieve acute neurological symptoms such as pain and paralysis [8].

Epidural angiolipoma is formed by primitive mesenchymal stem cells, mature adipocytes, and proliferative blood vessels in pathological state, it is divided into two subtypes: non-invasive and invasive. In comparison, there was no significant difference in age distribution between the two subtypes, both of which tended to occur in middle and old age. The common clinical symptoms are sensory dysfunction, motor dysfunction, tendon reflex changes or pathological signs, chest and back pain, and sphincter dysfunction, but the proportion of invasive chest and back pain was higher than that of non-invasive type. Imaging findings especially MRI are the most important method for preoperative identification of the two subtypes. MRI signal characteristics of invasive angiolipoma are basically the same as those of non-invasive angiolipoma, which are consistent with the imaging characteristics of fat and vascular components. The only difference is that invasive angiolipoma can detect bone destruction or erosion of surrounding soft tissues. Both of them

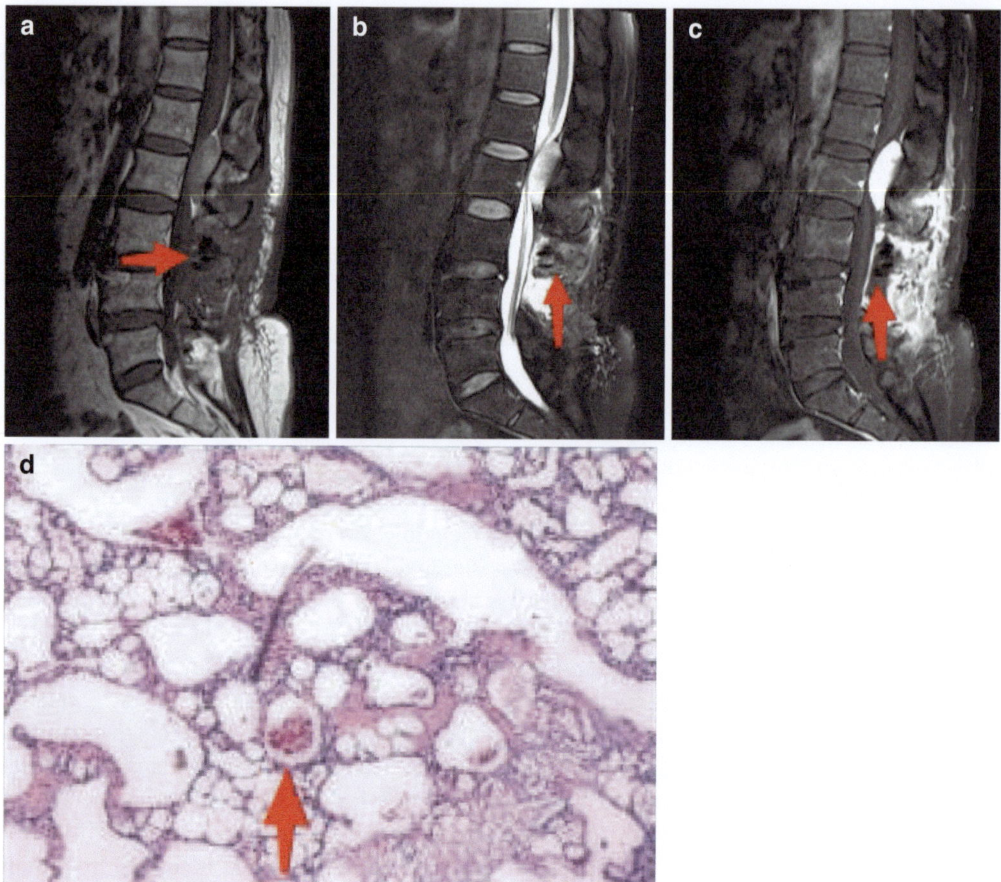

Fig. 28.3 (**a**) Preoperative MRI T1WI showed mixed long/short T1 signal under L1–2 spinal epidural, L3–5 epidural mixed signal, and the red arrow showed the last operation site; (**b**) preoperative MRI T2WI showed mixed long T2 signals under the epidural space of L1–2 spinal canal; (**c**) preoperative MRI sagittal enhancement showed L3–5 epidural mixed signal, red arrow showed dural enhancement at the last operation site, signal disorder in accessory area, and scar tissue formation was considered; (**d**) pathological examination showed that the tumor was composed of mature adipocytes and dysplastic blood vessels (HE 10 × 40). Abnormal blood vessel component shown by red arrow

show mature adipocytes and abnormal proliferative vascular components in postoperative histopathology (Fig. 28.3). Surgery is the best method for the treatment of epidural angiolipoma of the spinal canal and intraspinal epidural angiolipoma. Whether non-invasive or invasive, the operation should be completely removed as far as possible to preserve neural function, and the prognosis is generally good.

28.5 Diagnosis and Treatment of Intradural Lipoma

Intradural lipoma is commonly located in the intramedullary or around the nerve root, which is clinically divided into two types: (1) Lipoma below pia mater spinalis: it usually occurs in the thoracic and cervicothoracic spinal cord, the spinal cord and spine develop normally, and the pain in the corresponding area of the lesion segment is the first symptom; (2) Conus lipoma: it is often accompanied by low spinal cord and spinal canal insufficiency and subcutaneous fat pad. The main clinical manifestations are spasmodic weakness of one or both legs, malformation of ankle–toe joint, and sphincter dysfunction. These lipomas are not true tumors and are considered hamartomas [9].

Lipoma usually has tough texture, that has unclear boundary with spinal cord tissue, and is difficult to separate. Early operations are mainly limited to lipoma biopsy and palliative laminectomy decompression. With the rapid development of microsurgical technology and imaging and the application of intraoperative neuroelectrophysiological monitoring technology, the localization of intramedullary lipoma of spinal cord is more accurate, the protection of intraoperative nerve function is more perfect, and the application of surgical tools such as bone knife and laser knife has significantly improved the rate of successful surgical resection. Of course, the surgical purpose was mainly to relieve spinal cord compression and improve spinal cord function, so tumor resection was strictly limited to "intratumoral" (Fig. 28.4).

28.6 Minimally Invasive Techniques

The traditional surgical method for intraspinal tumors is laminectomy to expose tumors. Although this method is sufficient, it is highly traumatic, destroys the structure of the posterior column of the spine, affects the stability of the spine, and even induces spinal malformations. Fusion internal fixation may be required to rebuild spinal stability, but it may reduce spinal mobility, aggravate degeneration of adjacent segments, and also affect the judgment and operation of tumor recurrence [10]. Hemilaminectomy can reduce muscle dissection and preserve spinous process, contralateral lamina and supraspinous interspinous ligament, which is conducive to spinal stability. Microchannels maximize the use of anatomical space, providing the same spinal canal exposure with a smaller muscle dissection range and incision length than traditional retractors. The combination of hemilaminectomy and microchannel keyhole microsurgery can not only achieve the tumor resection effect of traditional microsurgery, but also further reduce the surgical trauma and reduce the damage to the spinal stabilization device (bone, ligament, and

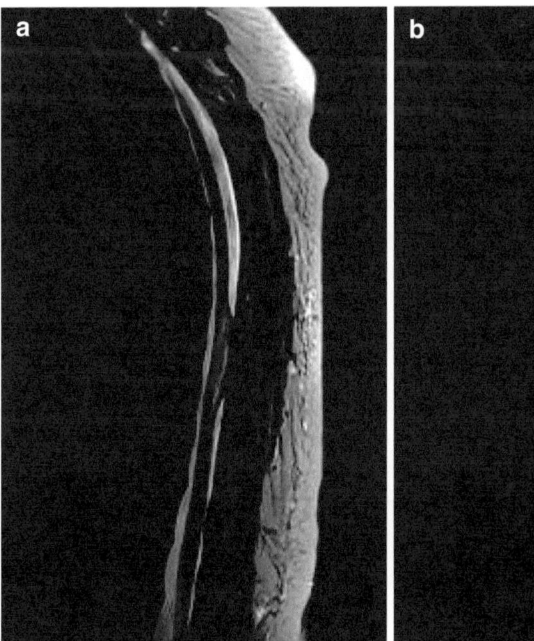
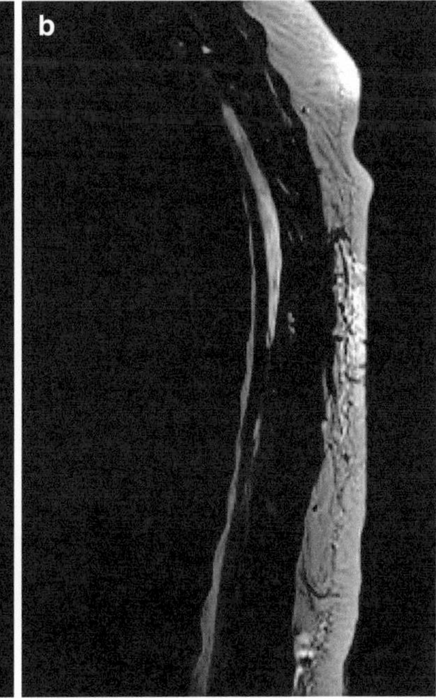

Fig. 28.4 (**a**) Preoperative MRI showed dorsal as well as caudal fat in relation to the neural placode; (**b**) postoperative MRI showing total/near total resection of the lipoma

muscle), so as to better maintain the stability of the spine, with less bleeding and postoperative reaction, and the advantages of rapid recovery, shorter hospitalization time [11].

In recent years, spinal endoscopy has been widely promoted and applied in China. It has become a routine technique in many centers. The limited and minimally invasive spine surgery has become a development trend of spine surgery, and spine endoscopy technology has gradually expanded from the initial application of simple lumbar disc herniation to lumbar spinal stenosis. The surgical site has been developed from the lumbar spine to the cervical and thoracic vertebrae. Surgical methods have changed from simple decompression to assisted fusion and orthosis under microscope. The diagnosis and treatment category had also rapidly expanded from spinal degenerative diseases to encompass spinal trauma, inflammation, malformation, and tumor [12]. Total spinal endoscopic surgery not only has the advantages of less trauma, less blood loss and low cost, but more importantly, this surgery adopts the method of stepwise expansion to separate one side of the paraspinal muscle and retain the spinous process in situ, which can better maintain the anatomical structure of the spine. Therefore, the operation has little influence on the stability of the spine. Compared with microscope, endoscopy can better solve the problems of visual angle and surgical operation affected by space stenosis [13]. Compared with open surgery, total spinal endoscopic surgery only grinds half of the lamina, leaving the spinous process in situ, narrowing the exposure range and the operation space, which has a certain impact on the sight range and operation freedom. At present, endoscopy is still two-dimensional imaging, compared with microscope three-dimensional imaging, stereoscopic display effect is not good. The unavoidable problem of this procedure is how to close the operative cavity tightly. Total endoscopic surgery is limited in space and difficult to suture, so it is difficult to complete strict dural repair well, which requires more improvement and exploration.

28.7 Postoperative Complications

At present, the largest literature report on spinal lipoma comes from 122 cases of lumbosacral lipoma including SC Bai from PLA General Hospital, among which the incidence rate of complications accounts for 14.8%. Including postoperative numbness (4.1%), new postoperative dyskinesia (3.3%), total sensory loss (1.6%), urination dysfunction and constipation (4.1%), cerebrospinal fluid leakage (0.8%), fat liquefaction of surgical incision resulted in no healing (0.8%) [14]. Lumbosacral lipoma is often complicated with spina bifida, and the spinal canal lipoma prolapses along with the dural at the spinal rift and connects with the subcutaneous adipose tissue. After surgical resection, the dural is difficult to be tightly sutured, that is, it faces high risks of cerebrospinal fluid leakage, subcutaneous fluid accumulation, and surgical incision infection. During the operation, artificial replacement materials or autologous fascia can be carefully sutured, and it is recommended that patients be prone after surgery to facilitate wound healing.

28.8 Conclusion

Gowers was the first to describe intraspinal lipoma in 1876 [15]. An earlier extensive review of more common lipomas was conducted by Crols et al. [16]. Although these lipomas are thought to be congenital lesions, adult patients are rare due to the often very insidious onset of symptoms and the restricted awareness and medical resources in underdeveloped areas. Despite long-delayed treatment, surgical intervention is still clearly favored, as neurological decline will continue without treatment. According to our surgical experience, the factors that determine the surgical strategies for this type of spinal lipoma are the patient's age and the location of the spinal lipoma, intramedullary or extramedullary, the number of lipomas attached to the spinal cord, and the relationship of lipomas to nerve roots. We suggest that the operation of cervical and thoracic lipoma should be carried out on the basis of adequate preoperative evaluation and patient education. Aggressive early surgery is recommended for children and adults with lumbosacral lipoma, and extended decompression of the lamina provides a better long-term advantage. However, the surgical indications and treatment strategies for spinal lipoma remain controversial [4, 14]. The long-term advantage of total resection over partial resection of lipoma also needs to be tested in further studies.

References

1. HA T. Intraspinal (intramedullary and subdural) lipoma. Chin J Contemp Neurol Neurosurg. 2019;19(02):131.
2. Pang D, Zovickian J, Oviedo A. Long-term outcome of total and near-total resection of spinal cord lipomas and radical reconstruction of the neural placode, part II: outcome analysis and preoperative profiling. Neurosurgery. 2010;66:253–72.
3. Pierre-Kahn A, Lacombe J, Pichon J, Giudicelli Y, Renier D, Sainte-Rose C, Perrigot M, Hirsch JF. Intraspinal lipomas with spina bifida: prognosis and treatment in 73 cases. J Neurosurg. 1986;65(6):756–61.
4. Arslan E, Kuzeyli K, Arslan EA. Intraspinal lipomas without associated spinal dysraphism. Iran Red Crescent Med J. 2014;16(5):e11423.
5. Chen S, Liu SL, Lin J. Diagnosis and surgical treatment of spinal epidural angiolipomas. Chin J Spine Spinal Cord. 2013;23(04):380–2.
6. Tateiwa D, Yamasaki R, Ariga K, Hayashida K, Wada E. An intraspinal extradural lipoma with spinal epidural lipomatosis: a case report and a review of literature. Surg Neurol Int. 2018;9:212.
7. Fogel GR, Cunningham PY, Esses SI. Spinal epidural lipomatosis: case reports, literature review and meta-analysis. Spine J. 2005;5(2):202–11.
8. Liu YD, Cao Y, Liu DL. Biological characteristics of epidural fat and its implications in clinic. Chin J Spine Spinal Cord. 2020;30(08):757–61.
9. Zhou LF. Contemporary neurosurgery. Shanghai: Fudan University Press of Shanghai; 2015. p. 866.
10. Raygor KP, Than KD, Chou D, et al. Comparison of minimally invasive transspinous and open approaches for thoracolumbar intradural-extramedullary spinal tumors. Neurosurg Focus. 2015;39(2):E12.
11. Guozhong L, Ma C, Wu C. Application of microchannel keyhole approach microscopic operation for intraspinal tumors. Chin J Minim Invasive Surg. 2019;19(06):494–7.
12. Ruan DK. Consideration on progressive expanding the indications of percutaneous endoscopic spine surgery. China J Orthop Trauma. 2021;34(11):991–3.
13. Xicai Y, Dakuan G, Liu WP, et al. Clinical research on endoscopic surgery for spinal intradural extramedullary space-occupying lesions. Chin J Minim Invasive Neurosurg. 2019;24(11):497–9.
14. Bai S, Tao B, Wang L, Yu X, Xu B, Shang A. Aggressive resection of congenital lumbosacral lipomas in adults: indications, techniques and outcomes in 122 patients. World Neurosurg. 2018;112:e331–41. https://doi.org/10.1016/j.wneu.2018.01.044.
15. Caram PC, Carton CA, Scarcella G. Intradural lipomas of the spinal cord; with particular emphasis on the intramedullary lipomas. J Neurosurg. 1957;14(1):28–42.
16. Crols R, Appel B, Klaes R. Extensive cervical intradural and intramedullary lipoma and spina bifida occulta of C1: a case report. Clin Neurol Neurosurg. 1993;95(1):39–43.

Part III

Incidental Findings of the Craniovertebral Junction, and Spinal Nerves and Peripheral Nerves

Jayesh Sardhara, Ashutosh Kumar,
Abhirama Chandra Gabbita, and Sanjay Behari

29.1 Introduction

Incidental atlantoaxial dislocation (AAD) remains a recondite entity. Even though the patient is asymptomatic, the presence of subtle clinical deficits, cord indentation, deformation, and alteration in cord signals intensities on imaging in the region of the tip of the odontoid process are essential indicators that establish the presence of incidental AAD. There is a lack of literature on exact incidence, means of diagnosis, and consensus on surgical indications for incidentally found asymptomatic AAD. Though normal at diagnosis, these subsets of patients are at high risk of new-onset severe neurologic and respiratory compromise even from minor trauma. The management strategy of incidental AAD is even sparsely described in the literature. The associated primary diseases in which AAD is commonly presented are congenital craniovertebral junction (CVJ) anomalies, rheumatoid arthritis (RA), syndromic AAD, os odontoideum, Chiari malformation (CM), and torticollis. Among them all, the most common variety is congenital AAD. We also aim to review the literature and summarize incidental AAD's management algorithm in this chapter.

J. Sardhara (✉) · A. Kumar · A. C. Gabbita ·
S. Behari
Department of Neurosurgery, Sanjay Gandhi Post
Graduate Institute of Medical Sciences,
Lucknow, India

29.2 Classification of AAD

Menezes had classified the congenital anomalies of CVJ into different malformations of occiput, atlas, and axis [1]. For all practical purposes, atlantoaxial instability (AAI) can also be classified into reducible and irreducible variety based on findings of dynamic X-ray neck in flexion and the extension positions. Goel classified AAD into three types according to the direction of the facet joint dislocation, type 1 (anterior AAD), type 2 (posterior AAD), and type 3 (central dislocation without any AAI). Type 2 and type 3 are usually detected incidentally [2].

AAD is defined as an abnormal increase in the atlanto-dental interval [ADI], the cut of more than 3 mm in adults, and more than 4.5 mm in the pediatric age-group [3]. The ADI assesses the displacement of the atlas relative to the axis in a two-dimensional (2D) plane. However, the displacements occur in a three-dimensional (3D) plane due to the coupled movements of the occiput, axis, and atlas relative to each other. Thus, this region's dislocations also need to be assessed in 3 different planes. These displacements often occur in combinations. They include the rotational dislocation and the coronal tilt of C1/C2 in different planes. Accordingly, we defined the congenital AAD in 3D according to the three Cartesian coordinates (X, Y, and Z axes) (Table 29.1). We identified the different multiplanar C1–2 displacements that can occur due to

Table 29.1 Definition of atlantoaxial dislocation (AAD) based on three-dimensional (3D) Cartesian coordinates (Sardhara et al.) [4]

	C1/2 dislocation in any one of these following axis or combinations is called AAD
1.	Along Z coordinate: translational dislocation [atlanto-dental interval >3 mm in adult or >4.5 mm in pediatric population less than 9 years of age.]
2.	Along with Y coordinate: central dislocation [presence of BI based on McCrae's line]
3.	Along X coordinate: rotational atlantoaxial dislocation and coronal tilt causing cervical torticollis (a) presence of rotation of axis in relation to atlas (>5°) and/or (b) coronal tilt: difference of atlantoaxial facet joint angle >10° bilaterally in the coronal plane
4.	Combination of above—displacement in all planes

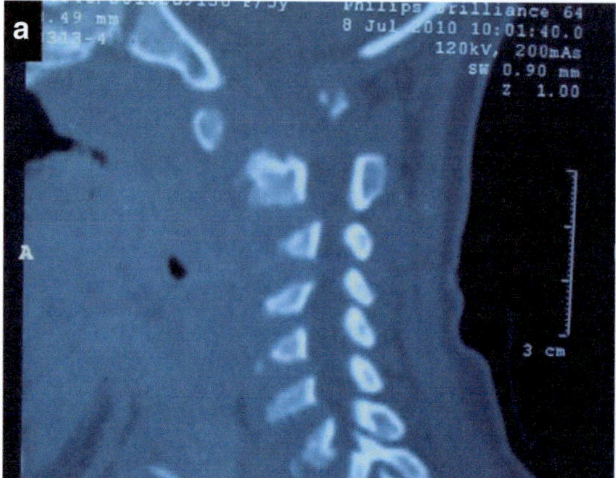

Fig. 29.1 A 8-year-child with Morquio syndrome presented with incidental atlantoaxial dislocation (AAD) (Type-1 AAD) on computed tomography (CT) (sagittal—**a** and coronal view—**b**) craniovertebral junction (CVJ) showing reducible C1/C2 instability with characteristic bullet shaped cervical vertebrae due to bony developmental anomalies

facet joint dislocations in all dimensions based on the 3D computed tomography (CT) evaluation. Based on various possible combinations of these dislocations, patients were classified into six types of C1–2 dislocations. Type I: Translational dislocation only (Figs. 29.1 and 29.2); Type II: central dislocation that consisted of pure basilar invagination (BI); Type III: translational with central dislocation (Fig. 29.3); Type IV: translational and rotational dislocation with coronal tilt.

Type V: central and rotational dislocation with coronal tilt; type VI: combined type of dislocation, that is, translational, central, and rotational dislocation with coronal tilt (occurring along all the three axes and in all 3 planes, respectively) that consisted of anteroposterior dislocation, BI, rotatory dislocation, and coronal tilt. Type 6 is the most common type of AAD (Fig. 29.4) and is often symptomatic. While type 1 is most common to present with incidental AAD [4].

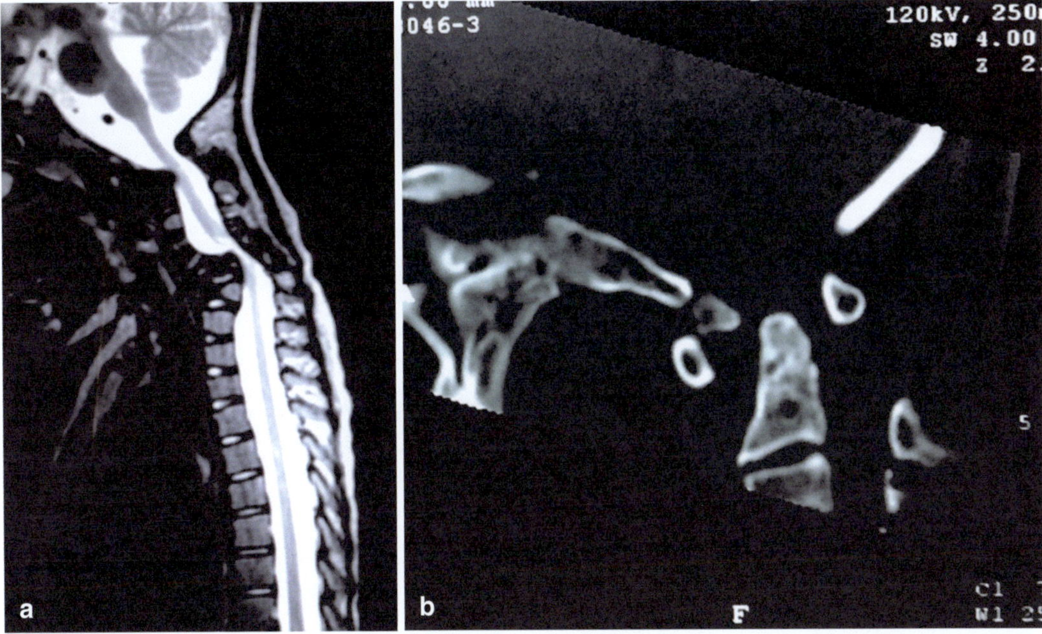

Fig. 29.2 Magnetic resonance imaging showing a patients of Larson syndrome and subaxial cervical kyphosis with incidentally found reducible AAD (type-1) (**a**). (**b**) Depicted CT CVJ of another reducible AAD with asymptomatic patient of os odontoideum (type-1)

Fig. 29.3 CT CVJ shown an image of irreducible AAD with basilar invagination (type-3)

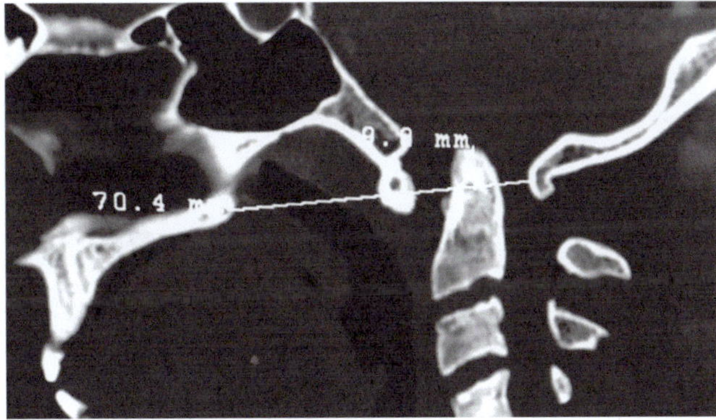

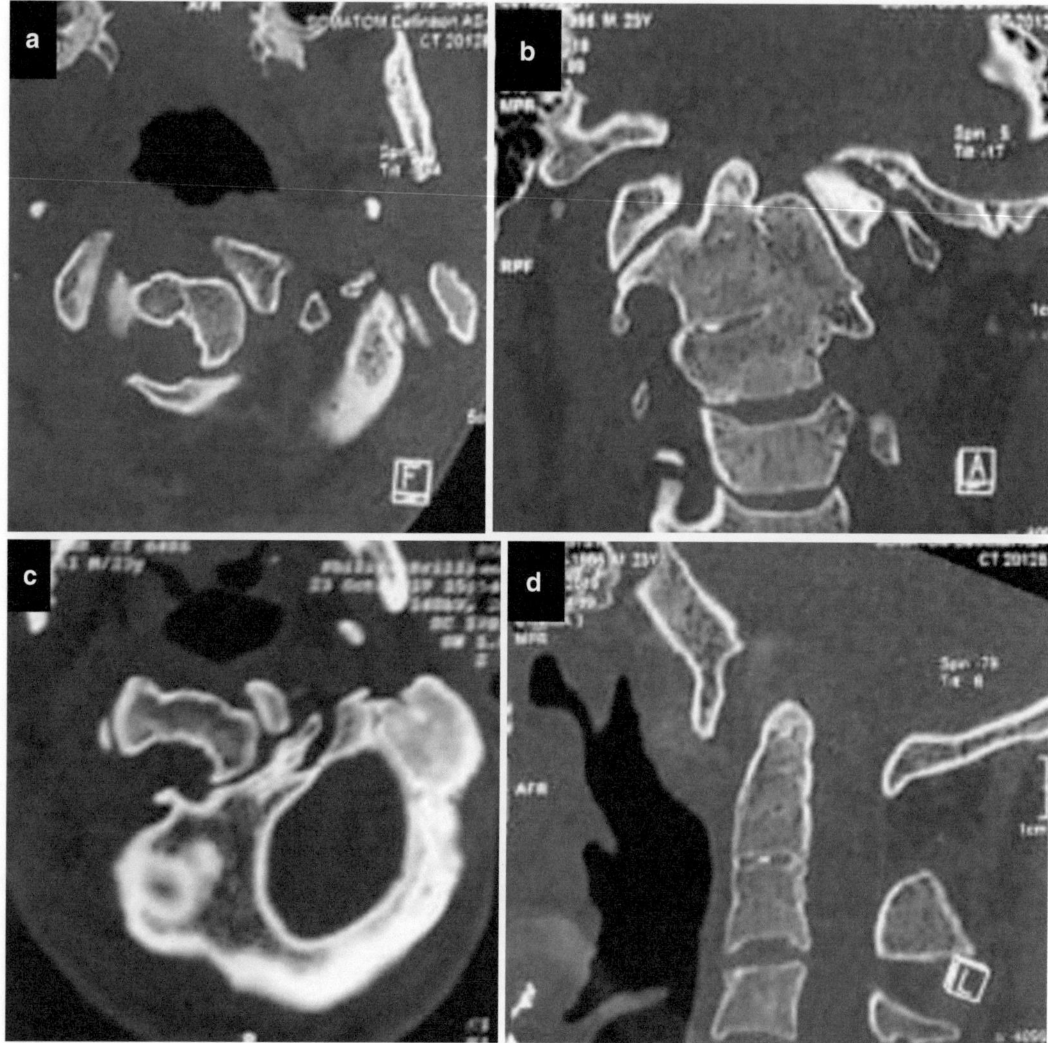

Fig. 29.4 A patients with incidental AAD with painless torticollis on evaluation CT shown combination of rotational dislocation (**a, c**), coronal tilt (**b**), and irreducible central with translational C1/C2 dislocation (**d**) [type-6 AAD]

29.3 Various Presentations of Incidental Atlantoaxial Dislocation

Patients with traumatic AAD complain of neck pain and limitation of movement (especially rotation) after neglected injuries to the neck. Cervical muscle spasms, tenderness, and torticollis may be found on physical examination. Patients with AAD related to congenital deformities in the CVJ often have a microtrauma history that may be obscure. Common symptoms include neck pain, limitation of neck movement, and numbness. Tuberculosis may destroy the lateral mass of the atlas, causing atlantoaxial instability and dislocation. Such a presentation is more commonly seen in children. Rotational dislocation can occur if the disease process destroys one side of the lateral mass. In such cases, the patient would complain of neck pain and develop torticollis [5, 6]. Tumors in the upper cervical vertebrae can also cause AAD. The symptoms include occipital and cervical pain that is usually continuous, progressive, more severe at night, and often accompanied by torticollis. Another type of AAD often found in children is spontaneous atlantoaxial subluxation (AAS), usually associated with pharyngeal or neck infection [7]. Continuous neck pain and limitation of cervical movement are early symptoms, which may gradually intensify.

Signs of incidental AAD are short neck, low hairline, limitation of neck motion, web neck, scoliosis, features of skeletal dysplasia, neck pain and posterior occipital headache, basilar migraine, hand or foot isolated weakness, sensory abnormalities, nystagmus (usually downbeat and lateral gaze) [8–13]. Vascular symptoms like intermittent attacks of change in consciousness, transient loss of visual fields, confusion, and vertigo appear in 15–25% of patients with CVJ anomalies. The phenomenon basilar migraine, which affects about 25% of children with basilar invagination (BI) and medullary compression, often involves compression of the vertebrobasilar arterial system.

29.4 Chiari Malformation with Atlantoaxial Dislocation

CM type 1 is defined radiologically as the descent of the cerebellar tonsils more than 5 mm (adults) or 3 mm (children) below the foramen magnum (FM). It is usually associated with hydrocephalus, syringomyelia (50–70%), and a spectrum of bony abnormalities such as platybasia, AAD, and BI [14]. The prevalence of CMs in the general population is estimated to be slightly less than 1 in 1000 [15]. These asymptomatic CMs are primarily of type 1. Sometimes these cases are co-existed with irreducible AAD and Goel type-2 BI. They are often detected coincidently among patients who have undergone diagnostic imaging for unrelated reasons, within which AAD can be an associated finding. There have been no epidemiologic studies reporting the exact incidence among children and adults.

The natural history of the untreated asymptomatic CM type 1 with associated AAD is mainly unknown. Whitson et al. published a prospective study of CM type 1 where they followed up the tonsil position over regular intervals in non-surgically managed children for up to 7 years. They concluded that neurologic findings did not change in the 52 children who met the inclusion criteria throughout the study. Although radiologic changes were common, no surgeries were performed solely because of radiologic change. Overall, the tonsil position on radiologic images remained stable in 50% of patients, was reduced by 38%, and increased in 12% of patients. A radiological resolution was seen in 12% of patients, and 24% of images showed some form of change in tonsil position. Therefore, they interpreted that CM in children is not a radiologically static entity but rather a dynamic one. These changes do not correlate with neurologic changes, symptom development, or the need for future surgery [16]. Similarly, Massimi et al. in 2011 had a similar observation in 13 children who remained asymptomatic, with stable or improved radiological picture. Three cases showed the appearance of symptoms: One did not require any treatment; the remaining two underwent endoscopic third ventriculostomy because of hydrocephalus, which is a possible consequence of CM type 1. However, this was a small series of cases to be inferred statistically [17]. Benglis et al. in 2011, published retrospective results of 124 cases with CM type 1, and most patients with CM type 1 who were followed up without surgery did not progress clinically or radiologically [18].

Although most patients with previously diagnosed asymptomatic CMs do not progress to neurologic deficits, some patients deteriorate, often acutely especially following trauma or hydrocephalus. Several authors have described sudden deaths; these may be postulated due to various reasons such as obstructive hydrocephalus and progression of symptoms after minor head trauma. Wan et al. in 2008 reported that minor head or neck trauma could precipitate the onset of symptoms in a small number of previously asymptomatic patients with CM type 1 [19]. Hofkes et al. in 2007 studied the cerebrospinal fluid (CSF) flow dynamics around the tonsillar ectopia and concluded that abnormal CSF flow pattern is significantly more often seen in patients with symptomatic CM type 1 than in patients with asymptomatic tonsillar ectopia [20]. Therefore, this may be possible to predict and confer surgical options for those with CSF flow disturbances.

There continue to be many variations in the management of the CM type 1. Nishizawa et al. in 2001 reported that the long-term clinical courses of patients with asymptomatic incidentally identified syringomyelia associated with CM type 1 were observed to be benign. Magnetic resonance imaging (MRI) parameters did not provide predictable values to recommend interventional surgery. Unless changes in neurologic or MRI findings are detected, early interventional surgery is not necessary [21]. Schijman et al. in 2004 published an international survey in which a consensus opinion was that no operation should be performed in asymptomatic patients with a CM type 1 unless there is associated syringomyelia. The CM decompression should be performed in patients with scoliosis when syringomyelia is present. This study also concluded that FM decompressive surgery should be done in patients with CM associated with scoliosis, even in the absence of syringomyelia [22]. A recent international survey of asymptomatic CM patients highlighted the summary of management [23]. According to that, that patients with isolated CM type 1 or with associated small (2 mm) syrinx, non-operative management are preferred by the majority of the neurosurgeons >90% and 65% consensus for respective conditions [23]. The majority of asymptomatic patients prefer non-operative management with CM or CM with small (2 mm) syrinx. Whereas, in the presence of a large syrinx (≥ 8 mm), approximately 80% recommend surgery. Therefore, a reasonable derivation is that patients who are not symptomatic and without syrinx or scoliosis need not be offered surgery, as the likelihood of progression of their symptoms is low.

In incidental cases, our protocol is expectant management with periodic clinico-radiological follow-up. We do not advocate any additional FM decompression apart from C1–C2 fixation in patients with CM and AAD/BI. In patients with CM with a normal C1–C2 relationship, we perform FM decompression without dural opening irrespective of the associated bony CVJ anomalies. In patients with symptomatic brainstem compression, in addition to FM decompression, C1–C2 joints are opened, distracted, and fixed. This brings about indirect ventral decompression and posterior CSF space opening due to FM decompression.

29.5 Rheumatoid Arthritis with Atlantoaxial Dislocation

Rheumatoid arthritis (RA) is well recognized as a chronic, progressive, systemic inflammatory disease primarily affecting synovial joints, resulting in disabilities. The cervical spine is frequently involved and potentially severe in patients with RA [24]. Collin et al. (1991), described in his case series that asymptomatic cervical spine subluxation in patients with RA is highly prevalent. Forty-nine percent of the patients showed evidence of atlantoaxial subluxation (AAS). Thirty-eight percent also showed evidence of AAI [25]. Kauppi et al. mentioned a 35% prevalence of AAI. Grauer et al. in their article, showed a 41% prevalence of incidental C1/C2 instability in rheumatoid patients planned for total hip or knee replacement [25, 26].

The C1/C2 joint is more prone to subluxation, most commonly anteriorly. Only 25% of patients with AAS have symptoms or signs, as mentioned by Arawwawala [27]. Younes et al. concluded that C1–C2 pannus was the most commonly found lesion (62.5%), followed by atlantoaxial subluxation (AAS, 45%). The most common AAS was anterior subluxation (25%), followed by lateral subluxation (15%), then by vertical, rotatory, and subaxial subluxations (10% each, respectively). C1/C2 involvement was found in 29 (72.5%) patients and was asymptomatic in 5 (17.2%) patients [28]. Standard dynamic X-ray views constitute the first-line imaging method of choice. The sensitivity and comprehensiveness of the assessment are significantly high with MRI. MRI and CT are usually reserved for selected patients [28].

29.6 Syndromic Atlantoaxial Dislocation

Syndromic association of CVJ anomalies is an infrequent developmental cause of AAI [29]. Eighty-four syndromes have been identified that involve the CVJ and affect the atlanto-axial stability. Morquio syndrome, Larson syndrome, Down syndrome, Marfan syndrome, acromesomelia, achondroplasia, Goldenhar syndrome, and spondyloepiphyseal dysplasia congenita are the common syndromes presented with incidental AAD.

Different genetic syndromes have unique variable mechanisms attributed to AAI. It includes segmentation failure, laxity of ligaments due to connective tissue abnormality, an abnormal collection of substance at upper cervical canal causing cord compression, and dysplastic odontoid process causing inefficacy of transverse ligaments resulting subsequently AAD [30]. Apart from the weakness of limbs, sensory loss, neck pain, and restricted movement, which is a more common presentation of non-syndromic AAD, comparatively in a syndromic group of AAD facial dimorphism, associated limb anomalies, and torticollis are unique features. Merits and demerits of prophylactic fusion to arrest cervical myelopathy progression and prevent sudden neurological deterioration by acute C1/C2 dislocation are variable based on individual syndromes.

Morquio syndrome is a type IV mucopolysaccharidoses characterized by deposition of mucopolysaccharides in connective tissue and cartilage ground substance. These glycosaminoglycans accumulate posterior to the dens, further decreasing the space available for the cord at this level [31]. Furthermore, AAI from odontoid hypoplasia is virtually universal in this condition. Holzgreve and coworkers described AAI in a review of 13 patients with Morquio syndrome [32]. In Morquio syndrome, Os odontoideum is considered a universal radiological feature (Fig. 29.1) [33]. As per Crockard, every Morquio patient should be screened and assessed for spinal cord compression between 3–8 years [31]. The objective of the treatment is to avoid neuro-logical damage or at least to arrest the progression of neurological disability. Transoral decompression and C1/C2 posterior fusion can be combined with significant anterior compression [34]. The resulting compression from the deposits and the AAI can result in debilitating, progressive myelopathy that has led some authors to advocate prophylactic occipitocervical fusion in selected cases [35, 36]. Thus, early cervical spine management with prophylactic fusion has been recommended to prevent cervical myelopathy and further complications [36]. Prophylactic fusion was reported to have relatively better neurologic consequences than fusions performed after neural compromise.

Down syndrome is easily recognized by the characteristic facial features, hypotonia, mental retardation, ligamentous laxity, and transverse palmar creases. AAI in Down syndrome has been described most since the initial publication by Tisher and Martel in 1965 [37]. The lack of attendant neurological symptoms and signs has resulted in the unfortunate belief that these children do not require surgical attention. Minor trauma and upper respiratory infection have resulted in severe neurological deficits in children with previously recognized pathologic instability without any intervention. In Down syndrome, the ligamentous laxity contributes to a high incidence of C0–C1 instability (10%) and C1–C2 luxation (15–20%) [38]. C1–C2 subluxation is stable in 44% of cases, and about 60% of these patients develop the precipitous onset of cervical medullary compression [39]. One-third of patients with Down syndrome have os odontoideum with AAI; 22% also have associated hypoplasia of the arch of the C1 with associated bifid anterior or posterior arches. Reducible basilar invagination mandates primary stabilization. With a sagittal plane excursion of more than 8 mm, AAI requires surgical attention [40]. Decompression is considered the primary treatment because of the narrow canal and CVJ instability; removal of the posterior arch of C1, widening of the occipital foramen, and occipitocervical fusion are required. An immunocompromised status (impaired monocyte and neutrophil chemotaxis, decreased phagocytoses, qualitative deficiency of T lymphocytes), which may have facilitated respiratory infections in the first hand in these patients, also leads to postoperative complications [33]. Rates of bone fusion may also be less in patients with down syndrome, probably because of deficient collagen synthesis, which contributes to bone graft pseudoarthrosis. It merits long-term immobilization in the postoperative period for at least 6 months [41]. Interestingly, posterior occipitocervical fusion results in the disappearance of the soft tissue thickening and normalization of dens development [31].

Larsen syndrome is a rare genetic condition of autosomal dominant or autosomal recessive inheritance. This connective tissue disorder is caused by mutations of the filamin B gene located on chromosome 3p14.3. Deformities of the cervical spine are most dangerous because of the risk of cord compression leading to paralysis and death [42] (Fig. 29.2). With time, cervical kyphosis and instability associated with this syndrome will progress rather than resolve. For this reason, the cervical spine should be imaged immediately after a diagnosis of Larsen syndrome. Management of cervical kyphosis and cervical instability depends on the patient's age, the severity of the kyphosis, and the severity of the syndrome. Anterior spinal fusions alone are not recommended in very young children with Larsen syndrome because of its high risk for spinal cord injury and arrest of anterior growth, eliminating the potential for kyphotic correction [43]. Posterior arthrodesis produces optimal results in patients with mild and flexible cervical kyphosis. However, anterior decompression and circumferential fusion are indicated in patients presenting with severe or rigid cervical kyphosis and myelopathic symptoms. The cervical spine should be immobilized via a postoperative halo vest after posterior spinal fusion or circumferential fusion [44]. Our experience includes two pediatric patients of Larson syndrome with reducible AAD (one had severe kyphosis), doing well after posterior fusion by sublaminar wiring. One infant patient with severe kyphosis had been planned for second-stage circumferential decom-pression and instrumented fusion for subaxial severe canal stenosis.

29.7 Incidental Os Odontoideum

In os odontoideum, the tip of the odontoid process is separated from the body of C2. Os odontoideum may be revealed as part of a workup for neck pain and/or neurological symptoms but is often found incidentally. Although, majority of spine surgeons agree that patients with signs or symptoms of neurological dysfunction should undergo stabilization, however, the role of surgical stabilization in asymptomatic patients and those with neck pain alone remains controversial.

In the guidelines published by Congress of Neurological Surgeons (CNS) and American Association of Neurological Surgeons (AANS), patients with os odontoideum, with or without C1–2 instability, patients without symptoms or neurological signs may be managed with clinical and radiographic surveillance. The authors also acknowledged that patients with C1–2 instability are at risk for future spinal cord damage and that surgical stabilization and the fusion of C1–2 are "meritorious" [45].

The literature of the natural history of os odontoideum is very sparse and dated. Various reports have presented evidence of patients treated conservatively without further incident. Fielding et al. reported a series of 35 patients, 8 of whom had no radiographic evidence of C1–2 instability and underwent conservative management [46]. Each of them remained asymptomatic at follow-up evaluation. All five asymptomatic patients with os odontoideum managed conservatively by Dai et al. remained stable at follow-up [47]. Spiering et al. analyzed 37 patients with os odontoideum [48]. Twenty patients were managed conservatively. In the study, patients with a minimal sagittal diameter (distance between the posterior border of the body of C-2 and the posterior atlantal arch on flexion) of <13 mm, had the greatest risk of developing permanent or progressive cord signs.

Sudden death and significant neurological morbidity with trivial trauma have been reported frequently in patients with a previously undiagnosed os odontoideum. Choit et al. published in their report about two children who each had an os odontoideum that had not been found on initial imaging and that caused subsequent morbidity [49]. More recently, Zhang et al. case series described ten patients with AAD with os odontoideum, including three who were asymptomatic and suffered a spinal cord injury [50]. Based on this, the authors advocated fusion and instrumentation for all patients with radiographically unstable os odontoideum, whether symptomatic or not. The incomplete odontoid process found in os odontoideum yields unstable C1–2 joint. It is highly fatal and can be disastrous to assume that the remaining weak supporting structures are strong enough to cope with the physiological loads and forces from even minor trauma.

29.8 Torticollis with Rotatory Atlantoaxial Dislocation

Rotatory AAD can manifest as painful spasms of the neck with painful torticollis in children or incidental findings as painless torticollis after minor trauma history [4]. It is essential to recognize atlantoaxial rotatory subluxation as there may be high risk due to underlying compromised C1/C2 complex that can cause neurological damage or even sudden death. Torticollis, in such cases, is the incidental sign but is a natural protective phenomenon in response to progressive C1/C2 instability and basilar invagination. Rotatory AAD can be subdivided into reducible or irreducible types as a practical surgical classification [51]. Reducible type rotatory AAD is classified as one where the dislocation reduces on dynamic images or after the application of cervical traction.

Using halo traction or cervical collar, mobile and reducible rotatory AAD can be treated by conservative observation for about 3 months. If, during the period, the rotatory dislocation reduces and remains reduced on dynamic imaging, there is no need for surgery [51]. Else, surgical fixation of the rotatory dislocation in a reduced position

should be carried out. For patients with "irreducible" rotatory dislocation, an attempt can be made to reduce the dislocation by surgical distraction (C1/C2 joint manipulation) and reduction by manual realignment of facets [4, 51]. 3-D model construction or 3-D CT scanning is the latest advance in the investigative modality. It can be most effective to diagnose and confirm rotational atlantoaxial dislocation, especially in patients with torticollis [4].

29.9 Management Strategy

The summary of the broad management strategy is described as an algorithm in Table 29.2.

White and Panjabi defined clinical instability as "the loss of the ability of the spine under physiological loads to maintain its pattern of displacement so that there is no initial or additional neurological deficit, no major deformity, and no incapacitating pain" [52]. For some patients with incidental AAD, everyday physiological loads are well tolerated and supported by the accessory structures. The potential loss following trivial trauma in conservatively managed patients could be more damaging than early surgical intervention. Especially in the case of younger patients, the hassles of daily life, like unavoidable physical interactions in school, while commuting, and at the workplace, cannot be avoided. Thus, a patient's age is critical in surgical selection for an incidentally discovered AAD. Young patients are more likely to need protection than older ones.

Patients with incidentally discovered AAD should be considered for surgery on a case-by-case basis while evaluating multiple factors, including clinical status, activity level, and radiological features predicting overt instability. All patients with neurological symptoms or significant neck pain with radiological confirmation of reducible AAD (overt C1/C2 instability) should undergo surgical stabilization. This mainly includes those patients who show evidence of radiographic instability at the atlantoaxial level, who are relatively young, and who have bone anatomy favorable for screw fixation should be strongly considered for surgery. Asymptomatic patients or irreducible AAD

Table 29.2 Management algorithm of incidental Atlantoaxial Dislocation (AAD)

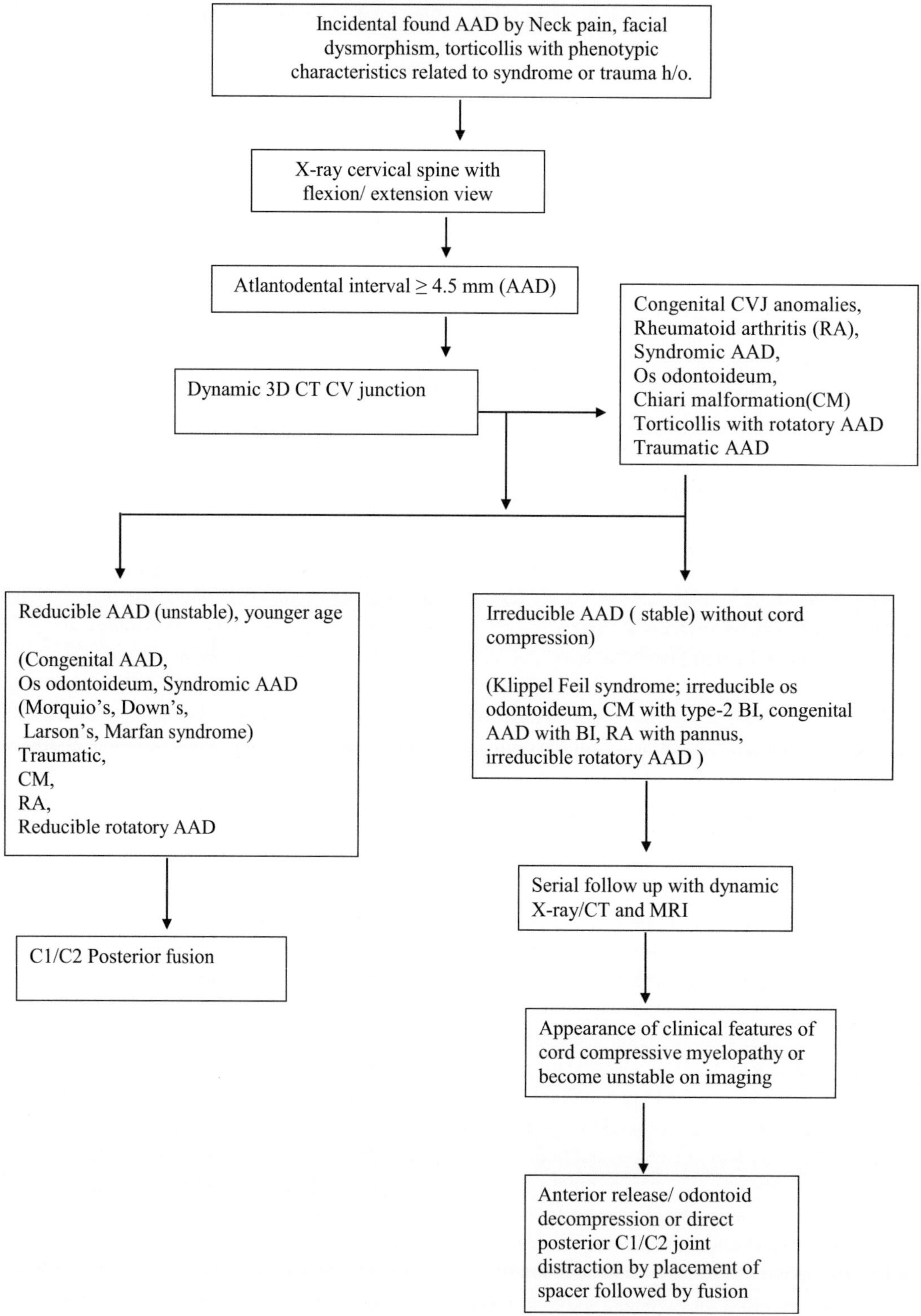

(fixed variety or covert atlantoaxial instability) without spinal cord compression may be evaluated with serial radiographs and clinical evaluations to detect whether instability or significant symptoms develop.

29.10 Surgical Techniques

Surgical techniques and fixation technology have evolved tremendously over the last several decades. The main objective of surgical treatment is atlantoaxial arthrodesis after complete reduction of C1/C2 facet joint dislocation to attain the physiological alignment and alleviate the compression from the spinal cord. Both anterior and posterior approaches have their own merits and demerits. The most widely used C1/C2 fusion method is the Goel and harms technique of C1 lateral mass and C2 pars screw and rod fixation done by posterior approach. Other posterior approaches are posterior wire and lamina clamp fixation, posterior transarticular screw fixation, posterior pedicle (lateral mass) screw and plate fixation, and C1/C2 distraction by application of spacer with C1/C2 fixation. The conventional transoral odontoidectomy for irreducible AAD and BI has recently been modified by endoscopic endonasal odontoid decompression and C1/C2 fixation. Transoral Anterior Reduction and Fixation with Plate and Anterior Cervical Transarticular Screw are the recently introduced techniques for surgical management of AAD.

29.11 Conclusion

Incidental AAI is a covert but highly lethal disease, and therefore it demands critical evaluation and management strategy. Asymptomatic and fixed variety of AAD can be treated conservatively under strict precaution. Further anticipation of progressive disease and instability must be carefully assessed by serial clinical and radiological follow-up. All patients with neurological symptoms or significant neck pain with radiological confirmation of reducible AAD (overt C1/C2 instability) should undergo surgical stabiliza-

tion by preferably posterior C1/C2 fixation technique. Posterior C1/C2 fusion is still the gold standard surgical method as surgical treatment of AAD.

References

1. Menezes AH, Ahmed R, Dlouhy BJ. Developmental anomalies of the craniovertebral junction and surgical management. In: Youmans and Winn neurological surgery. University of Iowa; 2017. p. 1856–70.
2. Goel A. Goel's classification of atlantoaxial "facetal" dislocation. J Craniovertebr Junction Spine. 2014;5:3.
3. Fielding JW, Cochran GV, Lawsing JF III, Hohl M. Tears of the transverse ligament of the atlas: a clinical and biomechanical study. J Bone Jt Surg Am. 1974;56:1683–91.
4. Sardhara J, Behari S, Sindgikar P, Srivastava AK, Mehrotra A, Das KK, et al. Evaluating atlantoaxial dislocation based on Cartesian coordinates: proposing a new definition and its impact on assessment of congenital torticollis. Neurosurgery. 2018;82:525–40.
5. Behari S, Nayak SR, Bhargava V, Banerji D, Chhabra DK, Jain VK. Craniocervical tuberculosis: protocol of surgical management. Neurosurgery. 2003;52:72–81.
6. Kumar A, Singh S, Dikshit P, Das KK, Srivastava AK. Occipital condyle syndrome in a case of rotatory atlantoaxial subluxation (type II) with craniovertebral junction tuberculosis: should we operate on "active tuberculosis?". J Craniovertebr Junction Spine. 2020;11:143–7.
7. Grisel P. Felix Dévé. Presse Med. 1951;59:1647–8.
8. Song D, Maher CO. Spinal disorders associated with skeletal dysplasias and syndromes. Neurosurg Clin N Am. 2007;18:499–514.
9. Henderson FC, Francomano CA, Koby M, Tuchman K, Adcock J, Patel S. Cervical medullary syndrome secondary to craniocervical instability and ventral brainstem compression in hereditary hypermobility connective tissue disorders: 5-year follow-up after craniocervical reduction, fusion, and stabilization. Neurosurg Rev. 2019;42:915–36.
10. Passias PG, Wang S, Kozanek M, Wang S, Wang C. Relationship between the alignment of the occipitoaxial and subaxial cervical spine in patients with congenital atlantoaxial dislocations. Clin Spine Surg. 2013;26:15–21.
11. Sobolewski BA, Mittiga MR, Reed JL. Atlantoaxial rotary subluxation after minor trauma. Pediatr Emerg Care. 2008;24:852–6.
12. Patel PR, Lauerman WC. Maurice Klippel. Spine. 1995;20:2157–60.
13. Speer MC, Enterline DS, Mehltretter L, Hammock P, Joseph J, Dickerson M, et al. Chiari type I malformation with or without syringomyelia: prevalence and genetics. J Genet Couns. 2003;12:297–311.

14. Rangari K, Das KK, Singh S, Kumar KG, Bhaisora KS, Sardhara J, et al. Type I Chiari malformation without concomitant bony instability: assessment of different surgical procedures and outcomes in 73 patients. Neurospine. 2021;18:126–38.

15. Sahu RN, Behari S, Sardhara JC. Management of incidental Chiari malformations. In: Progress in clinical neurosciences. p. 73–83.

16. Whitson WJ, Lane JR, Bauer DF, Durham SR. A prospective natural history study of nonoperatively managed Chiari I malformation: does follow-up MRI surveillance alter surgical decision making? J Neurosurg Pediatr. 2015;16:159–66.

17. Massimi L, Caldarelli M, Frassanito P, Di Rocco C. Natural history of Chiari type I malformation in children. Neurol Sci. 2011;32:275–7.

18. Benglis D, Covington D, Bhatia R, Bhatia S, Elhammady MS, Ragheb J, et al. Outcomes in pediatric patients with Chiari malformation type I followed up without surgery. J Neurosurg Pediatr. 2011;7:375–9.

19. Wan MJ, Nomura H, Tator CH. Conversion to symptomatic Chiari I malformation after minor head or neck trauma. Neurosurgery. 2008;63:748–53.

20. Hofkes SK, Iskandar BJ, Turski PA, Gentry LR, McCue JB, Haughton VM. Differentiation between symptomatic Chiari I malformation and asymptomatic tonsillar ectopia by using cerebrospinal fluid flow imaging: initial estimate of imaging accuracy. Radiology. 2007;245:532–40.

21. Nishizawa S, Yokoyama T, Yokota N, Tokuyama T, Ohta S. Incidentally identified syringomyelia associated with Chiari I malformations: is early interventional surgery necessary? Neurosurgery. 2001;49:637–41.

22. Schijman E, Steinbok P. International survey on the management of Chiari I malformation and syringomyelia. Childs Nerv Syst. 2004;20:341–8.

23. Singhal A, Cheong A, Steinbok P. International survey on the management of Chiari 1 malformation and syringomyelia: evolving worldwide opinions. Childs Nerv Syst. 2018;34:1177–82.

24. Alberstone CD, Benzel EC. Cervical spine complications in rheumatoid arthritis patients: awareness is the key to averting serious consequences. Postgrad Med. 2000;107:199–208.

25. Collins DN, Barnes CL, FitzRandolph RL. Cervical spine instability in rheumatoid patients having total hip or knee arthroplasty. Clin Orthop. 1991;272:127–35.

26. Neva MH, Häkkinen A, Mäkinen H, Hannonen P, Kauppi M, Sokka T. High prevalence of asymptomatic cervical spine subluxation in patients with rheumatoid arthritis waiting for orthopaedic surgery. Ann Rheum Dis. 2006;65:884–8.

27. Arawwawala D, Morgan P. Preoperative cervical spine X-rays for patients with rheumatoid arthritis. Br J Hosp Med. 2005;2007(68):56.

28. Younes M, Belghali S, Kriâa S, Zrour S, Bejia I, Touzi M, et al. Compared imaging of the rheumatoid cervical spine: prevalence study and associated factors. Jt Bone Spine. 2009;76:361–8.

29. Menezes AH. Craniovertebral junction database analysis: incidence, classification, presentation, and treatment algorithms. Childs Nerv Syst. 2008;24:1101–8.

30. Sardhara J, Behari S, Jaiswal AK, Srivastava A, Sahu RN, Mehrotra A, et al. Syndromic versus nonsyndromic atlantoaxial dislocation: do clinicoradiological differences have a bearing on management? Acta Neurochir. 2013;155:1157–67.

31. Stevens J, Kendall B, Crockard H, Ransford A. The odontoid process in Morquio-Brailsford's disease. The effects of occipitocervical fusion. J Bone Jt Surg Br. 1991;73:851–8.

32. Holzgreve W, Gröbe H, Von Figura K, Kresse H, Beck H, Mattei J. Morquio syndrome: clinical findings in 11 patients with MPS IVA and 2 patients with MPS IVB. Hum Genet. 1981;57:360–5.

33. Visocchi M, Fernandez E, Ciampini A, Di Rocco C. Reducible and irreducible os odontoideum in childhood treated with posterior wiring, instrumentation and fusion. Past or present? Acta Neurochir. 2009;151:1265–74.

34. Ashraf J, Crockard HA, Ransford AO, Stevens JM. Transoral decompression and posterior stabilisation in Morquio's disease. Arch Dis Child. 1991;66:1318.

35. White KK, Steinman S, Mubarak SJ. Cervical stenosis and spastic quadriparesis in Morquio disease (MPS IV). A case report with 26-year follow-up. J Bone Jt Surg Am. 2009;91:438–42.

36. Ransford AO, Crockard HA, Stevens JM, Modaghegh S. Occipito-atlanto-axial fusion in Morquio-Brailsford syndrome. A 10-year experience. J Bone Jt Surg Br. 1996;78:307–13.

37. Tishler J, Martel W. Dislocation of the atlas in mongolism: preliminary report. Radiology. 1965;84:904–6.

38. Spitzer R, Rabinowitch JY, Wybar KC. A study of the abnormalities of the skull, teeth and lenses in mongolism. Can Med Assoc J. 1961;84:567–72.

39. Menezes AH, Ryken TC. Craniovertebral abnormalities in Down's syndrome. Pediatr Neurosurg. 1992;18:24–33.

40. Menezes AH. Specific entities affecting the craniocervical region: Down's syndrome. Childs Nerv Syst. 2008;24:1165–8.

41. Segal LS, Drummond DS, Zanotti RM, Ecker ML, Mubarak SJ. Complications of posterior arthrodesis of the cervical spine in patients who have Down syndrome. J Bone Jt Surg Am. 1991;73:1547–54.

42. Muzumdar AS, Lowry RB, Robinson CE. Quadriplegia in Larsen syndrome. Birth Defects Orig Artic Ser. 1977;13:202–11.

43. Sakaura H, Matsuoka T, Iwasaki M, Yonenobu K, Yoshikawa H. Surgical treatment of cervical kyphosis in Larsen syndrome: report of 3 cases and review of the literature. Spine. 2007;32:E39–44.

44. Mummaneni PV, Dhall SS, Rodts GE, Haid RW. Circumferential fusion for cervical kyphotic deformity. J Neurosurg Spine. 2008;9:515–21.

45. Klimo P, Coon V, Brockmeyer D. Incidental os odontoideum: current management strategies. Neurosurg Focus. 2011;31:E10.
46. Fielding JW, Hensinger RN, Hawkins RJ. Os odontoideum. J Bone Jt Surg Am. 1980;62:376–83.
47. Dai L, Yuan W, Ni B, Jia L. Os odontoideum: etiology, diagnosis, and management. Surg Neurol. 2000;53:106–8.
48. Spierings EL, Braakman R. The management of os odontoideum. Analysis of 37 cases. J Bone Jt Surg Br. 1982;64:422–8.
49. Choit RL, Jamieson DH, Reilly CW. Os odontoideum: a significant radiographic finding. Pediatr Radiol. 2005;35:803–7.
50. Zhang Z, Zhou Y, Wang J, Chu T, Li C, Ren X, et al. Acute traumatic cervical cord injury in patients with os odontoideum. J Clin Neurosci. 2010;17:1289–93.
51. Goel A, Shah A. Atlantoaxial facet locking: treatment by facet manipulation and fixation. Experience in 14 cases. J Neurosurg Spine. 2011;14:3–9.
52. Panjabi MM, White AA 3rd. Basic biomechanics of the spine. Neurosurgery. 1980;7:76–93.

Ketan Desai, Sanjeev Pattankar, Rohan Roy,
and Alay Khandhar

30.1 Introduction

Peripheral nerve sheath tumors (PNSTs) are a subset of neuroepithelial tumors defined by their distinct anatomic location involving numerous nerves [1]. The benign neurogenic tumors, namely schwannomas and neurofibromas, of the spine and peripheral nerves are not uncommon and present with clinical symptoms like neurogenic pain, paresthesia, and local swelling [2]. In the majority of cases, the sensorimotor neurological deficit is mild to moderate. In contrast, the malignant PNST are invasive soft tissue sarcomas that present with rapidly progressive severe sensorimotor complaints and deficits [3].

The incidental findings, either related to neurogenic tumors or any other type of pathology, are commonly detected on radiological examination [4]. They are defined as abnormal findings not related to the chief complaints for which the radiological study is being done. The detection of incidental benign neurogenic tumors involving spinal and peripheral nerves is not common, and the exact incidence is not clearly known. These tumors can arise from sheaths of any peripheral nerve fibers in the body or any pluripotent cells of neural crest origins and grow unnoticed in any anatomical regions with dead spaces (actual/ potential) [5]. For obvious reasons, such tumors are more commonly found in the torso (chest, abdomen, pelvis, retroperitoneum, etc.) than in the extremities. There are isolated case series and case reports available in the literature [6–35]. The commonly reported locations of incidental benign neurogenic tumors are mediastinum, retroperitoneum, and lumbar spine [7, 12, 36]. The frequent use of high-definition radiological investigations like computerized tomography (CT) and magnetic resonance imaging (MRI) scans has led to an increased incidence of incidental tumor detection in the body, including spine and peripheral nerves [5, 37]. Hence, proper awareness of their clinical spectrum and a high degree of suspicion are necessary for the effective management of incidental PNSTs.

30.2 Incidentalomas: General Cause and Effect

The incidentally detected tumors are also known as incidentalomas, and the commonest amongst them are adrenal tumors of benign nature. The terminology used to describe such patients with incidentalomas is "VOMIT" (victim of modern imaging technology) [38]. The quality of imaging modalities, namely CT and MRI scans, has improved considerably; and the concept of "newer is better" is frequently applied in investi-

K. Desai (✉) · S. Pattankar · R. Roy · A. Khandhar
Department of Neurosurgery and Gamma Knife
Radiosurgery, P. D. Hinduja Hospital and Medical
Research Center, Mumbai, India

© The Author(s), under exclusive license to Springer Nature Switzerland AG 2023
M. Turgut et al. (eds.), *Incidental Findings of the Nervous System*,
https://doi.org/10.1007/978-3-031-42595-0_30

gating every clinical symptom (trivial/non-trivial), thereby giving rise to incidental findings. The rate of detection of incidental findings is directly related to the area of the radiological field that is targeted. The wider field of view of CT and MRI scans has led to better visualization of organs and tissues and, therefore, a higher probability of encountering additional incidental findings [39]. The MRI or CT scans of the abdomen and chest have a higher rate of detection of incidental findings than that of the brain, neck, and extremities.

The description of such an unexpected finding routinely triggers the utilization of additional medical healthcare facilities including tests, diagnostic procedures, and treatment protocols [37, 39]. This process has been called the "cascade effect." Barring a smaller percentage of patients who benefit from early detection of a sinister disease incidentally, such an uncontrolled "cascade effect" is known to pose an additional risk to most patients. All in all, the detection of incidentalomas can cause mental agony, incurring an extra financial cost and often surgical intervention that could have been otherwise avoided.

30.3 Incidentalomas: General Management Pitfalls

The protocol of dealing with the incidental findings, including those seen in spinal and peripheral nerves, is far from being settled. Often, there is a communication gap between the referring physician and the radiologist performing the radiological tests. This radiologist can end up giving more importance to the incidental finding, thereby inviting undue delay in the treatment of primary pathology [4, 5, 39]. A collaboration between clinicians and radiologists is essential to effectively deal with such incidental abnormalities and avoid unnecessary treatments. The clinicians and radiologists need proper awareness of such common incidentalomas, their natural histories, and desirable treatment strategies, to avoid any undesirable consequences.

As detection of incidental findings is sometimes beneficial to the patient in averting a major health catastrophe by prompt early treatment, it is up to the clinician to decide the significance and importance that needs to be attached to such incidental findings detected in radiological studies [5]. The reporting of incidental findings on the radiological study is of paramount importance as omission or non-reporting can have medicolegal implications [4]. It has also serious implications for the patients, with respect to their future medical and life insurance.

30.4 Peripheral Nerve Incidentalomas

The benign PNSTs, namely schwannomas and neurofibromas, are not uncommon. The reported incidence of symptomatic benign neurogenic tumors is 10–12% of all benign soft tissue neoplasms [1]. Whereas the incidence of neurogenic incidentalomas is not common. Incidental PNSTs are those tumors that have been diagnosed by chance, while the patient is being evaluated for some other pathology or during a routine health checkup. The common site for the incidental PNSTs is the lumbar spine, retroperitoneum, and mediastinum. Incidental PNSTs of the extremities are very rare with only a few isolated case reports, as most of them become symptomatic relatively early when compared with tumors in the abdomen and chest, as the space for expansion is limited. Also, sensory symptoms are early to manifest as majority of the nerves of the extremities are sensorimotor.

The lumbar spine MRI, which is commonly performed for back pain/lower limb sensorimotor complaints, is the most common radiological modality detecting incidentalomas in the peripheral nervous system in the lumbosacral, retroperitoneal, or pelvic regions (Fig. 30.1) [40]. Incidental intradural PNSTs and retroperitoneal/presacral PNSTs are often found when radiological investigations like MRI/CT scans are performed for suspected lumbar disc herniation, trauma, and spondylotic changes in the lumbar

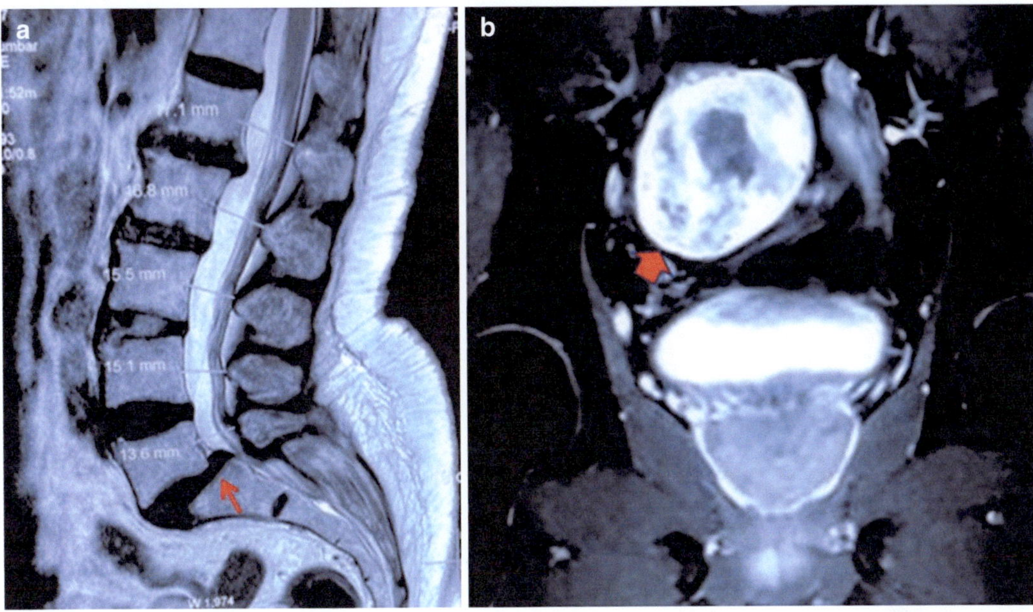

Fig. 30.1 Radiological images belonging to an elderly female who was investigated for a progressively worsening lower back pain and bilateral lower limb radiculopathy. (**a**) Magnetic resonance imaging (MRI) lumbosacral spine sagittal image revealed an anterior spondylolisthesis of L5 over S1 (red arrow), with pseudo disc herniation at L5–S1, and a L1–L2 disc bulge. (**b**) Gadolinium-enhanced coronal section of MRI scan found an incidental right lumbar plexus neurogenic, heterogeneously enhancing tumor (red arrowhead). A patient was surgically treated for the symptomatic L5–S1 listhesis and kept on follow-up for the incidental lumbar neurogenic tumor

spine [37, 40, 41]. These incidental PNSTs, due to their inconspicuous radiological features, are seen to mimic other commoner local pathologies in the respective anatomical regions. A confirmed diagnosis of any incidental PNST can only be obtained with histopathological analysis post-biopsy or surgery.

The retroperitoneal neurogenic tumor may present with vague abdominal complaints that are neglected by the patient. In the mediastinum, incidental paraspinal neurofibromas, schwannomas, and paragangliomas are detected following plain X-ray of chest done for routine body checkup or following investigations like MRI and CT scans done for chest complaints (Fig. 30.2) [12, 32, 35, 37]. The benign neurogenic tumors are also found in association with disc herniation in the cervical and lumbar spine [37, 40, 41]. Often there is confusion with respect to clinical diagnosis as both pathologies can present with similar clinical features. The overall detection of incidental findings on radiological investigations reported in the literature is 7–10% [37]. The rate of diagnosis of incidental neurogenic tumors in patients with suspected lumbar disc herniation is reported to be <0.05%. In patients with neurofibromatosis-1 (NF-1), incidental neurogenic tumors most commonly found are neurofibromas, and the risk of malignant transformation is relatively high. In the region of the abdomen and chest, the role of scout film of CT and MRI scans is very important as locating an incidental tumor helps in expanding the area of investigation. The incidental PNSTs can also be detected by detailed clinical examination. Incidental asymptomatic neurogenic tumors in the neck and extremities can be detected by simple palpation. A large retroperitoneal neurogenic tumor, like schwannoma and neurofibroma, can be detected by per abdominal and rectal examination.

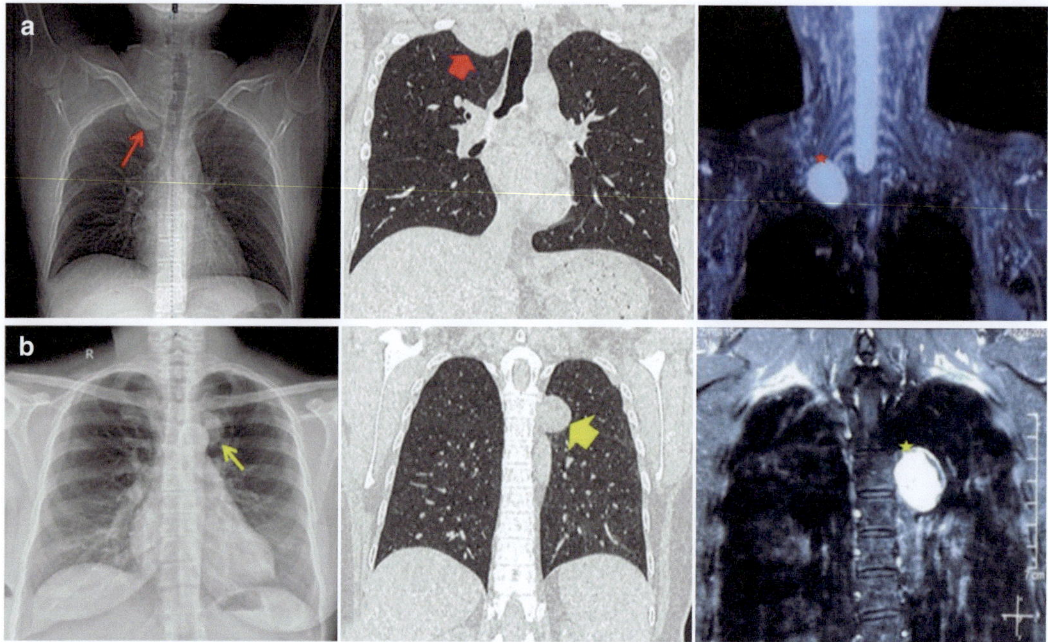

Fig. 30.2 Examples of incidental mediastinal peripheral nerve sheath tumors (PNSTs) seen in our clinical practice. (**A1–A3**) are the radiological images of a 32-year-old male, who underwent a chest X-ray (**A1**) as part of a routine health checkup. This resulted in picking up of an incidental PNST compressing the right lung apex (red arrow). This led to the "cascade effect," resulting in the patient getting a computed tomography (CT) thorax (**A2**; red arrowhead) and contrast-enhanced MRI (**A3**; red star), which confirmed the diagnosis. Patient was managed conservatively and kept on close follow-up. (**B1–B3**) are the radiological images belonging to a 30-year-old female, who during her COVID-19 infection was found to have a mediastinal shadow (yellow arrow) indenting onto the left medial upper lobe on chest X-ray (**B1**). She underwent CT thorax (**B2**; yellow arrowhead) and contrast MRI (**B3**; yellow star) which confirmed the diagnosis of incidental mediastinal PNSTs

30.5 Peripheral Nerve Incidentalomas: Varieties

A thorough review of literature on the topic of incidental PNSTs led us to hundreds of case reports published from multiple clinical disciplines. Depending on the tumor's anatomical location and proximity to nearby vital organs/structures, various clinical disciplines have reported such incidental occurrences to highlight nuances in their management. For presenting the available scientific information in a systematic way, we have subdivided incidental PNSTs into the following anatomical sub-groups:

- Neck and thoracic incidental PNSTs
  - Parapharyngeal [18]
  - Laryngeal [16]
  - Phrenic nerve schwannomas [34]
  - Mediastinal [26, 32]
  - Pleural schwannomas [35]
- Abdominal and retroperitoneal incidental PNSTs
  - Lumbar, sacral or lumbosacral plexus [19, 28, 36]
  - Gastric [11]
  - Appendiceal [8, 27]
  - Pancreatic [9, 20]
  - Miscellaneous (Colonic [17, 24], pilonidal [14], etc.)
- Genito-urinary incidental PNSTs
  - Prostate and peri-prostatic [6, 30, 31]
  - Uterine and cervix [29]
  - Vaginal [25]

Common incidental PNSTs found in the neck and thoracic region include parapharyngeal PNSTs, laryngeal PNSTs, phrenic nerve schwannomas, mediastinal PNSTs, and primary pleural schwannomas. Mediastinal PNSTs, accounting for 8% incidence of all the PNSTs in the body, are the most usually found incidental neck and thoracic neurogenic tumor [12]. Primary pleural schwannomas, arising from the autonomic nerve fiber sheaths, are relatively rarer. On the other hand, most schwannomas found in the neck region originate from the vagus nerve, or occasionally phrenic nerves/laryngeal nerves. Parapharyngeal PNSTs remain asymptomatic till they reach a size of ≥2.5 cm to present as an oropharyngeal or neck mass [18]. These, along with laryngeal and phrenic nerve PNSTs, are detected usually in MRIs done for cervical spine pathologies [16, 34].

Incidental abdominal and retroperitoneal PNSTs commonly comprise lumbosacral plexus tumors, gastric schwannomas, and other miscellaneous PNSTs. Though rare, retroperitoneal schwannomas account for 0.7–2.7% of all schwannomas [36]. As they are slow-growing tumors, with a large retroperitoneal space to occupy, they are asymptomatic and are often incidental radiographic findings. Among gastrointestinal (GI) PNSTs, gastric schwannomas arising from Auerbach's or Meissner's plexus are the most common [11]. These are routinely picked up by abdominal CT scans done for unrelated conditions. Appendiceal schwannomas are incidental findings during appendicectomies [27]. Sigmoid or colonic PNSTs are found incidentally during lower GI endoscopies [17, 24].

Many isolated case reports of genito-urinary PNSTs are available in the literature. Prostate and periprostatic incidental neurogenic tumors have been found to coexist in patients with prostatic carcinoma [6, 30, 31]. Rare entities like the cervix or uterine or vaginal PNSTs are known to be diagnosed during routine gynecological examination in peri or post-menopausal women [25, 29].

30.6 Peripheral Nerve Incidentalomas: Management

The management protocol in the incidental benign PNSTs is conservative, with close observation, and a wait-and-watch policy till it becomes symptomatic [5, 36, 37, 39]. This policy stands its ground in every case of benign PNST, immaterial of its anatomical location. The growth rate of incidental benign neurogenic tumors is not known, and they can remain static and asymptomatic for a significant period of time. The average estimated growth rate of a retroperitoneal schwannoma is reported to be 1.5–1.9 mm/year [36]. However, a close follow-up is necessary to detect any clinical worsening, increase in the size of the tumor, or signs of malignant transformation. The large incidental PNSTs need detailed radiological evaluation to rule out malignancy. In suspected cases of malignant PNST, a biopsy procedure should be definitely considered. Another indication for surgery in incidental PNSTs is a tissue diagnosis, especially in regions not feasible for biopsies, as differentiating them from local malignant pathological mimics is necessary. Most of these tumors require a multi-disciplinary approach to surgical management, as peripheral neurosurgeons are not well versed with these anatomical spaces.

It is also important to realize that missing or inadequately evaluating the incidental tumor can negatively impact a patient's care. Additionally, such errors can invite malpractice and medicolegal litigations. Reporting of incidental findings is part of the routine radiological reporting process. It is, therefore, mandatory to obtain clinical history and findings so that the focus on the primary problem is not missed. Both the clinicians and radiologists should share this responsibility for patients' benefit. Proper documentation and communication of the clinically relevant examination findings should be carried out by the clinicians. Radiologists should be consulted by clinicians before ordering tests in cases of ambiguity.

Reciprocally, it is the radiologist's responsibility to consult and convey the incidental findings to the clinicians before finalizing radiological reports.

Conflict of Interest The authors have no conflict of interest concerning reported materials or methods.

References

1. Maniker AH. Diagnostic steps, imaging, and electrophysiology. Neurosurg Clin N Am. 2004;15:133–44.
2. Desai KI. Primary benign brachial plexus tumors. Neurosurgery. 2012;70:220–33.
3. Desai KI. The surgical management of symptomatic benign peripheral nerve sheath tumors of the neck and extremities: an experience of 442 cases. Neurosurgery. 2017;81:568–80.
4. Brown SD. Professional norms regarding how radiologists handle incidental findings. J Am Coll Radiol. 2013;10:253–7.
5. Booth TC, Najim R, Petkova H. Incidental findings discovered during imaging: implications for general practice. Br J Gen Pract. 2016;66:346–7. https://doi.org/10.3399/bjgp16X685777.
6. Vamadevan S, Le K, Shen L, Ha L, Mansberg R. Incidental prostate-specific membrane antigen uptake in a peripheral nerve sheath tumor. Clin Nucl Med. 2017;42:560–2.
7. Mirpuri-Mirpuri PG, Álvarez-Cordovés MM, Pérez-Monje A. Schwannoma retroperitoneal. Semergen. 2012;38:535–8. https://doi.org/10.1016/j.semerg.2011.10.017.
8. Crispin MD. Appendiceal schwannoma: an incidental finding after Crohn's bowel resection. ANZ J Surg. 2019;89:E35–6.
9. Mourra N, Calvo J, Arrive L. Incidental finding of cystic pancreatic schwannoma mimicking a neuroendocrine tumor. Appl Immunohistochem Mol Morphol. 2016;24:149–50.
10. Kobayashi N, Kikuchi S, Shimao H, Hiki Y, Kakita A, Mitomi H, et al. Benign esophageal schwannoma: report of a case. Surg Today. 2000;30:526–9.
11. Mujtaba MA, Al Hillan A, Shenouda D, Hossain MA, Zurkovsky E. Incidental finding of gastric schwannoma in a renal failure patient—managed by a minimally invasive procedure: report of a rare case. Am J Case Rep. 2019;20:1241–4.
12. Shanmugasundaram G, Thangavel P, Venkataraman B, Barathi G. Incidental ancient schwannoma of the posterior mediastinum in a young male: a rare scenario. BMJ Case Rep. 2019;12:10–3.
13. Gelpi E, Vicente-Pascual M. Clinical Neuropathology image 1-2017: incidental schwannoma of the posterior root. Clin Neuropathol. 2017;36:3–4.
14. Bedir R, Semerci O, Güvendi GF. Incidental cutaneous microcystic/reticular schwannoma in pilonidal sinus. Balkan Med J. 2020;37:52–3.
15. Sozen E, Ucal YO, Kabukcuoglu F, Çelebi I, Dadas B. Temporal bone histopathology case of the month: an incidental middle-ear mass: Jacobson's nerve schwannoma. Otol Neurotol. 2012;33:37–8.
16. Tse A, Anwar B. Laryngeal schwannoma: excision via a laryngofissure approach. J Surg Case Rep. 2015;2015:rjv059.
17. Chelimilla H, Chandrala CK, Niazi M, Kumbum K. Incidental finding of isolated colonic neurofibroma. Case Rep Gastroenterol. 2013;7:369–75.
18. Mushi E, Winter S. Management of an incidental malignant peripheral nerve sheath tumour in the parapharyngeal space. J Laryngol Otol. 2013;127:104–6.
19. Eljack S, Rosenkrantz AB, Das K. CT and MRI appearance of solitary parapelvic neurofibroma of the kidney. Br J Radiol. 2010;83:108–10.
20. Duma N, Ramirez D, Young G, Nikias G, Karpeh M, Bamboat Z. Enlarging pancreatic schwannoma: a case report and review of the literature. Clin Pract. 2015;5:793.
21. Carroll C, Jagatiya M, Kamel D, Siddiqi J. A parapharyngeal space schwannoma arising from the vagus nerve: a case report. Int J Surg Case Rep. 2017;41:22–5. https://doi.org/10.1016/j.ijscr.2017.09.025.
22. Bhatia RK, Banerjea A, Ram M, Lovett BE. Benign ancient schwannoma of the abdominal wall: an unwanted birthday present. BMC Surg. 2010;10:1–5.
23. Leonard A, McCarthy LP, Pastor DM. When a polyp is not a polyp: incidental finding of a sigmoid schwannoma at first colonoscopic screening. BMJ Case Rep. 2018;2018:3–5.
24. Baig MMAS, Patel R, Kazem MA, Khan A. Schwannoma in the ascending colon, a rare finding on surveillance colonoscopy. J Surg Case Rep. 2019;2019:80518.
25. Park J-W, Hwang SO, Choi S-J, Lee BI, Park JH, Song E. Incidental diagnosis of vaginal schwannoma in a patient with thigh pain. Obstet Gynecol Sci. 2014;57:86.
26. Zisis C, Fragoulis S, Rontogianni D, Stratakos G, Bellenis I. Malignant triton tumour of the anterior mediastinum as incidental finding. Monaldi Arch Chest Dis. 2006;65:222–4.
27. Den Hartog T, Whitman C, Brozik M. Incidental schwannoma identified during laparoscopic appendectomy for acute appendicitis: a case report. S D Med. 2020;73:150–1.
28. Hartman J, Granville M, Jacobson RE. Two cases with incidental finding of large asymptomatic intradural lumbar tumors. Cureus. 2018;10(10):e3446. https://www.cureus.com/articles/14153-two-cases-with-incidental-finding-of-large-asymptomatic-intradural-lumbar-tumors
29. Tahmasbi M, Nguyen J, Ghayouri M, Shan Y, Hakam A. Primary uterine cervix schwannoma: a case report and review of the literature. Case Rep Pathol. 2012;2012:1–4.

30. Agrawal K, Sajjan RS, Gavra M, Fraioli F, Bomanji J, Syed R. Incidental neurofibroma on 18F-fluorocholine PET/MR. Clin Nucl Med. 2015;40:e455–6.

31. Dietrick B, Friedes C, White MJ, Allaf ME, Meyer AR. Incidental periprostatic schwannoma discovered during evaluation for prostatic adenocarcinoma. Urol Case Rep. 2020;31:101150. https://doi.org/10.1016/j.eucr.2020.101150.

32. Khan S, McElhaney N, Siddiqui F, Karki A. Incidental intrathoracic schwannoma post upper respiratory tract infection associated with Horner's syndrome: a case report. Respir Med Case Rep. 2020;30:101126. https://doi.org/10.1016/j.rmcr.2020.101126.

33. Choi JH, Yoo KH, Lee DG, Min GE, Kim GY, Choi TS. A case of incidental schwannoma mimicking necrotic metastatic lymph node from bladder cancer. Medicina (Kaunas). 2021;57:2–5.

34. García RLB, Jimenez J, Vargas N, Granados Á. Phrenic nerve schwannoma as an incidental intraoperative finding. Case report. Int J Surg Case Rep. 2022;91:106783.

35. Shoaib D, Zahir MN, Khan SR, Jabbar AA, Rashid YA. Difficulty breathing or just a case of the nerves? Incidental finding of primary pleural schwannoma in a COVID-19 survivor. Cureus. 2021;13:8–13.

36. Ogose A, Kawashima H, Hatano H, Ariizumi T, Sasaki T, Yamagishi T, et al. The natural history of incidental retroperitoneal schwannomas. PLoS One. 2019;14:e0215336. https://doi.org/10.1371/journal.pone.0215336.

37. Lumbreras B, Donat L, Hernández-Aguado I. Incidental findings in imaging diagnostic tests: a systematic review. Br J Radiol. 2010;83:276–89. https://doi.org/10.1259/bjr/98067945.

38. Hayward R. VOMIT (victims of modern imaging technology)—an acronym for our times. Bmj. 2003;326:1273.

39. Orme NM, Fletcher JG, Siddiki HA, Harmsen WS, O'Byrne MM, Port JD, et al. Incidental findings in imaging research. Arch Intern Med. 2010;170:1525–32. https://doi.org/10.1001/archinternmed.2010.317.

40. Kamath S, Jain N, Goyal N, Mansour R, Mukherjee K. Incidental findings on MRI of the spine. Clin Radiol. 2009;64:353–61.

41. Bapat MR, Rathi P, Pawar U, Chaudhary K. Intradural tumor and concomitant disc herniation of cervical spine. Indian J Orthop. 2011;45:74–7. https://doi.org/10.4103/0019-5413.73663.

Acquired Incidental Findings of the Brain and Spine

Namita Mohindra and Vivek Singh

31.1 Introduction

In recent years, awareness about health issues and diagnostic modalities has increased dramatically which has lead to an increase in imaging investigations, both for symptomatic and asymptomatic individuals who seek/self-refer themselves for screening investigations. Computed tomography (CT) scan involves radiation and has lower clarity as compared to magnetic resonance imaging (MRI) for central nervous system lesions, hence is less commonly performed without a specific indication.

MRI is increasingly being performed for diagnostic evaluation of patients as well as in research settings. The advancements in hardware of machines and improvements in software have lead to the development of more sensitive sequences which are capable of detecting very subtle findings. Hence incidental findings and normal variations are more frequently being encountered by radiologists and clinicians initiating a discussion on the relevance of these findings, potential impact on patients and ethical issues related to management.

Patients are apparently asymptomatic (for the lesion), and detection is potentially detrimental as the treatment may be beneficial or harmful. Risks need to be explained to volunteers in research settings and to subjects undergoing "routine health check-ups."

Guidelines for reporting (documentation) as well as further work-up/management need to be updated.

The new question which has emerged is whether to treat incidental findings or not and whether screening for such findings could be justified or not.

31.2 Definition of Incidental Findings

Incidental findings are broadly defined as "previously undetected abnormalities of potential clinical relevance that are unexpectedly detected and not related to the purpose of the scan" [1].

However, there is some discordance in literature regarding what entities could have "potential clinical relevance."

Morris et al. [2] defined incidental brain findings as "apparently asymptomatic intracranial abnormalities that were clinically significant because of their potential to cause symptoms or influence treatment." Further subdivision into neoplastic (benign and malignant tumors) and non-neoplastic categories was done (including cysts, structural vascular abnormalities, inflammatory lesions, and "other" such as hydrocepha-

N. Mohindra (✉) · V. Singh
Department of Radio-diagnosis, Sanjay Gandhi Post Graduate Institute of Medical Sciences, Lucknow, India

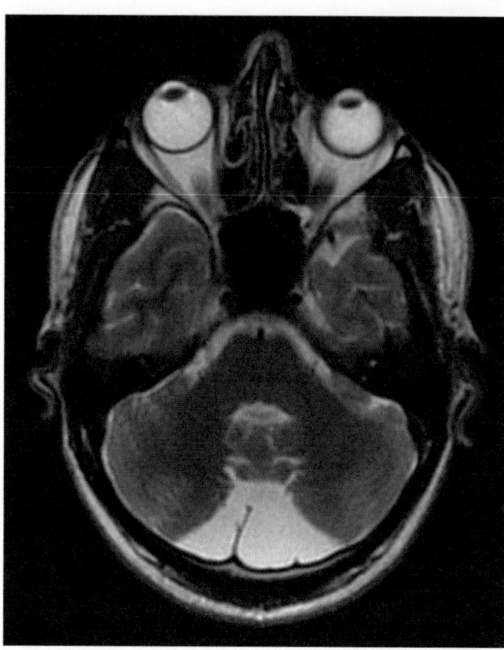

Fig. 31.1 Magnetic resonance imaging (MRI) T2 axial images showing mega cisterna magna

lus, Arnold-Chiari malformations, and extra-axial collections). Normal variants such as cavum septi pellucidi, large cisterna magna (Fig. 31.1), and ventricular asymmetry were excluded. Subclinical vascular pathological changes such as asymptomatic brain infarcts and white matter lesions were not classified as incidental findings due to their association with increasing age and uncertain role in causing symptoms [3, 4]. However these lesions are potentially clinically relevant due to increased risk of adverse neurological events associated with them [5–8].

Another definition used for research is "a finding that has potential health or reproductive importance which is discovered in the course of neuroimaging, but is beyond the aims of the study" [9].

31.3 Prevalence of Incidental Findings

Prevalence reported in literature is varied as it is influenced by the entities included as "incidental findings." In addition, the sequences used (stan-

dard versus high resolution) also affect the prevalence and types of findings detected. Differences in study population (healthy research volunteers versus general population versus patients who underwent MRI for various reasons), age-group of subjects, and the presence of co-morbidities such as diabetes mellitus, hypertension, myocardial infarction, and hyperlipidemia could also influence results (Table 31.1).

Katzmann et al. (1999) [10] reported a high prevalence of 18% incidental findings in 1000 healthy volunteers, probably because of a wide variety of incidental findings included (ranging from neoplastic, non-neoplastic lesions, unidentified bright objects in white matter, demyelinating lesions lacunae to simple sinus disease). A lower prevalence of age-related changes was found in the study probably as the mean age was 30 years. A prevalence of 1.1% was reported for clinically serious abnormalities such as brain tumors.

In a study on 2000 persons aged 46–97 years from the population-based Rotterdam study, in whom high resolution MRI was performed; asymptomatic brain infarcts were present in 7.2%, cerebral aneurysms (1.8%), and benign primary tumors (1.6%), mainly meningiomas. The prevalence of asymptomatic brain infarcts and meningiomas increased with age, as did the volume of white matter lesions, whereas aneurysms showed no age-related increase in prevalence [11]. Due to the older age-group and use of high-resolution sequences, more small aneurysms were identified in this study. Findings not considered clinically relevant [simple sinus disease, variations from norm-enlarged Virchow-Robin (VR) spaces, ventricular asymmetry, pineal cysts] were not reported.

In the meta-analysis by Morris et al. [2] (in which markers of cardiovascular disease white matter hyperintensities (WMHs), silent infarcts, and microbleeds were excluded), it was found that the *combined* prevalence of neoplastic and non-neoplastic incidental findings was 2.7% [neoplastic 0.7% and non-neoplastic 2% (1.1–3.1%)]. The prevalence of incidental brain findings was significantly more (4.3% v 1.7%,

Table 31.1 Prevalence of incidental findings in different studies

Study	Study population	Findings included	Excluded findings	Prevalence (%)
Katzmann et al. (1999) [10]	1000 Healthy volunteers, mean age 30 years	All incidental findings in head (intracranial and extracranial, e.g., sinus disease)	None	18
Vernooij et al. (2007) [11]	2000 volunteers aged 46–97 years	Asymptomatic brain infarcts, cerebral aneurysms Benign primary tumors	Normal variations Extracranial findings (e.g., sinus disease)	7.2 1.8 1.6
Morris et al. (2009) [2]	19,559 participants in 16 studies	Overall incidental findings		2.7
Morris et al. (2009) [2]	NA	Neoplastic and non-neoplastic findings (studies using high-resolution MRI)	Markers of cerebrovascular disease	4.3
Bos et al. (2016) [12]	5800 participants, mean age 64.9 years	Incidental findings which needed further work-up		3
Morris et al. (2009) [2]	NA	Neoplastic and non-neoplastic findings (studies using low-resolution MRI)	Markers of cerebrovascular disease	1.7
Kumpulainen et al. (2020) [13]	Birth cohort of 175 healthy infants	Subdural and intraparenchymal hemorrhages, cysts, and their co-existence	NA	7.4 (intracranial hemorrhages 6.9%)

$P < 0.001$) on high-resolution MRI sequences as compared to standard resolution sequences. Prevalence of neoplastic incidental brain findings increased with age.

31.4 Classification of Incidental Findings

1. Classification according to perceived need and urgency for further referral [10, 14].
   (a) No referral necessary (normal or common findings such as sinusitis).
   (b) Routine referral (those not requiring immediate further evaluation, but needing documentation, e.g., old infarcts).
   (c) Urgent referral (those needing non-emergent evaluation) e.g., low-grade astrocytomas.
   (d) Immediate referral required, e.g., acute subdural hematoma.

Prevalence of incidental findings was 18% in a study by Katzmann et al. [10] of which 15.1%

required no further referral; 1.8% routine referral; 1.1% urgent referral; and none required immediate referral. Prevalence of clinically serious abnormalities such as brain tumors was reported in 1.1% participants.

The problem with such a classification is that perceived needs for referral may differ and may change over time. Age of patient, size, or location of lesion and presence of co-morbidities may also influence decisions. Such a classification would also be dependent upon evolving knowledge about appropriate management and updated guidelines.

Recently a modification of this classification has been suggested [15] which addresses the relevance and severity of findings (based on prior studies [11, 16]). In this classification, age of patient, size, and location of lesions is taken into consideration while deciding documentation. The findings are divided into 3 categories: Category I-non-reportable; Category II, "reportable"—findings requiring additional medical clarification, and Category III, "actionable"—findings requiring emergency clarification.

Table 31.2 Classification of incidental findings according to etiology [2]

Non-neoplastic (prevalence ~2%, excluding markers of cerebrovascular disease)	Prevalence (%)	Neoplastic (prevalence ~0.7%)	Prevalence (%)	Markers of cerebrovascular disease
Arachnoid cysts	0.5	Gliomas	0.05	
Aneurysms	0.35	Lipomas	0.04	Silent infarcts
Cavernous angiomas AV malformation	0.16 0.35	Meningiomas	0.29	White matter hyperintensities
Definite demyelination Possible demyelination	0.06 0.03	Acoustic neuroma	0.5	Microbleeds
Extra-axial collection	0.04	Pituitary adenomas	0.15	

Findings such as solitary cerebral micro-hemorrhages; WMH (Fazekas grade 1); intracranial stenosis <50%; cavernous angiomas in non-eloquent areas, in older individuals without hemorrhage; meningiomas, calcified without perifocal oedema in older patients are considered Category I-"non-reportable."

Findings such as multiple cerebral micro-hemorrhages; WMH (Fazekas grade 2/3); radiological isolated syndrome; intracranial stenosis >50%; cavernous angiomas in other areas, in younger individuals or with hemorrhage; meningiomas with perifocal edema in younger patients or with hyperintense signals on T2W images and neoplastic masses including pituitary masses are considered Category II "reportable."

Areas of diffusion restriction; larger hemorrhages or neoplastic lesions accumulating contrast are categorized as Category III, "actionable" lesions requiring emergency clarification.

2. Classification according to etiology has also been used and the entities can be: (Table 31.2)
   (a) Non-neoplastic including structural vascular abnormalities
   (b) Neoplastic
   (c) Markers of cerebrovascular disease including white matter hyperintensities

From the radiologist's perspective, it is important to describe the specific MRI features to correctly diagnose the incidental findings, and discuss the situations in which additional MRI sequences are required for clarification of the incidental findings observed.

31.5 MRI Features of Incidental Findings in Brain and Their Differential Diagnosis

31.5.1 Ventricular System Asymmetries [15]

Ventricular asymmetry is found in 6–10% of all examinations and is generally considered clinically irrelevant. However, if the temporal horns are dilated and posterior horns are rounded with disproportionately prominent ventricles as compared to narrow cerebrospinal fluid (CSF) spaces, then a differential diagnosis of normal pressure hydrocephalus should be considered and clinically correlated for possible symptom triad of incontinence, gait disturbance, and mental decline. In cases with asymmetric dilatation of temporal horns, the differential diagnosis includes medial temporal sclerosis (MTS), however MTS is associated with history of epilepsy, hippocampal atrophy, or hyperintensity.

In cases where hydrocephalus is suspected, additional T2 or fluid-attenuated inversion recovery (FLAIR) axial images should be taken with sagittal T2W (or CISS) to rule out aqueduct obstruction.

31.5.2 Arachnoid Cysts [15]

Prevalence is 0.3–1.4%. There are no definite size criteria for calling "large" however, generally cysts of >3 cm size are considered large and symptomatic cysts require attention. Even small cysts need to be mentioned in reports as they may be asymptomatic but have a potential risk of enlarging if they continue to retain CSF. If epidermoid cysts are in the differential, then diffusion-weighted imaging (DWI) sequence should be done for clarification [17].

31.5.3 Pineal Cysts [15]

Pineal cysts are common (prevalence ~10%), generally <10 mm in diameter, and do not show signal suppression on FLAIR images. Larger cysts may cause headaches if they compress the tectal plate. Morphologically, it is not possible to differentiate cysts from pineocytomas. Contrast MRI may be done if signal characteristics are very inhomogenous.

31.5.4 Prominent Virchow_ Robin Spaces [15]

Dilated perivascular spaces (PVSs) are also known as VR spaces. There are no strict size criteria for defining this, but most authors use a threshold of 2–3 mm for calling enlargement of VR spaces. These findings are more commonly observed on the 3 Tesla MRI systems, typically as clusters of variable sized cysts in basal ganglia and cerebral white matter. They are fluid-isointense on all sequences with no signal alteration in the adjoining medullary layer on FLAIR images. They do not show restricted diffusion and do not enhance on post-contrast images (unless there is a pathological process spreading along them). Exceptions: giant/tumefactive PVS most commonly seen in the mesencephalon-thalamic region, and dilated anterior temporal PVS, may exhibit some T2/FLAIR signal abnormality but should remain stable over time.

Three subtypes of prominent VR spaces are described based on location: [18]

1. Type I appear along lenticulostriate arteries in the basal ganglia through the anterior-perforated substance.
2. Type II are found along the path of perforating medullary arteries, toward cortical gray mat-

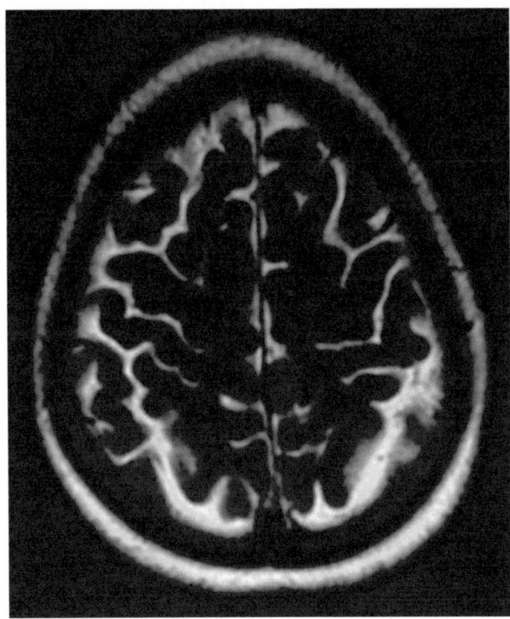

Fig. 31.2 MRI, T2W axial image of brain, showing prominent Vircow-Robin spaces and an extra-axial small T2-isointense lesion in left parafalcine region likely meningioma

ter over the high convexities, often asymmetrically involve one hemisphere (Fig. 31.2).
3. Type III appear in the midbrain at the ponto-mesencephalic junction surrounding penetrating branches of the collicular and accessory collicular arteries.

Differential diagnosis: This entity needs to be differentiated from other lesions such as:

(a) Chronic vascular and inflammatory insults: Chronic lacunar infarcts tend to be larger (often >5 mm), wedge shaped, and show a T2/FLAIR hyperintense rim. Similarly plaques of multiple sclerosis also show surrounding T2/FLAIR hyperintensity.
(b) Benign cysts such as neuroglial cysts (Fig. 31.3), arachnoid cysts, and choroidal cysts (depending on location), however these are usually solitary lesions, whereas dilated VR spaces are usually multiple, bilateral (occur in clusters).
(c) Low-grade cystic neoplasms such as pilocytic astrocytomas (Fig. 31.4), ganglioglio-

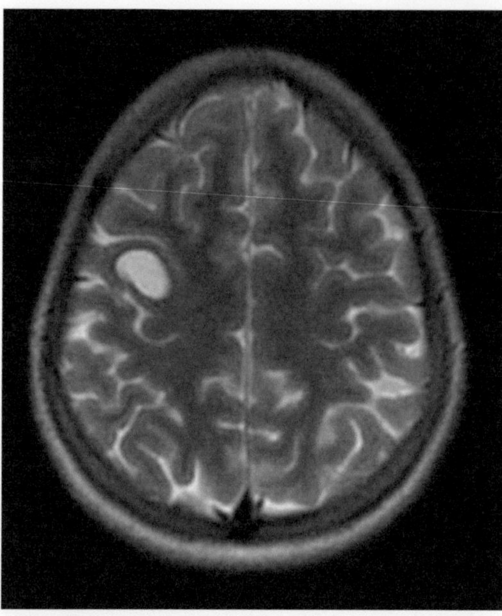

Fig. 31.3 MRI, T2W axial image showing a well-defined cerebrospinal fluid signal intensity lesion in right frontal lobe, neuroglial cyst

mas, and pleomorphic xanthoastrocytomas would contain solid enhancing component, restricted diffusion and perilesional oedema.

(d) Dysembryoplastic neuroepithelial tumors (DNET): In the temporal lobe, prominent VR spaces may be confused with DNETs which are benign, slow growing the World Health Organization (WHO) grade I tumors with characteristic "bubbly" cystic appearance. They show extensive associated T2/FLAIR signal abnormality and cause complex partial seizures. Minimal enhancement is noted in 20–30% of cases [19].

(e) Multinodular and vacuolating neuronal tumor which is a benign, mixed glial neuronal lesion seen as a subcortical cluster of tiny, cystic, nodular lesions with associated T2/FLAIR signal abnormality. It is usually seen in the deep cortical ribbon and superficial subcortical white matter in the high convexities and is associated with seizures in 30% of patients. It rarely shows progression or enhancement [20].

(f) Cystic infections such as neurocysticercosis and toxoplasmosis usually show peripheral ring enhancement. Typically cerebral toxo-plasmosis shows a "target sign" within the basal ganglia, corticomedullary junction, sometimes with intrinsic T1 shortening and/or susceptibility [21].

In addition, some disease entities such as cryptococcosis, chronic lymphocytic inflammation with pontine perivascular enhancement responsive to steroids, can spread via PVSs, with enhancement and characteristic MRI appearances.

31.5.5 Hemorrhages

Incidental intracranial hemorrhages (mostly subdural location) are relatively common among infants born by vaginal delivery and usually do not have clinical significance in asymptomatic neonates. They are unlikely to affect neurodevelopment scores in early life [13].

In adults, subdural hematomas (SDHs) or hygromas may be asymptomatic. Chronic subdural hematomas (cSDHs) are hypointense on T1W and T2W with blooming on SWI (Fig. 31.5). There is a consensus that cSDH if symptomatic and/or presenting with thickness greater than 1 cm should be drained [22].

31.5.6 Micro-hemorrhages

Micro-hemorrhages are intracerebral petechial hemorrhages seen as foci of blooming on susceptibility weighted imaging (SWI)/gradient echo (GRE) sequences. These are more often seen in older age, in higher tesla MRI systems (3 T > 1.5 T MRI), and in thin section SWI images as compared to thick section GRE images. Solitary foci have little relevance. Identification of 2 lesions is considered positive. In most cases, patients are asymptomatic, however, if multiple microbleeds are identified in an apparently healthy patient these are possible predictors of a cerebral vascular event [23]; and further evaluation for cardiovascular risk factors is indicated. Depending on the distribution, and extent of cognitive dysfunction, they could be indicators of underlying disorders. Lobar micro hemorrhages are commonly seen in cerebral

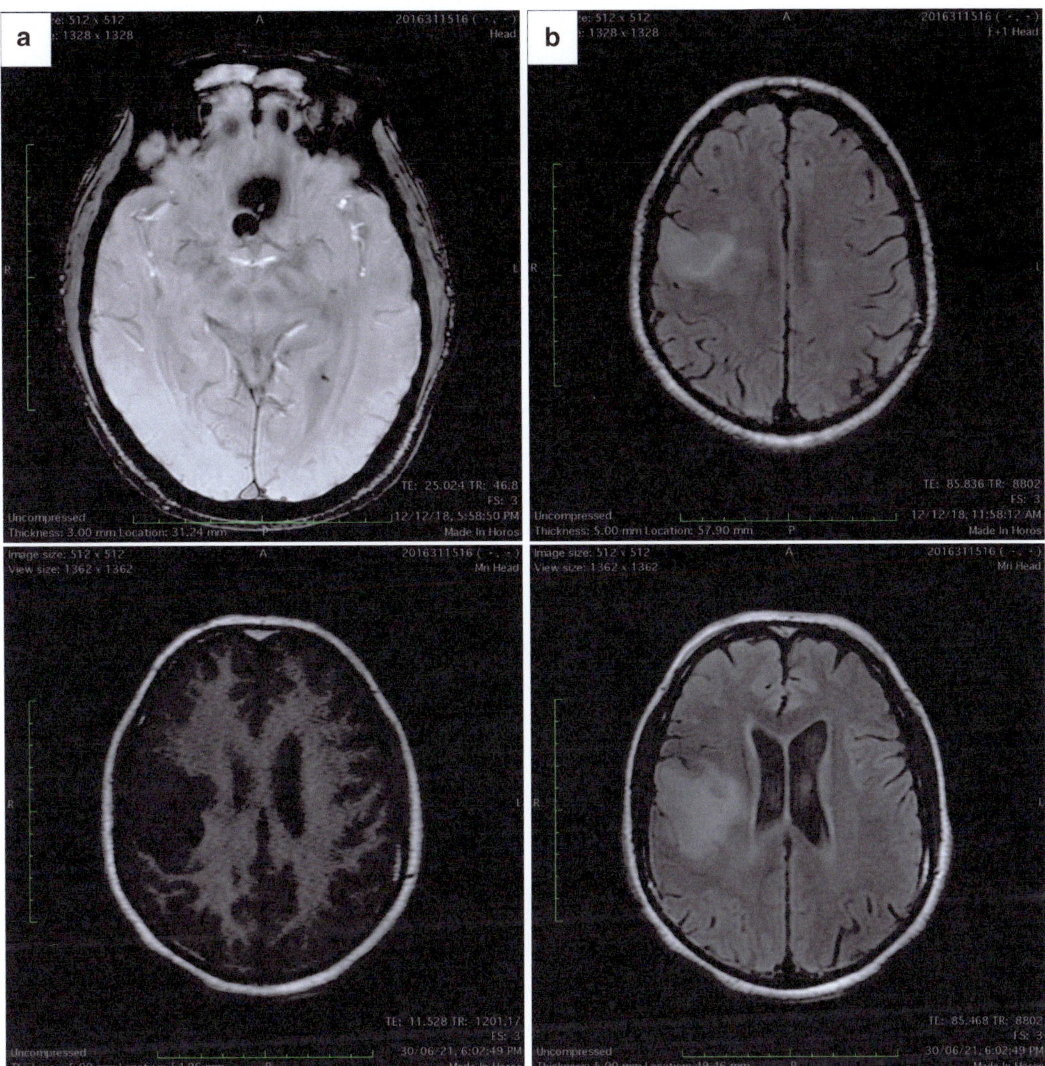

Fig. 31.4 (a) MRI, susceptibility-weighted angiography (SWAN) axial image showing coil mass in the anterior communicating artery (ACom) region with susceptibility artifacts. (b) T2-fluid attenuated inversion recovery (FLAIR) axial image of the same patient showing intra-axial T2/FLAIR bright mass in right frontal lobe with minimal mass effect in form of effacement of the adjacent sulcal spaces, likely a low-grade glioma incidentally detected. (a, b) Same lesion in above patient showed increase in size and some cystic component on further follow-up scans

amyloidosis, whereas deep and infratentorial location is more frequent with hypertensive arteriopathy.

31.5.7 Changes in the White Matter

T2 hyperintensities in white matter, called WMH, are commonly observed and require careful analyses for correct interpretation as the differentials vary with location, orientation, and signal characteristics on other sequences [24].

Leukoaraiosis (WMHs) is rarefaction of the white matter caused by damage to the medullary layer arteries [25].

On MRI, they are seen as patchy or flat hyperintensities on T2 and FLAIR images which spare the subcortical U-fibers.

Prevalence increases with age, and changes are more marked in persons with symptomatic

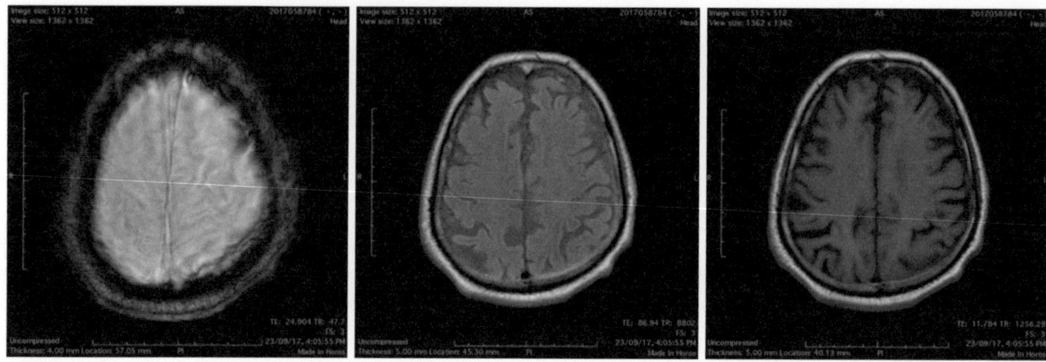

Fig. 31.5 (**a**) MRI, SWAN images showing thin subdural hemorrhage (SDH) along the left parietal convexity. (**b, c**) Axial FLAIR and T1W images showing incidentally detected thin SDH along the left parietal convexity

Fig. 31.6 MRI, axial FLAIR images showing incidentally detected symmetric peritrigonal FLAIR hyperintensities in a 30 year female

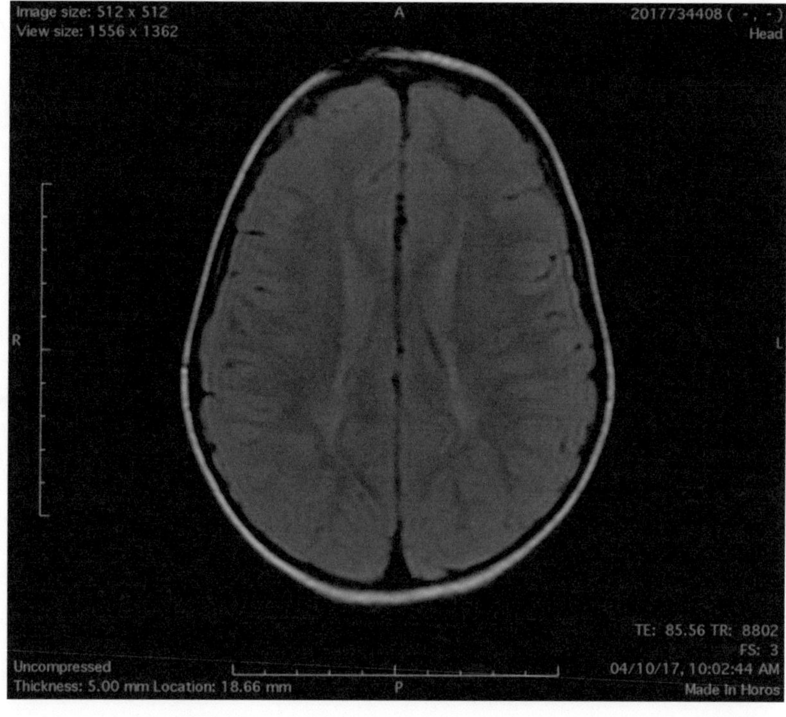

cerebrovascular disease or with cardiovascular risk factors. The Fazekas scale is used to classify them into 3 groups according to severity: Grade I: mild WMH, individual punctate lesions <10 mm; Grade 2: moderate WMH; individual lesions between 10 and 20 mm; Grade 3: severe WMH, confluent lesions; individual or confluent lesions >20 mm [26]. Patients with Grade 2 or 3 Fazekas changes should be evaluated for cardiovascular risk factors.

There is lack of clarity in literature regarding lesions which are bright on T2 and normal on T1W, whether they represent ischemic demyelination or ischemic necrosis (infarcts) [14].

Non-hemorrhagic infarcts are hyperintense T2-weighted images, and hypointense (almost similar to CSF signals) on T1-weighted images. The T1 hypointensity of infarcts distinguishes it from non-necrotic white matter disease [14]. Criteria for hemorrhagic infarcts are heterogeneously increased signal on T1 and heterogeneously hypointense signals on T2w images.

WMH in peritrigonal region (Fig. 31.6): These are frequently encountered and have a wide imaging differential diagnosis. In children, these could represent terminal zone of myelination which does not require any further work-up.

WMH in patients with migraine are found in around 40% cases (literature reports between 30 and 50% in various studies) and are mostly associated with severity and duration of migrainous headache [27].

WMH in patients with areas of SWI blooming may suggest these are related to the severity of underlying small-vessel pathology as shown by a stroke prevention study [28].

In a recent study [29], it was hypothesized that WMHs seem to play a role in the etiology of idiopathic normal pressure hydrocephalus (iNPH) before ventriculomegaly. It was found that apparently asymptomatic subjects with imaging characteristics of iNPH had subclinical cognitive decline.

31.5.8 Radiological Isolated Syndrome

In MRI, T2 or FLAIR hyperintensities identified in apparently healthy subjects (without neurological symptoms) which appear like demyelinating lesions, similar (in shape, size, and location) to those observed in multiple sclerosis the entity is called radiological isolated syndrome [30].

These are found in 0.1% of young people (15–24 years of age) [31] and approx. 40% of them develop neurological symptoms in the next 2–5 years, with 10% of them eventually meeting the diagnostic criteria for multiple sclerosis (MS) [32].

31.5.9 Vascular Changes

Stenosis is not reliably detected on routine anatomical sequences, they are identified on time-of-flight (TOF) magnetic resonance angiography (MRA) sequences and are likely to be overestimated by this method. A stenosis >50% is recommended to be reported and further evaluated especially if extensive WMH (Fazekas grade 2 or 3) is also noted [33].

31.5.10 Acute Incidental Infarcts

Most acute infarcts are symptomatic however, sometimes the symptoms are not correctly perceived by patient/relatives. Prevalence of acute incidental infarcts (AII) varies between 8 and 28% [34] and increases with age. They are hyperintense on T2W and FLAIR, hypointense on T1W, bright on DWI, and dark on apparent diffusion coefficient (ADC). After 72 h, they become subacute. Transient ischemic attack (TIA) and AII both are associated with increased risk of subsequent stroke, hence they should be immediately investigated further.

31.5.11 Aneurysms

Aneurysms are identified on TOF MRA sequences or T1W post-contrast images, sensitivity for detection of small lesions is high on TOF MRA [37]. Prevalence of aneurysms varies between 1 and 3% [11, 16], most often saccular, involving the basal cerebral arteries. More than 90% of unruptured, asymptomatic aneurysms found at angiography or autopsy are less than 10 mm in diameter [35].

Subarachnoid hemorrhage occurs if an intracranial intradural aneurysm, distal to the origin of the ophthalmic artery (for the ICA) or distal to the origin of the posterior inferior cerebellar artery (for the vertebral artery) ruptures.

Risk of rupture depends upon multiple factors including the size and location, co-morbidities such as hypertension, and history of smoking. Earlier an average of 5% risk of rupture was presumed [36] however individualized risk estimation models are being investigated, and current recommendation is to work-up an incidentally found aneurysm in a neurovascular set-up, regardless of age of patient or configuration of the aneurysm.

However, the American Heart Association has cautioned against screening for intracranial aneurysms in the general population [37].

31.5.12 Cavernomas

Cavernomas are low flow vascular malformations without any intervening brain tissue and show hemosiderin deposits and gliosis in the adjoining medullary layer. The estimated prevalence is 6%, and they may occur sporadically or post-radiogenically. In approximately 20% cases, they remain asymptomatic, most often they are supra-tentorial. MRI appearances-typical popcorn appearance on T2W images (with inhomogenous central core and hypointense rim and blooming on on GRE or SWI sequences). Incidental lesions can be monitored, except if located in brainstem when prompt action may be needed.

Developmental venous anomaly (Fig. 31.7) **and capillary telangiectasias** are developmental anomalies mostly benign and asymptomatic but large ones can be symptomatic.

31.5.13 Arterio-Vascular Malformation

It is the commonest cause of intracerebral hemorrhage in young adults though its prevalence is only 0.1%. They are classified according to the size, location, and type of venous drainage. Risk of hemorrhage depends on the above factors as well as the presence or absence of aneurysms in the feeder vessels. Thus, evaluation in a neuro-vascular center is recommended for deciding further management [38].

Calcified foci, probably representing healed granulomas may sometimes be detected incidentally. These appear hypointense on both T1 and T2 W sequences, with or without perifocal gliosis and show blooming on SWI.

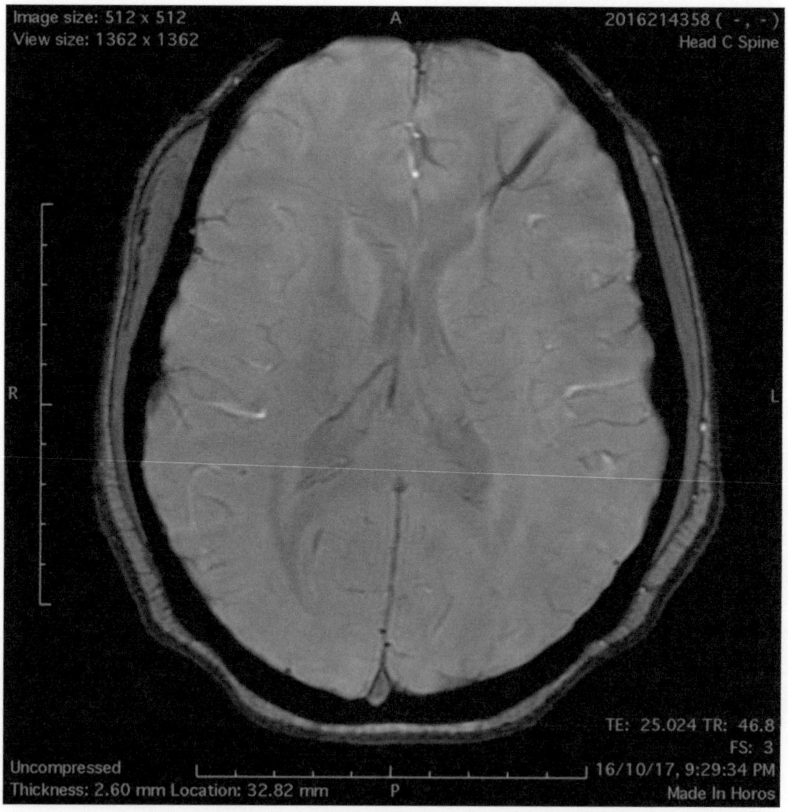

Fig. 31.7 MRI, axial susceptibility weighted image (SWAN sequence) showing developmental venous anomaly in left frontal lobe

31.5.14 Neoplastic Lesions

31.5.14.1 Meningiomas

These are extra-axial lesions with a prevalence of 0.5%. MRI appearance of meningiomas is iso-to minimally hypointense to cortex on T1W (Fig. 31.1), hyperintense on T2W images and show strong homogenous enhancement on post-contrast scans (Fig. 31.8). Sometimes a dural tail of enhancement may be seen.

Approximately 94% meningiomas remain asymptomatic, rate of growth is typically slow [39, 40] and about 63% do not grow [41]. 50% of all meningiomas are discovered at autopsy [42]. The presence of calcifications and T2 isointense signals to the cortex correlates with limited growth, whereas absence of calcifications and T2 hyperintense signals, perifocal edema in young patients are predictive of tumor growth [43]. Some authors suggest that small convexity meningiomas (<2 cm size) do not need follow-up [12].

Nevertheless, it is not possible to accurately predict which meningiomas may progress rapidly, hence some clinicians recommend repeat MRI yearly for 2–3 years to monitor the lesions for possible rapid growth [11].

31.5.14.2 Gliomas

Incidental gliomas are rare (prevalence 0.05%). They are typically hypointense on T1 and hyperintense on T2, FLAIR images with indistinct margins. In every suspected case, additional contrast enhanced MRI should be done in atleast 2 planes (or 3DT1 sequence should be obtained). High-grade tumors show enhancement and require further management (category 3), however low-grade tumors do not enhance and a neuro-oncological work-up for these should be done (category 2) [44].

It is not known whether early treatment with surgery, radiotherapy, or chemotherapy improves symptom free survival for patients with low-grade glioma [45].

31.5.14.3 Pituitary Tumors

Are usually adenomas found in 0.1% patients, are typically isointense to the normal pituitary on T2 and T1W images. Lesions <10 mm are termed micro-adenomas. They can be detected on post-contrast scans as hypo-enhancing lesions relative to the normal pituitary. Caution should be exercised while evaluating potential lesions as approx. 35–50% patients <35 years age may show an upward convexity of contour of pituitary gland. The maximum cranio-caudal dimensions of normal gland should not be >10 mm in sagittal images (except in pregnant or lactating women). Further endocrinological and neuro-ophthalmological investigation is recommended, (Category 2) even in cases of low growth tendency [46].

Other tumors such as acoustic neuromas (Fig. 31.9) and intracranial lipomas may also be seen rarely.

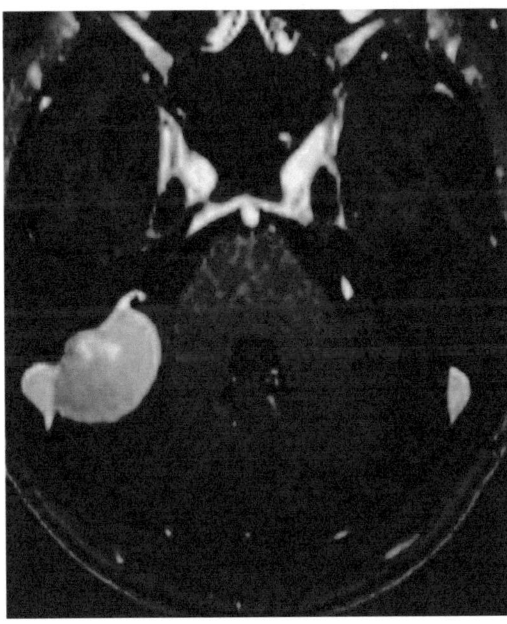

Fig. 31.8 MRI, T1 post-contrast image showing well-defined homogeneously enhancing extra-axial mass in the right cerebellopontine angle (CPA) region, likely meningioma

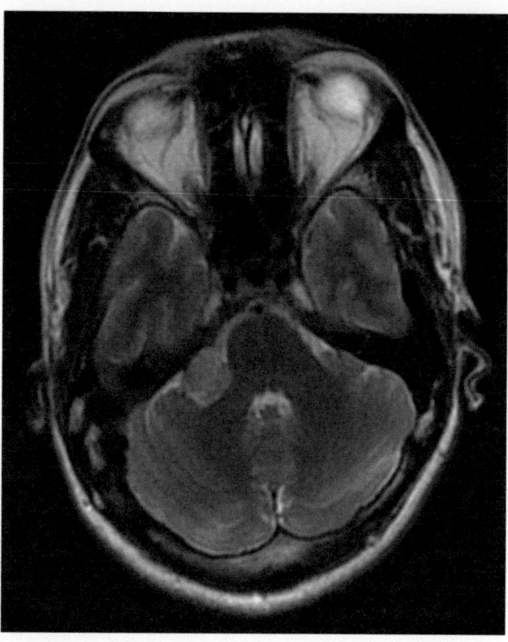

Fig. 31.9 MRI, T2 axial image showing another well-defined extra-axial mass in the right CPA region, likely schwannoma

31.6 MRI Features of Incidental Findings in Spine and Their Differential Diagnosis

Incidental findings in spinal imaging could be related to bony vertebral anomalies, spinal content anomalies, and outside the vertebral structures like adjacent organs seen on imaging (Table 31.3).

Prevalence of spinal incidental findings: there is heterogeneity in literature about the prevalence of spinal incidental findings it ranges from 8 to 30% depending upon the number and findings taken as incidental. Some authors have defined incidental findings as those identified outside the area of interest, which in spinal imaging would refer to findings other than disease related to vertebral column or spinal canal contents [47].

In this chapter, we will focus on spine and spinal content-related findings only. Some of the common vertebral bony abnormalities seen on radiological work-up are as follows:

Table 31.3 Incidental findings in spine

Vertebral			Spinal canal content abnormalities
Congenital malformations	Diffuse changes	Focal changes	
Abnormal segmentation (block vertebrae)	Osteoporosis	Vertebral hemangioma	Fatty filum terminale
Aberrant number of vertebra	Marrow reconversion	Lipoma-intraosseous	Extraspinal synovial cyst
Failure of chondrification or ossification	Degenerative	Degenerative endplate changes	Tarlov cyst
Synchondrosis mimicking fracture		Bone stress	Low lying cord
Absent pedicle		Paget disease	Fibrolipoma
Butterfly vertebra		Enostosis or "bone island"	Meningocele
Os odontoideum			
Spinal bifida occulta			

(a) **Block vertebra**—Common in cervical spine where two or more vertebra fail to segment. These are commonly associated with Klippel-Feil Syndrome and should be reported because cardiac and genitourinary anomalies associated with them need to be ruled out.

(b) **Aberrant number of vertebra**—Almost 20% of population have aberrant lumbar vertebrae and there exact numbering is important for spine surgical level demarcation.

(c) **Hemivertebra and butterfly vertebra** can be incidental but may lead to kyphoscoliosis. Butterfly vertebrae have sclerotic outline along the cleft that differentiates it from compression fracture.

(d) **Spina bifida occulta**—results from failure of fusion of neural arch ossification centers and its prevalence in general population is around 22%. Associated with many spinal anomalies like tethered cord, syringomyelia, genitourinary, and foot deformities but is not a very reliable indicator. It should be reported and be known before any spinal surgical intervention where failure to identify this can lead to complications injuring neural structures [48].

Vertebral hemangiomas are the most common benign spinal neoplasms with reported incidence ranging from 10 to 27% (based on imaging/autopsy). On MRI, they are hyperintense on T1 and T2W images and mostly suppress on fat suppression sequences. Around 1–2% of vertebral hemangiomas could be symptomatic causing pain or neurological symptoms. 1/3rd are multiple and mostly located in thoracolumbar region. Being highly vascular lesions they can bleed and extend into epidural space causing neurological symptoms due to cord compression. They can rarely cause burst fractures also [49].

Fatty filum terminale presents as linear fat signal (high intensity on T1W) within a normal sized filum terminale. If the size of filum is more than 2 mm, then intraspinal lipoma is suspected. Autopsy and radiological studies have reported its incidence to be 4–6% [50].

Tarlov cysts or perineural cysts have an incidence of 1–5% and are CSF filled structures within nerve root sheaths level, at dorsal root ganglion mostly in sacral region. These cysts are connected to the subarachnoid space of vertebral column and are mostly asymptomatic. Sometimes they may enlarge and cause nerve compression symptoms like pain, weakness, and sensory abnormalities [51].

Extraspinal synovial cysts incidence is around 1%, and these cysts can be seen in lumbar spine, adjacent to the facet joints and are formed as a result of degenerative changes. Though usually asymptomatic, they may cause pain and radiculopathy in few cases. Hemorrhage within the cyst can cause acute symptoms. They appear as hypo- to isointense on T1W and hyperintense on T2W MRI with cyst lining being hypointense on T2W. Contents could be variable in appearance due to hemorrhage or calcification within it [47].

Marrow infiltrative disorders—Abnormal marrow signal is identified as hypointense to adjacent paraspinal muscle or intervertebral disc on T1W MRI. On T2W sequence abnormal marrow shows bright signal not suppressed on fat sat sequences. Normal marrow conversion and reconversion under certain conditions do occur but if incidentally detected they should be reported and further imaging such as chemical shift imaging, DWI and ADC maps along with post-contrast MRI are done to ascertain the abnormality. There are studies which have shown incidental marrow abnormality on MRI led to bone marrow biopsies which detected hematological disorders. Prevalence of incidental detection of abnormal marrow signals on MRI is around 0.2%. It has been proposed that further evaluation in the form of hematological work-up should be done in cases of incidentally detected marrow signal abnormalities [52, 53].

Extramedullary hematopoiesis is commonly associated with myeloproliferative disorders. It may be seen during neurological work-up and is frequently located in paravertebral, epidural, and presacral regions, though all body parts can be involved. These are well-defined masses hyperintense (compared to adjacent muscles) on both T1 and T2W, due to fat contents within it. Sometimes they can be seen incidentally, without any pre-existing ailment. In one study, around 4% of extramedullary hematopoiesis were incidentally detected, and extensive investigation of these patients for occult malignancy and hematological disorders is still debated [54].

While evaluating spine many paraspinal, thoracoabdominal, and neck structures are seen which sometimes have incidental pathological findings both benign and malignant. Therefore, it is important to identify and able to judge whether the lesion requires any further investigation (e.g., solitary pulmonary nodule, pleural pathologies like effusion and thickening, soft-tissue sarcoma, aortic aneurysm, arterial dissections, paravertebral collection, paravertebral erythropoiesis) or just a mention in the report without necessarily needing further follow-up (e.g., simple renal cysts, small uterine fibroid, thyroid cyst, and nodule).

31.7 Concerns Regarding Detection and Documentation of Incidental Findings and Ethical Issues

There is shortage of evidence regarding further management of incidental findings. While a true negative MRI may be reassuring, the use of MRI as a screening modality is not likely to be very useful or cost-effective.

In such a scenario, knowledge about incidental findings is likely to trigger a cascade of further investigations, follow-up, and management decisions, plus an increase in costs. Apart from causing unexpected anxiety to the patient, there would be concerns regarding medical insurance or even employment.

Information regarding probability of incidental findings, especially if high-resolution MRI should be provided to subjects and the uncertainty regarding guidelines for further management also need to be explained/discussed.

Sometimes incidental findings may be more significant than the disease for which the patient is being investigated; hence appropriate emphasis should be laid, balancing the significance of findings to the gamut of investigations the patient might undergo for it. Incidentalomas may lead to timely intervention and prevent grave consequences. These do have medicolegal implications also as in one study they have stated around 47% of radiology lawsuits were due to missed diagnoses and it is important to identify the relevance of such findings [55].

31.8 Conclusion

The increase in number of MRI scans being performed (both for diagnostic work-up of symptomatic patients and screening of healthy individuals including research subjects) has lead to an increase in detection of incidental lesions. These are more prevalent with higher tesla MRI machines and with high-resolution sequences as compared to standard resolution sequences. A thorough knowledge of the classical imaging features of commonly encountered incidental findings and their imaging differentials is essential for guiding further work-up and management. It is also important to understand the significance of the incidental findings and when to label them as 'clinically relevant' or potentially serious.

References

1. Illes J, Kirschen MP, Edwards E, et al. Ethics: incidental findings in brain imaging research. Science. 2006;311:78.
2. Morris Z, Whiteley WN, Longstreth WT Jr, Weber F, Lee YC, et al. Incidental findings on brain magnetic resonance imaging: systematic review and meta-analysis. BMJ. 2009;339:b3016. https://doi.org/10.1136/bmj.b3016.
3. Cordonnier C, Al-Shahi Salman R, Wardlaw J. Spontaneous brain microbleeds: systematic review, subgroup analyses and standards for study design and reporting. Brain. 2007;130:1988–2003.
4. Vermeer SE, Longstreth WT Jr, Koudstaal PJ. Silent brain infarcts: a systematic review. Lancet Neurol. 2007;6:611–9.

5. Longstreth WT Jr, Manolio TA, Arnold A, et al. Clinical correlates of white matter findings on cranial magnetic resonance imaging of 3301 elderly people: the cardiovascular health study. Stroke. 1996;27:1274–82.

6. Vermeer SE, Prins ND, den Heijer T, Hofman A, Koudstaal PJ, Breteler MM. Silent brain infarcts and the risk of dementia and cognitive decline. N Engl J Med. 2003;348:1215–22.

7. Longstreth WT Jr, Dulberg C, Manolio TA, et al. Incidence, manifestations, and predictors of brain infarcts defined by serial cranial magnetic resonance imaging in the elderly: the cardiovascular health study. Stroke. 2002;33:2376–82.

8. Bernick C, Kuller L, Dulberg C, et al. Silent MRI infarcts and the risk of future stroke: the cardiovascular health study. Neurology. 2001;57:1222–9.

9. Wolf SM, Lawrenz FP, Nelson CA, Kahn JP, Cho MK, et al. Managing incidental findings in human subjects research: analysis and recommendations. J Law Med Ethics. 2008;36:219–48. https://doi.org/10.1111/j.1748-720X.2008.00266.x.

10. Katzman GL, Dagher AP, Patronas NJ. Incidental findings on brain magnetic resonance imaging from 1000 asymptomatic volunteers. JAMA. 1999;282:36.

11. Vernooij MW, Ikram MA, Tanghe HL, et al. Incidental findings on brain MRI in the general population. N Engl J Med. 2007;357:1821–8.

12. Bos D, Poels MM, Adams HH, Akoudad S, Cremers LG, Zonneveld HI, Hoogendam YY, Verhaaren BF, Verlinden VJ, Verbruggen JG, Peymani A, Hofman A, Krestin GP, Vincent AJ, Feelders RA, Koudstaal PJ, van der Lugt A, Ikram MA, Vernooij MW. Prevalence, clinical management, and natural course of incidental findings on brain MR images: the population-based Rotterdam Scan Study. Radiology. 2016;281(2):507–15. https://doi.org/10.1148/radiol.2016160218.

13. Kumpulainen V, Lehtola SJ, Tuulari JJ, Silver E, Copeland A, Korja R, Karlsson H, Karlsson L, Merisaari H, Parkkola R, Saunavaara J, Lähdesmäki T, Scheinin NM. Prevalence and risk factors of incidental findings in brain MRIs of healthy neonates—the FinnBrain Birth Cohort Study. Front Neurol. 2020;10:1347. https://doi.org/10.3389/fneur.2019.01347.

14. Bryan RN, Manolio TA, Schertz LD, Jungreis C, Poirier VC, Elster AD, et al. A method for using MR to evaluate the effects of cardiovascular disease on the brain: the cardiovascular health study. AJNR Am J Neuroradiol. 1994;15:1625–33.

15. Langner S, Buelow R, Fleck S, et al. Management of intracranial incidental findings on brain MRI. Fortschr Röntgenstr. 2016;188:1123–33.

16. Hegenscheid K, Seipel R, Schmidt CO, et al. Potentially relevant incidental findings on research whole-body MRI in the general adult population: frequencies and management. Eur Radiol. 2013;23:816–26.

17. Galassi E, Tognetti F, Gaist G, Fagioli L, Frank F, Frank G. CT scan and metrizamide CT cisternography in arachnoid cysts of the middle cranial fossa: classification and pathophysiological aspects. Surg Neurol. 1982;17(5):363–9.

18. Kwee RM, Kwee TC. Virchow-Robin spaces at MR imaging. Radiographics. 2007;27:1071–86.

19. Fernandez C, Girard N, Paz Paredes A, et al. The usefulness of MR imaging in the diagnosis if dysembryoplastic neuroepithelial tumor in children: a study of 14 cases. AJMR Am J Neuroradiol. 2003;24:829–34.

20. Alsufayan R, Alcaide-Leon P, de Tilly LN, et al. Natural history of lesions with the MR imaging appearance of multinodular and vacuolating neuronal tumor. Neuroradiology. 2017;59:873–83.

21. Masamed R, Meleis A, Lee EW, et al. Cerebral toxoplasmosis: case review and description of a new imaging sign. Clin Radiol. 2009;64:560–3.

22. Alves JL, Santiago JG, Costa G, Pinto AM. A standardized classification for subdural hematomas—I. Am J Forensic Med Pathol. 2016;37:174. https://doi.org/10.1097/PAF.0000000000000255.

23. Schrag M, Greer DM. Clinical associations of cerebral microbleeds on magnetic resonance neuroimaging. J Stroke Cerebrovasc Dis. 2014;23:2489–97.

24. Launer LJ, Berger K, Breteler MM, Dufouil C, Fuhrer R, et al. Regional variability in the prevalence of cerebral white matter lesions: an MRI study in 9 European countries (CASCADE). Neuroepidemiology. 2006;26:23–9.

25. Mok V, Kim JS. Prevention and management of cerebral small vessel disease. J stroke. 2015;17:111–22.

26. Pantoni L, Fierini F, Poggesi A. Impact of cerebral white matter changes on functionality in older adults: an overview of the LADIS Study results and future directions. Geriatr Gerontol Int. 2015;15:10–6.

27. Negm M, Housseini AM, Abdelfatah M, Asran A. Relation between migraine pattern and white matter hyperintensities in brain magnetic resonance imaging. Egypt J Neurol Psychiatry Neurosurg. 2018;54(1):24.

28. Roob G, Schmidt R, Kapeller P, Lechner A, Hartung HP, Fazekas F. MRI evidence of past cerebral microbleeds in a healthy elderly population. Neurology. 1999;52:991–4.

29. Engel DC, et al. Incidental findings of typical iNPH imaging signs in asymptomatic subjects with subclinical cognitive decline. Fluids Barriers CNS. 2021;18:37. https://doi.org/10.1186/s12987-021-00268-x.

30. Okuda DT, Mowry EM, Beheshtian A, et al. Incidental MRI anomalies suggestive of multiple sclerosis: the radiologically isolated syndrome. Neurology. 2009;72:800–5.

31. Forslin Y, Granberg T, Jumah AA, et al. Incidence of radiologically isolated syndrome: a population-based study. Am J Neuroradiol. 2016;37(6):1017–22. https://doi.org/10.3174/ajnr.A4660.

32. Okuda DT, Siva A, Kantarci O, et al. Radiologically isolated syndrome: 5-year risk for an initial clinical event. PLoS One. 2014;9:e90509.
33. Holmstedt CA, Turan TN, Chimowitz MI. Atherosclerotic intracranial arterial stenosis: risk factors, diagnosis, and treatment. Lancet Neurol. 2013;12:1106–14.
34. Saini M, Suministrado MS, Hilal S, et al. Prevalence and risk factors of acute incidental infarcts. Stroke. 2015;46:2722–7.
35. Rinkel GJ, Djibuti M, Algra A, van Gijn J. Prevalence and risk of rupture of intracranial aneurysms: a systematic review. Stroke. 1998;29:251–6.
36. Fiehler J. Unruptured brain aneurysms: when to screen and when to treat? Fortschr Röntgenstr. 2012;184:97–104.
37. Bederson JB, Awad IA, Wiebers DO, Piepgras D, Haley EC Jr, Brott T, et al. Recommendations for the management of patients with unruptured intracranial aneurysms: a statement for healthcare professionals from the Stroke Council of the American Heart Association. Stroke. 2000;31:2742–50.
38. Spetzler RF, Ponce FA. A 3-tier classification of cerebral arteriovenous malformations. Clinical article. J Neurosurg. 2011;114:842–9.
39. Olivero WC, Lister JR, Elwood PW. The natural history and growth rate of asymptomatic meningiomas: a review of 60 patients. J Neurosurg. 1995;83:222–4.
40. Nakamura M, Roser F, Michel J, Jacobs C, Samii M. The natural history of incidental meningiomas. Neurosurgery. 2003;53:62–70.
41. Yano S, Kuratsu J, Kumamoto Brain Tumor Research Group. Indications for surgery in patients with asymptomatic meningiomas based on an extensive experience. J Neurosurg. 2008;105:538–43.
42. Staneczek W, Janisch W. Epidemiologic data on meningiomas in East Germany 1961–1986: incidence, localization, age and sex distribution. Clin Neuropathol. 1992;11:135–41.
43. Chamoun R, Krisht KM, Couldwell WT. Incidental meningiomas. Neurosurg Focus. 2011;31:E19.
44. Shah AH, Madhavan K, Sastry A, et al. Managing intracranial incidental findings suggestive of low-grade glioma: learning from experience. World Neurosurg. 2013;80:e75–7.
45. Cavaliere R, Lopes MB, Schiff D. Low-grade gliomas: an update on pathology and therapy. Lancet Neurol. 2005;4:760–70.
46. Freda PU, Beckers AM, Katznelson L, et al. Pituitary incidentaloma: an endocrine society clinical practice guideline. J Clin Endocrinol Metab. 2011;96:894–904.
47. Park HJ, Jeon YH, Rho MH, Lee EJ, Park NH, Park SI, Jo JH. Incidental findings of the lumbar spine at MRI during herniated intervertebral disk disease evaluation. Am J Roentgenol. 2011;196(5):1151–5. https://doi.org/10.2214/AJR.11.7005.
48. Jean-Valery CEC, Walcott BP. Incidental vertebral lesions. Neurosurg Focus. 2011;31(6):E17.
49. Nguyen JP, Djindjian M, Gaston A, Gherardi R, Benhaiem N, Caron JP, Poirier J. Vertebral hemangiomas presenting with neurologic symptoms. Surg Neurol. 1987;27(4):391–7.
50. Brown E, Matthes JC, Bazan C 3rd, Jinkins JR. Prevalence of incidental intraspinal lipoma of the lumbosacral spine as determined by MRI. Spine (Phila Pa 1976). 1994;19:833–6.
51. Voyadzis JM, Bhargava P, Henderson FC. Tarlov cysts: a study of 10 cases with review of the literature. J Neurosurg. 2001;95:25–32.
52. Spierings J, van der Linden AN, Kuijper PH, Tick LW, Nijziel MR. Incidentally detected diffuse signal alterations of bone marrow on MRI: is bone marrow biopsy indicated? Neth J Med. 2014;72(7):345–8.
53. Shah GL, Rosenberg AS, Jarboe J, Klein A, Cossor F. Incidence and evaluation of incidental abnormal bone marrow signal on magnetic resonance imaging. Sci World J. 2014;2014:380814. https://doi.org/10.1155/2014/380814.
54. Fan N, Lavu S, Hanson CA, et al. Extramedullary hematopoiesis in the absence of myeloproliferative neoplasm: Mayo Clinic case series of 309 patients. Blood Cancer J. 2018;8:119. https://doi.org/10.1038/s41408-018-0156-6.
55. Brenner RJ, Lucey LL, Smith JJ, et al. Radiology and medical malpractice claims: a report on the practice standards claims survey of the Physician Insurers Association of America and the American College of Radiology. AJR Am J Roentgenol. 1998;171:19–22.

Incidental Lesions of the Brain with Potential Clinical Implications in Psychiatry

Sena Kısa Koç [ID], Ayla Uzun Çiçek, and Yavuz Yılmaz

32.1 Introduction

Incidental lesions are findings that are seen during a medical investigation or imaging in clinical practice and are recognized without any suspicion or clinical symptoms. While the frequency of these lesions can be up to 34% in the general population, 10% of them have been determined to be clinically significant in studies [1]. With the increase in imaging frequency and accessibility, an increase in the incidence of incidental lesions has been observed recently. However, discussions on how to manage an incidental lesion, its clinical consequences and its risks in terms of medical ethics have increased [1]. At the same time, the necessity of obtaining informed consent from the patients or volunteers participating in the studies is discussed before the brain magnetic resonance imaging (MRI) and cranial tomography imaging, the results of which incidental lesions can be detected and produced are discussed. The stress that may occur in the time required to reach a radiologist or neurosurgeon after the detection of the lesions

is important from a psychiatric point of view [2]. Imaging to be performed during the advanced examination and follow-up process should also be examined in terms of health economy and workforce [3].

32.2 Prevalence of Incidental Findings

According to a meta-analysis involving a total of 16 studies and 19,559 individuals [4], 2.7% of MRI scans showed incidental abnormalities. While this rate was 4.3% in high-resolution brain MRIs, it was 1.7% in clinically typical low-resolution brain MRIs. This meta-analysis also shown that the likelihood of finding malignant lesions rises with age [4].

In a study conducted in Rotterdam with the participation of 5800 volunteers [5], incidental lesions were detected at a rate of 9.5% (in 549 volunteers). Meningiomas and cerebral aneurysms account for more than half of this rate. These are followed by abnormalities of the pituitary gland (1.2%), and then arachnoid cysts (1.6%) [5]. In these studies, the imaging frequency of lesions can be found to be low, since contrast material is not used in imaging techniques [4, 5].

Meike W. Vernooij conducted additional research on this topic in 2007 [6]. In this study involving 2000 participants, brain infarcts (145

S. K. Koç (✉) · A. U. Çiçek
Department of Child and Adolescent Psychiatry, Faculty of Medicine, Cumhuriyet University, Sivas, Turkey

Y. Yılmaz
Department of Psychiatry, Faculty of Medicine, Cumhuriyet University, Sivas, Turkey

© The Author(s), under exclusive license to Springer Nature Switzerland AG 2023
M. Turgut et al. (eds.), *Incidental Findings of the Nervous System*,
https://doi.org/10.1007/978-3-031-42595-0_32

individuals) were the most prevalent incidental lesions, followed by cerebral aneurysms and benign primary tumors. Among the benign tumors, meningiomas were the most common [6].

In a study that included participants over the age of 65 [7], incidental lesions were found in MRI and computed tomography studies in 77.9% of the 503 participants, and only 22 individuals had worrisome lesions that required further investigation. 3.8% of them showed evidence of having neoplasm. Cysts were the most frequent type of these lesions [7].

32.3 The Ethics of Managing Incidental Findings

The discovery of incidental lesions has been more common as the use of imaging in both research and clinical practice has expanded. Therefore, ethical issues have begun to surface in this area. The detection of lesions can be advantageous for patients or research participants, but it can also be detrimental in several aspects. For instance, early discovery of a life-threatening lesions can extend the patient's life expectancy, whereas the anxiety that may arise during the follow-up of rare lesions can be deleterious [8]. Because of this follow-up process, patients who require urgent clinical imaging may have to wait longer to access imaging facilities.

When a lesion is discovered, the time it takes to reach a specialist may be extended, or an advanced examination may be required [2]. In this case, the patient's anxiety should also be taken into account. The patient may apply to a second or third doctor in these circumstances. This anxiety is more noticeable in the parents of younger patients [9], so they may be more willing to get opinions from more than one expert [10], because of this, the country's health care system may face workforce and financial challenges. Therefore, J. Kole and A. Fiesler, in the article they published in 2013 [2], recommended that information be given about the risk of incidental lesion detection and obtaining the patient's consent before the imaging studies to be performed.

32.4 Informing a Patient About Incidental Lesions

In a study involving 32 volunteers [11], patients were asked how they wanted to be informed that they had an incidental lesion. It was questioned whether they received adequate support. Thirty-two volunteers with incidental brain lesions participated in the study and were informed before brain MRI study. This study indicated that the doctor's notification approach had a substantial impact on the patient. Some patients stated that the first notifying doctor did not want to give detailed information about the diagnosis in order not to take risks. As a result, they reported experiencing anxiousness for one and a half months prior to meeting with a neurosurgeon. They complained that the stress of the waiting period had caused their arterial blood pressure to rise. In addition, some patients reported that their physicians delivered the news in a stressful way. They claimed that this strategy led patients to conjure up terrifying tales regarding the lesion. In addition, 91% of patients felt it was more comfortable to get bad news face-to-face as opposed to over the phone. 9% of the patients indicated that receiving news over the phone was not an issue. 48% of the patients thought that learning early what the diagnosis of the detected lesion might be, what the treatment possibilities were and what kind of results it might cause would be better for their stress management. On the other hand, 52% of them stated that they thought it would be more stressful to learn what the diagnosis of the detected incidental lesion could be and what kind of results it might cause [11]. In another investigation on this topic, [12] patients with incidental lesions from the Rotterdam trial were interviewed. The purpose of these interviews was to determine why the patients participated in the study, if they desired to hear about lesions detected at the conclusion of the study. The majority of participants believed that learning about the lesion was advantageous, citing health precautions or treatment as the most important reason for this. When the patients learnt about the lesions, several of them initially believed that the lesions would not impact them.

Others thought that if clinically insignificant lesions were not highlighted, their lives would be less stressful and they would have a better quality of life overall. Specifically, they said that their relatives were under a significant lot of stress in this regard. Some participants were unprepared for this news and reported experiencing severe stress and headaches in the first few months. Patients who said they did not experience shock upon hearing the news in the short term also reported that these incidental lesions had less of an impact on their lives in the long term. However, they stated that they were slightly stressed during the follow-up days. Particularly when a lesion that can be treated is discovered, participants report being pleased that the lesion was detected and reported to them. Some patients believed it would be preferable not to learn about the lesion, and they made statements such as, "Whenever I have a headache, I believe it may be related to this issue," and believed they had lost their independence. Volunteers stated that even if they were less affected, their families and relatives in their social environment experienced a great deal of stress as a result, and that they themselves endured very stressful periods, particularly for family members who had lost loved ones for similar reasons [12].

32.5 Meningioma Patients' Psychological Stress

In prevalence research on incidental lesions, benign tumors were determined to be the third most common cause [6]. Meningiomas were the most prevalent of these tumors. Asymptomatic meningiomas are identified in 1–2% of brain MRI examinations. With its slow growth and generally benign nature, it is observed more commonly and accidentally in the elderly, especially [13]. And it is more prevalent in females than males [14]. This frequency increases over time, especially with the increase in the frequency of imaging and the quality of the devices. After meningiomas are identified, they are often monitored or surgically removed. When both groups were compared to a healthy control group using the Distress Thermometer (DT) and Hospital Anxiety and Depression Scale (HADS), rates of anxiety and depression were found to be elevated. According to HADS, anxiety disorder was identified in 45% of patients post-op and in 42% of patients who were followed up, while depression was identified in 61% and 87%, respectively. Additionally, sleep problems were detected in 45 and 42%, respectively. As a result, the stress factor in meningioma patients is lower than in patients with other aggressive central nervous system tumors, although anxiety is discovered at a rate of 80% and depression is recognized at a rate of more than 90%. Especially in patients who are followed up, the rate of depression is higher. For this reason, further studies are needed to increase psycho-oncological support in meningioma patients [15].

32.6 Unruptured Aneurysms as Incidental Lesions

In the prevalence studies on incidental lesions, the second most common cause was found to be brain aneurysms. And the prevalence of unruptured aneurysms have grown as the number of recent check-ups have increased. Ruptured aneurysm has a significant mortality and morbidity rate (between 32 and 67% mortality at the period of bleeding). Anxiety may be caused by the possibility of aneurysm rupture in patients with incidentally identified aneurysms [16]. This anxiety may prompt the individual to seek treatment. There are two standard treatment modalities for unruptured aneurysms. These are endovascular coiling and surgical clipping method. It was determined that these treatments could cause negative outcomes including death in 8.8% and 17.8%, respectively. The treatment itself might present a greater danger to the participant's physical and mental health than the abnormality itself does [17]. The frequency of unruptured aneurysms is between 0.6 and 4.2% [18]. Despite the low frequency of these aneurysms, they are important in terms of high risk of mortality and morbidity after rupture. In a study conducted in China [19], the quality of life of patients with unruptured aneurysms was evaluated in terms of anxiety and depression. Detected incidental unruptured aneurysms in these patients were associated with high rates of depression, anxiety, and poor quality of life, especially when first detected. These have resulted in social isolation. After 5 years of observation, when these unruptured lesions are not treated, the anxiety and depression levels of the patients decrease and their quality of life improves, but when compared to the healthy control group, anxiety and depression remain high and social isolation is observed. In this study, it was observed that cognitive losses occur especially after 5 years of follow-up. Therefore, psychosocial support of patients and cognitive rehabilitation exercises are recommended after aneurysms are detected [19].

32.7 Stress in Newly Diagnosed Patients with Brain Tumors

It was determined that anxiety disorders resulting from brain tumors were more prevalent than other types. According to a study [20], sexual problems are one of the most prevalent issues in this regard, followed by fatigue and anxiety. In addition, it has been observed that anxiety is more prevalent in young people than in older people, and that this is reflected in the patients' functionality at the same rate. It is also known that suicidal ideation is more prevalent among oncology patients compared to the general population. In a study [21], 7.7% of patients with a brain tumor were diagnosed with severe depression, and 25.5% were diagnosed with moderate depression. It was determined that female patients are especially susceptible to this. Twenty-one percent of the patients (17 patients) reported having suicidal thoughts at least once during this process; two of these patients made a suicide plan, and this thought frequently crosses their minds. Even though patients with strong family support were identified in the study, rates of suicidal thinking and depression were discovered to be quite high. It has been observed that female patients, patients with a low level of education, and foreign nationals have a higher rate of depres-

sion and a greater risk of depression than others. In this study, frequent patient follow-up was recommended, particularly with regard to suicidal ideation [21].

32.8 Conclusion

The incidence of incidental lesion identification has increased as a result of the recent increase in imaging frequency, the technological advancement of imaging modalities, and the expansion of research on this topic. For this reason, additional research is required for the evaluation of the discovered lesions from an ethical, medical, and legal perspective. It has been suggested in some studies that the physician who initially evaluated the imaging should receive communication skills training prior to delivering the results to the patient [1].

Conflict of Interest There are no financial, personal, or professional interests related to this article.

References

1. Stip E, Miron JP, Nolin M, et al. Incidentaloma discoveries in the course of neuroimaging research. Can J Neurol Sci. 2019;46(3):275–9. https://doi.org/10.1017/cjn.2018.397.
2. Kole J, Fiester A. Incidental findings and the need for a revised informed consent process. AJR Am J Roentgenol. 2013;201(5):1064–8. https://doi.org/10.2214/AJR.13.11138.
3. Al-Shahi Salman R, Whiteley WN, Warlow C. Screening using whole-body magnetic resonance imaging scanning: who wants an incidentaloma? J Med Screen. 2007;14(1):2–4. https://doi.org/10.1258/096914107780154530.
4. Morris Z, Whiteley WN, Longstreth WT Jr, et al. Incidental findings on brain magnetic resonance imaging: systematic review and meta-analysis. BMJ. 2009;339:b3016. https://doi.org/10.1136/bmj.b3016.
5. Bos D, Poels MM, Adams HH, et al. Prevalence, clinical management, and natural course of incidental findings on brain MR images: the population-based Rotterdam Scan Study. Radiology. 2016;281(2):507–15. https://doi.org/10.1148/radiol.2016160218.
6. Vernooij MW, Ikram MA, Tanghe HL, et al. Incidental findings on brain MRI in the general population. N Engl J Med. 2007;357(18):1821–8. https://doi.org/10.1056/NEJMoa070972.

7. Boutet C, Vassal F, Celle S, et al. Incidental findings on brain magnetic resonance imaging in the elderly: the PROOF study. Brain Imaging Behav. 2017;11(1):293–9. https://doi.org/10.1007/s11682-016-9519-4.

8. Ells C, Thombs BD. The ethics of how to manage incidental findings. CMAJ. 2014;186(9):655–6. https://doi.org/10.1503/cmaj.140136.

9. Wright E, Amankwah EK, Winesett SP, Tuite GF, Jallo G, Carey C, Rodriguez LF, Stapleton S. Incidentally found brain tumors in the pediatric population: a case series and proposed treatment algorithm. J Neuro-Oncol. 2019;141(2):355–61. https://doi.org/10.1007/s11060-018-03039-1.

10. Gupta SN, Gupta VS, White AC. Spectrum of intracranial incidental findings on pediatric brain magnetic resonance imaging: what clinician should know? World J Clin Pediatr. 2016;5(3):262–72. https://doi.org/10.5409/wjcp.v5.i3.262.

11. Jagadeesh H, Bernstein M. Patients' anxiety around incidental brain tumors: a qualitative study. Acta Neurochir. 2014;156(2):375–81. https://doi.org/10.1007/s00701-013-1935-2.

12. CHC B, Van Bodegom L, Vernooij MW, Pinxten W, De Beaufort ID, Bunnik EM. The impact of incidental findings detected during brain imaging on research participants of the Rotterdam Study: an interview study. Camb Q Healthc Ethics. 2020;29(4):542–56. https://doi.org/10.1017/S0963180120000304.

13. Kalasauskas D, Keric N, Abu Ajaj S, von Cube L, Ringel F, Renovanz M. Psychological burden in meningioma patients under a wait-and-watch strategy and after complete resection is high-results of a prospective single center study. Cancers (Basel). 2020;12(12):3503. https://doi.org/10.3390/cancers12123503.

14. Wiemels J, Wrensch M, Claus EB. Epidemiology and etiology of meningioma. J Neuro-Oncol. 2010;99(3):307–14. https://doi.org/10.1007/s11060-010-0386-3.

15. Goebel S, Mehdorn HM. Development of anxiety and depression in patients with benign intracranial meningiomas: a prospective long-term study. Support Care Cancer. 2013;21(5):1365–72. https://doi.org/10.1007/s00520-012-1675-5.

16. Otawara Y, Ogasawara K, Kubo Y, Tomitsuka N, Watanabe M, Ogawa A, Suzuki M, Yamadate K. Anxiety before and after surgical repair in patients with asymptomatic unruptured intracranial aneurysm. Surg Neurol. 2004;62(1):28–31. https://doi.org/10.1016/j.surneu.2003.07.012.

17. Royal JM, Peterson BS. The risks and benefits of searching for incidental findings in MRI research scans. J Law Med Ethics. 2008;36(2):305–14. https://doi.org/10.1111/j.1748-720X.2008.00274.x.

18. Winn HR, Jane JA Sr, Taylor J, Kaiser D, Britz GW. Prevalence of asymptomatic incidental aneurysms: review of 4568 arteriograms. J Neurosurg. 2002;96(1):43–9. https://doi.org/10.3171/jns.2002.96.1.0043.

19. Su SH, Xu W, Hai J, Yu F, Wu YF, Liu YG, Zhang L. Cognitive function, depression, anxiety and quality of life in Chinese patients with untreated unruptured intracranial aneurysms. J Clin Neurosci. 2014;21(10):1734–9. https://doi.org/10.1016/j.jocn.2013.12.032.

20. Goebel S, Stark AM, Kaup L, von Harscher M, Mehdorn HM. Distress in patients with newly diagnosed brain tumours. Psychooncology. 2011;20(6):623–30. https://doi.org/10.1002/pon.1958.

21. Hickmann AK, Nadji-Ohl M, Haug M, Hopf NJ, Ganslandt O, Giese A, Renovanz M. Suicidal ideation, depression, and health-related quality of life in patients with benign and malignant brain tumors: a prospective observational study in 83 patients. Acta Neurochir. 2016;158(9):1669–82. https://doi.org/10.1007/s00701-016-2844-y.

Medicolegal and Ethical Aspects of Incidental Neurological Findings

Mehmet Turgut

33.1 Introduction

The term "incidental neurological finding" called "neurological incidentaloma" is used to describe a neurological finding of the brain and spine that was discovered outside the scope of any study, but is of potential significance to the individual [1]. As covered in detail in other parts of the book, with the advent of non-invasive imaging tools such as computed tomography (CT) and magnetic brain imaging (MRI) in clinical practice, incidental findings of the brain and spine are reported in 2–18% of cases for non-tumoral abnormalities and 0.5–3% for tumoral lesions [2–5]. Moreover, it has been reported that incidental findings of the brain and spine are higher in children, the elderly, and in women [5]. The incidence of incidental neurological findings on MRI was found to be 2.7% in adults and 16.4% in children [6]. In clinical practice, asymptomatic incidental findings of the brain include arachnoid cyst, Chiari malformation, vascular lesions (aneurysm, cavernoma, etc.), meningioma, glioma, and lesions involving the pituitary gland [2, 7, 8]. Among these, surgical intervention is not necessary for some meningiomas and aneurysms that are <5 mm in size [9, 10]. Incidental findings involving the pituitary gland are pituitary adenomas and Rathke cleft cysts where no further imaging follow-up is necessary in the presence of a Rathke cleft cyst, in contrast to a solid pituitary mass in which a radiological follow-up should be within 6–12 months and neurosurgery and/or endocrine consultation is necessary because of the risk of mass effect to surrounding structures as a result of growth or bleeding, called "pituitary apoplexy." Moreover, as described in detail in other chapters of the book, various incidental lesions of the spine include syringohydromyelia, ventriculus terminalis, filum terminale lipoma, perineural cysts, vertebral hemangioma, butterfly vertebra, and block vertebrae.

Today it is vital to develop guidelines on how laboratory physicians, including neuropathologists and microbiologists, and/or neuroradiologists will report their incidental findings regarding the brain and/or spine to the referring physicians, including primary care or family physicians, emergency room physicians, neuroradiologists, neurologists, and neurosurgeons, and/or their patients. The purpose of this chapter is to provide an overview of the current management of incidental findings of the brain and spine, called "neurological incidentalomas," and the medicolegal and ethical aspects of cases with these findings, exemplified in the case scenarios. As described below with examples, undiagnosed

M. Turgut (✉)
Department of Neurosurgery, Aydın Adnan Menderes University Faculty of Medicine, Efeler, Aydın, Turkey

Department of Histology and Embryology, Aydın Adnan Menderes University Health Sciences Institute, Efeler, Aydın, Turkey

and/or undisclosed and/or mishandled incidental findings of the brain and spine often result in medical malpractice suits.

33.2 Management Strategy for Incidental Findings of the Brain and Spine

Nowadays, the detection of any asymptomatic incidental neurological finding in a patient who is undergoing diagnostic testing for unrelated reasons is a common occurrence. For clinical specialists, including primary care or family physicians, emergency room physicians, neuroradiologists, neurologists, and neurosurgeons, there is an increased risk of a false negative or positive error in cases with incidental neurological findings of the brain and spine where false negative ones may aggravate the disease, while false positive ones will unduly stress the patient and his/her relatives [11, 12]. Importantly, some authors have suggested consulting an expert before explaining an incidental neurological finding to an individual [1, 13]. Undoubtedly, both knowledge of management guidelines for incidental findings of the brain and/or spine and the proper handling of such cases by neurosurgeons, neurologists, and neuroradiologists are very important issues [1, 14, 15]. Therefore, in such cases, the additional requirement for further expert consultations and new diagnostic studies of previously detected incidental neurological findings is increasing in frequency. However, there is currently no established management strategy for incidental findings of the brain and spine.

Unfortunately, during daily clinical practice, it is possible to overlook and/or ignore these findings under the intense working conditions in the hospital and that can cause serious harm and even death of the patient. Every neuroradiologist should diagnose and report an incidental finding regarding the brain and/or spine to the relevant responsible physician, although other medical professionals managing the patient also have an obligation to report such findings. In cases where further investigation, follow-up or consultation

from another medical specialist is also required, serious consequences may arise if there is a delay in the diagnosis in such cases. Therefore, it is now clear that protocols and guidelines for identifying incidental neurologic findings must be established and trained medical professionals should address incidental findings of the brain and/or spine. However, there is still an uncertainty, resulting in some ethical and legal consequences for different approaches [7, 16]. It is anticipated that guidelines and algorithms regarding incidental neurological findings will be useful for decision-making for patients with such asymptomatic but potentially clinically important incidental neurological findings and in medicolegal/ethical problems [17].

33.3 Obligations of Medical Professionals Regarding Incidental Findings of the Brain and Spine

As a rule, the responsible physician who requests imaging of brain and/or spine such as CT and/or MRI for his/her patient's complaints has the obligation to inform them of the presence of any incidental neurological finding. Unfortunately however, the patient is often discharged from the hospital and goes home before the requested study report is issued, and the physician does not inform his/her patient, and their physicians and other health professionals who see the patient later assume that he/she has been previously informed. Such incidental findings of the brain and/or spine, which can be quite important, can often be related to the examinations requested without the knowledge of the principal responsible physician due to reasons such as shift changes, or on occasion the results of the examination may be lost. However, the obligation to carefully review all the test results of the patient belongs to the physician who requested the examination or is primarily responsible for supervising the examinations. In order to diagnose any incidental neurological finding, not only the final findings of the patient, but also all neuroradiological examination results should be carefully reviewed.

If the attending physician is hasty and careless, he/she may miss these findings and their details. In some cases, oral information regarding the neuroradiological images or neuropathological findings of the patient may later change in the final report, and such alterations may be missed by the attending physician due to the lack of communication between health professionals and may lead to various diagnostic problems regarding the brain and spine.

33.4 Medicolegal and Ethical Issues Regarding Incidental Findings of the Brain and Spine

In recent years, because of a variety of diagnostic methods routinely used to obtain high-resolution imaging of the brain and spine, it is a frequent practice to identify incidental abnormalities of the brain and/or spine [5]. Even today, however, there is still not a uniform set of guidelines regarding management of incidental neurological findings, and the vast majority of health professionals including physicians do not have enough information regarding how to deal with them [1]. In clinical practice, various legal and ethical questions arise in these cases as to whether these normally healthy individuals should be informed, and if so, how, and then, when should it be done [5]. Unfortunately, however, there is no standard approach regarding the management of incidental neurological findings for which a general consensus has been reached by all participants [14]. Therefore, the proper handling of incidental findings of the brain and/or spine still poses a unique challenge in clinical practice [5].

In medicine, there are certain ethical principles, known as "no harm," "general salvage" and "mutual benefit and indebtedness" "the Declaration of Helsinki" and "Nuremberg Law," that are cornerstones for the current ethical regulations involving human research including informed consent, analysis for positive risk and benefit, and right of withdrawal without any negative effect [5, 18]. Additionally, the following medicolegal perspectives are also important for the approach to incidental findings of the brain and/or spine lesions: legal liability, fiduciary duties, tort law, and contract law [5]. The most important ethical and medicolegal issues related to the management of incidental neurological findings are discussed below.

33.4.1 Legal Principles

In the presence of any incidental neurological finding, the following primary laws regarding the issue of legal liability should be considered: (1) The concept of tort law, which consists of eliminating a wrong done to a person for compensation with monetary compensation; (2) The concept of contract law, which consists of contracts consisting of agreements to which the law applies, and (3) The concept of bailment law, which consists of transfer of ownership of goods by the owner to another person [5].

33.4.2 Ethical Principles

Basic ethical principles regarding incidental neurological findings are as follows: (1) first, not to harm, called *"primum non nocere,"* meaning information of the individual regarding incidental neurological findings and the assessment of the harm and risks to reduce the harm and unnecessary fear and anxiety; (2) general duty to help and rescue; and (3) mutual benefits and owing [5, 19].

33.4.3 Informed Consent

33.4.3.1 Informed Consent Forms
Although incidental neurological findings can be perceived as potential risks and harms, there are no clear standard protocols for the disclosure of incidental findings of the brain and/or spine [5]. To the best of my knowledge, there are a total of 13 different strategies for the handling of incidental neurological findings between different centers [5, 14, 20]. Theoretically, a standard research protocol for disclosure of incidental

neurological findings should include the following points: the disclosure of incidental findings to individuals, the skills and training in disclosing incidental neurological findings, the possibility of false positives in incidental neurological findings and their potential harm to individuals, and the necessity of referral for expert opinion and proper management of incidental findings of the brain and/or spine [5]. As a rule, the disclosure and interpretation of any incidental finding of the brain and/or spine are unethical unless participants choose not to know such findings [5]. In clinical practice, the vast majority of consent forms usually include the participant(s) choice to be informed about the finding, the participant(s) choice to inform their physician of the findings, the participant(s) choice for disclosure of risks about the finding and all known and foreseeable risks, including rare and remote ones [5].

33.4.3.2 Patient's and Parents' Right to Information

From a legal perspective, in informed consent cases, the plaintiff should prove that a reasonably prudent patient in the plaintiff's situation would refuse treatment if he/she was aware of the risks that the defendant had failed to disclose through negligence. As a rule, an ethical question exists whether patients should be informed about incidental findings of the brain and/or spine which do not require any treatment, even though they may cause considerable concern to patients and/or their relatives [21]. As a rule, the consequences of not disclosing incidental neurological findings to patients and/or their relatives should be carefully evaluated by specialists and as a precaution, an informed consent should be obtained before beginning the imaging study [21].

33.4.4 Practical Approaches

Initially, it should be noted that some incidental findings of the brain and/or spine carry the potential for unnecessary expense and harmful concern for individuals [5]. Individuals should be asked if they wish to be informed about any incidental neurological finding and their consent should be

obtained [5]. No legal responsibility for possible pathologies exists if individuals choose not to be informed about incidental findings of the brain and/or spine [5].

33.5 Case Scenarios of Malpractice and Ethical Violation Due to the Negligent Management of Incidental Findings of the Brain and Spine

The case scenarios of malpractice related with the negligent management of incidental findings of the brain and/or spine that are described below in detail will be useful for the correct diagnosis and appropriate management for physicians from various disciplines, including primary care or family physicians, emergency room physicians, neuroradiologists, neurologists, neurosurgeons, and any other involved health professionals.

33.5.1 Missed or Delayed Diagnosis and Treatment

Case 1 *A claim was settled against an emergency room physician and a neurosurgeon, alleging that it caused a delay in the diagnosis of his incidental disease and inadequate treatment.*

A brief case scenario may be as follows: "*A 48-year-old man was admitted to the emergency room with the complaint of headache for 2 weeks, associated with nausea, vomiting, and confusion for 3 days ... And CT scan report revealed the presence of 'a recurrent neoplasm' in which an MRI will be appropriate, but unfortunately an MRI was never ordered by the emergency room physician ... An MRI requested by a neurosurgeon 2 months later demonstrated that the tumor had progressed, but the report of the MRI was not conveyed to the patient ... One month later, the man went to her neuro-oncologist for the complaints of severe headaches and a new CT scan confirmed the progression of the tumor seen on the previous MRI ... Then, the patient filed a mal-*

practice lawsuit against the emergency room physician, alleging that it caused a delay in the diagnosis of his disease and inadequate treatment."

In this case scenario, there was a delay in the diagnosis of the incidental neurological lesion and in the ability to manage it properly. As expected, the expert will confirm negligence in the failure to inform about the incidental neurological lesion (recurrent neoplasm) on the CT scan by emergency room physician. As a matter of fact, 4 months later, the MRI examination, which was later requested by a neurosurgeon, confirmed this diagnosis. Unfortunately, the tumor had progressed, but the report of the MRI was not conveyed to the patient by the neurosurgeon. One month later, the man went to her neuro-oncologist for the complaint of headaches and a new CT scan confirmed the progression of the tumor seen on the previous MRI. Most likely, if these failures had not occurred, the patient would have recovered without any neurological deficit. From a medicolegal point of view, it is obvious that these failures lead to the patient's severe neurological impairment.

With the increased use and sensitivity of imaging studies including CT and/or MRI, there has been a marked increase in the number of incidental neurologic findings identified. In particular, emergency room physicians make a preliminary reading for the radiological studies, but various incidental neurological findings may be encountered in the last reading made by a neuroradiologist the next day [22]. In such cases, the measures that can be taken to reduce the legal liability of emergency physicians are as follows: (1) It should not deviate from the common and consistent policy of consensus for the emergency department, (2) A copy of the radiology interpretation associated with incidental neurological findings should be given to the patient, and the follow-up of the primary care physician should be recommended.

Case 2 *A claim was settled against an emergency room physician and a neuroradiologist for the negligence regarding management of an incidental neurological finding.*

A brief case scenario may be as follows: *"A 64-year-old male patient was admitted to emergency department of the hospital with complaints of headache, dizziness and vision, and was admitted to be examined and treated .... Both CT and MRI studies of brain and cervical spine were requested by the emergency room physician for the patient's primary symptoms. In the study reports written by the neuroradiologist, it was stated that there were no significant findings other than 'the lump' that was detected as an incidental finding in the neck region of the patient. The emergency room physician assumed that the patient would later be referred to the relevant specialists and they would inform the patient about the follow-up of this incidental finding. After about 6 months, the existing lump got bigger and it was understood that the mass was a kind of malignancy in the neuro-oncology department. He accused the physicians of not including the findings in his radiological reports ... The patient filed a medical malpractice lawsuit against all medical team members, including the emergency room physician, the neuroradiologist, and other health professionals, who were responsible for the diagnosis and treatment of his disease, who saw him and thought they should warn him about this ..."*

In this case scenario, there was a "failure to diagnosis and begin treatment of malignancy" in a man presenting with a lump in the neck region. As anticipated, the expert report from an emergency room physician or the neuroradiologist will confirm the presence of negligence about the management of the patient in the form of "failure to diagnosis and begin treatment of malignancy." It is expected that such a patient will be diagnosed and referred to the relevant specialist physician who will carry out the treatment without delay. From the legal point of view, all health personnel, including the physicians, have the obligation to provide the necessary care to the patient for whom they are responsible for examination and treatment in accordance with professional standards. If they harm their patients due to practices contrary to current professional standards, they may face medical malpractice lawsuits, which is called "medical negligence" in the public opinion. It is accepted that every health personnel, especially physicians, knows that appropriate patient care, important information in the tests performed, should be communicated to the patient, and that more measures should be taken and followed in order to protect the patient's health. As in the case scenario above, it is negligent to assume otherwise and responsible personnel assume that others will perform this task.

Theoretically, from the legal point of view, in the following situations, there will be a corresponding liability for compensation for a medical malpractice associated with a condition that can be prevented or treated with early diagnosis and appropriate treatment: (1) Failure to notify the patient of incidental neurological findings detected in the scan performed by the emergency room physician, neuroradiologist, or another physician working in the hospital; (2) A delay in the diagnosis of the emergency room physician or neuroradiologist or others on duty in the hospital, thus causing the progression of the disease or the need for long-term treatment.

33.5.2 Misdiagnosis of Chiari Malformation as Epileptic Seizure Causing Delayed Treatment

Case 1 *A claim was settled against neurologists for "misdiagnosis" and "delayed treatment" of a patient with a Chiari malformation as an epilepsy.*

A brief case scenario may be as follows: "A 22-year-old boy had been evaluated by an neurologist for falling seizures, which were interpreted as seizures about 10 years ago ... He had been diagnosed as 'epilepsy' based on his EEG report and an antiepileptic drug was started and MRI of the brain was requested by another neurologists upon the insistence of the patient's family As a result, it was said that 'Chiari malformation' was detected as an incidental neurological finding by a neuroradiologist that the family did not need to worry about.... Lastly, when the child's parents took the child to a neurosurgeon, however, they learned that severe

Chiari symptoms were present, that neurologists did not notice, and that there was a syrinx that could cause permanent paralysis .... Surgically, a decompressive craniectomy was performed and the patient returned to his life.... Despite the stopping of antiepileptic treatment, the child did not have a fall seizure and thus the diagnosis of epilepsy was confirmed to be incorrect."

In this case scenario, it is obvious that the patient's surgical treatment was delayed due to the neurologist's insufficient medical knowledge that Chiari malformation could cause a fall and thus require surgical intervention. Therefore, as expected, an expert report from the consulting neurologist or neurosurgeon will delay the surgical treatment and confirm the negligence regarding the patient's treatment. Based on neurological examination and imaging findings, neurologists treating such a patient would be expected to be able to make the differential diagnosis between Chiari malformation and epilepsy and then refer him to a neurosurgeon for surgical treatment. Otherwise, the patient and his relatives may be subject to a lawsuit against the neurologist with the allegation of malpractice.

33.5.3 Ethical Violation in the Management of Cerebral Stroke by an Orthopedic Surgeon

Case 1 *An allegation of ethical violation has been filed against an orthopedic surgeon because of management of a patient with ischemic brain infarction without filling out the consent form.*

A brief case scenario may be as follows: "A 75-year-old man was admitted to a local hospital for his osteoarthritic hip pain and incidental ischemic vascular changes was found in his right parietal lobe on brain MRI study, inspite of absence of any complaint or any neurological deficit ... Considering the presence of cardiac arrhythmias and diabetes comorbidity in his medical history, orthopaedic surgeon decided to disclose the incidental neurological findings to him in anticipation of further management and without his consent and without issuing any consent form for further advice and guidance he contacted the his family physician to explain to him what happened … As expected by the orthopaedic surgeon, he was admitted again to a tertiary hospital because of development of neurological deficit 3 days later and the definitive diagnosis of ischemic infarction in the right parietal lobe was confirmed. He was discharged from the hospital to home 2 weeks later following stabilization with antiplatelet and anticoagulant therapy … During his follow-up of 1 year, complete recovery in neurological functions was achieved."

In this case scenario, there was no medical defect in the follow-up of the patient with ischemic stroke by the orthopedic surgeon. In the beginning, however, there was an ethical violation due to lack of consent form issuance. As explained in detail above, the consent form should be issued and the possibility of incidental neurological findings should be addressed in a clear and understandable way in the consent form for further advice and guidance. In this form, a clear documentation of the individual's willingness to be informed about incidental neurological findings should also be available and knowledge of legal and ethical guidelines and protocol regarding disclosure is also vital for all health personnel including physicians. As a rule, the possible consequences of incidental neurological findings should be carefully evaluated by specialists before the findings are disclosed to patients and/or their relatives and as a precaution an informed consent should be obtained at the beginning before imaging study.

33.6 Comment Upon Case Scenarios Regarding Incidental Findings of the Brain and Spine

Today, it is well-known that detection of any asymptomatic incidental finding of the brain and spine in a patient who is undergoing any kind of diagnostic testing for unrelated reasons is a common event. Unfortunately, undiagnosed and/or undisclosed and/or mishandled incidental findings of the brain and spine often result in medical malpractice suits. In conclusion, differential diagnosis is very important because all of these diagnoses may hinder the correct management of patients.

As noted in the case scenarios given above, the vast majority of malpractice related to the negligent management of incidental findings of the brain and/or spine includes misdiagnosis or delayed diagnosis and/or medical errors in the management of the patients by physicians, that include primary care or family physicians, emergency room physicians, neuroradiologists, neurologists, and neurosurgeons. In fact, the case scenarios described above stress the importance of proper handling of incidental findings of the brain and/or spine according to basic ethical and legal principles because they still poses a challenge in clinical practice.

"Medical malpractice" has been defined as *"damage caused by the physician not performing the standard, up-to-date practice during treatment, lack of skills or not giving the treatment to the patient"* by World Medical Association (WMA) [23–26]. For a legal malpractice claim to be appropriate, it must include an injury resulting from negligence that causes significant harm to the patient or from breach of medical treatment accepted as a standard of care by a medical center, physician, or other healthcare professional as a result of errors in diagnosis, treatment, and aftercare management, as specified by the American Board of Professional Liability Attorneys (ABPLA) [27, 28]. Unpublished reports in clinical practice show that it is possible to encounter numerous instances of negligence that could result in litigation, including not asking for appropriate tests to make a correct diagnosis, not recognizing the patient's symptoms, misreading or ignoring laboratory results, not making a correct diagnosis or misdiagnosis, unnecessary surgical intervention, various surgical errors, incorrect medication or dose administration, misdiagnosis, poor follow-up, and early discharge of the patient from the hospital, etc.

While the physician fulfills his obligation to manage the patient in accordance with the authority of the physician's contract, he is certainly not medicolegally responsible for not achieving the desired result; however, he is responsible for the damages arising from carelessness in his care, efforts, actions, and behaviors to achieve this result [25–28]. More importantly, the physician should act carefully and be responsible for even the slightest mistake [26]. Therefore, in situations that cause uncertainty, the physician is obliged to carry out investigations that will eliminate the uncertainty, even at a minimum level, and to take preventive measures in the meantime [25, 26]. As a legitimate demand, the patient has the right to expect his/her physician, who is a member of the health profession, to show meticulousness and vigilance at every stage of the treatment.

In the case scenarios presented under the three main titles listed above, as a result of delays in diagnosis, inadequacy in neuroradiological and clinical management, health professionals including primary care or family physicians, emergency physicians, neuroradiologists, neurologists, and neurosurgeons. As a precaution of failure regarding medical and ethical principles, every medical professional should at least be alerted to the appropriate management of these patients. In fact, in many countries around the world, including the United States, it is possible that such cases could be the subject of lawsuits against doctors for alleged maltreatment. It should not be forgotten that the duty of the physician is not to act with the guarantee of completely healing the patient, but the physician has to continue the follow-up treatment of the patient with the utmost care and attention. Finally, it should be emphasized that patients and their relatives should be informed about the possible risks and benefits of surgical intervention.

33.7 Conclusion

In conclusion, undiagnosed and/or undisclosed, and/or mishandled incidental findings of the brain and/or spine often result in medical malpractice suits and they are sources of claims of error regarding medical malpractice against medical professionals. In medicine, incidental neurological findings are diagnoses or situations unrelated to the original medical problems. Therefore, the physicians must take such findings into account and act quickly because such findings have the potential for medical malpractice if they are not taken into account. In this chapter, an update on the many case scenarios in which incidental neurological findings are detected in their imaging studies of the brain and/or spine was provided for the practicing clinicians. From an ethical perspective, the principles of management, including primum non nocere, the duty to help and rescue, and the balance of mutual benefit versus indebtedness should be considered in the presence of incidental findings of the brain and/or spine. Legally, every case with incidental neurological finding should be evacuated according to fiduciary duties, tort law, contract law, and surety law. From a legal point of view, as a rule, if a person has suffered disability and material loss due to any undiagnosed and/or unexplained, and/or mishandled incidental neurological finding, or if a person has encountered a situation such as disability or death, he/she will have the right to material and moral compensation as well as criminal liability against the physicians who treat him/her. Even today, however, management of incidental neurological findings in imaging is still not a resolved topic and health professionals may be faced with a serious medical malpractice act in cases with incidental lesions of the brain and/or spine, as a result of any negligence and carelessness.

References

1. Wolf SM, Paradise J, Cagaanan C. The law of incidental findings in human subjects research: establishing researchers' duties. J Law Med Ethics. 2008;36:361–83.
2. Bos D, Poels MMF, Adams HHH, Akoudad S, Cremers LGM, Zonneveld HI, Hoogendam YY, Verhaaren BFJ, Verlinden VJA, Verbruggen JGJ, Peymani A, Hofman A, Krestin GP, Vincent AJ, Feelders RA, Koudstaa PJ, van der Lugt A, Ikram MA, Vernooij MW. Prevalence, clinical management, and natural course of incidental findings on brain MR

images: the population-based Rotterdam scan study. Radiology. 2016;281(2):507–15.

3. Illes J, Kirschen MP, Edwards E, Bandettini P, Cho MK, Ford PJ, Glover GH, Kulynych J, Macklin R, Michael DB, Wolf SM, Grabowski T, Seto B. Practical approaches to incidental findings in brain imaging research. Neurology. 2008;70(5):384–90.

4. Katzman GL, Dagher AP, Patronas NJ. Incidental findings on brain magnetic resonance imaging from 1000 asymptomatic volunteers. JAMA. 1999;282(1):36–9.

5. Leung L. Incidental findings in neuroimaging: ethical and medicolegal considerations. Neurosci J. 2013;2013:439145.

6. Dangouloff-Ros V, Roux C-J, Boulouis G, Levy R, Nicolas N, Lozach C, Grevent D, Brunelle F, Boddaert N, Naggara O. Incidental brain MRI findings in children: a systematic review and meta-analysis. Am J Neuroradiol. 2019;40(11):1818–23.

7. Morris Z, Whiteley WN, Longstreth WTJ, Weber F, Lee Y-C, Tsushima Y, Alphs H, Ladd SC, Warlow C, Wardlaw JM, Salman RAS. Incidental findings on brain magnetic resonance imaging: systematic review and meta-analysis. BMJ. 2009;339:b3016.

8. Wrensch M, Minn Y, Chew T, Bondy M, Berger MS. Epidemiology of primary brain tumors: current concepts and review of the literature. Neuro-Oncology. 2002;4(4):278–99.

9. Islim AI, Mohan M, Moon RDC, Rathi N, Kolamunnage-Dona R, Crofton A, Haylock BJ, Mills SJ, Brodbelt AR, Jenkinson MD. Treatment outcomes of incidental intracranial meningiomas: results from the IMPACT cohort. World Neurosurg. 2020;138:e725–35.

10. Wiebers DO. Unruptured intracranial aneurysms: natural history, clinical outcome, and risks of surgical and endovascular treatment. Lancet. 2003;362(9378):103–10.

11. Kirschen MP, Jaworska A, Illes J. Subjects' expectations in neuroimaging research. J Magn Reson Imaging. 2006;23:205–9.

12. Kumra S, Ashtari M, Anderson B, Cervellione KL, Kan L. Ethical and practical considerations in the management of incidental findings in pediatric MRI studies. J Am Acad Child Adolesc Psychiatry. 2006;45:1000–6.

13. Underwood E. When a brain scan bears bad news. Science. 2012;338:455. https://doi.org/10.1126/science.338.6106.455.

14. Illes J, Kirschen MP, Karetsky K, Kelly M, Saha A, Desmond JE, Raffin TA, Glover GH, Atlas SW. Discovery and disclosure of incidental findings in neuroimaging research. J Magn Reson Imaging. 2004;20:743–7.

15. Lawrenz F, Sobotka S. Empirical analysis of current approaches to incidental findings. J Law Med Ethics. 2008;36:249–55.

16. Hitzeman N, Cotton E. Incidentalomas: initial management. Am Fam Physician. 2014;90(11):784–9.

17. Berlin L. The incidentaloma: a medicolegal dilemma. Radiol Clin N Am. 2011;49(2):245–55.

18. Rits IA. Declaration of Helsinki, recommendations guiding doctors in clinical research. World Med J. 1964;11:281.

19. Scanlon TM. What we owe to each other. Cambridge: Harvard University Press; 1998.

20. Palmour N, Affleck W, Bell E, Deslauriers C, Pike B, Doyon J, Racine E. Informed consent for MRI and fMRI research: analysis of a sample of Canadian consent documents. BMC Med Ethics. 2011;12(1):1.

21. Hoggard N, Darwent G, Capener D, Wilkinson ID, Griffiths PD. The high incidence and bioethics of findings on magnetic resonance brain imaging of normal volunteers for neuroscience research. J Med Ethics. 2009;35(3):194–9.

22. Thompson RJ, Wojcik SM, Grant WD, Ko PY. Incidental findings on CT scans in the emergency department. Emerg Med Int. 2011;2011:624847.

23. Arıkan M, Kalkan E, Erdi F, Deniz M, İzci E. The distinction between cases and malpractice-complications in medical law: the perspectives of the senior students of the faculty of medicine and the faculty of law, problems and suggestions for solution. Türk Nöroşir. 2016;26:40–8.

24. Birtek F. Complication-malpractice distinction in terms of medical interventions. İstanbul Barosu Dergisi. 2007;81:1997–2007.

25. Hakeri H. Distinction between malpractice and complication in medical law. Toraks Cerrahisi Bülteni. 2014;1:23–8.

26. Kök N. Malpractice and complication distinction. In: Kalkan E, Serel TA, Yılmaz EN, editors. Legal guide for physicians. Ankara: Sage Publishing; 2018. p. 109–39.

27. Bal BS. An introduction to medical malpractice in the United States. Clin Orthop Relat Res. 2009;467(2):339–47.

28. Marcus P. Book review of medical malpractice law: a comparative law study of civil responsibility arising from medical care. Hastings Int Comp Law Rev. 1981;5:235–43.

Conclusions

The discovery of an asymptomatic lesion in the brain or spine can be potentially devastating. Is it just an incidental radiological entity with no potential consequences? Is it a benign, slow growing lesion, which may need to be addressed when there is a perceived growth in the lesion? Is it benign but in a relatively inaccessible region of the brain or spine, with the potential to cause further issues related to compression of nearby vital areas or by cerebrospinal pathway obstruction? Or is the incidental lesion a harbinger of a malignant entity, with the potential to cause significant symptomatology in the future?

The lesion may be a congenital, post-traumatic, infective, neoplastic, or vascular entity. From an academic standpoint, it may just be a scientific curiosity, requiring only a prolonged follow-up. For the individual concerned who harbors the lesion, however, the psychological trauma of "waiting and watching"; the financial cost of repeated imaging to serially assess the "hanging Damocles' sword," in anticipation of the dreadful day when the treating doctor will pronounce that the lesion is growing, and therefore needs to be addressed with therapeutic or surgical intervention; and the exasperation at discovering that the erudite doctor, whose immense professional knowledge, he/she innately trusts, also does not have a decisive answer for addressing the newly discovered lesion, are real-time issues with devastating consequences.

This book helps to ally these very apprehensions. It has focused upon the commonly occurring asymptomatic lesions and attempts to provide well-defined standard protocols that define the current state of knowledge regarding these entities. Each chapter defines one entity and has a stand-alone character. Thus, the doctor as well the patient may focus on the particular entity that interests them. For the student of neurosurgery, the book attempts to list all those lesions that may be asymptomatic at a given point of time but may require clinical considerations in the future that he/she should be aware of during the decision-making process. For the regular readers of science and medicine, who are focusing on this book based on their desire to quench scientific curiosity, and who are not particularly weighed down by the onerous task of having to take a medical decision for one particular patient, this book provides a focus on a wide spectrum of asymptomatic lesions that may coexist without causing any harm, that may grow and spread, that may be potentially harmful, or that may cause a sudden clinical deterioration. The book also helps to define the prophylactic as well as therapeutic interventions that may be immediately required or should be kept in mind for the future. Khaled Hosseini in his outstanding book " A Thousand Splendid Suns" stated, "Of all the hardships a person had to face, none was more punishing than the simple act of waiting." This book helps to breakdown, into a few logical scientific steps, the protocols for the person who has just made the devastating discovery of having an asymptomatic lesion in his/her

© The Editor(s) (if applicable) and The Author(s), under exclusive license to Springer Nature Switzerland AG 2023
M. Turgut et al. (eds.), *Incidental Findings of the Nervous System*,
https://doi.org/10.1007/978-3-031-42595-0

brain or spine and has to wait in trepidation to understand what the consequences of its existence within him/her are. Ralph Waldo Emerson once said, "Knowledge is the antidote to fear." The editors hope that the knowledge that emerges from this compendium of asymptomatic lesions of the central nervous system will help to allay this very ignorance and fear in the affected patients and also help their treating doctors in developing logical treatment protocols for their future.

Index

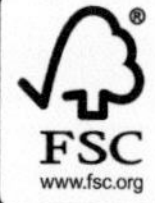

If you have any concerns about our products,
you can contact us on
ProductSafety@springernature.com

In case Publisher is established outside the EU,
the EU authorized representative is:
Springer Nature Customer Service Center GmbH
Europaplatz 3, 69115 Heidelberg, Germany

Printed by Libri Plureos GmbH
in Hamburg, Germany